Pediatric Skills

for Occupational Therapy Assistants

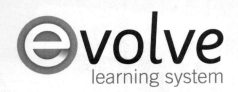

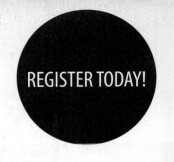

To access your free Evolve Resources, visit:

http://evolve.elsevier.com/Solomon/pediatricskills/

Evolve Resources for Solomon & O'Brien: Pediatric Skills for Occupational Therapy Assistants, 3rd edition, offers the following features:

- **Reference lists with links to PubMed abstracts**

- **Learning activities**
  Wordplay games using terms from the chapter key terms

- **Video clips**
  Case-based video clips

- **Review questions**
  Chapter by chapter questions help students prepare for exams

Evolve Instructor Resources for [Solomon & O'Brien: Pediatric Skills for Occupational Therapy Assistants, 3e] offers the following features:

- **Instructor's Resource Manual**

- **PowerPoint lecture slides**

- **Test bank**
  Multiple choice questions, including answers help instructors create exams

Pediatric Skills

for Occupational Therapy Assistants

3rd EDITION

JEAN W. SOLOMON, MHS, OTR/L

Occupational Therapist
Berkeley County School District
Moncks Corner, SC

JANE CLIFFORD O'BRIEN, PHD, OTR

Associate Professor
Occupational Therapy Department
Westbrook College of Health Professions
University of New England
Portland, Maine

Illustrations by Morgan Midgett
With 30 Contributing Authors

ELSEVIER
MOSBY

3251 Riverport Lane
St. Louis, Missouri 63043

Pediatric Skills for Occupational Therapy Assistants ISBN: 978-0-323-05910-7
Copyright © 2011 by Mosby, Inc., an affiliate of Elsevier, Inc.

Notices

Previous editions copyrighted
Library of Congress Cataloging-in-Publication Data

Pediatric skills for occupational therapy assistants / [edited by] Jean
W. Solomon, Jane Clifford O'Brien.—3rd ed.
    p. ; cm.
  Rev. ed. of: Pediatric skills for occupational therapy assistants /
Jean W. Solomon, Jane Clifford O'Brien. 2nd ed. c2006.
  Includes bibliographical references and index.
  ISBN 978-0-323-05910-7 (pbk. : alk. paper)
  1. Occupational therapy for children. 2. Occupational therapy
assistants. I. Solomon, Jean W. II. O'Brien, Jane Clifford. III.
Solomon, Jean W. Pediatric skills for occupational therapy assistants.
  [DNLM: 1. Occupational Therapy—methods. 2. Adolescent Development.
3. Adolescent. 4. Child Development. 5. Child. WS 368]
  RJ53.O25P435 2011
  618.92'89165—dc22
  2010033835

Acquisitions Editor: Jolynn Gower
Developmental Editor: Lindsay Westbrook
Publishing Services Manager: Catherine Jackson
Project Manager: Sara Alsup
Design Direction: Teresa McBryan
Designer: Jessica Williams

Printed in

Last digit is the print number: 9 8 7 6 5 4 3 2 1

In memory of First Lt. Keith Heidtman, Sept. 2, 1982 - May 28, 2007,
and to the men and women of the 2nd Squadron,
6th Cavalry Regiment of the 25th Infantry Division.

Contributors

Lisa Baillargeon MS, OTR/L
Occupational Therapist
Greenbriar Terrace Healthcare
Peoplefirst Rehabilitation
Nashua, New Hampshire

Diana Bal, MHS, OTR/L
Occupational Therapist
Berkeley County School District
Moncks Corner, South Carolina

Allyson Barry, MS, OTR/L
Staff Therapist
Sundance Rehabilitation
Massachusetts

Kathleen Bauer, MA, OTR
Senior Occupational Therapist
St. Mary's Hospital for Children
Bayside, New York

Katherine Michaud, MS, OTR/L
Occupational Therapist

**Patricia Bowyer, EdD, MS, OTR/L,
    FAOTA**
Associate Professor and Associate Director
School of Occupational Therapy-Houston
College of Health Sciences
Texas Woman's University
Houston, Texas

Gilson J. Capilouto, Ph.D, CCC-SLP
Associate Professor
Division of Communication Sciences
    and Disorders
College of Health Sciences
University of Kentucky
Lexington, Kentucky

**Ricardo C. Carrasco, PhD, OTR/L,
    FAOTA**
Chairman, FiestaJoy Foundation, Inc.
Winter Park, Florida

Nancy E. Carson, MHS, OTR/L
Assistant Professor
Division of Occupational Therapy
College of Health Professions
Medical University of South Carolina
Charleston, South Carolina

Patty Coker-Bolt, PhD, OTR/L
Assistant Professor
Medical University of South Carolina
College of Health Professions
Division of Occupational Therapy
Charleston, South Carolina

Michelle Desjardins, MS, OTR/L
USC/WPS Sensory Integration Certified
Pediatric Clinical Specialist
Interim Coordinator of Clinical
    Fieldwork Education OT/PT/SLP
Interactive Metronome Certified
New Hampshire Deaf-Blind Advisor
Northeast Rehabilitation Hospital
Department of Pediatric Rehabilitation
    Services
Salem, New Hampshire

Gwendolyn J. Duren, MSOTS
Occupational Therapy Department
Westbrook College of Health Professions
University of New England
Portland, Maine

Katie Fortier, MS, OTR/L
Occupational Therapist
Country Rehabilitation and Nursing
    Center
Newburyport, Massachusetts

Teressa Garcia-Reidy, MS, OTR/L
Occupational Therapist
Fairmount Rehabilitation Programs
Kennedy Krieger Institute
Baltimore, Maryland

**Nadine Kuzyk Hanner, AHS, OTA,
    MSOT, OTR/L**
Occupational Therapist
Private Practice
Summerville, South Carolina

Caryn Birstler Husman, MS, OTR/L
Occupational Therapist, Community
    Occupational Therapy Clinic
Adjunct Professor
Occupational Therapy Department
Westbrook College of Health Professions
University of New England
Portland, Maine

Monica Keen, MS, OTR/L
Adjunct Professor
OTA Department
Trident Technical College
North Charleston, South Carolina

Jessica M. Kramer, PhD, OTR/L
Assistant Professor
Department of Occupational Therapy
Boston University
Boston, Massachusetts

Chou-Hsien Lin, MS, OTR/L
Occupational Therapist
Rehabilitation Services
Aroostook Medical Center
Presque Isle, Maine

Dianne Koontz Lowman, EdD
Associate Professor, Director of Distance Education and
Academic Performance, Occupational Therapy
Virginia Commonwealth University
Richmond, Virginia

Angela Chinners Marsh, AHS COTA/L
Occupational Therapy Assistant, Special Education
Department, Charleston County School District
Charleston, South Carolina

Erin C. Naber, PT, DPT
Senior Physical Therapist
Fairmount Rehabilitation Programs
Kennedy Krieger Institute
Baltimore, Maryland

Randi Carlson Neideffer, AA, AHS COTA, MSOT OTR/L
Occupational Therapist
Special Education Department
Charleston County School District
Charleston, South Carolina

Dawn B. Oakley, MS, OTR
AVP of Rehabilitation
St. Mary's Hospital for Children
Bayside, New York

Gretchen Parker OTR/L ret.
Lexington, South Carolina

Dana Rothschild, MA, OTR/L
Academic Fieldwork Coordinator
Trident Technical College
Private Practice
Charleston, South Carolina

Susan A. Stallings-Sahler, Ph.D., OTR/L, FAOTA
Associate Professor of Occupational Therapy
Brenau University
Gainvesville, Georgia
and
President, Sensational Kids Pediatric Rehabilitation, Inc.
Martinez, Georgia

Julie Savoyski, MS, OTR/L
Asperger's Association of New England
Life Management Assistance Program
Watertown, Massachusetts

Barbara J. Steva, MS, OTR/L
Occupational Therapist
University of New England
Community Occupational Therapy Clinic
Biddeford, Maine

Melissa A. M. Stevens, MS, OTR/L
Occupational Therapy Clinical Advisor
New Hampshire

Kerryellen Griffith Vroman PhD, OTR/L
Assistant Professor
Occupational Therapy Department
College of Health and Human Services
University of New Hampshire
Durham, New Hampshire

Harriet G. Williams, PhD
Professor and Director
Lifespan Motor Control Laboratories
Arnold School of Public Health
University of South Carolina
Columbia, South Carolina

Pamela J. Winton, PhD
Senior Scientist and Director of Outreach
FPG Child Development Institute
Research Professor, School of Education
University of North Carolina - Chapel Hill
Chapel Hill, North Carolina

Robert E. Winton, MD
Psychiatrist
Durham, North Carolina

PREVIOUS EDITION CONTRIBUTORS

Melissa A. Fullerton, MS, OTR/L

Gloria Graham, MA

Karen Howell, PhD, OTR/L

Lise M.W. Jones, MA, OTR, SIPT Certified

Paula Kramer, PhD, OTR, FAOTA

Peggy Zaks Machover, MA (Psychology)

Cindy Timms Mathena, MS, OTR/L

Paula Mccreedy, MEd, OTL

Paula Murrill, B.A., COTA/L

Donna Newman, BS, AAS, COTA

Angela M. Peralta, AS, COTA

Susan Stockmaster

Sharon Kalscheuer Suchomel, OTR

Joyce A. Wandel, MS, OTR/L

REVIEWERS

Patty Coker-Bolt, PhD, OTR/L
Assistant Professor
Medical University of South Carolina
College of Health Professions
Division of Occupational Therapy
Charleston, South Carolina

Christine Blake, CHT, OTR/L
Carolina Hand Therapy, Inc.
Mt. Pleasant, South Carolina

Robert Hunter, B.S., M.S.
Biology Instructor
Atlana, Georgia

Foreword

The occupational life of children fascinates parents, grandparents, siblings, teachers (and complete strangers). As infants and children reach into the world with their bodies and minds, they establish a foundation for engaging in occupation throughout the lifespan. Achievement of normal developmental milestones, coupled with opportunities to explore and practice skills in diverse contexts and environments, ensures that most children reach adulthood as occupational beings prepared to assume adult roles. Occupational therapy practitioners, however, typically don't work with these "normal" children, but instead they address the challenges faced by children whose physical or other disabilities interfere with successful occupational engagement. Occupational therapy for children requires broad and deep knowledge of human development, medical and psychiatric conditions, activities of daily living, school and work, social and educational systems theory, and foundational occupational therapy theories and concepts. This is a tall order.

The third edition of *Pediatric Skills for Occupational Therapy Assistants* more than meets this challenge, as it expands on the successful plan of the previous two editions. The authors and their competent roster of contributors have updated the references and integrated the *Occupational Therapy Practice Framework: Second Edition*. They provide new chapters on emerging practice areas and on community and social systems. They retain and expand the student-friendly features and clear organization that have made this a useful basic textbook for occupational therapy assistant (OTA) education.

Throughout the text, vivid case examples illustrate principles. Samples of documentation are interwoven with the cases, making the connection explicit. Boxed "clinical pearls" provide smart and serious advice to the novice. Practical tips, specific strategies and guidelines give a clear and concrete sense of clinical practice. Engaging classroom and homework activities offer faculty and students ideas for application of concepts and techniques.

Multiple detailed examples illustrate the separate and complementary roles of the occupational therapist (OT) and the OTA. A systems perspective and recognition of the multiple viewpoints of diverse stakeholders (parents, teachers, etc.) affords students an excellent model for beginning practice in pediatrics.

Pediatric practice for the OTA continues to expand, while basic entry-level education for the OT has moved to the master's degree level. Different and complementary texts are needed for the two levels of practitioner. The third edition of *Pediatric Skills for Occupational Therapy Assistants* provides more than the foundation content required by the Accreditation Council for Occupational Therapy Education for educational programs for the OTA. This text prepares the OTA to work as a partner with the OT at entry level and beyond. It's clear to me that this new edition will serve students well, and will remain a resource for graduates and advanced OTA practitioners to consult with confidence during clinical practice.

Mary Beth Early, MS, OTR/L
Professor, Occupational Therapy Assistant Program
Department of Natural and Applied Sciences
LaGuardia Community College
City University of New York
Long Island City, New York

Preface

This book has been written for the occupational therapy assistant (OTA) student and the certified occupational therapy assistant (COTA) working in the pediatric practice settings. The language is consistent with the *Occupational Therapy Practice Framework* (2nd edition). Emphasis is on concrete, practical information that may readily be used by students, COTAs, and entry-level registered occupational therapists (OTRs) who work with children and adolescents. Theories, frames of reference, and practice models are introduced and integrated into the content so that they can be easily applied. When possible, the text differentiates between the roles of the COTA and the OTR. The term occupational therapy practitioner refers to OTRs and COTAs, and is used during discussions of procedures that can be performed by either.

All of the chapters contain the following elements: outline, key terms, objectives, summary, review questions, and suggested activities. Each chapter begins with an outline to provide readers with information about the topics included in the chapter. The list of key terms contains important words that the author(s) want readers to understand. These key terms are listed in the order in which they appear in the chapter. The chapter objectives concisely outline the material readers will learn from studying the chapter. A summary at the end of each chapter re-emphasizes the key points of the chapter and review questions help readers synthesize the information presented. Suggested activities, also found at the end of each chapter, are designed to reinforce information presented in the chapter and can be completed individually or in small groups.

Boxes, case studies, vignettes, tables, and figures are used throughout the chapters to reiterate, exemplify, or illustrate specific points. "Clinical Pearls" refer to words of wisdom based on the clinical expertise of the chapter author(s), and are also included. The Clinical Pearls contain helpful hints or reminders that have been consistently useful for occupational therapy practitioners working with children and youth. Several chapters include appendices useful in clinical practice.

The first five chapters present an overall framework for the book. Chapter 1 presents information about recommended pediatric curriculum content, selected practice models, and COTA supervision and service competency. The next four chapters present information about systems—family, medical, educational, and community—in which occupational therapy practitioners who work with children and youth practice.

The next part of the book serves as a foundation for clinical practice by presenting typical development. Chapter 6 provides an overview of the periods and principles of normal development and the development of occupational performance. Chapter 7 presents information about normal development in the areas of occupation, while chapter 8 examines typical development of occupational performance skills. Chapter 9 describes the uniqueness of adolescence and the journey into adulthood.

Chapter 10 presents an overview of the occupational therapy process in the context of the *Occupational Therapy Practice Framework* (2nd edition). An overview of anatomy and physiology for the pediatric practitioner is covered in Chapter 11.

Chapters 12 through 16 describe the etiology, signs, and symptoms of pediatric conditions/disorders that an OT practitioner may encounter including specific chapters outlining pediatric health conditions, psychosocial conditions, obesity, intellectual disability, and cerebral palsy. A chapter on positioning and handling techniques follows the chapter on cerebral palsy, since the information is applicable to the intervention with children and adolescents who have abnormal postural mechanisms (such as those who have cerebral palsy).

Chapters 18 through 21 examine specific areas of intervention of primary importance to OT practitioners and include specific strategies for the intervention of activities of daily living (ADL) (Chapter 18), instrumental activities of daily living (Chapter 19), play and playfulness (Chapter 20) and handwriting (Chapter 21). Each chapter provides readers with intervention techniques and case studies to make application clear.

Chapters 22 and 23 provide readers with techniques and tools to use in practice. Chapter 22 provides readers with an overview of the use of therapeutic media, including a variety of specific activities to use with children and adolescents. Chapter 23 describes motor control and motor learning principles as they are used with children and youth as specifically related to fine motor skills.

The last several chapters explore specialized areas of pediatric practice. Chapter 24 explores sensory processing and integration. Chapter 25 presents an overview of the Model of Human Occupation and its use in pediatric practice. Chapter 26 describes the process of assistive technology. Chapter 27 reviews types of orthoses, orthotic fabrication and kinesio taping. The final chapter examines the use of animals in therapy and provides ideas to incorporate animals into practice with children and youth.

This book has evolved from many years of teaching pediatric skills to students. The third edition includes four new chapters to reflect new areas of practice, including chapters on community systems, obesity, Model of Human Occupation, and instrumental activities of daily living. All chapters have been revised and updated to reflect current practice. The talent of the contributing authors is impressive and reflects expertise from many areas. We are grateful to the authors, reviewers, and contributors for their wisdom and skill.

Jean W. Solomon
Jane Clifford O'Brien

Acknowledgments

We have had the opportunity to work with many talented people on this third edition. The authors come from various areas of the country and represent a wide range of practice areas. They are talented and dedicated professionals who are passionate about the care of children and youth who have special needs. The authors have extensive clinical experience and knowledge that they have shared with the readers. It was fun and exciting reconnecting with colleagues and friends who participated in this project.

We appreciate the hard work of the Elsevier editorial and production staff—Kathy Falk, Jolynn Gower, Lindsay Westbrook, Rohini Herbert, and Sara Alsup.

Contents

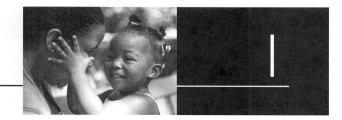

Scope of Practice

JEAN W. SOLOMON

JANE CLIFFORD O'BRIEN

CHAPTER *Objectives*

After studying this chapter, the reader will be able to accomplish the following:

- Describe the Centennial Vision of the American Occupational Therapy Association (AOTA).
- Describe the basics of the *Occupational Therapy Practice Framework: Domain and Process*, 2nd edition, and its relationship to clinical practice.
- Recognize eight subject areas in which entry-level certified occupational therapy assistants need to have general knowledge.
- Describe the four levels at which registered occupational therapists supervise occupational therapy assistants.
- Define service competency and give examples of ways it may be obtained.
- Discuss AOTA's Code of Ethics and apply the code to case scenarios.
- Define and give examples of the different types of scholarship.

KEY TERMS

Centennial Vision

Occupational Therapy Practice Framework: Domain and Process (2nd edition)

Levels of supervision

Service competency

AOTA's Code of Ethics

Scholarship

CHAPTER OUTLINE

Centennial Vision

Occupational Therapy Practice Framework

The Occupational Therapy Process

Roles of the Occupational Therapist and Occupational Therapy Assistant

Qualifications, Supervision, and Service Competency

QUALIFICATIONS

SUPERVISION

SERVICE COMPETENCY

AOTA's Code of Ethics

Scholarship

Summary

This chapter provides an overview of occupational therapy (OT) practice with children and adolescents. The chapter begins with a discussion of the subject areas important in pediatric OT curriculum followed by a description of the Centennial Vision of the American Occupational Therapy Association (AOTA), with respect to issues of children and youth. To understand the OT process, a review of the *Occupational Therapy Practice Framework: Domain and Process, 2nd edition,* is provided. Using case examples, the authors provide descriptions of levels of supervision and service competency requirements. The scope of OT practice with children and adolescents would not be complete without an understanding of the AOTA Code of Ethics. Lastly, the authors emphasize life-long learning scholarship.

During the past 20 years, significant changes have occurred in the provision of pediatric OT services.[2,3,8] Numerous federal laws that expand the services available to infants, children, and adolescents who have special needs or disabilities have been implemented. Approximately 20% of all OT assistants (OTAs) work in pediatric settings.[12] OT practitioners provide pediatric services in medical settings such as outpatient clinics and hospitals, as well as in community settings such as schools, homes, and daycare centers.[12] Because numerous practitioners work with infants, children, and adolescents, it is important that both entry-level occupational therapists and OTAs have a solid foundation in pediatrics.

The AOTA has identified eight subject areas that must be included in any pediatric OT curriculum.[4,8] An entry-level OT practitioner must have knowledge in the following areas:

Normal development: OT practitioners working with children who have special needs or atypical development patterns must have a firm foundation in the knowledge of normal development in order to understand children and base interventions.

Importance of families in the OT process: Families are the most consistent participants on the pediatric team. Understanding the needs of families and children is essential to the therapeutic process.

Specific pediatric diagnoses: Pediatric OT practitioners use knowledge of specific pediatric diagnoses to determine which tools and methods are the most appropriate for assessment and intervention.

OT practice models (i.e., frames of reference): Understanding models of practice and frames of reference is necessary for organizing and developing interventions based on evidence from the profession. Knowledge of the principles and techniques allows practitioners to develop interventions for children with a variety of diagnoses.

Assessments appropriate for a child who has a specific disability or diagnosis: OT practitioners work with children with a number of different diagnoses. Therefore, OT practitioners must be knowledgeable about a variety of assessments to determine the specific needs of children. Assessments may also be used to measure outcomes of interventions.

Age-appropriate activities: OT practitioners working with children need to adjust therapy activities to suit the age and developmental needs of a particular child. Thus, knowledge of a range of age-appropriate activities is essential to practice.

Differences among systems in which OT services are provided: OT services are provided in a variety of settings. These settings exist within systems that have different missions. OT practitioners work within these settings and design interventions to meet the needs of their clients as well as those of the system. For example, children receiving services in a public school system require educationally relevant therapy goals and objectives, whereas children receiving services in a hospital require medically necessary goals and objectives.

Assistive technology: OT practitioners who work with infants, children, and adolescents who have disabilities or special needs must have knowledge of the range of assistive technologies that promote safe and independent living.

CENTENNIAL VISION

In 2017, the profession of OT will be 100 years old. AOTA has adopted a **Centennial Vision** that recognizes OT as a science-driven and evidence-based profession that continues to meet the occupational needs of clients, communities, and populations. AOTA is actively promoting OT practitioners to assume leadership roles and contribute to outcome databases that support evidence-based practice.[1]

The centennial vision addresses areas of pediatric practice, including the health and wellness of children and youth (including programs to prevent childhood obesity), and the psychosocial needs of children and youth.[7] AOTA, through its vision, suggests that practitioners continue to provide evidence of the importance of occupation and intervention.[1] The vision encourages practitioners to become leaders in the profession and to support the profession through participation in AOTA, scholarship (at many different levels) and clinical practice.[1]

The **Occupational Therapy Practice Framework (OTPF)** defines both the process and domain of occupational therapy.[6] Subsequent chapters discuss the OT process and domain in detail.

OCCUPATIONAL THERAPY PRACTICE FRAMEWORK

The OTPF was developed to assist practitioners in defining the process and domains of OT.[6] The OTPF is designed to be used by occupational therapists, certified occupational therapists, consumers, and health care providers. Figure 1-1 illustrates the framework.

The OTPF defines the process of OT as a dynamic, ongoing process that includes evaluation, intervention, and outcome. *Evaluation* provides an understanding of the clients' problems, occupational history, patterns, and assets.[6] *Intervention* includes the plan (based on selected theories, models of practice, frames of reference, and evidence), implementation, and review. *Outcome* refers to how well the goals are achieved. The domain of OT practice is occupation, defined as "activities . . . of everyday life, named, organized, and given value and meaning by individuals and a culture. Occupation is everything people do to occupy themselves, including looking after themselves, enjoying life, and contributing to the social and economic fabric of their communities." [11 (p.32)]. See Figure 1-2 for an illustration of the process. Occupation is viewed as both a means and an end.[6] Using occupation as a means includes such things as participating in school activities to improve the ability to function in school; it follows the "learning by doing" philosophy. Occupation is also viewed as an end in that the goal of therapy sessions is to enable the child to function in his or her occupations. For example, therapy sessions focusing on handwriting skills are intended to improve the child's ability to function in an academic occupation. The OTPF defines the areas of occupation as activities of daily living (ADLs), instrumental activities of daily living (IADLs), education, work, play, leisure, and social participation.[6] Clinicians examine performance skills (motor, processing and communication) and patterns (habits, routines, roles) associated with areas of occupation. Clinicians analyze the demands of activities and client factors required for an occupation in order to develop intervention plans. However, the OTPF focuses on the occupation instead of its components. Equally important is an examination of the contexts and environments in which an occupation occurs. According to the OTPF, these contexts and environments are cultural, personal, temporal, virtual, physical, and social (Table 1-1). Contexts influence how an occupation is viewed, performed, and evaluated. For example, when considering the temporal context, practitioners would expect differences in social behavior between a 2-year-old toddler and 6-year-old child.

THE OCCUPATIONAL THERAPY PROCESS

The OT practitioner uses a model of practice to organize her thinking and chooses a frame of reference to design interventions based on a child's needs and the family's needs (refer to Chapter 10 for specifics on model of practices and frames of reference). The frame of reference helps the practitioner decide what to do during therapy sessions. The OT process begins when a referral for OT services is made by a parent, physician, teacher, or other concerned professional. The occupational therapist decides whether the referred client should be screened, which helps determine whether the client will benefit from OT services.[3,8,9] If the screening shows that the child is likely to benefit from OT services, then the practitioner performs an evaluation. The occupational therapist determines the areas to be evaluated and may assign portions of the evaluation to an OTA. The evaluation process helps the occupational therapist identify the child's strengths and weaknesses. Long-term goals and short-term objectives are established on the basis of the OT practitioner's

AREAS OF OCCUPATION	CLIENT FACTORS	PERFORMANCE SKILLS	PERFORMANCE PATTERNS	CONTEXT AND ENVIRONMENT	ACTIVITY DEMANDS
Activities of Daily Living (ADL)*	Values, Beliefs, and Spirituality	Sensory Perceptual Skills	Habits	Cultural	Objects Used and Their Properties
Instrumental Activities of Daily Living (IADL)	Body Functions	Motor and Praxis Skills	Routines	Personal	Space Demands
Rest and Sleep	Body Structures	Emotional Regulation Skills	Roles	Physical	Social Demands
Education		Cognitive Skills	Rituals	Social	Sequencing and Timing
Work		Communication and Social Skills		Temporal	Required Actions
Play				Virtual	Required Body Functions
Leisure					Required Body Structures
Social Participation					
*Also referred to as *basic activities of daily living (BADL)* or *personal activities of daily living (PADL)*.					

FIGURE 1-1   Aspects of Occupational Therapy's Domain. All aspects of the domain transact to support engagement, participation, and health. This figure does not imply a hierarchy. (From the American Occupational Therapy Association: Occupational therapy practice framework: Domain and process, 2nd edition, *Am J Occup Ther* 62(6):625–683, 2008.)

EVALUATION

Occupational profile—The initial step in the evaluation process that provides an understanding of the client's occupational history and experiences, patterns of daily living, interests, values, and needs. The client's problems and concerns about performing occupations and daily life activities are identified, and the client's priorities are determined.

Analysis of occupational performance—The step in the evaluation process during which the client's assets, problems, or potential problems are more specifically identified. Actual performance is often observed in context to identify what supports performance and what hinders performance. Performance skills, performance patterns, context or contexts, activity demands, and client factors are all considered, but only selected aspects may be specifically assessed. Targeted outcomes are identified.

INTERVENTION

Intervention plan—A plan that will guide actions taken and that is developed in collaboration with the client. It is based on selected theories, frames of reference, and evidence. Outcomes to be targeted are confirmed.

Intervention implementation—Ongoing actions taken to influence and support improved client performance. Interventions are directed at identified outcomes. Client's response is monitored and documented.

Intervention review—A review of the implementation plan and process as well as its progress toward targeted outcomes.

OUTCOMES (Supporting Health and Participation in Life Through Engagement in Occupation)

Outcomes—Determination of success in reaching desired targeted outcomes. Outcome assessment information is used to plan future actions with the client and to evaluate the service program (i.e., program evaluation).

FIGURE 1-2 Process of Service Delivery. The process of service delivery is applied within the profession's domain to support the client's health and participation. (From the American Occupational Therapy Association: Occupational therapy practice framework: Domain and process, 2nd edition, *Am J Occup Ther* 62(6):625–683, 2008.)

TABLE 1-1

Definitions of Contexts*

CONTEXT	DEFINITION	EXAMPLE
Cultural	Customs, beliefs, activity patterns, behavior standards, and expectations accepted by the society of which the individual is a member. Includes political aspects, such as laws that affect access to resources and affirm personal rights. Also includes opportunities for education, employment, and economic support.	Ethnicity, family attitude, beliefs, values
Personal	"[F]eatures of the individual that are not part of a health condition or health status."[1] Personal context includes age, gender, socioeconomic status, and educational status.	25-year-old unemployed
Temporal	"Location of occupational performance in time."[2]	Stages of life, time of day, time of year, duration
Virtual	Environment in which communication occurs by means of airways or computers and an absence of physical contact.	Realistic simulation of an environment, chat rooms, radio transmissions
Physical	Nonhuman aspects of contexts. Includes accessibility to and performance within environments having natural terrain, plants, animals, buildings, furniture, objects, tools, or devices.	Objects, built environment, natural environment, geographic terrain, sensory qualities of environment
Social	Availability and expectations of significant individuals, such as spouse, friends, and caregivers. Also includes larger social groups that are influential in establishing norms, role expectations, and social routines.	Relationships with individuals, groups, or organizations; relationships with systems (political, economic, institutional)

*Context refers to a variety of interrelated conditions within and surrounding the client that influence performance.
[1] World Health Organization: International classification of functioning, disability and health (ICF), Geneva, Switzerland, 2001, WHO.
[2] Crepeau E, Cohn E, Boyt-Schell B: *Willard and Spackman's occupational therapy*, 11th edition, Philadelphia, 2009, Lippincott Williams and Wilkins.
Adapted from the American Occupational Therapy Association: Occupational therapy practice framework: Domain and process, 2nd edition, *Am J Occup Ther* 62:625–683, 2008.

interpretation of the assessment. In collaboration with the OTA, the occupational therapist develops an intervention plan based on these goals and objectives.[2] Depending on the client's progress and periodic reassessments, the plan is implemented and modified. The intervention is designed to address the goals and objectives based on a selected frame of reference. When deciding on a frame of reference, clinicians consider the diagnosis, client's age and stage in life (e.g., toddler, adolescent, adult), setting, their clinical expertise, and current evidence-based research, as well as the client's goals. Clinicians must keep themselves informed about current research and intervention strategies to develop effective interventions for the children they serve. The client is discharged when all of the goals and objectives have been met or if the occupational therapist decides that services should be discontinued. (For a more detailed discussion of the OT process, see Chapter 10).

ROLES OF THE OCCUPATIONAL THERAPIST AND OCCUPATIONAL THERAPY ASSISTANT

The occupational therapist is responsible for all aspects of the OT process and supervises the occupational therapy assistant (OTA). The extent to which the OTA is supervised by the occupational therapist depends on a variety of factors, including the knowledge, skill, and experience of the OTA. In any case, occupational therapists and OTAs are both considered *OT practitioners*, and therefore they share the responsibility of communicating with each other about their clients.[3,9]

QUALIFICATIONS, SUPERVISION, AND SERVICE COMPETENCY

Entry-level OTAs must meet basic qualifications to practice in the field of OT. As they gain experience by working with occupational therapists, OTAs require less supervision and gradually become more competent at providing occupational therapy services.[3]

Qualifications

Entry-level OTAs meet specific qualifications, which include having successfully completed course work in an accredited OTA program and having passed the certification examination administered by the National Board for Certification in Occupational Therapy (NBCOT).[3] In addition, OTAs must meet specific requirements established by OT regulatory boards in their respective states and obtain a license if required by state law.

Supervision

Four **levels of supervision** have been delineated by AOTA: close, routine, general, and minimal. *Close* supervision is direct, daily contact between the OTA and the occupational therapist at the work site. *Routine* supervision is direct contact between the OTA and the occupational therapist at the work site at least every 2 weeks and interim contact through other means, such as telephone conversations or e-mail messages. *General* supervision is minimum direct contact of 1 day per month and interim supervision as needed. *Minimum* supervision is that provided on an "as needed" basis. It is important to note that individual state OT regulatory agencies may require stricter guidelines than those established by AOTA. Stricter state guidelines supersede those of AOTA.[2,3,8,9]

The level of supervision that OTAs require varies with their level of expertise. AOTA defines three levels of expertise: entry, intermediate, and advanced.[3] OTAs' progress from one level to another is based on their acquisition of skills, knowledge, and proficiency and not on their years of experience. Entry-level OTAs are typically new graduates or those entering a new practice setting and have general knowledge of the population or setting but limited experience. Intermediate-level OTAs have acquired a higher level of skill through experience, continuing education, and involvement in professional activities. Advanced-level OTAs have specialized skills and may be recognized as experts in particular areas of practice. Although the extent to which a particular OTA is supervised varies according to the individual, the level of supervision generally falls into one defined by AOTA based on the OTA's expertise. An entry-level OTA requires close supervision, an intermediate-level OTA requires routine or general supervision, and an advanced-level OTA requires minimum supervision (Table 1-2).[3]

Service Competency

Levels of supervision are closely related to establishing **service competency**. AOTA defines service competency as "the determination, made by various methods, that two people performing the same or equivalent procedures will obtain the same or equivalent results."[2,3,8,9] Service competency is a means of ensuring that two individual OT practitioners will have the same results when administering a specific assessment, observing a specific performance area or component, or providing intervention. Communication between the OTA and the occupational therapist is an essential part of the entire OT process but is especially important when

TABLE 1-2

Supervision of the Occupational Therapy Assistant

LEVEL OF SUPERVISION	TYPE OF SUPERVISION
Close	Direct and daily contact; on-site supervision
Routine	Direct and regularly scheduled contact; on-site supervision
General	Indirect supervision as needed and direct contact once a month or as mandated by state regulatory board
Minimum	Direct and indirect supervision as needed or as mandated by state regulatory board

establishing service competency. Occupational therapists must be sure that they and the OTAs are performing assessments and intervention procedures in the same way. Once an occupational therapist has determined that an OTA has established service competency in a certain area, the OTA may perform an assessment or intervention procedure (within the parameters of that particular area) without close supervision by the occupational therapist. Ensuring service competency is an ongoing mutual learning experience.[3]

AOTA has specific guidelines for establishing service competency. For standardized assessments and intervention procedures that require no specific training to administer, the occupational therapist and OTA both perform the procedure. If they obtain equivalent results, the OTA may be allowed to administer subsequent procedures independently. For assessments and intervention procedures requiring more subjective interpretations, direct observation and videotaping are valuable tools that can be used to establish service competency. These tools allow practitioners to observe a client performing a particular task and compare their individual interpretations of the performance. Likewise, an occupational therapist can videotape a client, have an OTA watch the tape, and compare and contrast the observations that have been made. If the occupational therapist and the OTA consistently have similar interpretations, the OTA has established competency in observing and interpreting the particular area of performance.[2,3,8,9] Specific examples of establishing service competency are provided below.

Videotaping

Teresa, an OTA, used the biomechanical approach to intervention while providing care for Abigail, a 10-month-old child who had experienced a brachial plexus injury at birth. Before working with Abigail, Teresa reviewed a videotape of her supervising occupational therapist treating another child with a brachial plexus injury. Her discussion of the tape with the occupational therapist revealed that she understood the intervention procedures used. Abigail's next therapy session, which was led by Teresa, was videotaped. The occupational therapist watched the tape and observed that Teresa carefully positioned the child and successfully carried out the intervention plan. The occupational therapist determined that Teresa had established the service competency needed to treat Abigail. The occupational therapist and Teresa agreed that as part of the ongoing learning process, each month they would videotape and subsequently discuss one of Abigail's intervention sessions.

Co-treatment

Raja, a 4-year-old boy, diagnosed with cerebral palsy, recently received a nerve block to decrease flexor tone in his right arm. Since then, he was being treated by Alejandro, the occupational therapist. Alejandro recently asked Richard, an OTA, to assist him in treating Raja. Richard prepared for the co-treatment by reading about nerve blocks and carefully observing Alejandro's one-on-one intervention session with Raja. Richard asked pertinent questions and expressed a keen interest in working with Raja. After several successful co-treatment sessions in which Alejandro and Richard obtained equivalent outcomes from the procedures used, Alejandro assigned Raja's case to Richard. Richard then received only general supervision from Alejandro because he demonstrated service competency while working with Raja.

Observation

Missy, an OTA, used the rehabilitative approach to treat Dewayne, a 6-year-old who had had an amputation below the elbow. Before becoming an OTA, Missy had volunteered regularly at Shriner's hospital (on the unit which specialized in trauma and burn cases) and she had observed many clients being fitted with prostheses and had frequently assisted the therapists. After graduating as an OTA, she was hired to work in the OT department at Shriner's hospital. As an OTA, she worked closely with an occupational therapist, who developed intervention plans for clients with injuries similar to those of Dewayne. Missy also observed and assisted in administering the department's Prosthetic Checklist, which is designed to assess the care, application, and use of prostheses. Missy began working with Dewayne when the child was fitted for his first prosthesis at the age of 3. The occupational therapist observed Missy administering the procedures on the Prosthetic Checklist; their findings were equivalent. When Dewayne was fitted with a new prosthesis, the occupational therapist was confident that Missy could independently complete the checklist procedures accurately. Missy demonstrated service competency in administering the assessment.

AOTA'S CODE OF ETHICS

In 2005, the Representative Assembly of AOTA approved the Occupational Therapy **Code of Ethics**.[5] An updated version of the code of ethics was approved by the Representative Assembly in 2010. This new code was tailored to better address the ethical concerns of the profession.[5a] This is a public statement of the principles used to promote and maintain high standards of conduct by all occupational therapy personnel. The Code of Ethics is based on seven principles:

- Beneficence
- Nonmaleficence
- Autonomy and confidentiality
- Social justice
- Procedural justice
- Veracity
- Fidelity

Beneficence refers to the benefit of services to consumers. For example, if a child is not progressing or benefitting from OT services, then discontinuation of services would be considered an ethical decision. *Nonmaleficence* refers to the principle of not inflicting or imposing harm on consumers. The OT practitioner avoids activities or interventions that may hurt the child or adolescent. For example, the practitioner carefully observes the child's response to multisensory inputs and is alert to prevent sensory overload. The principles of *autonomy* and *confidentiality* relate to the rights and privacy of consumers. OT practitioners actively involve consumers in the intervention process and respect and uphold the consumer's rights to privacy and confidentiality. The principle of *social justice* refers to providing fair and equitable OT services for all clients.[5a] Thus, OT practitioners must make sure that all clients receive the same level of services despite such things as their ability level, socioeconomic status, or culture. For example, the OT practitioner does not schedule more sessions just because the parent's insurance will cover the cost, rather the practitioner schedules sessions based upon the child's needs. The principle of *procedural justice* necessitates that OT practitioners comply with state and federal laws and the AOTA's policies. Furthermore, this principle ensures that practitioners provide OT services in accordance with established policies and procedures. In terms of the relationship between the occupational therapist and the OTA, procedural justice ensures that supervision is provided within the required guidelines established in state laws. *Veracity* means honesty in all professional matters. Practitioners are adhering to the principle of veracity when they accurately document services provided, including the child's progress. Veracity also includes being honest about one's professional qualifications and level of competency. *Fidelity* refers to respect, fairness, discretion, and integrity. In practice, practitioners are following the principle of fidelity when they provide the same quality of care to all consumers, regardless of payment schedules, culture, or disability. OT practitioners are expected to adhere to the profession's code of ethics at all times.[5]

SCHOLARSHIP

Occupational therapy practitioners must be life-long learners to be competent in the provision of services. **Scholarship** is a form of leadership and enables practitioners to expand their knowledge base and to maintain competence. Scholarship involves the dissemination of findings, either formally or informally. OT practitioners may choose a variety of options for disseminating their findings, including in-service training, conference presentations, poster sessions, publications, journal club discussions, and informal networking. Practitioners may choose to network with others by using Internet technology, such as blogging. Scholarship may involve formal learning, for example, by taking courses. Some practitioners may wish to demonstrate knowledge through practical application.

Boyer defines the types of scholarship as: discovery, integration, application, and teaching.[10] *Discovery* scholarship includes work that contributes to the body of knowledge of a profession, thus increasing evidence-based practice options. For example, searching the literature to review various intervention methods is a form of discovery scholarship.

Integration scholarship involves interpreting and synthesizing research findings to identify linkages across disciplines. Exploring interventions used in physical therapy, speech therapy, or education and relating those findings to OT is a form of integration scholarship.

Frequently, OT practitioners are interested in applying professional knowledge to solve clinical problems and to assess outcomes. This type of scholarship is called *application* scholarship.

OT practitioners frequently educate others and family members on intervention techniques and, as such, are interested in examining their teaching effectiveness. *Teaching* scholarship is used to determine how the client best learns. It is also used when OT faculty and practitioners examine how the OTA student learns in the classroom and while on fieldwork.

OT practitioners are encouraged to actively engage in scholarly activities at various levels on a regular basis. For instance, participation in a journal club to discuss a particular client group, laws, or systems in your state offers scholarship opportunities to practitioners. Presenting new interventions or interesting findings at state conferences or through in-service training is often helpful in refining ideas. Engaging in a variety of scholarship activities benefits practitioners as well as clients.

SUMMARY

This chapter presented an overview of pediatric OT practice beginning with an overview of the AOTA Centennial Vision and how it relates to OT practice with children. An overview of the OTPF was followed by a discussion of the OT process. The role of the occupational therapist and the OTA were defined throughout the chapter, with an emphasis on the qualifications, supervision, and service competency requirements for the entry-level OTA. Examples throughout the chapter illustrated how levels of supervision, and service competency are used in the delivery of OT services within the realm of the OTPF. A discussion of the AOTA Code of Ethics was presented, using pediatric case examples to reinforce key concepts. Finally, the authors defined scholarship, providing examples to illustrate how OTAs can contribute to the professions' work in pediatrics.

References

1. American Occupational Therapy Association: *AOTA's centennial vision: shaping the future of occupational therapy.* Available at: http://www.aota.org/nonmembers/area16. Accessed March 5, 2010.
2. American Occupational Therapy Association: Guidelines for documentation of occupational therapy. *Am J Occup Ther* 62:684–690, 2008.
3. American Occupational Therapy Association: Guidelines for supervision, roles, and responsibilities during the delivery of occupational therapy services. *Am J Occup Ther* 63(6):707–803, 2009.
4. American Occupational Therapy Association: Occupational therapy assistant model curriculum, September 2008. Available at: http://www.aota.org. Accessed June 2, 2010.
5. American Occupational Therapy Association: Occupational therapy code of ethics. *Am J Occup Ther* 59(6):639–642, 2005.
5a. American Occupational Therapy Association: Occupational therapy code of ethics and ethical standards, 2010. Available at: http://www.AOTA.org. Accessed June 2, 2010.
6. American Occupational Therapy Association: Occupational therapy practice framework: domain and process, ed 2. *Am J Occup Ther* 62:625–683, 2008.
7. American Occupational Therapy Association: Psychosocial aspects of occupational therapy. *Am J Occup Ther* 58:669–672, 2004.
8. American Occupational Therapy Association: Scope of practice. *Am J Occup Ther* 58:673–677, 2004.
9. American Occupational Therapy Association: Standards of practice for occupational therapy. *Am J Occup Ther* 59:663–665, 2005.
10. Boyer EL: *Scholarship reconsidered: priorities of the profession,* San Francisco, 1997, Jossey-Bass.
11. Law M et al: Core concepts of occupational therapy. In Townsend E, editor: *Enabling occupation: an occupational therapy perspective,* Ottawa, Canadian Association for Occupational Therapists, pp 29–56. 2002
12. American Occupational Therapy Association: Occupational therapy salaries and job opportunities continue to improve: 2006 AOTA workforce and compensation survey. *OT Practice,* September 25, 2006.

Recommended Reading

Crepeau E, Cohn E, Boyt-Schell B: *Willard and Spackman's occupational therapy,* ed 11, Philadelphia, 2009, Lippincott Williams & Wilkins.
Hussey S, Sabonis-Chafee B, O'Brien J: *Introduction to occupational therapy,* ed 3, St. Louis, 2007, Mosby.
Sladyk K, Jacobs K, Macrae N: *Occupational therapy essentials for clinical competence,* Thorofare, NJ, 2009, Slack, Inc.

REVIEW Questions

1. List and describe five content areas in which a pediatric OT practitioner needs to have knowledge while working with children and adolescents.
2. Describe the guidelines for evaluation and intervention discussed in the OTPF.
3. What is service competency? How is it established?
4. Describe the various types of scholarship that would enhance practice.
5. Define the seven ethical principles, and provide a clinical example of each.

SUGGESTED *Activities*

1. Interview an OTA or an occupational therapist who works in pediatrics. The focus of the interview should be supervision and service competency. Questions might include the following:
   (a) Which courses in school have proved to be the most useful to you as a pediatric OT practitioner?
   (b) How many years of clinical experience do you have?
   (c) What is the level of supervision that you receive (OTA) or give (occupational therapist)? What are the means by which this occurs?
   (d) How is service competency established between the occupational therapist and the OTA in your workplace?

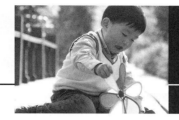

2

Family Systems

PAMELA J. WINTON

ROBERT E. WINTON

CHAPTER *Objectives*

After studying this chapter, the reader will be able to accomplish the following:

- Describe why it is important for an occupational therapy practitioner to have knowledge of and skills related to working with families.
- Describe the differences between prescriptive and consultative professional roles.
- Understand the way a therapy program for a child always has an impact on the family unit.
- Describe the key concepts of family systems and life cycle theories and the roles of these concepts in interventions for children.
- Recognize and appreciate that all families have unique ways of adapting and coping with life events and that effective therapy builds on these existing coping strategies.
- Describe several communication strategies that an occupational therapy practitioner can use to promote familial–professional partnerships.

KEY TERMS	CHAPTER OUTLINE

Domain

Client-centered

Prescriptive

Consultative

Morphostatic principle

Morphogenetic principle

Equifinality

Consultative and prescriptive
professional roles

Life cycle

Normative life cycle events

Non-normative life cycle
events

Adaptation

Resources

Perceptual coping strategies

Acknowledgment

The Importance of Families

*Current Issues Affecting Occupational Therapy Practitioners
and Families*

CHANGES IN POLICIES AND SERVICE DELIVERY MODELS

EXPANSION OF PRACTITIONERS' ROLES

DEMOGRAPHIC CHANGES IN THE AMERICAN POPULATION

IMPLICATIONS FOR PRACTICE

Family Systems Theory

DESCRIPTION

GENERAL SYSTEMS THEORY CONCEPTS

IMPLICATIONS FOR PRACTICE

Family Life Cycle

DESCRIPTION

IMPLICATIONS FOR PRACTICE

Family Adaptation

DESCRIPTION

IMPLICATIONS FOR PRACTICE

Essential Skills for Successful Interventions with Families

Summary

Margarita Sanchez, 3 years old, has been diagnosed with pervasive developmental delays and mild-to-moderate cerebral palsy. She lives in a small apartment with her paternal grandmother, great aunt, parents, and three siblings who are 11 months, 5 years, and 6 years of age. When Heather McFall, the occupational therapy (OT) practitioner, arrives for a routine visit, she learns that Margarita's mother has not been working with Margarita on the toilet training program that was discussed during the last visit. Heather had recommended that they start the program because she thought it was important that Margarita be toilet trained in time to begin a public school prekindergarten program in the fall. After some discussion, it becomes apparent that in the winter Mrs. Sanchez is unable to deal with the wet, soiled clothes that invariably accompany a toilet training program. After further discussion, Heather and Mrs. Sanchez agree to wait until the weather gets warmer to begin toilet training. During their conversation, Heather also realizes that she needs to plan a time for the Sanchez family to visit the prekindergarten class and see what they think of the program. Although Heather is enthusiastic about the academic and social experiences that Margarita would have in the class, Mrs. Sanchez seems hesitant and uncharacteristically quiet when they talk about the program. Heather has learned that Mrs. Sanchez tends to become quiet when she has reservations about an idea.

As Heather leaves the apartment, she thinks about her relationship with the family and how it has developed during the 2 years she has been working with Margarita. At the beginning of the relationship, Heather was often frustrated by Mrs. Sanchez's seeming disinterest in, or inability to follow through with, some of the home program ideas that Heather introduced. She had fretted and fumed but tried to help Mrs. Sanchez see the importance of taking Margarita's needs seriously and devoting the necessary time to therapy. It was only after discussing the case with a colleague that Heather realized she had departed from the guidelines of the 2008 Occupational Therapy Practice Framework (OTPF).[2] She had gotten caught up in her own expertise in the **domain** of OT and had strayed from a **client-centered*** consultative process.

As Heather recalls this, she laughs to herself as she recognizes that she has "done it again" with regard to the toilet training directive. She is also happy that she has recovered her client-centered role and has helped Mrs. Sanchez develop a plan that incorporates some of her ideas into the family routines. Mrs. Sanchez's silent response also has clued her in to the fact that she had departed from the client-centered consultative role related to the preschool issue. She resolves that on the next visit she will attempt to remain client centered as she revisits the idea of preschool.

THE IMPORTANCE OF FAMILIES

The vignette of Margarita and her family underscores the reason it is important for OT practitioners to understand family systems. Box 2-1 contains the key reasons for using a family-centered approach in early intervention when working with young children who have disabilities.

Families have the most significant environmental influence on a young child's life and development. As evident in the case study presented above, the majority of Margarita's time is spent with her family. If the family members are not convinced of the benefits of therapy or are unable to find time to carry out the intervention plan, optimal improvement in Margarita's case is unlikely to occur. As interventionists, OT practitioners enter children's lives for relatively brief periods. Family members are the "constants" in most children's lives.

The OT practitioner may function in two distinct roles in his or her involvement with a family—**prescriptive** and **consultative**. When working directly with the child, the OT practitioner functions primarily in the prescriptive and directive role; when working with the family, he or she functions primarily in the consultative role. Consulting with the family on the possibility of achieving the desired goals for the child and for the family builds collaboration and trust, which are key ingredients for intervention success with families.

CLINICAL *Pearl*

Developing a trusting and collaborative relationship with families is a key ingredient for intervention success.

BOX 2-1

Reasons Families Are Important

- A family has a significant environmental influence on a young child's life and development.
- Interventions with children inevitably affect the family.
- Laws and current service delivery models promote a family-centered approach.
- Professional organizations, including the American Occupational Therapy Association, have identified the areas of competency and created recommended guidelines for working with families.

---

* The Occupational Therapy Practice Framework: Domain and Process[2] defines the term "client" as the individual or the individual within the context of a group (i.e., a family). The terms "client-centered" and "family-centered" are used interchangeably in this manuscript.

Interventions with children have an inevitable impact on the life of the family; therefore, interventions are most effective when the family is consulted and invests in the development of the treatment plan. Margarita's story reveals the importance of considering the whole family with regard to the intervention plan. It also illustrates the advantages of the occupational therapist functioning in a family-centered, consultative role, one that acknowledges and supports a family's central function in the design and implementation of intervention plans. Margarita's therapist learned the importance of this concept when she recalled her initial failed attempt to help the family institute a toilet training program and again while introducing the idea of preschool for Margarita.

The family-centered approach is also the focus of many current laws and health care delivery models. Public Law 99-457, which was passed in 1986 (IDEA, Part C), is considered revolutionary because of its emphasis on the central role a family plays in interventions with young children. This law and its subsequent interpretations have altered the way in which services for young children are planned and delivered. Some of the highlights of the early intervention component of the law include the following: (1) families are mandated co-leaders on state-level advisory boards that make recommendations about the way in which service systems are designed; (2) family concerns, resources, and priorities guide the development of individual intervention plans; (3) families play an important role in children's assessments and evaluations; and (4) families have certain rights to confidentiality, record keeping, notification, and other procedures related to the programs and agencies that serve their children. The law ushered in additional changes that ultimately benefit families, such as promoting interdisciplinary and interagency collaboration. The importance of collaboration among agencies and disciplines became apparent when numerous stories surfaced about various health care professionals providing conflicting advice and recommendations to families with regard to their children with disabilities.[6]

Professional organizations, including the American Occupational Therapy Association (AOTA), have identified particular areas of competency and recommended certain guidelines to emphasize the importance of practitioners having the skills and knowledge necessary to work effectively with families.[1] The dramatic changes in the relationship between families and professionals, which were catalyzed by Public Law 99-457, as well as the increased focus on the importance of families in all human service organizations did not develop overnight. The existing workforce has had to develop new collaboration and communication skills. University and community college training programs have had to retrain their faculties and upgrade their curricula in order to prepare students adequately for the newly defined pediatric roles (Box 2-2).[3] Professional organizations have supported the changes by creating recommended practice guidelines and areas of competency.

BOX 2-2

American Occupational Therapy Association Guidelines for Curriculum Content in Pediatrics

ACADEMIC AND LEVEL I FIELDWORK
Family Systems Theory
The way families operate as units, the impact of diverse cultures and child-rearing patterns on family life, and differences in child rearing

Family Life Cycle
Critical stages of family life and parenting

Family Ecology
The way family systems operate in society, including the immediate community and the state and federal systems

Effects of Disabilities on Families
The emotional and social impact of an infant, toddler, child, or youth with disabilities on the parents' and family's life

Effects of Family and Environment on Children With Disabilities
The impact of different family styles and environments on an infant, toddler, child, or youth with disabilities

Role of Occupational Therapy
The role of the occupational therapist in helping a family assess their concerns and priorities for intervention; the use of self-reporting instruments in OT

LEVEL II PEDIATRIC FIELDWORK
(FOR ENTRY-LEVEL PRACTICE)
Rapport
The way to establish rapport with caregivers; the role of the occupational therapist as a partner in treatment planning

Collaboration
Strategies for having collaborative consultations with infants, toddlers, children, or youths with disabilities and their caregivers

Adapted from the American Occupational Therapy Association Commission on Education: *Guidelines for curriculum content in pediatrics*, Bethesda, MD, 1991, The Association.

CURRENT ISSUES AFFECTING OCCUPATIONAL THERAPY PRACTITIONERS AND FAMILIES

Changes in Policies and Service Delivery Models

As mentioned previously, policies and legislation passed in the last 15 years have affected service delivery models and recommended OT practices. The resulting changes have included emphasis on the following approaches to service delivery.

- Interdisciplinary and family-centered approaches are used when planning and implementing interventions.
- Children who have disabilities are included in regular educational settings.
- Therapists act as consultants, providing pediatric treatment that is integrated into the children's regular routines and natural environments instead of using "pull out therapy"* (Figure 2-1).

Expansion of Practitioners' Roles

Recent changes in service delivery and implementation have resulted in an expansion of the OT practitioners' roles. Their duties now also include the following:

- Assessing family interests, priorities, and concerns
- Observing and gathering information about the daily routines of children and families in their homes and in the classrooms

---

* "Pull out therapy" is therapy not provided in the context of a child's daily routine.

- Gathering and sharing information with families about development and intervention strategies
- Implementing therapy in collaboration with parents, caregivers, and general educators

Demographic Changes in the American Population

In addition to changes in laws, policies, and recommended practices, the demographic makeup of the children being served has also changed. Nearly half of the children in the United States under the age of 5 years are racial or ethnic minorities.[5] In contrast, although the American population is becoming more diverse, the members of professional organizations such as AOTA and the American Speech and Hearing Association (ASHA) are predominantly Caucasian.[1,4]

Implications for Practice

The myriad changes taking place in the OT environment affect service delivery and implementation in numerous ways, including the following:

- OT practitioners are more likely than ever to be working with children and families whose cultural backgrounds and native languages are different from their own. They may need to use translators or interpreters. They must develop the ability to appreciate and respect cultural differences, which may mean developing an awareness of their own cultural identities, the acknowledgment of inherent biases and values, and knowledge of other cultures.

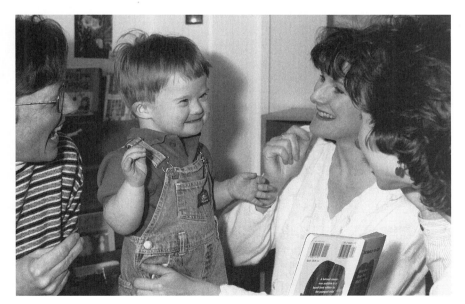

FIGURE 2-1 Therapist Working With the Mother, Child, and Early-Childhood Teacher at a Daycare Center. This is an example of interdisciplinary collaboration and embedding therapy into the daily routine. (Courtesy Don Trull, FPG Child Development Institute, University of North Carolina—Chapel Hill, Chapel Hill, NC.)

- Young children who have disabilities are more likely than ever to be in regular early childhood and educational programs. OT practitioners must be able to embed therapy into the daily routines of home, child-care, and regular educational settings and must develop expertise in consulting with early childhood teachers, families, and other specialists.
- OT practitioners need the knowledge and skill to work as members of interdisciplinary teams, which requires interpersonal, communicative, and collaborative skills.
- OT practitioners must obtain information on a wide range of community-based programs and services, both specialized and generic, to meet the individual needs of the various families and children with whom they work.

FAMILY SYSTEMS THEORY
Description

Family systems theory is a core framework for guiding interactions with families. It is a group of ideas that describe the many ways that individuals in families are connected across time and space,* and its implications for the families with whom practitioners work are far reaching. Developing and increasing an understanding of the family as a system significantly affects the way practitioners working with families perceive their own roles, determine which potential outcomes are positive, and perceive family changes. The core concepts of family systems theory are provided in Box 2-3.

General Systems Theory Concepts

Each living system (including family), to be recognizable as such, must have some order, no matter how undesirable or chaotic it appears to an outside observer. The maintenance of this order has been named the **morphostatic** (form maintenance) **principle**. Examples

---

* The definition of family in this chapter is inclusive: ". . . two or more people who regard themselves as a family and who perform some of the functions that families typically perform. These people may or may not be related by blood or marriage and may or may not usually live together."[8]

BOX 2-3

Family Systems Theory Concepts

MORPHOSTATIC PRINCIPLE

Like all systems, family systems are organized with recognizable feedback loops and "rules." These "rules" may be ones that are consciously recognized and spoken by family members but most are nonverbal and shared assumptions of family functioning. An example of a spoken "rule" is: "In our family, parents always inquire about his or her child's day and the child always responds." An example of a nonverbal "rule" is a parent expressing anger at a child and the child withdrawing to avoid conflict. Deviation from either pattern by the parent or the child would be met with corrective (morphostatic) action. Failure of the parent to inquire or the child to respond in the first instance would draw the immediate attention of the other, wondering if there was a problem. In the second example, an arguing response could be met with increasing anger from the parent until the child finally withdraws; if the parent fails to respond angrily to an "infraction," the child might escalate the misbehavior until the angry response occurs.

MORPHOGENETIC PRINCIPLE

Families do evolve; that is, they change. Just as a child grows and develops, families do, too. In the examples above, the parent who usually asks how his or her child's day was might get caught up in work or in taking care of a younger sibling and not be available when the now older and more independent child arrives home. The child might start volunteering information about his or her activities without being asked. In the latter example, the child, as he or she grows older and gains experience outside the family, may see this as undesirable and no longer be willing to continue the sequence. Either the parent or the child will initiate a conversation that leads to an agreement to make changes in the sequence.

EQUIFINALITY

This concept is, in many ways, a subset of the morphogenetic principle. Simply stated, it says that any system can change in an infinite number of ways. If we again take the second example above, a positive change was described. Another version might be that the now 16-year-old boy becomes increasingly belligerent, gets into a physical fight with his dad, and either runs away or is kicked out of the house. Even in this extreme example, it is important to recognize that the "family" continues and the notion of equifinality still applies. The child could become addicted to drugs, with the parents forever grieving, or he could eventually get into the military, receive the GI bill, do well in college for a couple of years, and be reunited with his family, who then support him through graduate school and he subsequently wins the Nobel prize. Equifinality does not imply an endpoint but, rather, a series of way stations in the life of a family. For the OT practitioner, it is the most important idea, one of hope and optimism.

for families include daily family rhythms such as meals, bedtime, expectations for bathing, greetings or departures, and affectionate naming. At the same time, these systems have a capacity for change, which has been named the **morphogenetic** (form-evolving) **principle.** Examples for families include gaining or losing a member through marriage, divorce, birth and death, and the shifting roles of members through marriage, school progression, or aging. Change is possible only through the introduction and assimilation of new information into the system, such as gaining or losing members.

A feature of the form-evolving (morphogenetic) aspect of living systems is their capacity to evolve along different paths and yet arrive at a given "destination." It implies that no single past event predicts a system's current form, nor does any specific current event specifically predict a future form. This has been named **equifinality.** The practitioner will see families that are similar in many ways but whose lives have been affected in dramatically different ways by the introduction of a child with special needs. A clear example is one in which the family seems to have been drawn closer together, in contrast with that in which the family has become emotionally disconnected.

Implications for Practice

The OT practitioner is an agent for bringing new information into the system. In addition to the core knowledge (the domain of the profession) the practitioner brings, he or she must develop communication skills to help the family assimilate this new information. To do so, the OT practitioner is guided by these two basic ideas: (1) "I must acknowledge and accept current family form and function" (support the current form); and (2) "I must ally myself with the system's capacity for change" (support the assimilation of the new knowledge I bring). These ideas form the basis for the consultative role.

The OT practitioner leverages his or her ability to support change by eliciting from the family its desired outcomes and integrating his or her ideas into a collaborative plan aimed first and foremost at achieving the family's goals. This is truly family-centered practice, with the family being the client and the OT practitioner being a consultant rather than a prescriptive interventionist.

A major goal in working with families is establishing a trusting relationship, particularly with key members. One of the first steps in establishing trust is to identify the outcomes family members desire. Given that different family members have different priorities, helping them find verbal expression for outcomes that everyone can endorse builds that trust in a powerful way. Sometimes families simply have the basic desire to help their children grow and develop. Regardless of whether a family's goals are vague, it is important to acknowledge the ways family members perceive the current situation and priorities while helping them agree on goals.

CLINICAL *Pearl*

The first step in a successful intervention is identifying what the family hopes to accomplish.

CLINICAL *Pearl*

Intervention efforts should begin with a clarification and acknowledgment of the way in which family members perceive their situation and define their priorities, however unfocused their goals may seem.

The second step in building a trusting relationship is developing strategies for accomplishing the family's agreed-upon goals. The strategies should be developed in collaboration with the family to ensure adherence to its beliefs and daily living patterns. In the case of Margarita, Heather began the intervention process by working with the mother, which, given her key role, was the appropriate way to begin establishing a trusting relationship. However, even if she had successfully consulted with the mother at the previous visit to determine that toilet training was a desirable goal for the family, she departed from the consultative role when she decided on the timeline for Margarita's toilet training. Instead, once the family had endorsed the idea, Heather could have consulted with Mrs. Sanchez about the practical realities and timing of implementing the training. To implement the toilet training even more powerfully, she could have included the father, grandmother, and aunt in developing strategies once they had endorsed these ideas as desired goals. This would have avoided some of the constraints created by Mrs. Sanchez's already complex life. Because Heather had failed to include the other family members in the planning process, she missed some opportunities to support the intervention/change process. Fortunately, Heather was able to shift out of the prescriptive and directive role, which had previously led to frustration.

Margarita's story illustrates a common occurrence—the professional role of the OT practitioner as the prescriber of intervention clashing with existing family functioning. This can significantly reduce the efficiency and effectiveness of any intervention. The paradox is that families desire professional expertise and assistance and it is hard for practitioners to resist the temptation to take a directive role. At the same time families do not like being told what exactly to do by someone else, especially as interventions may disrupt family routines and behaviors. Some families can be creative and take a prescribed intervention and weave it into existing family routines, beliefs, and daily living patterns, but many will do less well or discard the intervention altogether. Staying in a consultative role is key to intervention success. The OT practitioner helps families integrate the interventions that move them toward the agreed-upon goals and into their daily living patterns as well as they can. As the consultant, the OT practitioner not only helps the families integrate new intervention strategies but also helps them troubleshoot those aspects of the plan that they were unable to actually accomplish. "Trying harder" rarely works. Changing the process, the goals, and the timeline, however, are all reasonable adaptations to current family functioning. With this approach, families are more likely to take full advantage of the practitioner's expertise. OT practitioners who are able to relinquish their felt power as experts and provide consultation in a truly family-centered fashion are often able to make the most of their professional skills and expertise.

CLINICAL *Pearl*

The likelihood of families following through with intervention plans depends on the extent to which those plans are constructed to fit within families' existing routines, beliefs, and patterns of family life.

OT practitioners should also be aware that success with a family is an evolving process. As in the case of Heather, the only real mistake is the one that is not recognized. An easy way to enhance the family's trust is to consult with them on intervention plans gone awry. Being truly curious to learn about the family and collaborating with the family to add or change elements in a plan not only improve the odds of success but also further the family's acceptance of the therapist. Developing a trusting relationship with families takes time. Differences in cultural and linguistic backgrounds and heritages also influence how quickly and easily relationships are formed, but adhering to the consultative role does accelerate the process.

FAMILY LIFE CYCLE
Description

Another concept covered in the AOTA *Guidelines for Pediatric Curriculum Content*[3] is the family **life cycle**. Like individuals, families also go through normal or typical developmental phases. No consensus exists on the number of phases that should be considered, which is not surprising considering that family development is a fluid process and not a discontinuous series of steps. Critical stages of the family life cycle are those involving life transitions: birth, marriage, leaving home, and death.

Perhaps one of the most important points about the phases of the life cycle is the fact that moving from one phase to another causes stress and requires the family to adapt. Stress is completely normal and necessary for the evolution (morphogenesis) of the family system. Life cycle changes bring about changes in the needs, interests, roles, and responsibilities of each family member. For instance, becoming a parent entails learning a whole new set of skills and alters the relationships between the parents and among the parents and their extended family and friends. Families can often benefit from the extra support of friends, neighbors, or extended family members during life cycle transitions.

Children who have disabilities have special needs and undergo numerous stressful life cycle events. These events may include unexpected hospitalization for a lengthy period, unusual and sometimes painful treatments, and participation in special education and early intervention programs. These events often involve new relationships with numerous different professionals. Forming new relationships, especially when individual choice does not exist (as when a practitioner is assigned a case), can be stressful. In the case of Margarita, the arrival of an OT practitioner in the Sanchez household created a certain degree of stress. As Heather, the therapist, shifted into a more consultative role, the stress of intervention was no longer dealt with by dropping the prescribed intervention and changing nothing (morphostatic principle); rather, the intervention (toilet training) was integrated into a family plan for change that was endorsed, at least in its timing, by Mrs. Sanchez and was therefore more likely to succeed (adhering to the morphogenetic principle).

Watching a child miss typical milestones can create stress for a family. For instance, the realization that a child has not started walking or talking by the appropriate age can be very stressful. In Margarita's case, the fact that her younger 11-month-old sister had begun to walk whereas the 3-year-old Margarita had not, clearly highlighted the ongoing and unexpected stress caused by Margarita's extended dependency for basic functions such as feeding and toileting.

Because certain events—for example, frequent hospitalizations, participating in OT interventions, or not reaching important milestones—are not **normative life cycle events** (i.e., the usual or expected transitional events), families experiencing these events have fewer people with whom to share their experiences. For instance, the parents of adolescents often find it helpful to share "war stories" with other parents about transitional events, for example, teaching the adolescent to drive. The majority of the parents of adolescents can relate to the challenges and triumphs associated with this event. Research has shown that sharing experiences and getting support from family, friends, and neighbors are effective strategies for dealing with stress.[6] However, few parents can relate to **non-normative life cycle events** (not the usual or expected transitional events), such as the experience of raising a child who will never be able to walk.

Implications for Practice

The life events that have been described are somewhat arbitrary and obviously overlap, so they are grossly inadequate representations of the wide range of family experiences that exist. Cultural factors can also affect how these events and life stages are perceived and experienced. For example, is it acceptable for an adult child to be living with his or her parents? In the case of many Caucasian families, this situation would be perceived as a failure on the part of the child, whereas this may be normal in many Hispanic families. Practitioners tend to attach meanings, usually rooted in their own backgrounds, beliefs, and experiences, to the phases of the family life cycle. This tendency can potentially put practitioners at odds with certain families. This is illustrated in the case study about Margarita. Heather, with her Anglo-Saxon values, recommended that Margarita attend the prekindergarten program in a public school because she thought it would enhance Margarita's social and cognitive development. Mrs. Sanchez became quiet when Heather made that suggestion, something that Heather came to recognize as a sign of disagreement. Perhaps the Sanchez family considered it unusual for children to attend any school at such a young age, or they may have preferred a neighborhood parochial school with several bilingual nuns on the staff.

Being sensitive to family transitional events (normative and non-normative) is also important. Events such as the death of a parent, an adult child leaving home, and a job transition can all take the time and attention of the family away from intervention efforts. Consider the big picture when working with a family. Family-centered consultation is clearly preferred under such circumstances.

During non-normative transitional events, the families of children who have disabilities sometimes find it extremely helpful to be connected with each other. They can share information, similar experiences, and methods of coping. Parent-to-parent programs exist in many communities, and research has demonstrated their helpfulness.[7]

FAMILY ADAPTATION
Description

In what ways do families adapt to unexpected events, such as the birth of a child who has developmental delays? Crises, which are brought on by overwhelming stress, are not always negative. Families are living systems that evolve in response to internal events (e.g., illness, death, birth, emancipation) and external events (e.g., the loss of a job, a move to another city, the involvement of the OT practitioner). Like all living things, families are generally adaptive (the morphogenetic principle) by nature. Although serious crises can precipitate alcoholism, separation or divorce, or family violence, in some cases they can enable rapid positive changes, such as recommitment to a marriage or resolution of a long-standing conflict. For many years, research on the families of children with disabilities was focused on family dysfunction, stress, and pathology. However, in recent years research has revealed what some families had been saying for years: Despite the stress caused by their child's disability, dealing with the disability strengthened the family or changed it in some positive way.[8]

Families react and adapt to crises in individualized and unique ways. Family **adaptation** is affected by the interaction of family **resources** (e.g., time, money, and friends) and perceptions (the way events are defined). Social support plays an extremely important role in family and individual well-being. For the families of children with disabilities, the informal support of the extended family, friends, and neighbors appears to be more important than the formal support received from professionals and institutions. Of course, an important factor is the way families define their resources. In the previously mentioned Sanchez family, the extended family is a source of positive support for Margarita's parents, whereas in other families, a mother-in-law or an aunt living in the home could be a source of additional stress.

In addition, the way families define and understand a particular event, such as the birth of a child with a disability, is an important component of family adaptation. Specific **perceptual coping strategies** are listed in Box 2-4.

At times therapists get impatient with families who seem to ignore or minimize problems. Although it may be tempting to be judgmental in these situations, it is important to recognize that these families are using their own coping strategies. Families adapt as a whole, and this adaptive capacity should be supported. OT practitioners should not assess a given situation and assign direct responsibility to any specific factor. For example, a practitioner cannot accurately assume that George, a 6-year-old who cannot tie his shoes, would be able to if only he had started OT therapy at age 3. Too many other variables are relevant. For example, family financial

Perceptual Coping Strategies

PASSIVE APPRAISAL
Ignoring a problem and hoping it will go away

REFRAMING
Redefining a situation in ways that make it more manageable

DOWNWARD COMPARISON
Identifying a situation that is worse than your own

USE OF SPIRITUAL BELIEFS
Using philosophical or spiritual beliefs to make sense of and find meaning in a situation

demands, time constraints, and emotional strain may have been significant factors when George was 3. Beginning OT at that age could have forced George's father, who had just overcome his drinking and spousal abuse problems, to regress. In turn, this could have caused George to regress and lose his toileting skills. No individual, not even an OT practitioner, can conceive of all the potential positive outcomes and all the ways to achieve those outcomes (equifinality). Families and OT practitioners have attitudes and biases about the causes of problems and the possibilities of overcoming them. Nevertheless, the adaptive potential of a family as a whole is unlimited, and remembering this can help families as well as OT practitioners achieve the best possible outcomes.

Implications for Practice

When meeting a family for the first time, it is important to be interested in learning about the unique ways in which the parents have been adapting to their child's disability—the ingenious ways that they cope in their daily lives. In the story about Margarita Sanchez, Heather regained this curiosity and interest when she recognized Mrs. Sanchez's indirect feedback, that is, her quietness, which indicated that Heather had shifted from the consultative role.

CLINICAL *Pearl*

When meeting a family for the first time, it is important to express curiosity and interest in the unique ways in which they are adapting to their child's disability without judging and evaluating.

It is also important to use and support existing resources in families' lives. OT practitioners sometimes get so excited about specialized support services that they forget about generic support services such as churches, neighborhood playgrounds, and community recreation centers that are closer to home. If OT practitioners are not careful, their clients may suddenly realize that they have lost touch with neighbors and friends because of the time spent taking their children to specialized programs far from home. They could end up in a specialized world inhabited mainly by professionals.

Families must carry out daily tasks to perform their basic functions.* Family routines must be considered when home therapy programs are developed; otherwise, time-consuming programs that simply cannot be done within the parameters of the daily household routines and time schedule may be prescribed.

ESSENTIAL SKILLS FOR SUCCESSFUL INTERVENTION WITH FAMILIES

For OT practitioners, having good communication skills is just as important as having the proper knowledge to treat a client. Some essential communication skills include the following:

- *Solution-focused curiosity and interest*: People generally have an extremely positive response to practitioners who are nonjudgmentally interested in them and their situations. The focus should be on strengths, achievements, and desires rather than on the traditional problems and deficits. This "solution focus" allows the practitioner to support the adaptive (morphogenetic) potential of the family while not challenging or criticizing its current status. In the example of the Sanchez family, it would be better that Heather asks Mrs. Sanchez, "What have you found that works best for feeding Margarita?" rather than "What problems do you encounter when feeding Margarita?"
- *Collaborative goal setting*: A family that has requested or been referred for OT services has some goals, even if only vague ones, that they hope the services will help achieve. The practitioner may have a very different idea of what the goals should be. Collaborating with the family to clarify and develop a common set of goals helps practitioners efficiently and effectively manage the treatment planning process. Staying close to the agreed-upon plan while being willing to change the plan as family needs evolve builds trust, and family members perceive the therapist as being interested in helping them achieve *their* goals. For example, after

---

* Family functions include activities related to education, recreation, daily care, affection, economics, and self-identity.[8]

introducing herself, Heather could ask Mrs. Sanchez about Margarita and what she hoped to accomplish by getting involved in the early intervention program. Asking "What are Margarita's biggest problems?" is a deficit-oriented approach. Stating "I think we should work on Margarita's toilet training so that she is ready for kindergarten" could slow the development of a relationship between Heather and the Sanchez family. Carefully eliciting and acknowledging the family's wishes would create a solid basis for working with them. Starting with the family's hopes, dreams, and moments of pride reinforces the capabilities and competence of its members. After listening carefully to Mrs. Sanchez's expressed wishes for Margarita, Heather could say something like "So, you aren't sure about what you want to accomplish, but no matter what we do, Mrs. Sanchez, you want Margarita to feel like she is a part of the whole family." If Mrs. Sanchez nodded and smiled, Heather would know that she had identified a primary goal of the Sanchez family. She would keep that as a major feature of the treatment planning process.

CLINICAL *Pearl*

Build on family strengths, dreams, and hopes. When talking with families, ask "how" rather than "why" questions. Ask them to describe rather than explain situations. Instead of trying to establish some sort of linear cause-and-effect relationship among different factors, try simply to understand the relationships among events, people, and situations.

- **Acknowledgment**: "Solution-focused curiosity and interest" and "collaborative goal setting" are skills that are grounded in the central communicative tool known as **acknowledgment**, which practitioners can use to assure their clients that what they are saying is being heard and understood. OT practitioners can acknowledge the clients with whom they are speaking by providing appropriate feedback. This feedback can be in the form of verbal repetition or confirmation of the clients' statements (e.g., "So you have lived here for 5 years" or "I see"), nonverbal body movements (e.g., nodding the head, sitting forward with an interested expression), or paraverbal cues (e.g., "uh-huh" or "mm-hmm").

- *Continuity*: An OT practitioner's arrival and departure are the most important moments of contact with a family. At both times, the practitioner should be solution focused or future oriented. When arriving at the home, the practitioner is attempting to establish or re-establish positive rapport with the family. After discussing any relevant events that have taken place since the previous visit, the practitioner elicits from the family a desired outcome for that visit or restates an agreed-upon goal to guide activities during the current visit. When departing from the home, the practitioner and family identify events that will or may take place before the next visit as well as discuss a potential goal for the next visit. It can be difficult and frustrating for a practitioner to leave after a visit in which little progress has been made. In such a case, it is often helpful to leave the family with some "homework" related to their goal—to look for and note circumstances that relate to it—so that the practitioner can use the information as a stepping stone for the next session. For example, imagine that the parents want their daughter to be able to dress independently and have identified their daughter using the zipper of a dress as their goal; however, the goal seems unreachable, and little progress is being made. Their OT practitioner could ask them to pay attention to the circumstances under which their daughter attempts to touch or play with the zipper. The visit can then end on a more positive note, with the family having to focus on a smaller goal.

SUMMARY

Family systems theory provides a useful framework for thinking about families and the ways in which they operate. The challenges and triumphs of parenting a child who has a disability are similar to others that even families without children with disabilities face. An important factor in determining whether families can successfully adapt to these challenges is the strength and support of their relationships with other key individuals. An OT practitioner is one of these key players—a person who has the opportunity to make a difference in the life of a family through a sensitive, individualized intervention approach.

References

1. American Occupational Therapy Association: *AOTA 1995-96 member update*, Bethesda, MD, 1996, American Occupational Therapy Association.

2. American Occupational Therapy Association: *Occupational therapy practice framework: domain and process*, ed 2, Bethesda, MD, 2008, American Occupational Therapy Association.

3. American Occupational Therapy Association Commission on Education: *Guidelines for curriculum content in pediatrics*,

Bethesda, MD, 1991, American Occupational Therapy Association.

4. American Speech-Language-Hearing Association: *We can do better: recruiting, retaining, and graduating African-American students*, Rockville, MD, 1995, American Speech-Language-Hearing Association.

5. U.S. Census Bureau: *American community survey data*. Available at: http://www.census.gov/acs/www/Products/index.html. Accessed November 4, 2009.

6. Simons R: *After the tears: parents talk about raising a child with a disability*, San Diego, 1987, Harcourt Brace.

7. Singer GH et al: A multi-site evaluation of parent-to-parent programs. *J Early Intervention* 22:217, 1999.

8. Turnbull AP et al: *Families, professionals and exceptionality: positive outcomes through partnership and trust*, ed 5, Upper Saddle River, NJ, 2006, Merrill-Prentice Hall.

Recommended Reading

Turnbull AP et al: *Families, professionals and exceptionality: positive outcomes through partnership and trust*, ed 5, Upper Saddle River, NJ, 2006, Merrill-Prentice Hall.

Winton PJ, Brotherson MJ, Summers JA: Learning from the field of early intervention about partnering with families. In Cornish M, editor: *Promising practices for partnering with families in the early years*, Greenwich, CT, 2009, Information Age Publishing.

REVIEW *Questions*

1. What are three current societal trends that impact the work of the OT practitioner? Describe the impact of these trends on OT pediatric practice.
2. Describe three key concepts related to family systems theory and the implications of these concepts for OT practitioners.
3. Explain why non-normative transitional events may be more stressful than normative transitional events.
4. With the information provided on family systems and family adaptation, explain why it is important to individualize therapy programs for children and families.
5. What are four communication strategies that could be used during the initial home visit with a family?

SUGGESTED *Activities*

1. Spend some time with a child with special needs in his or her natural environment (e.g., home, neighborhood). Observe the various activities taking place. Keep a list of the ways different therapy activities could be embedded in these routines. Imagine the way therapy concepts could be introduced to the parents and then implemented. Write these ideas down.

2. Talk with the families of children with disabilities and with OT practitioners. Ask each group to describe the characteristics of an OT practitioner that they think are important. Take notes, and summarize the comments. Compare the comments of the two groups. Create a personal list of the skills and competencies of an effective OT practitioner.

## 3

Medical System

DAWN B. OAKLEY

KATHLEEN BAUER

CHAPTER *Objectives*

After studying this chapter, the reader will be able to accomplish the following:

- Describe occupational therapy practice in a medical system.
- Identify and discuss the components (i.e., settings and key members) of a pediatric medical system.
- Differentiate among pediatric acute care, subacute care, long-term care, and home care medical settings.
- List five commonly assessed areas of function in a pediatric medical-based occupational therapy evaluation.
- Differentiate among the multidisciplinary, transdisciplinary, and interdisciplinary styles of collaboration.
- Discuss the roles of the occupational therapist and the occupational therapy assistant during the process of intervention and documentation in a pediatric medical system.
- Discuss medical reimbursement issues and payment options for pediatric medical services.
- Identify the important challenges faced by a medical-based pediatric OT practitioner.

KEY TERMS

CHAPTER OUTLINE

Medical Care Settings

NEONATAL INTENSIVE CARE UNIT
PEDIATRIC INTENSIVE CARE UNIT
SUBACUTE SETTING
HOME
LONG-TERM CARE FACILITY

Models of Medical Care

Moving Through the Medical System Continuum

Role of Occupational Therapy in the Pediatric Medical System

ROLE OF THE OCCUPATIONAL THERAPY PRACTITIONER
ROLE OF THE OCCUPATIONAL THERAPY ASSISTANT
NEONATAL INTENSIVE CARE UNIT
STEP-DOWN NURSERY, PEDIATRIC INTENSIVE CARE UNIT, AND SUBACUTE SETTINGS
SUBACUTE, LONG-TERM, AND HOME CARE SETTINGS

Team Collaboration

Documentation

Reimbursement

Challenges for Occupational Therapy Practitioners Working in the Medical System

INFECTION CONTROL
CHARACTERISTICS OF AN EFFECTIVE HEALTH CARE PROVIDER
LEGAL AND ETHICAL CONSIDERATIONS IN A MEDICAL CARE SYSTEM

Summary

MEDICAL CARE SETTINGS

A medical system includes many team members, including children, families, specialists, generalists, nurses, physicians, physical therapists, child life or therapeutic activity therapists, speech and language pathologists, and occupational therapists. A **pediatric medical care system** comprises a group of individuals (professional, paraprofessional, and nonprofessional) who form a complex and unified whole dedicated to caring for children who are ill (Box 3-1).[9] This environment may initially be overwhelming to an entry level OT practitioner.

Comprehensive pediatric medical care occurs over a continuum of various settings, including: neonatal intensive care unit (NICU), step-down nursery or pediatric intensive care unit (PICU), subacute setting, the home, or a residential (long-term care) facility.

Neonatal Intensive Care Unit

The NICU is needed for infants after complicated births. The goal of the NICU team is to address the **acute** or extremely severe symptoms or conditions of such infants so that they can become physiologically stable (i.e., maintain a stable body temperature, heart rate, and respiratory rate).

The medical team closely monitors the medical status of NICU clients. A neonatologist serves as the leader of the NICU team (Figure 3-1). In addition to conducting a neonatal assessment, the neonatologist consults with the other professionals on the medical team about the specific needs of the infant. The following conditions may indicate that an infant should be admitted to the NICU:

1. Cyanosis—an infant who turns blue because of insufficient oxygen
2. Bradycardia—a heart rate of less than 100 beats per minute (bpm)
3. Low birth weight (LBW)—a weight of less than 2500 g
4. Very low birth weight (VLBW)—a weight of less than 1500 g
5. Extremely low birth weight (ELBW)—a weight of less than 750 g

When presented with an infant who has one or more of these conditions, additional medical team members take part in consultations and provide further examinations. Pulmonologists (lung specialists), cardiologists (heart specialists), gastroenterologists (digestive specialists), neurologists (brain specialists), social workers, and respiratory therapists are some of the additional medical team members who may be needed to address the needs of infants in the NICU.

Pediatric Intensive Care Unit

When the medical team determines that the infant has met certain physiologic requirements, the infant is moved out of the NICU. If the infant still requires some form of hospital-based medical care, the infant can be transferred to a step-down nursery or pediatric intensive care unit (PICU) (Figure 3-2). In addition to continuing to address the infant's acute symptoms, the goals of the PICU team are to attempt to wean the infant from external sources of medical support and, when applicable, provide sensorimotor stimulation. As the infant is moved from one unit to another, additional team members may be required, and the services of certain other members may no longer be needed. For example, in the PICU, the infant's medical team leader is no longer a neonatologist; it is a pediatrician.

Subacute Setting

As an infant's condition improves, he or she may no longer require the level of care provided in a PICU; however, the infant may not yet be ready to be discharged home. In this instance, the infant may be transferred to a **subacute** setting (Figure 3-3). The medical needs of the infant, as well as the desires of the infant's primary caregivers affect this decision. The goals of the subacute team are to provide appropriate medical treatment while continuing to wean the infant off medical supports and carrying out development-based therapeutic interventions.

Home

As an infant's status improves, discharge plans are formulated. The issue of where the infant goes after being discharged is discussed with the infant's primary caregivers. Going home is the ultimate goal for infants in acute, step-down nursery, and subacute settings. Once at home, the goals are to facilitate caregiver and infant bonding and promote the continued acquisition of developmentally appropriate skills.

The infants receive medical care through scheduled clinic and outpatient hospital-based visits (Figure 3-4). The coordination of an infant's nursing, therapy, and equipment needs are often transitioned to a community-based **home care** agency. These agencies monitor clients' medical needs and coordinate home-based therapeutic services. The age of the client determines where the services are provided. Infants and young children usually receive home-based services. As children mature, their services may remain at home, or they may transition to an outpatient clinic or community-based early intervention (EI) or Early Head Start setting.

BOX 3-1

Key Pediatric Medical Terms

CARDIOLOGIST
A physician specializing in the treatment of heart disease

CIVILIAN HEALTH AND MEDICAL PROGRAM OF THE UNIFORMED SERVICES (CHAMPUS)
CHAMPUS provides supplemental benefits to those in the uniform services direct medical care system. The program pays for medical care given by civilian providers to eligible persons, who include the retired members of the United States uniformed services and their dependants, the dependants of deceased members of the military, and the dependants of members of the North Atlantic Treaty Organization (NATO) when the NATO member is stationed in or passing through the United States on official business. The CHAMPUS program is spelled out in 32 CFR, section 1. The program is administered by the Department of Defense.

CIVILIAN HEALTH AND MEDICAL PROGRAM OF THE VETERANS ADMINISTRATION (CHAMPVA)
The federal program administered by the Defense Department for the Veterans Administration that provides care for the dependants of totally disabled veterans. Care is given by civilian providers.

DEVELOPMENTAL PEDIATRICIAN
A pediatrician with specialized training in the milestones of typical childhood development

GENETICIST
A person who specializes in genetics

HMO/PPO
Health maintenance organization/preferred provider organization

MEDICAID
The federal program that provides health care to indigent and medically indigent persons (i.e., those who cannot afford to pay their medical bills and qualify for Medicaid for medically related services). Although it is partially federally funded, the Medicaid program is administered by the states, in contrast to Medicare, which is funded and administered at the federal level by the Health Care Financing Administration (HCFA). The Medicaid program was established in 1965 by an amendment to the Social Security Act under a provision entitled Title XIX—Medical Assistance.

NEONATOLOGIST
A pediatrician with 3 years of advanced education who specializes in the treatment of neonates and premature infants

NEUROLOGIST
A physician who specializes in nervous system diseases

OPHTHALMOLOGIST
A physician who specializes in the treatment of eye disorders

ORTHOPEDIST
A specialist in orthopedics

PEDIATRICIAN
A physician who specializes in the diagnosis and treatment of illnesses and dysfunctions in children

PEDIATRIC NURSE PRACTITIONER
A registered nurse who provides primary health care to children (e.g., Jane Grey, R.N., P.N.P.). Special preparation is required.

PHYSIATRIST
A physician who specializes in physical medicine

PHYSICAL THERAPY ASSISTANT
A technical health care worker trained to carry out physical therapy procedures under the supervision of a physical therapist

PULMONOLOGIST
A physician who is trained and certified to treat pulmonary diseases

RADIOLOGIST
A physician who uses X-rays or other sources of radiation for diagnosis and treatment

REGISTERED PHYSICAL THERAPIST
A health care worker who has successfully completed an accredited physical therapy education program and passed a licensing examination. A registered physical therapist is legally responsible for evaluating, planning, conducting, and supervising a physical therapy program using rehabilitative and therapeutic exercise techniques and physical modalities.

SPEECH AND LANGUAGE PATHOLOGIST
An individual who is educated and trained to plan, direct, and conduct programs to improve the communication skills of children and adults with language and speech impairments caused by physiologic factors, articulation problems, or dialect. A speech and language pathologist can evaluate programs and may perform research related to speech and language problems.

Adapted from Slee V, Slee D: *Slee's health care terms*, ed 3, St Paul, MN, 1996, Tringa Press; Thomas CL, editor: *Taber's cyclopedic medical dictionary*, ed 18, Philadelphia, 1997, FA Davis.

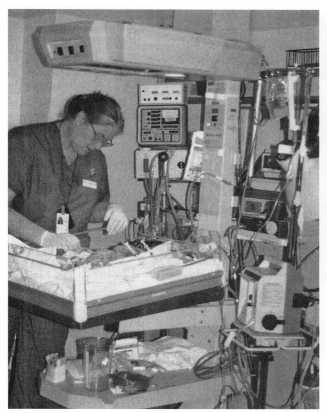

FIGURE 3-1 The neonatal intensive care unit can be an overwhelming environment. (From Parham LD, Fazio LS: *Play in occupational therapy for children*, ed 2, St Louis, 2009, Mosby.)

CLINICAL *Pearl*

Practitioners must respect the families' values, beliefs, and customs while providing home-based occupational therapy (OT) services for children.

Long-Term Care Facility

During discharge planning, some primary caregivers may decide that they are unable to handle their child's specific medical needs. In these cases, residential (**long-term care**) facilities are options available to them. The goals of the long-term care team are to provide appropriate medical care and carry out appropriate therapeutic interventions. An example of a therapeutic intervention is providing sensorimotor stimulation to prevent the development of contractures and prevent or minimize losses in range of motion.

MODELS OF MEDICAL CARE

In addition to the practice setting, occupational therapy (OT) practitioners need to be aware of the model of medical care under which services are being provided.

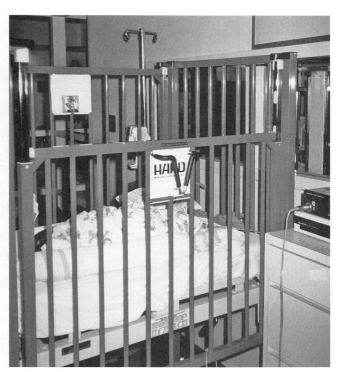

FIGURE 3-2 Infants are transferred to a step-down nursery or pediatric intensive care unit when they have the ability to maintain satisfactory physiologic functioning. (Courtesy Dawn B. Oakley and Kathleen Logan-Bauer, Bayside, NY.)

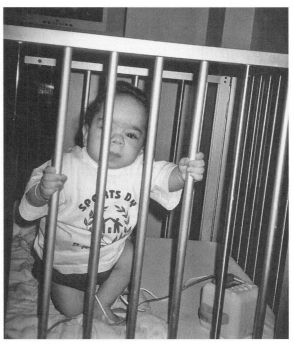

FIGURE 3-3 As infants become medically stable, they are discharged and transferred to a subacute or home care setting. A commercially available device is often all that is necessary to monitor the infants when they are alone. (Courtesy Dawn B. Oakley and Kathleen Logan-Bauer, Bayside, NY.)

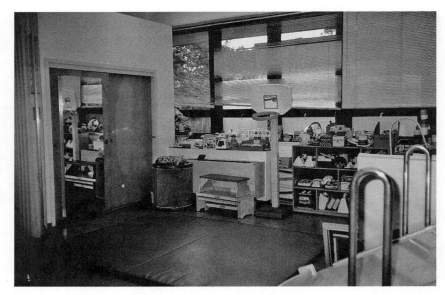

FIGURE 3-4 Occupational therapy outpatient hospital-based clinic. (Courtesy Dawn B. Oakley and Kathleen Logan-Bauer, Bayside, NY.)

The increased number of uninsured or underinsured children and families has resulted in the expansion of medical care practice outside of the more traditional arena (i.e., inpatient, center-based care). The models of pediatric service delivery have been broadened to include the stages of medical service provision. Federal programs, such as early interventions, involve the primary care physician as a vital member of the treatment team. In addition, therapy, nutrition, social work, and other services are provided under this federally mandated (state-governed) program to assist with meeting first-level (primary) medical care needs. One of the components of a primary medical care model is education. Pediatric primary care is strongly grounded in the understanding that caregivers must receive assistance in order to recognize the need for routine and follow-up medical care. Practices such as immunizations, vaccinations, regularly scheduled checkups, and ongoing monitoring of chronic conditions are all examples of strategies that are used under the primary care model to promote and support health in children. All medical personnel who provide services under this model of care are responsible for participating in the educational process.

The **second-level (secondary)** medical care model involves the follow-up that occurs once a child has become ill. In these instances, the caregiver receives guidelines to prevent further contamination of the child or others within the household or community. This level of medical care involves caregiver education, focusing on caregiver recognition of the importance of adherence to guidelines regarding care, sanitation, dispensing medication, and observation for signs of improvement or worsening of a condition. This level of care is more intense than in the primary care model. The increased level of medical care is provided to prevent the necessity of tertiary medical care.

The third-level (tertiary) medical care model involves the need for hospitalization. At this point in the medical care continuum, serious concerns have arisen regarding involvement of the child's body system(s) and that additional body systems will be affected by primary or secondary causes associated with the child's illness. This model continues to involve caregiver education; however, a greater level of responsibility for the child's recuperation is dependent on interventions provided by medical personnel.

The next section of this chapter focuses on a discussion of the continuum of medical care service options. The information gained from medical care models aids in the development of the pediatric knowledge base necessary to provide medical-based interventions.

MOVING THROUGH THE MEDICAL SYSTEM CONTINUUM

The extent to which a child is involved in the medical system continuum changes as the child's circumstances change. For example, a child may be admitted to an acute care facility because of an acute illness. The child may be subsequently discharged and return home but then be admitted to a long-term care facility because of extenuating circumstances at home. This is just one example of the way a child's involvement in the pediatric medical care system can change. The case study below follows the progression of one child through the pediatric medical care settings.

CASE *Study*

Daniel was delivered by a cesarean section with vacuum extraction because of fetal distress after 33 weeks of gestation. At birth, he was limp and cyanotic, with a heart rate of less than 100 bpm. No respiratory effort was noted at birth. Daniel's birth weight was 200 g. He required mechanical ventilation for the first 3 days of life. Daniel was weaned to nasal continuous positive airway pressure (CPAP) from days 3 to 18. He was intubated again on day 25 for gastrostomy tube placement.

Three days after the gastrostomy tube placement, Daniel was transferred to a step-down nursery. After the transfer, consultation requests were made to the staff geneticist, a physiatrist, and rehabilitation services.

After Daniel spent 30 days in the step-down nursery, the medical team and his parents determined that he should be discharged and transferred to a subacute facility. The responsibility for Daniel's treatment was then assumed by the subacute facility.

After Daniel spent 1 year as an inpatient at the subacute facility, the medical team and Daniel's parents decided that he was ready to be discharged and return home. Daniel was transferred from inpatient, medical-based care to outpatient, home-based care. As noted in the case study, when a pregnant mother has an emergency delivery, some degree of pediatric medical care is often required to treat birth-related trauma to the infant. In addition, children may need pediatric medical care for accidental injuries, neurologic and musculoskeletal traumas, and complications resulting from genetic defects.

ROLE OF OCCUPATIONAL THERAPY IN THE PEDIATRIC MEDICAL SYSTEM

CLINICAL *Pearl*

Childhood is filled with many typical developmental stages and events. The normal developmental progression can be negatively affected by atypical experiences and events, such as prolonged hospitalization.

The prolonged hospitalization of an infant or child is not a normal event. A hospitalization of more than a few days puts a typical child at risk for some degree of developmental delay. For example, to develop meaningful social and emotional bonds, infants and children need to be comforted and held by other human beings. Children and infants who are hospitalized typically are not held as often as those who are not in a hospital. These children and infants may have difficulty developing the social and emotional skills needed for successful interactions with members of their families and their peers.

The perceived or actual presence of developmental delays warrants the provision of OT and other rehabilitative services. Perceived deficits are those that may not yet be present but are known to be associated with a particular condition, such as Down syndrome. Perceived deficits can also be temporary developmental delays resulting from atypical experiences and events. The fundamental principle of OT is to promote optimal performance in each of the areas of occupation: play/leisure, activities of daily living (ADLs), instrumental activities of daily living (IADLs), social participation, and education. Pediatric medical-based OT practitioners use play activities to facilitate the acquisition of age-appropriate developmental skills (e.g., gross motor, fine motor, cognitive).

Role of the Occupational Therapy Practitioner

Medical-based OT practitioners are either occupational therapists or occupational therapy assistants (OTAs). Occupational therapists are responsible for providing the overall framework for medical-based services. Collaboration between OT practitioners is essential and is facilitated by the OTA's knowledge of the occupational therapist's responsibilities, which include conducting screenings and evaluations, formulating and carrying out daily intervention plans, and documentation. The OTA's responsibilities include formulating and carrying out daily intervention plans and documentation. OTAs also assist with or conduct portions of the pediatric medical-based screening and contribute to the pediatric medical-based evaluation.

After receiving a referral from a physician, medical-based pediatric **screening** and **evaluation** are usually completed by the occupational therapist within 24 hours and 72 hours, respectively. The screening and evaluation are conducted by means of formal and informal measurement tools as well as through clinical and parental observations. Throughout the assessment process, a medical-based OT practitioner should be aware that certain factors, such as time, the severity of the illness, and the overall stress associated with being in a hospital environment, may mask a child's true abilities in a given performance area.

The deficits that are identified during screening and evaluation are addressed in a medical intervention plan. An occupational therapist formulates the long-term goals and short-term objectives that will guide the intervention plan. The medical intervention plan is developed either solely by an occupational therapist or jointly by an occupational therapist and an OTA. The medical intervention plan is an outline of the activities and tasks that are used during treatment sessions.

The OT practitioner initiates OT interventions only when the medical stability of a child has been determined. Medical stability is used to determine the manner in which services are provided and how often they are provided. The goals of the intervention plan should be gradually integrated into the child's environment. Intervention strategies are designed to increase the child's functional level.

Role of the Occupational Therapy Assistant

As mentioned previously, medical-based pediatric OT services are provided to promote optimal function in hospitalized children. OTAs are prepared to play a role in the provision of these services. The responsibilities of the OTA are dictated by the facility in which the services are being provided. The typical responsibilities of an OTA include conducting an initial developmental screening, collaborating with another OT practitioner on an evaluation, planning interventions, updating goals, and collaborating with others on the discharge plan.

OTAs working in the pediatric medical setting understand that client factors impact their provision of services. The plan of care developed for a child admitted to a medical setting also incorporates information reflecting a child's preadmission status as well as his or her current status. This information, along with the child's medical diagnosis and medical course, is used to develop goals that will lead to discharge. Clinicians gather information regarding the preadmission status to develop an understanding of a child's baseline performance in the following areas:

- Cognitive (level of alertness, orientation, behavior, moods, activity level, memory, attention to task)
- Sensory (visual, auditory, oral, tactile, vestibular, gustatory, pain)
- Neuromuscular system (extremity movements and limitations, strengths, weaknesses, prior injuries/ surgeries, presence or absence of age-appropriate reflexes)
- Cardiovascular and respiratory systems (blood pressure, breathing patterns, prior activity and fatigue levels)
- Voice/speech/respiration (verbal or nonverbal communication, quality of voice, ability to sustain conversation)
- Digestive/metabolic (eating, absorption, energy return on caloric intake), skin (intact, abrasions, cuts, wounds, injection or access sites)
- Elimination function (output schedule, level of independence)[3]

Experienced OTAs evaluate this information on the basis of their understanding of the connections that exist among body systems, body structures, and function. Their knowledge surrounding the interrelatedness of body systems and how strengths or deficits in one

system affect the performance of another assist in the development of an appropriate plan of care (inclusive of objectives and goals that maximize a child's optimal level of occupational performance).[3]

Neonatal Intensive Care Unit

Only highly qualified allied health professionals perform NICU-based intervention. The therapists who work in the NICU are required to have advanced education and certification in NICU-based treatment. For example, therapists in the NICU must have a thorough knowledge of life signs, which are key indicators of the infant's status (e.g., color, respiration rate, body temperature, extremity movement). Changes in these indicators are noted by the therapist through sight, hearing, and touch. A role for the OTA in the provision of NICU services has not been identified.[1] If an OT practitioner would like to work with this special client population, he or she should obtain the necessary education and certification required to ensure that treatment is provided safely and appropriately.

Step-Down Nursery, Pediatric Intensive Care Unit, and Subacute Settings

Providing intervention in a step-down nursery or PICU also requires related experience to ensure the provision of the most appropriate treatment. However, unlike the situation in the NICU, OTAs with appropriate educational training may be able to receive on-the-job training qualifying them to assume a role in providing medical services in the step-down nursery and PICU.[1]

OTAs working in the step-down nursery or PICU require additional education and on-the-job training because the infants and children admitted to these units may still have serious medical problems. An OTA working in one or both of these settings may participate in the screening, evaluation, and intervention of the clients. The initiation of screening or an intervention might distress an infant or child who is in the step-down nursery or PICU. Therefore, the OT practitioner must carefully monitor clients, be sensitive to indications of distress, and be prepared to respond appropriately.

During the initial screening and assessment, the OTA is introduced (oriented) to the client's case. Each client is evaluated to establish a functional physiologic baseline (e.g., respiratory rate, heart rate, oxygen saturation level). Clients must be constantly evaluated during daily intervention sessions to ensure that they remain within the physiologic range that was established according to their baseline functioning levels.

The NICU, PICU, and subacute pediatric care settings can be intimidating because of the intricacies associated with these settings. The provision of services in these areas is typically reserved for the experienced clinician. As noted previously, the NICU and PICU are not traditionally entry-level placements for the beginning OTA. However, an experienced OTA can provide services in a PICU or subacute setting with appropriate supervision by an occupational therapist. One of the steps that lead toward becoming an experienced OTA is the development of a pediatric medical knowledge base.

The knowledge necessary to work in these areas is made up of three components: (1) an understanding of the equipment, (2) an understanding of the standards of care that govern operations in these settings, and (3) an understanding of medical status signs that will guide the provision of therapeutic services. The level of care required by the children admitted to one of these settings is high, and the status of these children is monitored regularly. Children may also need scheduled medication(s). The equipment found in these settings varies depending on the population of children being served. Some examples of the equipment found in these settings are shown in Box 3-2.

Some examples of standards of care include adherence to treatment guidelines (where and when treatment can occur), sign-out practices (children's locations must be recorded at all times), medical supervision (treatment must be provided in accordance with medical orders), and

caregiver/parental expectations (guardian expectations and goals are included in the development of a comprehensive plan of care). Clinicians providing services in these settings must accommodate all of these factors.

In addition to the equipment that monitors the children's status, a clinician needs to perform ongoing monitoring to assess their readiness to receive therapy services or their ability to tolerate specific therapeutic interventions. Once a clinician has the opportunity to develop a level of comfort for service provision in the medical setting, he or she will develop a site-specific medical status checklist. Box 3-3 shows a medical status checklist for an entry-level clinician working with a child.

The checklist serves only as a general guideline. The clinician and child share the ultimate responsibility of determining whether a therapeutic intervention

---

BOX 3-2

Equipment Examples

APNEA MONITORS
Monitor respiration

INTRAVENOUS LINES/TUBES
Pass through the skin and into the veins

PULSE OXIMETER
Measures pulse and oxygen saturation levels, that is, the amount of oxygen found in the blood

FEEDING TUBES
Oral tubes can be placed in the mouth and empty into the stomach; nasal tubes can be placed in the nose and empty into the stomach; and gastrointestinal tube (GT) can be placed in the abdomen and empty into the stomach.

ULTRAVIOLET LIGHTS
Light ray frequencies used to treat illness

WARMING BLANKETS/LIGHTS
Temperature control coverings (may be placed directly over a protective covering on the body or above a bed) used to assist in the maintenance of body temperature

Adapted from Venes D: *Taber's cyclopedic medical dictionary,* ed 21, Philadelphia, 2009, FA Davis.

BOX 3-3

Medical Status Checklist

HEALTH STATUS
Should be well enough to receive therapy services

HEART RATE
Should be within child-specific, established guidelines

OXYGEN SATURATION
Levels
Should be within child-specific, established guidelines

Color
Should be within typical shading, as demonstrated by the child when not in distress

SKIN TEMPERATURE
Should be warm to the touch unless child presents with a condition that affects internal temperature regulation

BREATHING PATTERN
Should be typical of the child when not in distress (i.e., based on either age-appropriate or diagnosis-related breathing patterns)

AFFECT
Should confirm that presenting behavior is typical of a child

SLEEP–WAKE CYCLE
Should confirm that existing patterns have not been interrupted

MOVEMENT PATTERNS
Should demonstrate movement patterns that are part of the child's repertoire and those that are fostered by the introduction of therapeutic interventions

is being tolerated. Since it is not uncommon for medically fragile children to experience distress when they are moved or touched, clinicians need to develop monitoring ranges that are acceptable for treatment.

Subacute, Long-Term, and Home Care Settings

OTAs must be trained in medical-based pediatric therapy to provide services in the PICU, subacute, long-term, and home care settings. Working in a subacute, long-term, or home care setting is different from working in a step-down nursery or PICU setting in that an experienced OT practitioner may not be required to work under the direct supervision of an occupational therapist. The clients in these settings are typically more medically stable than those in the NICU, step-down nursery, or PICU. However, OTAs working in these settings must be familiar with the signs of physiologic distress and be prepared to respond properly.

TEAM COLLABORATION

Team collaboration is important in any medical setting, but it plays a particularly essential and integral part of medical and therapeutic intervention in pediatric care. Before the initiation of a therapeutic intervention, OT practitioners consult with the physicians and nurses assigned to the client's care and obtain updates on the status of their clients. Areas of particular importance include medications, physiologic stability, nutritional status, and sleep patterns. OT practitioners may obtain this information from written reports and during rounds and medical team meetings.

Consultations among medical team members facilitate collaboration. Team members may use one of four types of collaborative style: (1) **multidisciplinary**, (2) **interdisciplinary**, (3) **transdisciplinary**, or (4) "individual-versus-group" sessions (Table 3-1).[5,8]

CLINICAL *Pearl*

For a transdisciplinary team to be effective, the team members must trust and respect each other so that they are comfortable with role release (i.e., relinquishing certain professional duties to other team members).

DOCUMENTATION

The OT practitioner's ability to clearly document the events that occur in a pediatric medical setting is crucially important. Documentation is used for many purposes, including updating others on client status, justifying the necessity for OT services, and explaining requests for supplies and reimbursements.

An OT practitioner who works in a pediatric medical care system should know the types of documentation that exist and the reasons these documents are necessary. OT practitioners usually complete a medical-based screening or assessment of the infant initially. A screening helps determine whether a thorough evaluation is needed. In some medical care settings, a more detailed assessment is the second step in the documentation process. In other medical care settings, the assessment form is the initial document completed by a practitioner. Screenings and evaluations include medical history, general observations, gross motor function, fine motor function, visual and perceptual function, cognitive function, sensory function (when applicable), ADL function, summary and recommendations, frequency, and long- and short-term goals. Box 3-4 contains an example of a medical evaluation that outlines a client's strengths and weaknesses. The information is used to establish baseline functioning, thereby delineating the parameters for improvement.

Documentation in a medical care setting is required by accrediting and licensing agencies. The medical record is a legal document. If the occupational therapy process is not documented, then OT services did not occur. Entries in a medical record should be concise, clear, accurate, complete, and chronologically ordered. The Health Information Portability and Accountability Act (HIPAA) protects a client's medical information, otherwise known as *patient health information*.[7] In certain medical care facilities, standardized assessments are administered during the evaluation phase of the OT process.

An example of a standardized pediatric assessment is the WeeFIM (UB Foundation Activities, Inc, Queens, NY).[11] The WeeFIM is a functional assessment that is used to describe a child's performance during essential activities; it is used to measure those activities that children can actually carry out and not what they may merely be capable of doing. The assessment can be used to clarify a child's functional status, provide information for team conferences, facilitate goal planning, and provide information on burden-of-care issues, that is, those issues related to the person who is meeting the child's basic needs (i.e., eating, bathing, dressing, grooming, transferring, moving, and toileting).[10,11] The WeeFIM also provides a uniform language that practitioners should use when measuring and documenting the severity of disabilities and outcomes of pediatric rehabilitation as well as habilitation. It allows practitioners to measure disability types as well as determine the amount of help a child needs to perform basic activities. The assessment is conducted by direct observations or through interviews with the caregiver and can be used in inpatient and outpatient settings (Box 3-5); however, it is not meant to be used as the *only* diagnostic tool.

TABLE 3-1

Methods of Team Collaboration

APPROACH	DESCRIPTION
Multidisciplinary	The multidisciplinary approach evolved from a medical model in which multiple professionals evaluated the child and make recommendations.[3] Professionals who use this type of approach may be directly or indirectly involved with the child and family but do not necessarily consult or interact with each other. Assessment, goal setting, and direct intervention may be carried out by each professional with a minimum of integration across disciplines.[4]
Interdisciplinary	The interdisciplinary approach to treatment is cooperative and interactive. A team comprising professionals from several disciplines (who are often at the same location) have frequent direct involvement with the child and collaborate with each other on the child's care program. Although the evaluations are performed independently by each discipline, program planning is carried out by group consensus, and goals are set collaboratively between the professionals and the parents. This approach allows the child and the family to receive coordinated services and benefit from the expertise of professionals from several disciplines.[6]
Transdisciplinary	Although the transdisciplinary approach involves collaboration among various disciplines, one team member is usually designated to intervene directly, and the other team members act as consultants. This approach was developed on the assumption that families benefit more from having their intervention programs provided by one primary professional rather than multiple professionals. All team members contribute to assessment and program planning, and then the designated person implements the plan while consulting with other members of the team. Therefore, the transdisciplinary model enables health care professionals to perform tasks that are normally outside the scope of practice of their discipline. Implementation of this model requires professionals to be comfortable with role release, or relinquishing some or all of their professional duties to another professional. During this process the team members must share information and exchange responsibilities.[8]
"Individual-versus-group" sessions	The "individual-versus-group" session approach is used to encourage frequent team member collaboration. It allows for informal and impromptu communication between two or three team members. During team collaboration, information is exchanged about the child's status. Specific information is shared so that members can compare notes, which, in turn, serves to improve the treatment approaches of the members of the individual disciplines.[10]

Adapted from Case-Smith J, Allen AS, Pratt PN: Arenas of occupational therapy services. In Case-Smith J, Allen AS, Pratt PN, editors: *Occupational therapy for children*, ed 3, St Louis, 1996, Mosby.

After the initial screening or assessment has been completed, the OT practitioner notes the child's progress and changes in the status over time. The progress is recorded in the form of a daily note, weekly progress note, or monthly progress note in a narrative or in the **SOAP-note** format (see Chapter 10). SOAP stands for Subjective information (general statements concerning the child by the caregiver or child), Objective information (what is done), Assessment (effect of interventions), and Plan (what will be done). (See *Physical Dysfunction: Practice Skills for the Occupational Therapy Assistant* for a clear, concise description of common medical documentation).[6] An example discharge note based on the SOAP format for the case study on Daniel, cited earlier, might be as follows:

S

Nursing reports that Daniel is in a "great mood" today and drank 8 ounces of formula this morning.

O

Daniel is a 14-month-old male who presents with a diagnosis of prematurity, bronchopulmonary dysplasia, and a gastrointestinal tube (GT) placement. Daniel receives OT, physical therapy (PT), and speech therapy (ST) services twice weekly for 30 minutes each. He is medically stable and receives his nutrition by way of a combination of oral and overnight GT feedings.

At present, Daniel is alert and oriented to person and place. He is able to cruise with contact guard. He demonstrates right and left unilateral hand skills (active grasp and release in response to verbal prompts). Daniel is able to attend to light-up/auditory toys for approximately 45 seconds with moderate cueing. He tolerates hand-over-hand assistance to participate in cause-and-effect activities in approximately 75% of the trials.

BOX 3-4

Medical-Based Occupational Therapy Education

ST. MARY'S HOSPITAL FOR CHILDREN INITIAL OCCUPATIONAL THERAPY EVALUATION

Name: Kevin   *Unit*: CUW
DOB: 7/13/02   *Sex*: Male
Medical Record #: 12345
Diagnosis: Duchenne muscular dystrophy
2/28/10: Doctor's orders received. Full evaluation with recommendations to follow.

MEDICAL HISTORY

Kevin, 7 years and 8 months old, has Duchenne muscle dystrophy. On 3/21/2006, he underwent a spinal fusion and multiple tendon releases. He was subsequently placed in two long-leg casts with bars. Kevin was born at 36 weeks' gestation and weighed 5 lb 5 oz. Kevin was a healthy child until he was diagnosed with Duchenne muscular dystrophy at age 5.

GENERAL OBSERVATIONS

Kevin is a thin, frail male child, who has an overall decreased affect. He has a scar from spinal surgery that extends from approximately T1/T2 to his coccyx. He is able to verbalize his needs by speaking in a soft, high-pitched voice, Kevin is able to visually track objects in all planes. He is seated in a reclined wheelchair with his lower extremities elevated and in a spica cast.

GROSS MOTOR FUNCTION

Kevin has hypotonicity throughout his trunk and upper extremities. He is able to transition from the prone position to the supine position, and vice versa. Kevin requires significant assistance to maintain the sitting posture. He exhibits pectus excavation, bilateral scapular winging, a kyphotic posture, and bilateral rib flaring.

UPPER EXTREMITY FUNCTION

Passive range of motion (PROM) is WNL (within normal limits). Gonometric active range of motion (AROM) measurements are as follows:

	RIGHT	LEFT
Shoulder flexion	No ROM at either shoulder; uses compensatory techniques (e.g., climb arms on chest)	
Elbow flexion	Flexes both elbows in a gravity-eliminated plane	
Wrist extension	0–30 degrees	0–25 degrees
Wrist flexion	0–60 degrees	0–55 degrees
Ulnar deviation	0–30 degrees	WNL
Radial deviation	0–20 degrees	WNL
Supination	WNL	WNL
Pronation	WNL	WNL

Courtesy Kathleen Logan-Baucer, Bayside, NY.

CLINICAL *Pearl*

Always remember a child and his or her diagnosis are not one and the same (i.e., Yes: Jack is a child, who presents with autism. No: Jack is an autistic child).

CLINICAL *Pearl*

The WeeFIM is a tool that can be used for the efficient assessment and documentation of progress.

A

Daniel presents with developmental delays in the areas of advancing postural control, bilateral hand function, eye-hand coordination, and attention to a task, which interfere with his ability to engage in self-care, social participation, and play.

P

Daniel would benefit from home-based OT services to promote his continued improvement in the areas of independent mobility/transition, in-hand manipulation, visual perception, and sustained attention skills needed for engagement in self-care, play, and social participation. Daniel was referred to the early intervention (EI program).

BOX 3-5

WeeFIM Instrument Rating Guidelines

INPATIENT
Within 72 Hours of Admission
WeeFIM admission assessment must be completed.

Within 72 Hours of Discharge
WeeFIM discharge assessment must be completed.

Within 80 to 180 Days of Discharge
WeeFIM follow-up assessment must be completed. Interim WeeFIM assessments (between admission and discharge) may be performed at the facility's discretion.

OUTPATIENT
During Initial Contact
WeeFIM admission assessment must be completed. Additional WeeFIM assessments may be performed at the facility's discretion.

At Time of Discharge
WeeFIM discharge assessment must be completed.

Adapted from Uniform Data Systems for Medical Rehabilitation: *WeeFIM system workshop,* Queens, NY, 1988, UB Foundation Activities, Inc.

BOX 3-6

Letter of Equipment Justification

RE: Frankie
Diagnosis: Severe tracheomalacia, gastroesophageal reflux, and supraventricular tachycardia
Medicaid #: GF12345U
DOB: 7/12/2009

TO WHOM IT MAY CONCERN:
Frankie is a 10-month-old male who had severe tracheomalacia, gastroesophageal reflux, and supraventricular tachycardia at birth. He has decreased head and postural control as well as tracheotomy.

Current equipment: Currently Frankie does not have any equipment.

Equipment ordered: One Panda stroller with swivel-front wheels, a combined sun/rain hood, and foot straps.

Justification: Frankie is an active, alert, and oriented 10-month-old male with decreased head and trunk control, which affects his ability to assume and maintain independent, upright postural sets. Frankie's inability to maintain an upright and erect posture places him at risk for occluding his tracheostomy and limits his ability to achieve his full respiratory capacity. These limitations affect his endurance and gas exchange.

A Panda stroller will assist Frankie with maintaining a neutral posture, which will facilitate his mechanical efficiency and therefore improve his endurance for maintaining an upright position. Improvement in his endurance will increase his upper extremity use, which will foster the acquisition of age-appropriate fine motor skills. The stroller will help prevent bony deformities and joint contractures, thereby preventing the need for future surgeries. Frankie's ability to swallow and digest will also be improved if he can maintain a neutral position. A neutral position allows Frankie to use gravity to help him carry out the previously stated functions.

Thank you in advance for your assistance with this matter.

Therapist's signature   Therapist's signature

Physiatrist's signature

Courtesy: Nechama Karman, Dawn B. Oakley, Queens, NY, 1996.

Progress notes are important for justifying interventions, continuing services, and planning discharge. OT practitioners should record clearly and concisely the therapeutic interventions and the child's responses to them. They must also document the justification for specialized equipment. Insurance sources may approve or deny a request based on an OT practitioner's ability to justify the necessity for the requested item. OT practitioners can justify the necessity for equipment by identifying the ways in which its use will benefit the child's level of functioning. For example, OT practitioners may discuss how the equipment will improve respiratory, cardiac, musculoskeletal, esophageal, and gastrointestinal functions. OT practitioners should emphasize how the equipment helps the child in terms of safety as well. See Box 3-6 for an example of a letter of justification. The letter includes information on the way the requested equipment will improve the child's ability to function in the areas of respiration, trunk control (musculoskeletal), endurance (cardiac and respiratory), and swallowing and digestion (physiologic).

REIMBURSEMENT

Medical-based treatment is reimbursed by a variety of sources, including private insurance companies, Medicaid, the Civilian Health and Medical Program of the Uniformed Services (CHAMPUS), the Civilian Health and Medical Program of the Veterans Administration (CHAMPVA), health maintenance organizations (HMOs), and preferred provider organizations (PPOs) (see Box 3-1). Many of these sources require specific documentation to justify the services rendered. An OT practitioner should be aware of the general billing requirements and documentation for each source.

For example, private insurance companies, HMOs, and PPOs require frequent documentation to justify the initiation and continuation of services. In certain instances, specific clinics and vendors must be used. A hospital social worker or case manager is the best source of information regarding insurance requirements and coverage.

Charitable organizations are another reimbursement source. They are usually nonprofit companies or organizations that raise funds to be given to other nonprofit organizations. A charitable organization makes a donation to a pediatric institution or agency, which, in turn, deposits the donation into an appropriate general fund. The agency then determines the way to distribute these funds to pay for the specific expenses of individual children.

CHALLENGES FOR OCCUPATIONAL THERAPY PRACTITIONERS WORKING IN THE MEDICAL SYSTEM

There are unique challenges faced by OT practitioners working in various settings in the medical care system. The number of specialties that are included in the pediatric medical care system may be challenging. In addition to rehabilitative services (e.g., OT, PT, ST), a variety of specialized service personnel constitute the system, including radiology technicians, medical laboratory technicians, audiologists, pharmacists, dietitians, orthotists, and recreational therapists. A medical-based OT practitioner has to become familiar with other pediatric disciplines and their roles in the medical institution. This knowledge facilitates the team collaboration process.

OT practitioners must have extensive knowledge of medical terminology when working in medical systems. The terminology can initially seem overwhelming. However, the study of the basic word roots and common diagnoses used in pediatric medical practice helps practitioners develop this much-needed knowledge base. A good reference source for medical terminology is *Mosby's Medical, Nursing, and Allied Health Dictionary*.[4]

A successful medical-based OT practitioner participates in continuing education activities on a regular basis and may become certified in advanced pediatric practice skills such as sensory integration and neurodevelopmental treatment. The medical field is a dynamic system, and therefore OT practitioners must keep up with developments in current assessment techniques, interventions, and medical equipment.

Children with certain conditions such as pneumonia, asthma, diabetes, and cerebral palsy may be admitted to hospitals frequently.[10] These children may develop episodes of acute illness or the need for corrective surgery. OT practitioners must be aware that children who are frequently hospitalized require a different approach to treatment to maintain a sense of continuity with the aspects of their lives outside the hospital. The OTA draws upon the components of the models of practice (such as the Model of Human Occupation (MOHO) and Developmental models) to assist in the development of therapeutic intervention plans that integrate the children's preadmission habits, routines, and roles with their current levels of performance. The integration of all performance patterns will aid in motivating the child to work toward goals that will lead to discharge and to resuming prior admission status after discharge from the hospital setting.

Practitioners working in medical care systems frequently have to address issues related to palliative care. Children who have been diagnosed with terminal illnesses may be treated in a medical care setting or home setting and may require OT services. The focus of OT intervention services for children diagnosed with terminal illnesses varies depending on their status. Initially, the OT practitioner may focus on the restoration or maintenance of function related to the child's or caregiver's ability to carry out prediagnosis performance skills. As the child's status declines, the focus of therapy services may shift to the maintenance and integration of energy conservation techniques that assist in easing the performance of independent or assisted performance skills. The clinician may also integrate the use of treatment modalities that allow the caregiver's and child's memories to be recorded in a permanent manner as a source of future comfort for the family after the child dies. As a child enters the final stage of life, the OT practitioner may focus on ensuring that the child is comfortable and positioned to interact with the environment. The clinician providing services works closely with the caregiver and the child to provide opportunities for meaningful occupations and interactions.

Infection Control

Infection control is the responsibility of every OT practitioner, who must follow universal precautions when working with any client. These precautions are expressed as a set of rules, which were instituted by the Centers for Disease Control (CDC) in 1985 to address concerns regarding the transmission of the human immunodeficiency virus (HIV) and the hepatitis B virus (HBV) to health care and public safety workers. When health care workers face the risk of being exposed to blood, certain other body fluids, or any other fluid visibly contaminated by blood, they must assume that all persons with whom they come in contact may be infected with HIV or HBV and therefore follow these precautions at all times.

All professionals working within medical care settings must adhere to infection control practices. One of the first lines of defense against the spread of infection is proper hand washing. Medical care settings provide detailed orientation sessions to educate employees on practices to prevent the spread of infection. Some medical facilities employ a nurse who is responsible for overseeing infection control. This nurse monitors the status of communicable infections, assists in the quarantine of an infected child, caregivers, or medical personnel, and works to prevent the spread of contagious infections to other medically compromised children. Health care professionals use protective equipment (e.g., masks, eye shields, gloves, and gowns) to prevent the spread of infection. Policies and procedures for the appropriate disposal of waste materials (i.e., diapers, soiled linens, blood, or other body fluid spills) must be followed to prevent further infection.

Hand Washing

Hand washing is the single most important component of infection control. Hands should be washed before and immediately after working with a client or whenever a person comes into contact with any type of body fluid. Hands should be washed when gloves are removed.

Use of Gloves

Gloves should be used by OT practitioners when there is a possibility of coming into contact with infected material or exposure to body fluids (e.g., during oral motor intervention, which requires the OT practitioner to place fingers in a child's oral cavity, or when changing diapers). Gloves should also be worn by OT practitioners who have scratches on or breaks in their skin.

Cleaning of Equipment and Toys

OT practitioners need to maintain equipment and toys in good, clean working order. Although equipment and toys are not sterilized after children use them, all of these items should be properly cleaned. OT practitioners can also require that families provide the children's favorite toys for use during therapy. They can educate the families about the safest and most effective methods of cleaning their children's toys.

According to the U.S. Department of Labor, Occupational Safety and Health Administration (OSHA), facilities and agencies must provide their workers with policies and procedures for cleaning and disinfecting.[12] These procedures are beyond the scope of this chapter. It is the responsibility of practitioners to become familiar with their facilities' policies and procedures for disinfecting.

Hepatitis B Vaccination

The OSHA standard regarding bloodborne pathogens requires employers to offer a free three-injection hepatitis B vaccination series to all employees who are exposed to blood or any other potentially infectious material during their routine duties. This policy includes OT practitioners and other health care workers. Vaccinations must be offered within 10 days of initial assignment to a job in which exposure to blood or other potentially infectious materials can be "reasonably anticipated."[12]

Characteristics of a Successful Health Care Provider

Certain characteristics promote the success of a health care provider in a medical care setting. OT practitioners working in medical care settings must possess people skills, including compassion, empathy, honesty, and proper manners, along with the ability to effectively communicate and actively listen to clients and team members. The pace of a medical care setting is fast. OT practitioners who exhibit high energy level, actively pursue new knowledge, and feel confident in expressing their findings to other team members will find success in a medical care setting. Articulating sound clinical reasoning skills to team members and family and being willing to listen to others' ideas is beneficial, especially when working with children, their families, and other health care providers.[7] Successful OT practitioners in medical care settings exhibit advanced technical skills and knowledge of current techniques, assessments, as well as documentation guidelines. Importantly, they respect other team members' time, opinions, and professional expertise and are also able to advocate for clients and families.

Legal and Ethical Considerations in a Medical Care System

Laws are a set of rules that govern practices in a variety of settings, including pediatric medical care settings. Laws set the minimum standards for the protection of consumers who receive medical care. If a health care provider performs an illegal act, then the offense is punishable by fines, imprisonment, and/or loss of license.[7] Health care professionals may be fined, suspended, expelled from a profession, or even face prison sentences for breaking laws. Acts that may be punishable by law include billing for services that were not provided, improper billing procedures, or providing a treatment modality that one is not qualified to perform (e.g., in some states, proper certification is required for the performance of certain modalities).

Each health care professional has a national organization that has adopted a code of ethics to govern the behavior of its members and establish standards of care for the profession. Pediatric OT practitioners are encouraged to be active members of the American Occupational Therapy Association (AOTA). All OT practitioners are expected to abide by the AOTA's Code of Ethics (See Chapter 1 for an overview of the code of ethics). In general, the AOTA Code of Ethics provides guidelines for ethical practice that include the following:[2]

- Beneficence
- Nonmaleficence
- Autonomy and confidentiality
- Social justice
- Procedural justice
- Veracity
- Fidelity

These seven principles provide the standards of practice related to competence (therapy skills and abilities), honesty (as related to the provision of care and interactions with others), and clear communication (as related to services provided and interactions with peers, patients, and caregivers).[2] For example, the principle of autonomy and confidentiality suggest that it is every OT practitioner's responsibility to ensure confidentiality for each patient and to allow patients to make decisions about their intervention plans.

SUMMARY

The pediatric medical care system is composed of individuals dedicated to caring for children with various illnesses. The five major settings in the pediatric medical care system are (1) the NICU, (2) the step-down nursery or the PICU, (3) the subacute care setting, (4) the residential or long-term care setting, and (5) the home-based care setting. Specific goals are addressed for each of these settings. Depending on their needs, infants or children are transferred from one setting to another for treatment.

Because long-term hospitalization is not a typical event in an infant's or child's life, it can hinder their development. As early as 1947, this fact prompted members of the medical community to identify a role for hospital-based OT services. Although OT practice in certain settings requires an advanced level of skill, medical-based OT services can generally be carried out by competent occupational therapists or OTAs.

Medical-based OT services should be provided in a way that promotes team collaboration, even when it is specific to an institution or facility. The four most common team collaboration approaches are (1) multidisciplinary approach, (2) transdisciplinary approach, (3) interdisciplinary approach, and (4) "individual-versus-group" sessions.

Appropriate documentation facilitates the collaboration process. Although documentation requirements vary depending on the regulations of each institution, they commonly include screenings, evaluations, treatment plans, progress notes, letters of justification, and discharge summaries. The OT practitioner's ability to clearly document medical-based objectives and progress has a direct impact on an institution's reimbursement rate and the client's ability to receive requested services and equipment.

The complex nature of the pediatric medical care system poses a unique challenge for medical-based OT practitioners because they are required to possess not only the basic OT skills but a working knowledge of the pediatric medical specialties, the ability to use and interpret pediatric medical terminology, and information about the frequent changes in the pediatric health care environment, including information about legal and ethical issues.

References

1. American Occupational Therapy Association: Guide for the supervision of occupational therapy personnel in the delivery of occupational therapy services. *Am J Occup Ther* 53,592–594, 1999.
2. American Occupational Therapy Association: Occupational therapy code of ethics and ethical standards, 2010. Available at: http://www.AOTA.org. Accessed June 2, 2010.
3. American Occupational Therapy Association: Occupational therapy practice framework: domain and process, ed 2. *Am J Occup Ther* 62(6):625–703, 2008.
4. Anderson KN: *Mosby's medical, nursing, and allied health dictionary,* ed 6, St. Louis, 2002, Mosby.
5. Dudgeon BJ, Crooks L: Hospital and pediatric rehabilitation services. In Case-Smith J, O'Brien J: *Occupational therapy for children,* ed 6, St. Louis, 2010, Mosby, pp 785–811.
6. Jabri J, Dreher JM: Documentation of occupational therapy services. In Early MB, editor: *Physical dysfunction: practice skills for the occupational therapy assistant,* ed 2, St. Louis, 2005, Mosby.
7. Judson K, Harrison C: *Law and ethics for medical careers,* ed 5, New York, 2010, McGraw-Hill.
8. Oakley D, Bauer-Logan K: *Traumatic brain lecture series,* Queens, NY, 1996, St. Mary's Hospital for Children.
9. Slee V, Slee D: *Slee's health care terms,* ed 3, St. Paul, MN, 1996, Tringa Press.
10. Venes D: *Taber's cyclopedic medical dictionary,* ed 21, Philadelphia, 2009, FA Davis.
11. Uniform Data System for Medical Rehabilitation: *WeeFIM system workshop,* Queens, NY, 1988, UB Foundation Activities.
12. U.S. Department of Labor, Occupational Safety and Health Administration: *Bloodborne facts: hepatitis B vaccination—protection for you,* Washington, DC, U.S. Department of Labor, Occupational Safety and Health Administration. 2010

REVIEW *Questions*

1. When might a child be transferred from one medical setting to another?
2. Which functional areas are assessed in a pediatric medical-based OT evaluation?
3. In what ways do the multidisciplinary, transdisciplinary, and interdisciplinary models of collaboration differ?
4. In what ways could a medical practitioner's documentation have an impact on the treatment and equipment needs of a child?
5. Why is continuing education an important aspect of medical-based OT practice?

SUGGESTED *Activities*

1. Create three examples of a narrative or SOAP note based on three observations of children in a natural setting (e.g., schoolyard, playground).
2. Purchase and review flash cards of common roots of medical terms.
3. Visit children in a hospital. Ask them about the things they like to do when they are at home or play a game with them. What did you learn from them?

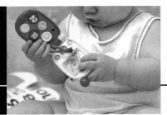

4

Educational System

DIANA BAL

CHAPTER *Objectives*

After studying this chapter, the reader will be able to accomplish the following:

- Identify the federal laws that govern the provision of educational services to children with disabilities.
- Explain the formation and function of an individual educational program team.
- Explain the process involved in an individual educational program.
- Compare and contrast the roles of the occupational therapist and the occupational therapy assistant in the school setting.
- Distinguish between the medical and educational models for occupational therapy service delivery.
- Describe the techniques for working with teachers and parents in schools.
- Differentiate between direct, monitoring, and consultation levels of occupational therapy service delivery.

KEY TERMS

Free appropriate public education

Least restrictive environment

Due process

Inclusion model

Related services

Individuals with Disabilities Education Act

Individual educational program

No Child Left Behind Act

Individual educational program team

Exceptional educational need

Individualized family service plan

Role delineation

CHAPTER OUTLINE

Practice Settings

Federal Laws
EDUCATION OF THE HANDICAPPED ACT (PUBLIC LAW 94-142)
REHABILITATION ACT AND THE AMERICANS WITH DISABILITIES ACT
PUBLIC LAW 99-457
INDIVIDUALS WITH DISABILITIES EDUCATION ACT
NO CHILD LEFT BEHIND ACT

Rights of Parents and Children

Identification and Referral

Evaluation

Eligibility

Individual Educational Program
TIPS FOR WORKING WITH PARENTS
TIPS FOR WORKING WITH TEACHERS
TIPS FOR PROVIDING INTERVENTION IN THE CLASSROOM

Transitions

Roles of the Occupational Therapist and the Occupational Therapy Assistant

Clinical Models Versus Educational Models

Levels of Service
DIRECT SERVICE
MONITORING SERVICE
CONSULTATION SERVICES

Discontinuing Therapy Services

Summary

One third to one half of occupational therapy (OT) practitioners work with children; public school systems are the second largest employers.[4] Despite these statistics, OT practitioners in public schools often find that they work alone, with a limited support network. This is especially true in rural areas, where one practitioner may provide therapy services to several small school districts or a cooperative educational service area. Being a member of an educational team requires that practitioners broaden their focus on the ways children function in their families, communities, and schools. This mode of thinking contrasts with the traditional medical model of "evaluate and treat," with its focus on the disabilities or limitations of children.[7] As part of a multidisciplinary educational team, OT practitioners working in school systems interact with a variety of people. They must therefore possess specialized technical skills and have knowledge of the educational system, current special education laws, and regulations.[3,8] OT practitioners must apply their knowledge and intervention skills in the context of a school setting while communicating effectively with parents* and educators.

*In the chapter the term *parents* is used in the general sense and refers to the legal guardian who is the child's primary caregiver and is responsible for the child's well-being. For example, the "parent" may be a grandparent, aunt, uncle, or even a friend of the family.

PRACTICE SETTINGS

Occupational therapists working in the public school setting collaborate with teachers and special educators. They work with the student in the classroom whenever possible. Sometimes taking the student to a separate room might be the optimal learning situation for the student (Figure 4-1). OT practitioners develop strategies to facilitate educational goals. Strategies and suggestions may be provided to the teacher to better enhance the student's learning.

FEDERAL LAWS

Pediatric OT services are mandated by law.[4] Box 4-1 summarizes the laws that have an impact on OT services in public school systems. Education is an important occupation of children. As such, OT clinicians working in school systems have the opportunity to directly impact the child's occupation. They are afforded the luxury of seeing the results of their interventions daily within the context for which it is intended. Their role is to improve the child's ability to function within that environment; they must become skillful in advocating the needs of the children within the contexts of the setting and the laws.

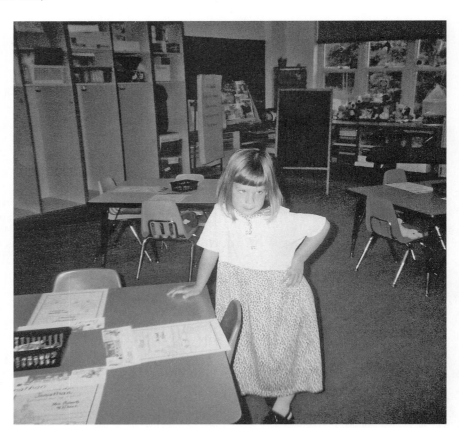

FIGURE 4-1 Working with a child in a separate room may help facilitate educational goals.

BOX 4-1

Summary of Federal Laws That Affect Occupational Therapy in Educational Settings

1973
Public Law 93-112, Section 504 of the Rehabilitation Act
- Discrimination against people with disabilities when offering services is prohibited.

1975
Public Law 94-142: Education for All Handicapped Children Act (renamed Education of the Handicapped Act [EHA])
- All children have the right to free and appropriate public education.

1986
Public Law 99-457, Part H (added to EHA)
- Birth-to-Three services should be equal in all states and counties.

1990
Americans With Disabilities Education Act
- In areas of public services, discriminatory practices against individuals with disabilities by employers are prohibited.
- EHA is renamed Individuals with Disabilities Education Act (IDEA).

1997
- IDEA is revised (IDEA-R).
- Part H of IDEA-R is renamed Part C.

2001
- No Child Left Behind stresses the use of scientifically based or evidence-based programs and practices.

Education of the Handicapped Act (Public Law 94-142)

In 1975, the U.S. Congress passed the Education of the Handicapped Act (EHA) (Public Law 94-142) requiring schools to provide **free appropriate public education** (FAPE) to all children from 5 to 21 years of age.[5,8,9] Children with special needs have the right to have their educational programs geared toward their unique needs, regardless of the nature, extent, or severity of their disabilities. In 1986, the law was amended so that public schools could be responsible for providing educational services to children at 3 years of age.

Provisions under this law guarantee children the right to be educated in the **least restrictive environment** (LRE) and receive other services that may be required

for them to benefit from their educational program. The law also outlines parents' and children's rights and the legal course of action. Parents have the right to **due process**—that is, voluntary mediation and impartial hearing—to resolve differences with the school that cannot be resolved informally.

Least Restrictive Environment

The right to be educated in the LRE allows a student who has special needs to be educated in a regular classroom whenever possible.[4,9] He or she is entitled to interact with peers who do not have disabilities. Before this law was enacted, students with disabilities were placed in special schools with other students who had disabilities, or they were placed in self-contained classrooms in a separate school building with no opportunity to interact with typically developing peers.

The LRE guidelines provided the impetus for the development of mainstreaming and **inclusion models** (i.e., models in which children with disabilities are able to spend time in regular classrooms). School personnel determine whether a student who has a disability can receive an appropriate education in a regular classroom with the aid of support services and necessary modifications. The team considers whether the child can benefit from any time in a regular classroom. The spirit of the EHA requires that schools provide an entire continuum of services to those students with special needs.[2,6,9] For some students, this may mean placement in a regular classroom that has been modified to meet their needs (e.g., one that has been equipped with positioning devices). For other students, it may mean placement in a regular classroom that allows them to go to a resource room for assistance from a special education or resource teacher. Some students need specialized instruction from a special education teacher, and they spend most of the day in the self-contained classroom but are integrated into a regular classroom for certain classes or activities. Students who have difficulty transitioning from one area to another can benefit from reverse mainstreaming, where the regular education students come into the special education classroom during certain courses.

Related Services

According to the EHA, schools are required to provide special, or related, services as necessary for the student to benefit from the educational program. These services include transportation, physical therapy (PT), OT, speech therapy (ST), assistive technology services, psychological services, school health services, social work services, and parent counseling and training.[5,9] Except for ST, these services are available only to a student classified as a special education student. ST is a "stand-alone" service, which means that a student who does not receive special education services may receive speech therapy.

Rehabilitation Act and Americans With Disabilities Act

The educational rights of children with disabilities are protected by two additional federal laws: Section 504 of the Rehabilitation Act (1973) and the Americans With Disabilities Act (ADA)(1990).[2,9] Section 504 of the Rehabilitation Act stipulates that any recipient of federal aid (including a school) cannot discriminate when offering services to people with disabilities. The ADA prohibits discriminatory practices in areas related to employment, transportation, accessibility, and telecommunications. A student with a disability who is not eligible for special education services but requires reasonable accommodation in his or her regular educational program may be eligible to receive related services under these laws. To be eligible, the student must have a condition that "substantially limits one or more major life activities," with learning being a major life activity.[2]

CASE *Study*

Jack is a 5 year old with spina bifida. He attends a regular kindergarten class and is able to perform academic activities in a manner equal to his peers. Jack comprehends the information provided, but due to the diminished strength and endurance caused by his disability, he is slower than others in completing his work. Jack needs to be catheterized two times a day by the nurse. Jack qualifies for related services under section 504 of the Rehabilitation Act. Specifically, the following accommodations will allow Jack to use educational services:

1. He must complete 50% of his work in class; other work will be sent home.
2. He will have extra class time to complete work whenever possible.
3. Classroom supplies will be readily available and placed in front of him before a task begins.
4. OT will be provided to increase strength and endurance for academic functions.
5. A peer or an adult will accompany him when he leaves the classroom.

Public Law 99-457

Public Law 99-457, which was passed in 1986, added Part H (which is now known as Part C) to the EHA. This law mandates services for preschoolers with disabilities and provided the impetus for the development of early intervention services for infants and toddlers from birth to 3 years of age.

Although the specific policies, procedures, and timelines for Birth-to-Three programs vary from those of the public school setting, both systems follow a similar framework that includes identification and referral, evaluation, determination of eligibility, development of the **individual educational program** (IEP) or individual family service plan (IFSP), and transitions.

Individuals With Disabilities Education Act

The EHA was renamed the Individuals With Disabilities Education Act (IDEA) in 1990; it was revised in 1997 and is now known as IDEA-R. This act encourages OT practitioners to work with children in their classroom environment (inclusion) and provide support to the regular education teacher (integration). It also encourages schools to allow students with disabilities to work toward meeting the same educational standards as their peers. IDEA-R changed the process for the identification, evaluation, and implementation of IEPs. Table 4-1 contains a comparison of the IDEA and the IDEA-R. For example, the occupational therapist and the occupational therapy assistant (OTA) can assist in the evaluation of the student to determine the need for the acquisition of a device that allows the child to remain in a regular classroom. The practitioner may consult with others on positioning, train team members, and consult with others on strategies to increase the likelihood of success in the classroom. The role of the occupational therapist under IDEA-R is to assist children with special needs so that they can participate in educational activities.

No Child Left Behind Act

The No Child Left Behind Act (NCLB) was enacted in 2001 in order to improve teaching standards and the student's learning results. NCLB supports the use of scientifically based practices by professionals working in the educational setting. Therefore, educators and OT practitioners are required to consider research when selecting instructional or interventional practices. Schools must report *adequate yearly progress* through a single accountability system that applies the same standards to all students. These standards are based on each state's academic achievement standards. Teacher quality and paraprofessional competencies are also parts of this Act, yet it does not specifically address the competencies of related services such as OT.[10] OT practitioners need to collaborate and consult with the team to prioritize the student's needs. Therapy is integrated into the classroom and provides consistent follow-through. Student-centered Individualized Educational Plan (IEP) goals and objectives enhance success in the educational environment (Figure 4-2).[10]

TABLE 4-1

Comparison of IDEA and IDEA-R

FORMER IDEA	IDEA-R
TEAM NAMES M-team (multidisciplinary team)	IEP team
REGULAR EDUCATION TEACHERS Works with students other than those with learning disabilities; not involved with special education students	Participation on IEP team
MEETINGS **Numerous meetings** Two meetings: (1) an M-team meeting to determine eligibility, and (2) a separate IEP and placement meeting to determine services and program	One meeting
Placement meeting Possible parental involvement	Required parental involvement
REPORTS M-team summary with minority report; if a member of the team disagrees with the eligibility findings, that member can submit a dissenting report	Single report of IEP team's determination of eligibility; no minority report
CONSENT Not required for re-evaluation	Parental consent for re-evaluation
MEDIATION Not available	Mediation (a voluntary process in which an impartial person helps schools and families reach agreement on issues related to the identification, evaluation, and educational placement of the child and provision of a free, appropriate public education without going through a due process hearing)
SPECIAL NEEDS TERMINOLOGY Handicapping condition, or handicap	Disability
PARENTS' RIGHTS Sent six times	Sent three times

IEP, Individual educational plan; *IDEA*, Individuals with Disabilities Education Act; *IDEA-R*, IDEA, revised.

RIGHTS OF PARENTS AND CHILDREN

The IDEA-R outlines several procedural safeguards for children with disabilities and for their parents. These procedures are detailed in the United States Code of Federal Regulations, Title 34, Subtitle B, Chapter III, Part 300. To summarize, the safeguards include notifying parents of all proposed actions, obtaining consent to evaluate, allowing parents to attend IEP team meetings, and providing the right to an independent evaluation and the right to appeal school decisions in front of an impartial hearing officer.[9] The IDEA-R requires that school districts inform parents of their rights in a written format.

IDENTIFICATION AND REFERRAL

Children are frequently referred for special programs by physicians and health care professionals. Screening clinics offered by agencies, schools, and early intervention programs aid in identifying children who need special

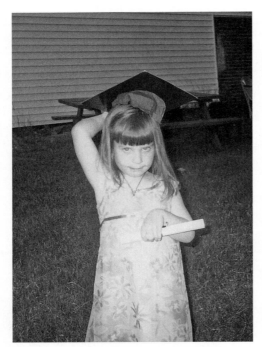

FIGURE 4-2   Education is an important occupation.

education services. Referrals are made to the appropriate agency (e.g., Child Find, early intervention clinic, or public school system). Once a referral is made, the responsible agency determines whether screening or an evaluation is needed.

Once children enter the school system, teachers often identify those who experience difficulty meeting educational expectations. Children receiving special education services may be referred to OT, or a child may qualify for services under Section 504. The **individual educational program team** (e.g., parent, teacher, special educator, OT clinician) determines a student's need for services (including OT). Children needing assistance with fine motor skills typically require evaluation by an occupational therapist. Likewise, students showing cognitive skill deficits require evaluation by a special educator; those with speech and language issues are referred to a speech therapist. The professional members are responsible for evaluating these children and determining whether they would benefit from related services. The interdisciplinary team collaborates and reviews the needs of students to determine their eligibility for related services.

EVALUATION

After a referral for OT services is received and parental consent is obtained, an evaluation can be initiated. (Some state and Medicaid conditions require a physician's order as a prerequisite to initiating these services.)

Evaluations measure the student's abilities at that particular time. Therefore, it is important to consider the viewpoint of everyone involved with the student, including teachers and parents. Knowledge of the student's strengths and needs may be gained from consultation with the teacher, parent, child, and staff. Standardized tests and clinical observations provide important information. State, local, and school policies may dictate what type of assessment will be used. However, clinicians must consider the child's needs in choosing an assessment. Observation of the child in the classroom, cafeteria, playground, and bathroom provides information about his or her functional skills.[1] Many children are able to perform certain activities in a quiet one-on-one situation but have difficulty generalizing or modulating them in a busy classroom. Students may also perform better when they are not aware that someone is watching or observing. Consultation with the teacher is key in identifying the specific problems and needs of the student. A questionnaire or referral form completed by the teacher is helpful to the team. The occupational therapist is responsible for completing the evaluation (with input from the OTA), interpreting the information, and presenting the report to the IEP team. The skills of the student should be reassessed before different objectives are formulated for a new IEP. Students are re-evaluated as needed or if requested by the parents, teachers, or team members. They must be re-evaluated at least every 3 years.

ELIGIBILITY

The IEP team determines the student's eligibility once all evaluations are completed. Eligibility for services in public schools is based on **exceptional educational need (EEN)**. The IEP team must consider all of the information obtained through the evaluations in order to determine whether the disability or condition interferes with the student's ability to participate in an educational program and whether the student needs related services to benefit from an educational program.[5,9] The presence of a disability does not necessarily mean that a student cannot participate in the regular educational program; nor does it mean that the student has an EEN.

CASE *Study*

For example, consider Mary, an 8-year-old girl in Grade 2, who had been diagnosed with cerebral palsy (left hemiplegia). Her parents requested an evaluation through the school district, which, in turn, conducted an IEP team evaluation and meeting to determine whether she was eligible for OT services. The team members' evaluation revealed that Mary had age-appropriate learning and thinking skills (cognition) and communication skills, although she sometimes drooled and spoke unclearly. Mary walked independently, moved around the building, and independently performed classroom tasks (e.g., printing, managing materials such as books and paper/pencil). Observations from team members led to the conclusion that she interacted well with her teachers and classmates and was an active participant in the classroom. The OT practitioner reported that Mary had mild spasticity in her left upper extremity, decreased control (isolation and precision) of her left upper extremity, and difficulty with bilateral tasks but that she successfully compensated for these factors and could participate in all classroom activities. She played with other children on the playground and handled self-feeding well. Mary participated in regular gym classes. She was independent in toileting.

The IEP team determined that while Mary had a documented disability (cerebral palsy), it did not interfere with her ability to receive an appropriate education. Therefore, an EEN did not exist and OT services were not required for Mary to participate in and benefit from her educational program. If Mary's family thought that she would benefit from OT services to resolve issues related to her muscle tone, range of motion (ROM), fine motor skills, and bilateral coordination skills, the family could seek and secure OT services in a clinic on an outpatient basis. For a child to be eligible to receive OT services in the public school setting, the services and goals must be educationally relevant.

INDIVIDUAL EDUCATIONAL PROGRAM

For school-age children (3 to 21 years of age) who receive special education services, an IEP is developed to outline the goals and objectives for the school year. It is a written plan as well as a process. The IEP team consists of the student's parent(s) or caregivers, regular education teacher, special education teacher or provider, a representative of the school district who is knowledgeable about the general curriculum, an individual who can interpret the instructional implications of evaluation results (i.e., the way certain factors may affect the student's ability to learn), and related services personnel. The representative of the school district, frequently given the title of local education agency (LEA) representative, may be the principal. The LEA representative is responsible for making sure that the programs outlined on the IEP are followed through in the educational environment. The person who interprets the evaluation results is often the school psychologist or a clinical psychologist. The student may be present at the meetings. The parents may invite anyone they wish to be present, such as a private therapist or parent advocate. If the family brings a lawyer to the IEP meeting to assist

with the process, then the school district may also bring a legal representative.

When developing the IEP, the team considers all evaluation results and the extent of the student's educational needs.[5] Goals, objectives, and methodologies (service and frequency) are developed at the meeting. The IEP is reviewed at least annually or sometimes more frequently if requested or necessary. The format of the IEP varies by state and school district. Box 4-2 contains information that must be included in an IEP. (See the Appendix to Chapter for a sample IEP form.[4])

BOX 4-2

Components of an Individual Educational Plan

- Statement of a child's present level of educational performance, including the way the child's disability affects his or her involvement in the general curriculum or age-appropriate activities
- Statement of measurable annual goals, including short-term objectives related to increased involvement and progress in the general curriculum and other (non)educational needs, such as those involving social and extracurricular activities
- Description of special education and related services and supplementary aids and services
- Description of program modifications or support to be used by school personnel to enable the child to attain goals; involvement and progress in general curricular, extracurricular, and nonacademic activities; and education and participation in activities with other children, both with and without disabilities
- Explanation of the extent to which the child will not participate in the regular classroom and Individual educational plan (IEP) activities with children who do not have disabilities
- Statement of any individual modifications needed for the child to participate in formal assessments of student achievement (e.g., statewide or districtwide tests)
- Projected date for beginning services and educational modifications; anticipated frequency, location, and duration of services
- Transition services, including linkage with other agencies
- Statement of the way that progress toward annual goals is measured
- Descriptions of methods to regularly inform parents of their child's progress (at least as often as the parents of children without disabilities are informed)

Sometimes when a child enters school at age 3 years, he or she already has a written **Individualized Family Service Plan** (IFSP). This document is the result of the collaboration between the parents and the Birth-to-Three program professionals and is reviewed every 6 months. IFSPs emphasize the family's goals for the child, whereas an IEP focuses on educational goals that the student works on in school and is reviewed annually (Box 4-3). Both documents require the parents to accept all or a portion of the recommended services. The parents or the school district have the option of going to due process if the team is unable to agree on the program or services recommended for the child. Children receiving special services are given progress notes with each report card.

The data collection sheets detail the child's objectives, frequency of performance in selected tasks, and success to date (Figures 4-3 A and 4-3 B). This information is used to document the child's progress in quarterly reports. Performance is measured in a variety of contexts, with the goal being integration. Progress notes include information from the data sheets and rely on consultation and collaboration with teachers and staff to ensure that the performance represents actual achievement in the occupation (e.g., education).

CLINICAL *Pearl*

Occupational therapy (OT) objectives embedded in the special education teacher's goals and objectives are reinforced by other team members. As a result, everyone on the team is responsible for the goals and objectives of the individual educational program (IEP).

BOX 4-3

Components of an Individual Family Service Plan

The format of the written plan may differ from program to program, but an Individual Family Service Plan (IFSP) must contain the following information:
- Child's current level of development
- Summaries of evaluation reports
- Family's concerns
- Desired outcomes (goals)
- Early intervention services and support necessary to achieve outcomes
- Frequency of, method for providing, and location of services
- Payment arrangements (if any)
- Transition plan

Tips for Working With Parents*

1. Parents know their child! Listen to what they have to say, and try to address their concerns. They may not know why their child is behaving in a particular manner (professionals may help with this), but they are aware of the behaviors.

2. Parents and caregivers may not be used to the language professionals use in meetings. Present information in layman's terms so that explanations are not needed. For example, say, "John has trouble getting around without tripping or bumping into things" instead of "John has dyspraxia."

3. Parents attending IEP meetings may be nervous and feeling uncomfortable. Put them at ease by beginning the meeting asking them what they hope to achieve from the meeting or what they see as their child's strengths.

4. IEP team meetings frequently highlight the child's weaknesses and present only briefly the child's strengths. Begin your report with the child's strengths; follow it by describing problem areas, with a plan for how to address these concerns.

5. Try to speak with parents before your evaluation. Ask them what they see at home and how they view the situation. This will help provide a focus for your evaluation and insight into the child.

6. When discussing the child's performance, be clear about what has been tried in the classroom and how it has or has not worked. This gives the team information on future goals, objectives, and intervention strategies.

7. Parents may become frustrated with a long list of problems. Order the list of problem areas in such a way that the most important issues may be targeted immediately for intervention. You can always address other problems later.

8. Ask the parents what works or does not work at home. You may be able to provide them with strategies to help their child, or they may be able to help you with strategies. Children benefit when both the parents and professionals are working on the same page.

9. Provide suggestions and/or strategies for helping the child function within the classroom. Using a previously developed list is acceptable, but make sure you have individualized it to the child. Use his or her name. Remember that any written information sent to others is a reflection of you. You do not want to give the parents the impression that you are too busy to work with their child.

---

*Tips provided by Jane O'Brien and Diana Bal

Name _____**Sample**_____

Date:	8/9	8/16	8/23	8/30	9/6	9/13
4 out of 9 pieces	1/9	2/9	1/9	2/9	N	2/9
Snip	1 snip	1 snip	1 snip	1 snip	N	1 snip
Scissor correctly	No	No	No	No	N	No
Drink—consecutive swallows	1 swallow	2 swallows	1 swallow	1 swallow	N	2 swallows
Spillage	Top half of shirt	Top half of shirt	Top half of shirt	Top half of shirt	N	Top quarter of shirt
Finger feed	10% chips	30% chips, pears	25% chips, pears, cheese	30% chips, cookies, pears	N	25% chips, pears, cheese

B

N, No school.

FIGURE 4-3 A   An example of a data collection sheet for therapy.

10. Follow up with the parents. Sending letters home with the child, e-mail messages, or brief phone calls let the parents know that you are working with them to help their child. Keep information confidential and protected. For example, there are some things you do not want to e-mail, but letting the parents know that "John had a great day in OT" is always welcomed.

Tips for Working With Teachers*

1. Most importantly, remember that the OT practitioner's job in a school setting is to help the child function within the classroom. The teacher is in charge of the classroom. Therefore, the OT practitioner must observe the teacher's style, rules, and classroom expectations before designing the intervention for a specific child.

2. Spend time in the classroom without making suggestions or judging the teacher.

3. Ask the teacher what he or she sees as the problem areas for the child. Ask the teacher how you could help the child function better within the classroom.

4. Prioritize strategies for the teacher. He or she must work with the entire class, so providing them with one or two effective strategies for a child is sufficient. You can always add more later.

5. Provide the teacher with short written strategies, and follow up as necessary.

*Tips provided by Judy Cohn, MS, ED, and Jane O'Brien

Name Sample

Date:	9/16	10/19	11/17	1/7	2/9	3/17	4/27	5/.
1. Will place 5 out of 9 pieces in an individual inset puzzle with minimal assistance	30% with 1 5% with 2	40% with 2 10% with 2						
2. Will snip with scissors 5 times, placing scissors in hands correctly with minimal assistance	5% with 1 and assistance for placement	25% with 1						
3. Will drink from a cup with consecutive swallows— no spillage.	10% front of shirt wet	15% minimal wet on shirt						
4. Will finger feed. Identify food:	24% chips	30% fries, pears, cheese						

A

FIGURE 4-3 B, cont'd An example of a data collection sheet for the individual educational plan in the appendix.

6. Respect the teacher's time. Teachers get very few breaks during the day. Discussing a child over lunch may seem like a good solution to the OT practitioner but may add stress to the teacher's day and not allow for a much-needed break. Another solution may be to ask to lead a 1-hour "handwriting" seminar for the entire class every Friday morning. The OT practitioner can work with the entire class, targeting the needs of a small group at the same time. This provides a break for the teacher and helps build rapport while benefiting the entire class.

7. E-mails and short notes are effective means of communication with teachers.

8. Help determine good child–teacher fits. Once a clinician understands the style and expectations of a classroom, he or she can assist in the placement of children with special needs. For example, some teachers are extremely organized and may work best with children who have difficulty with organization. Other children require flexibility and accommodation.

9. Present yourself to teachers as a resource. For example, providing them with writing kits full of activities to enhance writing skills, fine motor games, visual motor games, or crafts that may be easily implemented into the classroom may be helpful. Clinicians may lead morning exercises or warm-ups to address the sensory needs of the students while modeling activities for teachers.

10. Help teachers out by using OT resources. Establish a relationship between the nearby OT school. College students are frequently looking for projects that may help teachers and schools. Box 4-4 lists some examples of projects that may assist teachers and OT students.

11. Provide solutions to teachers concerning children with special needs. Gain their trust through collaboration, which works best by listening, discussion, and follow-through. Team members must be able to critically analyze their work and look for alternative solutions.

BOX 4-4

Projects That May Assist Teachers and Students in Programs for the Occupational Therapist and the Occupational Therapy Assistant

- Design a fine-motor kit for a classroom of first graders.
- Develop games associated with spring.
- Make pieces of equipment, toys, or other items needed for the classroom (positioning equipment must be checked out by the clinician).
- Develop a finger-puppet show (to improve finger individuation) based on a book (to encourage reading).
- Participate in a health fair at a local school.
- Volunteer for story time; find a book about children with special needs.
- Volunteer for a field trip or evening workshop.
- Develop teacher/parent handouts with strategies for children with organizational problems.
- Organize a teacher appreciation day.

12. Use layman's terms when speaking with teachers. It is best to describe the observed student's behavior in simple language rather than by using medical or psychological terms to describe behaviors. Speaking about what one observes limits misunderstanding. For example, instead of saying, "John is tactually defensive, which is why he has trouble modulating his behavior," say, "John does not like to be touched by other children unexpectedly; he finds this type of contact annoying, which is why he may hit other children." Then the OT clinician can provide a solution (e.g., allow John to be in the back of the line. Sometimes he will also want to be in the front of the line. When John is the "line leader," observe carefully and ask him to lead the way from the front. You do not want John to feel left out and never be allowed to be the line leader).

Tips for Providing Intervention in the Classroom*

1. Develop a good rapport with the teacher before providing intervention in the classroom. Be aware of the teacher's style, rules, routine, and classroom expectations.

2. Discuss with the teacher what you would like to do. Decide on a time that this fits in with other classroom activities. Be open to adjusting your plan to fit in with the teacher's agenda.

3. Working in small groups makes the intervention less obvious and intrusive.

4. Keeping a regular schedule allows the class to feel comfortable with you.

5. Walk into the classroom at a nondisruptive time (e.g., after the bell rings, when the children are settling down). It is not helpful if you interrupt quiet reading or testing to work with a child.

6. Provide intervention as the child participates in the activities. For example, a child with poor handwriting may complete a worksheet by repeating correct strokes during writing practice. The OTA or occupational therapist may help a child with hand movements to a song while standing by and providing trunk stabilization so that the child can move his or her arms.

7. Providing intervention in the classroom requires the OT practitioner to adjust the intervention so

---

* Tips provided by Judy Cohn, MS, ED, and Jane O'Brien

that the child can be successful at the activities. For example the teacher may choose the activities while the OT practitioner adapts and grades the activities. This requires OT practitioners to be flexible and "think on their feet." It is important that the OT practitioner has the child's goals and objectives firmly in his or her mind.

8. Flexibility is easily achieved when the OT practitioner is aware of the child's goals and objectives. If the classroom activity changes, the OT practitioner may select a different goal for the session. Once the OT practitioner is clear about the desired objective, he or she may adapt and modify the activity to address it.

9. Depending on the teacher, child, and classroom setting, it may be wise to schedule breaks for intervention in the classroom. The OTA may want to schedule direct service intervention on a monthly basis to allow the teacher a break from having someone enter the classroom. This must be included in the IEP.

10. Be responsible for developing a weekly lesson for the entire class. Attend the class at the same time (for consistency) and work from the teacher's lesson plan. For example, if the first-grade class is learning about animals, the OTA could design an entire session on animals. Students could make animal noises and walk like an animal (gross motor), match animal cards of mothers and cubs (visual perceptual), pick out animal shapes (fur for a bear, slippery snakeskin) (stereognosis), and make an animal craft (cutting, drawing, coloring) (fine motor).

11. Communicate clearly with the teacher. The OTA could e-mail the teacher to let her know the plan for the following week. It is important to be respectful of the teacher by being well-prepared for the class and letting her know in advance if you are unable to attend a class. It would be very helpful to the teacher if you have all the materials prepared (along with the lesson plan) in case you are unable to attend.

12. Ask for and accept feedback. Set up a system whereby the teacher can give you feedback. Make changes based on the feedback, and follow up with suggestions of your own. Teachers are more likely to listen to you if they feel you are listening to them. Be sure to ask how the children responded to your sessions. Some of these sessions may make the children more attentive for the rest of the day, whereas others may cause the children to become restless.

CASE *Study*

Tamara, an OTA, intended to work with Jovan in his first-grade classroom during art class. The objective for the session was for Jovan to hold a crayon with a static tripod grasp and imitate a circle. However, when Tamara entered the classroom, the teacher informed her that the art class had been canceled; they were now involved in playing "Simon Says" and other inside games because it was raining and the kids were all "wound up." Instead of insisting that Jovan participate in the scheduled art activity, Tamara decided to incorporate Jovan's second goal of improving postural control for writing activities. She quickly changed her intervention to facilitate the trunk and upper arm strengthening required for writing. Tamara asked the teacher if she could be the leader of the game. The teacher appreciated the break after a hectic rainy morning. Tamara led the activities for the entire class and provided hands-on help to Jovan as needed. The children performed arm pushups, wheelbarrow walks, crab walks, and sit-ups, among other physical activities. Jovan was proud of himself because he knew how to do the crab walk and got to show the others. Tamara ended the session by asking the children ("Simon says") to sit in their seats, put their heads down, count quietly to 20, and then look up. This helped quiet the children. The teacher enjoyed seeing the variation of "Simon Says" activities. Tamara explained that these were great pre-handwriting activities and that all the children could benefit from them. Tamara agreed to write them down for the teacher.

TRANSITIONS

Children undergo various transitions from infancy to 21 years of age. Students' services and programs change as they enter and leave the Birth-to-Three program and the public school system. A transition plan includes steps that should be taken to support students and their families as they go through these changes so that the transitions can be smooth and successful. Transition planning informs families about the different services and agencies available.

When a student reaches age 14, transition services such as vocational education and job coaches are discussed with the student and the family to help in identifying his or her interests and preferences. Students nearing the age of majority (sometimes at age 17) are informed of their rights under the IDEA-R. The family is notified that all rights accorded to parents transfer to the student but that they will continue to receive required parental notices. For the parents to retain their rights, they must be recognized as the student's legal guardians by the courts.

ROLES OF THE OCCUPATIONAL THERAPIST AND THE OCCUPATIONAL THERAPY ASSISTANT

Occupational therapists and OTAs have related but distinct roles in the educational setting. A successful partnership between the two ensures effective and efficient use of education and training, encourages creativity, and promotes professional growth and respect.[3] All OT services provided in the educational setting must comply with federal and state regulations. Additionally, professional standards of practice help occupational therapists and OTAs with **role delineation** in the educational setting. OT practitioners must work together to provide the best possible service to the child.

OT practitioners may be employed directly by the local educational agency (school district) or contracted through a local hospital, health care agency, or private practice. Those employed by the local educational agency must comply with the supervision and employment practices of the school district's structure. If the OT services are contracted through another agency (e.g., a hospital or health care agency), the practitioners are considered employees of that agency and may be supervised by one of its employees. Supervision guidelines and expectations should be closely coordinated between the employer and the local educational agency. In either situation, all licensing and state regulations regarding caseload and supervision standards must be followed.[3,5]

The occupational therapist is legally responsible for all aspects of the OT process. OTAs are responsible for providing services within their established level of competence. Professional supervision is a partnership that requires communication and mutual responsibility to clarify competencies and responsibilities. The practice standards established by the American Occupational Therapy Association (AOTA) delineate levels of supervision (see Chapter 1). The required level of supervision depends on many factors such as the OTA's level of experience and service competency, the complexity of the evaluation and therapy methods used, and the current practice guidelines and regulations of the state or local educational agency. Supervision in a school district can often be a challenge because of the large number of schools and the geographic distance. Having the occupational therapist and OTA work together in the same school at the same time allows ongoing supervision of and communication with the OTA. Occupational therapists are ultimately responsible for service performance.[3] If an occupational therapist is not comfortable with an OTA's performance of a particular task, it should no longer be delegated to the OTA. Likewise, an OTA who is not comfortable performing a certain task

is responsible for communicating this concern to the supervising occupational therapist.

Each of the practitioners has a role in screening and evaluation, IEP formation, treatment planning, and intervention. During the evaluation, occupational therapists determine which data are collected and the tools and methods to be used. OTAs can assist with data collection by making clinical observations and administering and scoring tests within their service competency level. Occupational therapists are responsible for analyzing, interpreting, and reporting information verbally and in writing. During the IEP formation, OTAs assist with developing goals and may attend the IEP meeting (under the direction of an occupational therapist) to report the findings and recommendations. Although OTAs do not interpret the findings or negotiate changes in levels of service or goals, they may suggest changes or reevaluation. OTAs are responsible for communicating observations, ideas, interpretations, and suggestions.

For the intervention phase, OTAs must first demonstrate service competency to the occupational therapist. Then they are responsible for developing intervention activities related to the goals and objectives (after initial direction from an occupational therapist). OTAs provide intervention aimed at improving children's occupations ranging from printing, cutting with scissors, using a keyboard, and performing lunchroom activities to managing clothing for toileting or recess. The OTA also collaborates and works with the teacher and other school personnel on appropriate positioning of the student and determining which materials or methods can be used in the classroom to increase the student's ability to participate successfully. The OTA is responsible for informing the occupational therapist of changes in the student's environment and providing current data regarding his or her performance.[3]

OTAs may be responsible for collecting data to establish evidence-based intervention. Since the domain of OT is occupation, the collected data must address occupation. Although goals and objectives must be measurable, practitioners must ensure that they are also meaningful to children, families, and educators. See Table 4-2 for a sample of goals and intervention activities. By collecting data on activities that are valued by educators, families, and children, practitioners support the importance of the profession. Goals and objectives that are too far removed from the actual occupation may be measurable, but if they are not meaningful much time is wasted. For example, consider the following goal: Marcie will cross the street with 75% accuracy. Although this goal is measurable, it is not meaningful and is, in fact, dangerous. Her mother's comment is: "What about the 25% of the time that she does not meet this goal?" Another commonly written goal states the following: "Mike will bring a spoon halfway to his mouth." As this

TABLE 4-2

Sample School-Based Goals and Intervention Activities

GOAL	ACTIVITY
Sam will write four sentences with 80% accuracy (spelling, legibility)	Hand strengthening, warm-up exercises Compensatory techniques, including lap top, frequency words available, Benbow Hand program, adaptive writing tool
Sam will remember to write all his assignments in his daily planner, with verbal reminders from the teacher for 10 school days	Teacher and parent will begin by reminding him. Clinician adds a fun game to the assignment; if Sam remembers it, he gets a reward (i.e., bring in a picture of you and your pet).
Sam will participate in regular gym class, with modifications made as needed	Clinician will consult with gym teacher to provide modifications as necessary. Occupational therapy clinician will consult with gym teacher about games and activities that the whole class may benefit from (e.g., parachute games, relay races, "Simon Says," dancing, etc.).

goal is written, Mike does not even get any food during mealtime. A better goal would be as follows: "Mike will bring a spoon to his mouth; the first half of the distance will be hand over hand, and he will complete the second half of the distance 7 out of 10 spoonfuls." OTAs can assist the occupational therapist in developing measurable and meaningful goals by describing the behaviors in the context of the classroom. Once the goals are established, the OTA may be responsible for collecting and recording the data on a regular basis.

CLINICAL MODELS VERSUS EDUCATIONAL MODELS

Providing OT services in an educational setting requires a shift in thinking and a change in philosophy from the clinical (medical) model. OT clinicians are traditionally trained under a medical model that views services for children based on dysfunction and its underlying components. In this model, therapists evaluate and treat physical problems, while environmental factors that can support or hinder a child's performance are not a primary concern. The focus of a medical model is the remediation of the underlying components of dysfunction and the removal of pathologic processes so that development can continue.[8,9]

In the school system, the practitioner evaluates the student's performance in the classroom to determine if physical, emotional, or behavioral aspects interfere with the student's ability to perform the tasks that are required to be performed by all students. The student's abilities are described in functional terms (rather than in terms of disability or diagnosis) and the capacity to meet classroom demands.[5,9]

Federal, state, and local educational agency regulations have established guidelines for the provision of OT services in the school system.[5] Box 4-5 contains questions to assist clinicians in determining whether a student

BOX 4-5

Determining the Need for Occupational Therapy in the School

- Does the child have an exceptional educational need (EEN)? Because occupational therapy (OT) is a related service, the child must have an EEN or qualify under Section 504 of the Rehabilitation Act to be eligible to receive OT services provided by the school system.
- Does the evaluation indicate the need for OT services? The evaluation may consist of standardized tests, portfolio reviews, classroom and school environment observations, and consultations with parents and teachers.
- Does the child demonstrate a significant delay in motor, sensory or perceptual, psychosocial, or self-help skills compared with the established norms of other children of the same age? A significant delay is one that is >1 SD (standard deviation) below the norm and affects school performance.
- Is OT a related service that may be required for the child to benefit from and participate in an educational program? Factors that affect the answer to this question include the child's program, other related services received, and the demands of the classroom, the child's level of function, and the potential for improvement or skill development.
- Does the child require the specialized skills of an OT practitioner, or can tasks and interventions be carried out by other personnel? For example, a teacher may be able to help a child learn eating skills by using adaptive equipment provided by an OT practitioner.

needs OT services and which level of service is recommended. Having an EEN designation and significantly delayed skills does not necessarily mean that a student should receive OT services in school; this is especially true for older students with severe cognitive deficits.

Practitioners working in schools may serve more children by working with them in groups. This provides peer support and is a natural part of school. Consulting with the teacher and classroom staff helps resolve many problems and may have an impact on many children. The OT practitioner may become more directly involved if a student's skills deteriorate or the OT practitioner thinks that a short period of direct service will help the student become more independent.

CLINICAL *Pearl*

Goal writing is much easier if the clinician takes the time to ask the teacher, parent, or child what they hope to get out of the occupational therapy (OT) sessions. Start out with very broad questions (e.g., "What would you like to do better?" "What is causing you trouble in school?" "What is interfering with the child's ability to learn?"), and then ask specific questions (e.g., "What aspects of reading are causing you trouble?" "What about your writing: Is it a problem?" "Do you tire easily?" "Is it messy?" "Do you have trouble holding the pencil?" "What does the child do in class that interrupts others?"). Continue until you have a clear visual picture of what the child hopes to accomplish. Make the goals as specific as possible without losing focus. Write the goals in simple terms so that all team members can understand them.

Although OT practitioners working in schools can bill Medicaid for educationally related services, Medicaid was created to provide medical and health-related services for the financially needy. However, it pays for health services for those who are eligible and is not dependent on where the services are provided. When therapy is provided in the school, it decreases the student's absence from school and is thus an effective way to provide medical care related to the education of children.

Consider the previous example of Mary, the 8-year-old girl with left-sided hemiplegia. Using a medical model, the OTA working in an outpatient clinic might design activities to address muscle tone, range of motion (ROM), strength, and isolated muscle control for fine motor skills. Intervention sessions would focus on refining performance skills. Conversely, because Mary was able to perform in the classroom and complete tasks at an age-appropriate level, OT services were not recommended for her in the school setting. Mary's mild motor impairments do not interfere with her educational goals.

Although children with medical conditions or diagnoses may benefit from OT in the school setting, the emphasis is to help children function in the classroom, gym, cafeteria, and playground. Providing services in an LRE often means working in the classroom. OT practitioners provide educationally relevant services, which makes the practitioners part of the educational team. In recent years, educational agencies and third-party payers have increased their requests for OT clinicians to use outcome-based practices in pediatric settings. Practitioners identify and treat problem areas, quanitify functional performance, and consider multiple factors including neuromuscular and psychosocial processes, the student's potential for improvement, social skills, environmental demands, and family priorities.[8,9]

CLINICAL *Pearl*

Occupational therapy (OT) services are most integrated when provided in the classroom. An informal exchange of ideas and effective intervention strategies naturally evolve among team members when the OT practitioner works with children in their classrooms. This allows for the carryover of strategies and changes that allow children to be successful in school.

LEVELS OF SERVICE

OT services can be delivered through direct service, monitoring, or consultation. The members of the IEP team decide on which service delivery level is appropriate for each child. Therapy emphasizes the child's ability to perform in the school environment rather than in the therapy room.[11] IDEA mandates that the child participate in the regular curriculum to the maximum extent possible, so therapy in the classroom is recommended whenever possible. OT plays a supportive role in helping the student participate and benefit from the special education program. This requires continuous collaboration between the teacher or other school staff member and the therapist.

In the classroom, paraprofessionals (such as teacher aides) benefit from training on and explanations of ways to work with children with special needs. For example, the OTA can teach and model how to perform proper body mechanics while lifting and handling a child with a severe disability. In addition, explaining to the staff how to feed, dress, and position children with various diagnoses is essential to carrying out integrated services and creating a safe educational environment.

Direct Service

With direct services, the OT practitioner works with the student so that he or she can acquire a skill. Direct therapy may be conducted one on one with the child or in a group setting; the time and frequency depend on the needs of the child.

For example, an OT clinician working with several students in a regular Grade 2 class could treat the children in the classroom during the regularly scheduled handwriting time. The OTA would be present for the handwriting session and work directly with the children designated in the IEP. Before the handwriting session, the OTA may encourage warm-up exercises. The entire class may do these exercises, but the OTA pays particular attention to the children under the IEP. While the students work on assignments, the OTA may review posture, provide cues for beginning the assignment, help with pencil grip, and provide verbal or tactile feedback, among other strategies. Direct service requires collaboration with the parent or teacher for follow-through and optimal learning. Clinicians who work as partners with teachers show the most success in this type of approach.

Monitoring Service

OT clinicians following monitoring services create programs for the child that the teacher, other staff member, or family can follow. The OT practitioner contacts them frequently so that the program can be updated or altered as necessary. The personnel who follow the program are well trained and need to have a clear understanding of its goals. Clinicians provide simple activities to be followed in a safe manner without the presence of a qualified practitioner. Billing procedures or state regulations may not acknowledge the monitoring service. Under this service, the clinician is responsible for ensuring that the child's goals are met.

Consultation Services

Consultation services are provided when the occupational therapist's expertise is used to help other personnel achieve the child's objectives. OT clinicians may contact others only once or on an as-needed basis as set up by the team. Ongoing contact with the teacher or caregiver may be necessary. Consultation services are useful for adapting task materials or the environment, designing strategies to improve posture and positioning, or demonstrating how to handle a situation.

For example, an OT practitioner may consult with the teacher about a sensory diet for a student who needs help organizing sensory input. The clinician would work together with the teacher to create sensory diet suggestions for the child in the classroom. Equipment such as a weighted vest, trampoline, vibrator, and weighted lap pad would be purchased or made for the student's and staff's use as necessary. Sensory diet suggestions could be outlined for the staff to use with the student on a daily basis.

Table 4-3 is an example of an outline with sensory strategies that could be provided to the teacher. The practitioner would then consult with the staff to set up a daily schedule of sensory diet needs, which could be adjusted as necessary.

DISCONTINUING THERAPY SERVICES

Discharging a child from OT services can be difficult because of the rapport that has been established among the child, family, and practitioner. Children may be discharged from OT when all of the intervention goals and objectives have been accomplished or therapy is not resulting in the desired changes. In cases of plateauing (i.e., the child does not make any progress toward the goal), the child may benefit from working with another therapist or an alternative approach. If possible, clinicians should avoid discharging a child from therapy when he or she is undergoing a transition, such as changing schools. Frequently, a child is eased out of therapy by decreasing the quantity and going from direct therapy to consultation service to discharge.[7] Children may require consultation on positioning when undergoing physical changes. Any change in service (including frequency) is discussed with the IEP team (including parents). For example, students entering middle school may not have had refined fine motor and self-care skills addressed. Service delivery is a dynamic process that requires flexibility and adaptability to the changing needs of the school and the child. Consultation with the teacher will help serve the child's needs in an effective manner. If this type of delivery does not work, the practitioner may decide to provide direct service. It is helpful to explain to parents the dynamic nature of OT services and the IEP process.

> **CLINICAL *Pearl***
>
> Remember that the teacher is the manager of the classroom. The occupational therapy (OT) practitioner is a guest, and his or her presence should not disrupt the routine.

> **CLINICAL *Pearl***
>
> Adolescents may need occupational therapy (OT) consultation to discuss their strengths and weaknesses for vocational activities. Children entering high school may benefit from consultation with an OT practitioner about study habits, strategies to succeed, and issues surrounding physical changes.

TABLE 4-3

Sensory Strategies for Brian

WHAT IT LOOKS LIKE FOR BRIAN	SENSORY DIET
TACTILE SENSE	
Seeks touch and deep pressure	Provide deep pressure
Seeks touch by touching objects and people around him	Provide weighted vest or weighted lap pad
Likes and seeks soft, silky material	Provide silk-like sheets or clothing
	Place a piece of silk on his seat
	Provide a piece of silk to calm Brian
VESTIBULAR SENSE	
Seems to seek vestibular movement by spinning or rocking	Equipment suggestions: swing, rocking chair, etc.
	Activity suggestions: "Sit and move" chair cushion
Gets overstimulated by activities in the environment	Encourage Brian to go to the quiet area in the corner of the room
	Have Brian rock in the rocking chair
PROPRIOCEPTIVE SENSE	
Seeks high impact by touching other people	Equipment: weights, joint compression, vibration, etc.
Pushes himself against other people	Provide weighted vest, joint compression, and vibration
AUDITORY SENSE	
Very sensitive to noise	Work in noiseless environment
	Try mufflers or headset to decrease noise
	Play quiet ocean sounds in the background
	Try rhythmic sounds, like a metronome
Easily distracted by sound	Keep verbal cues to a minimum and avoid extraneous noise
VISUAL SENSE	
Easily distracted by objects	Decrease visual distractions
Gets easily overstimulated by too much visual stimulation	Remove visual distractions from the wall; work in a cubicle

SUMMARY

OT practitioners must possess technical knowledge and skills as well understand child development, family systems, learning theory, community resources, and current federal and state regulations. Although there are federal regulations that dictate broad policies, OT practitioners must keep abreast of state regulations and local educational agency procedures to ensure compliance in all areas.

Communicating and working as a team is key to school-based practice. Practitioners must be prepared to discuss OT knowledge in a language that educators and families understand. Successfully functioning as part of a team requires the members to value the educational philosophy and listen carefully to parents and teachers.

Practitioners working in schools have the unique opportunity to help children function in the place where they work (school). Incorporating therapy into classroom activities takes skill and negotiation. Practitioners may need to "think outside the box" and provide therapeutic activities in a busy, crowded classroom. OT practitioners are responsible for modeling and teaching skills to others so that the educational staff can provide services to children on a daily basis. Clinicians working in educational settings analyze children in terms of their ability to perform occupations in the school, family, and community rather than in terms of their deficits in performance components. By working with a team of dedicated professionals, clinicians may improve a child's ability to learn, socialize, and function in school.

References

1. American Occupational Therapy Association: Occupational therapy practice framework: domain and process, ed 2. *Am J Occup Ther* 62(6):625–703, 2008.
2. American Occupational Therapy Association: *Occupational therapy services for children and youth under IDEA*, Rockville, MD, 1997, American Occupational Therapy Association.
3. American Occupational Therapy Association: Roles of occupational therapists and occupational therapy assistants in schools. *Am J Occup Ther* 41:798, 1987.
4. American Occupational Therapy Association Pediatric Curriculum Committee: *Guidelines for curriculum content in pediatrics*, Rockville, MD, 1991, American Occupational Therapy Association.
5. Bober P, Corbett S: *Occupational therapy and physical therapy: a resource and planning guide*, Madison, 1996, Wisconsin Department of Public Instruction.
6. Carver C: Crossing the thresholds. *OT Practice* 3:18, 1998.
7. *Daniel RR v. State Board of Education*, 874 F, 2d, 1036, 1989.
8. Kramer P, Hinojosa J: *Frames of reference for pediatric occupational therapy*, ed 2, Baltimore, 1999, Williams & Wilkins.
10. Martin E, Martin R, Terman D: The legislative and litigation history of special education. *Future Child* 6:25, 1996.
11. Swinth Y, Handley-More D: Update on school-based practice. *OT Practice* 8:22, 2003.

REVIEW *Questions*

1. What are some of the federal laws that have an impact on the provision of OT services in the public school system?
2. Which factors determine whether a child is eligible to receive OT services in a school setting?
3. In what ways do therapy services provided according to an educational model differ from those provided according to a medical model?
4. In what ways do the roles of an occupational therapist and an OTA differ in a school setting?

SUGGESTED *Activities*

1. Visit or volunteer in a public school, and observe the various programs and environments that have been developed for students with special needs, such as a learning disabilities resource room and a self-contained classroom.
2. Be politically aware and active. Keep abreast of changes in local, state, and federal laws. Participate in public hearings, and contact legislators when laws affecting the provision of OT services are being debated.
3. Volunteer with an occupational therapist or an OTA in the public school system to understand ways to integrate therapy services in the regular classroom.

CHAPTER 4 APPENDIX

Individual Educational Program

SCHOOL DISTRICT OF REEDSVILLE

Meeting Type	**x** Initial	___ Annual Review	___ Interim	_____Reevaluation
	__ Special Review	__ Extended School Year		_____Transition

Name: Brian IEP	**Birthdate:**	3/20/05
Social Security number: _____	**Medicaid number:** _____	
Sex: _____M_____	**Grade:** ₋₁(preschool)	

Primary disability: <u>Preschool</u>   **Other disabling conditions:** <u>Speech and language</u>

Date of meeting: <u>May 17, 2009</u>   **Anticipated annual review:** May 17, 2010
Time of meeting: 7:30 AM   **IEP initiation date:** August 9, 2009
Location of meeting: Lincoln Elementary School   **IEP ending date:** May 30, 2010

Present Levels of Performance

Area: Cognitive   **Method: Brigance**   Date: 5/10/2009

Findings: Brian follows verbal directions and sometimes chooses to disobey.

Brian has little interest in books, turning several pages at once. Brian enjoys routine songs and has begun to use his own hands to imitate gross arm motions to the music. Brian will touch eight body parts, match color, and sort by color. He picks out a named color for 10 colors.

Area: Fine motor   **Method:Peabody Developmental Motor Test (fine motor subtest) Therapist Observation**   Date: 5/10/2009

Findings: Brian is able to string beads with encouragement to stay on task. He tolerates textures such as lotion and shaving cream for short periods of time. He is able to tear paper into strips after minimum setup and throws beanbags into a target. Brian scribbles spontaneously but is unable to imitate strokes.

Area: Fine motor   **Method:Peabody Developmental Motor Test (gross motor subtest) Therapist Observation**   Date: 5/10/2009

Findings: Brian ambulates independently in the school and on uneven surfaces. He is able to ascend and descend the stairs with his hand held on or with the support of the railing. Running patterns are very immature, and he requires moderate assistance to play on outdoor playground equipment. Brian becomes hesitant and somewhat anxious or fearful of having his feet off a supporting surface. He continues to be hesitant and reluctant to try new sensorimotor activities, but with reassurance he will participate momentarily. Brian is able to throw and catch a medium-size ball.

CHAPTER 4 APPENDIX—cont'd

Individual Educational Program

Area: Language	Method: Brigance/Therapist Observation	Date: 5/10/2009

Findings: Brian says ``sss" for ``yes." He shakes his head for ``no." He waves bye-bye and shows affection with hugs and an ``aww" sound. Recently, Brian has been responding to requests to name an object with a one-syllable grunt.

Brian will participate in a group with picture symbol (pic/sym) exchange. He will also use a cheap talk device with eight pictures. He can produce the consonants /m/ and /p/ and the vowels /o/ and /a/. He has attached meaning to them in groups and stories.

Area: Self-help	Method: Brigance/Therapist Observation	Date: 5/10/2009

Findings: Brian is able to drink from a sipper cup without assistance but not able to consecutively swallow. He continues to be resistant to the feeding process but has broadened his variety of foods. Recently, he has been using a spoon on his own to feed himself.

Area: Social skills	Method: Brigance	Date: 5/10/2009

Findings: Brian watches other children play near him and may attempt to join in. He laughs and dances as he watches others play. Brian searches for hidden objects that he wants. He works with an adult for 10 minutes on activities. Brian begins to put things away at cleanup time when given prompts and gestures.

Strengths: Brian matches and sorts colors. He also picks out 10 named colors. Brian can follow one-step verbal directions. He says ``sss" for ``yes" and shakes his head for ``no."

How does the student's disability affect involvement and progress in the general curriculum?

Not applicable for preschool because there are no other 3 year olds present in the school setting.

How does the student's disability affect his or her participation in appropriate activities?
Brian has delays in language development, which require small-group instruction or teaching of curriculum at a slower pace.

Related Services

(Goals, objectives, and levels of performance are required for all related services other than routine or maintenance types, which require descriptions of the service. However, if an instructional activity is involved, the goals, objectives, and levels of performance are required.)

Service	Description	Minutes	Frequency	Instructional
Speech-language	Group	60	Weekly	Yes
Occupational therapy	Direct individual	30	Weekly	Yes
Physical therapy	Direct individual	30	Weekly	yes
Transportation	Special education bus	N/A	Daily	No

CHAPTER 4 APPENDIX—cont'd

Individual Educational Program

Special Factors

The IEP team has considered these special factors.

Yes No

X   The strengths of the student and the concerns of the parents for enhancing the education of their child.

X   The results of the initial evaluation or most recent evaluation of the student.

X   As appropriate, the result of the child's performance on any general state or district-wide assessment program.

X   In the case of a student whose behavior impedes his or her learning or that of others, the strategies, including positive behavioral interventions, strategies, and supports to address that behavior if appropriate.

X   In the case of a student with limited English proficiency, the language needs of the student as such should relate to the student's IEP.

X   In the case of a student who is blind or visually impaired, provide for instruction in and the use of Braille unless the IEP team determines, after an evaluation of the student's reading and writing skills, needs, and appropriate reading and writing media (including an evaluation of the student's future needs for instruction in and the use of Braille), that this instruction is not appropriate for the student.

X   The communication needs of the student, and in the case of a student who is deaf or hard of hearing, consider the student's language and communication needs, opportunities for direct communication with peers and professional personnel in the student's language and communication mode, academic level, and the full range of needs, including opportunities for direct instruction in the student's language and communication mode.

X   Whether the student requires assistive technology devices and services.

X   If, in considering these factors, the IEP team determines that a student needs a particular device or service (including an intervention, accommodation, or other program modification) in order for the student to receive FAPE, the IEP team must include a statement to that effect in the student's IEP.

LRE Documentation—Preschool Student

How does the nature and severity of this child's disability support placement in a separate (self-contained) class for children with disabilities?

A regular education curriculum is not appropriate at this time because Brian has not met prerequisite skills.

How would this child's presence in a regular preschool class/program substantially and consistently disrupt the performance of his or her classroom peers?

Brian needs individualized instruction to a degree that requires an excessive amount of teacher time, taking time away from the needs of nondisabled students.

What interventions were attempted in the home or preschool environment to facilitate this child's participation in a regular preschool class/program?

Location	Intervention	Begin	End	Results
Special education	Individual assistance	9/05/2009	5/05/2010	Moderately successful, but requires additional time
Assemblies	Individual assistance	9/05/2009	5/10/2006	Moderately successful, but requires shorter time
Cafeteria	Individual assistance	9/05/2009	5/10/2006	Moderately successful, but requires moderate assistance

CHAPTER 4 APPENDIX—cont'd

Individual Educational Program

What opportunities for interacting with nondisabled peers are to be provided for this child?

Activity	With Whom	Where	Minutes	Frequency
Assemblies	Nondisabled students	Auditorium	30	As provided
Lunch	Nondisabled students	Cafeteria	30	Daily
Playground	Nondisabled students	Playground	20	Daily

Based on this child's complete IEP and the IEP/staffing committee's consideration of each option listed on the continuum below, the appropriate placement for this child is:

Self-contained; in a separate (self-contained) class established primarily for children with disabilities

The school is at another location: Lincoln Elementary School

Physical education will not take place because 3 year olds do not participate in physical education.

Transition services will not be discussed at this time because the child is under the age of 14 and has not reached the age of majority.

Extended School Year (ESY) will be discussed at a future date.

Testing Participation

Based on this student's present level of performance and his or her goals and objectives, the student will not participate in any statewide and/or districtwide testing that other students in his or her grade level are taking at grade -1.

Promotion/Retention

Are alternative promotion/retention standards required?
Yes Brian must complete 70%pc of IEP objectives, with consideration given to chronological age.
Reporting to Parents
Progress toward annual goals will be reported to parents every 9 weeks through progress reports and will be measured by:
Accomplishment of short-term objectives

Modifications to Regular Education

What supplementary aids and services will be provided to the student, or on behalf of the student, for his or her advancement toward the attainment of the annual goals and participation in academic, nonacademic, and extracurricular activities in the general education curriculum and environment? Describe specific supplementary services/program modifications or support to be provided and indicate the anticipated location(s).

Individual Educational Program

Supplementary Services/Program Modifications or Support

Supplementary Aids

Area: Augmentative communication | Location: Special education | Min: 30 | Frequency: Daily
Aid: Cheap talk
Description: Used to say his name, friends, choose activity

Area: Augmentative communication | Location: Special education | Min: 30 | Frequency: Daily

Description: Picture symbol exchange to choose activity and indicate needs

LRE Recommendations

Minutes/week in special education: 720

Minutes/week in regular education: 0

Individual Educational Program Goals and Objectives for Brian IEP

Assessment area: Cognitive

Goal: Brian will increase his cognitive abilities by completing these short-term objectives.

Location(s)	Person(s) Responsible	Goal Type(s)
Special education	Special education teacher	Academic

Short-Term Objectives	Criteria	Assessment Method	Critical
Brian will identify 16 named body parts by (1) touching or 2) pointing.	80%	Classroom observation	No
Brian will identify 10 named pictures or objects by (1) touching or (2) pointing.	80%	Classroom observation	Yes

Assessment area: Fine motor

Goal: Brian will improve his fine motor skills by accomplishing 80% of the following short-term objectives.

Location(s)	Person(s) Responsible	Goal Type(s)
Special education	Special education teacher	Academic
	Occupational therapist	Related service

CHAPTER 4 APPENDIX—cont'd

Individual Educational Program

Short-Term Objectives	Criteria	Assessment Method	Critical
Brian will put 5 out of 9 pieces in an individual inset puzzle with (1) minimum assistance or (2) independently.	80%	Classroom observation	No
Brian will snip 5 times with regular or adapted scissors, placing the scissors in the hand correctly with (1) minimum assistance or (2) independently.	80%	Classroom observations	No

Assessment area: Gross motor

Goal: Brian will improve his gross motor skills by accomplishing 80% of the following short-term objectives.

Location(s)	Person(s)Responsible	Goal Type(s)
Special education	Special education teacher	Academic
	Physical therapist	Related service

Short-Term Objectives	Criteria	Assessment Method	Critical
Brian will access and play on the playground equipment independently and safely.	80%	Classroom observation	No
Brian will ascend a small set of stairs without the use of a railing or support.	80%	Classroom observations	No

Assessment area: Language

Goal: Brian will improve his language skills by accomplishing 80% of the following short-term objectives.

Location(s)	Person(s) Responsible	Goal Type(s)
Special education	Special education teacher	Academic
	Speech-language pathologist	Related service

Short-Term Objectives	Criteria	Assessment Method	Critical
Brian will communicate a desire to stop an activity by selecting pictures/symbols representing all done or stop.	80%	Classroom observations	No
Brian will follow unfamiliar one-step directions when given visual and verbal prompts.	80%	Classroom observations	Yes

Individual Educational Program

Assessment area: Self-help

Goal: Brian will improve his self-help skills by accomplishing 80% of the following short-term objectives.

Location(s)	Person(s) Responsible	Goal Type(s)
Special education	Special education teacher Occupational therapist	Academic Related service

Short-Term Objectives	Criteria	Assessment Method	Critical
Brian will drink independently from a cup, demonstrating consecutive swallows and no spillage.	80%	Classroom observations	Yes
Brian will finger-feed himself the food of the adult's choice without overreactions.	80%	Classroom observations	Yes

[a] Assessment area: Social skills

Goal: Brian will improve his social skills by accomplishing 80% of the following short-term objectives.

Location(s)	Person(s) Responsible Goal	Goal Type(s)
Special education	Special education teacher	Academic

Short-Term Objectives	Criteria	Assessment Method	Critical
Brian will participate in simple games such as Ring Around the Rosy during circle time.	80%	Classroom observations	Yes
Brian will share a toy with another child with (1) minimum assistance or (2) independently.	80%	Classroom observations	No

Individual Educational Program
Committee Members

The individuals listed below have attended the IEP/LRE meeting and participated as equal members in the development of this IEP.

By the signature below we agree with the educational and related services to be provided to this student as delineated in this IER. Our LRE recommendations and this student's placement are based on the completed IEP and the regulations under the Individuals with Disabilities Education Act.

Disability: **Preschool**   Placement: **Self-contained**

CHAPTER 4 APPENDIX—cont'd

Individual Educational Program

Attendee	Representing	Signature	Date
Sue Jump	Speech-language pathologist		
Jill Johnson	Physical therapist		
Stephanie Marks	Special education teacher		
Virginia Gray	Occupational therapist		
Rebecca White	Regular education teacher		
Debbie Smith	LEA representative		

_____ I have attended the IEP/ LRE meeting and have participated as an equal member of the committee in developing this IEP and determining the least restrictive environment and placement for my child.

_____ I have read the IEP/LRE documents or had them read to me and understand their contents.

_____ I agree with the educational and related services to be provided to my child as delineated in the IEP.

_____ I have received a copy of the IEP/LRE documents.

_____ I understand the IEP/LRE process.

Signature of Parent/Level Guardian/Surrogate Parent   MM   DD   YY

FAPE, Free appropriate public education; *IEP*, individual educational program; *LEA*, local education agency; *LRE*, least restrictive environment.

5

Community Systems

NANCY CARSON

CHAPTER *Objectives*

After studying this chapter, the reader will be able to accomplish the following:

- Understand the difference between community-based practice and community-built practice.
- Understand the importance of therapeutic use of self in providing services in the community and in building community partnerships.
- Identify the different service delivery methods occupational therapy practitioners may utilize in community settings.
- Identify the different community systems in which occupational therapy practitioners work.
- Understand the influence of public health on community interventions.
- Identify the challenges to providing services in the community.

CHAPTER OUTLINE

Community-based Practiceand Community-built Practice

Therapeutic Use of Self

Public Health Influence

Community Mental Health Movement

Community Occupational Therapy Interventions

Challenges in Practice in Community Systems

Summary

The delivery of occupational therapy (OT) services has expanded far beyond the traditional medical model that served the majority of clients in the past. As health care expands to meet the unique needs of an increasingly diverse society, the treatment setting has changed in order to address the needs of the clients more efficiently. This requires OT services to be provided in a **community** setting in which the child lives, learns, plays, or is otherwise occupationally engaged. It should be a setting that is accessible and appropriate for the client and which allows for successful intervention to occur (Figure 5-1).

Occupational therapists and occupational therapy assistants (OTAs) can provide services to children and adolescents in many community systems or community-oriented service delivery models. Community systems can include schools, preschools, after-school programs, daycare centers, faith-based programs, community recreational programs, community mental health centers, community health clinics, camps, group homes, residential care facilities, shelters for the homeless, and home health agencies. Any type of facility outside of the traditional medical model presented in a hospital or clinic setting that provides health-related programs or services to individuals in the community can be considered a community system. Any organization that offers programs or services in the context of one or more community settings can be thought of as a community system as well. A variety of service delivery models may exist within each of these community systems, too, and may include services such as individual therapy, group therapy, skill-building, coaching, mentoring, family education and training, teacher or caretaker education and training, and program consultation.

COMMUNITY-BASED PRACTICE AND COMMUNITY-BUILT PRACTICE

In order to understand how clinicians practice in these settings and how this may differ from traditional hospital-based practice, it is necessary to define a community. Understandably, *community* is a broad term with many definitions. One definition of *community* is "a person's natural environment, that is, where the person works, plays and performs other daily activities."[22] Another definition for community is "an area with geographic and often political boundaries demarcated as a district, county, metropolitan area, city, township, or neighborhood . . . a place where members have a sense of identity and belonging, shared values, norms, communication, and helping patterns."[9] Two definitions to articulate service delivery models help further understand the practice of OT in community systems. **Community-based practice** is defined as "skilled services delivered by health practitioners using an interactive model with clients" and **community-built practice** is "defined when skilled services are delivered by health practitioners using a collaborative and interactive model with clients."[22]

Community-based practice is initiated by the medical model and results from referrals from other health care workers. Community-built practice has a **public health** perspective that focuses on health promotion and education. Treatment involves defining the community and working with the community in a variety of ways to support the client and enhance occupational functioning (Figure 5-2). While both types of community practice emphasize an interactive model, it is community-built practice that involves

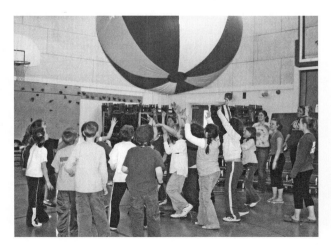

FIGURE 5-1 Wellness in the community: OT students promote physical activity and give back to the community by organizing fun games for children.

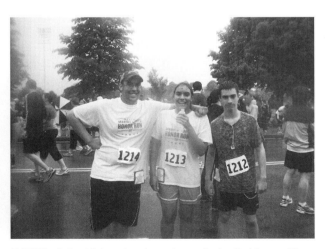

FIGURE 5-2 High school students (Jack Cuthbert, Cilana Cuthbert, and Scott O'Brien) give back to the community by running a race in honor of those who serve.

collaboration and a strong emphasis on empowerment and wellness.[22]

It is imperative that the OT clinician be aware of the community systems in which the client is engaged. Even if services are not provided in the context of a community agency, the environmental implications of the communities in which the child interacts on a daily basis must be considered to allow for optimal occupational functioning and health. The definition of **health** provided by the World Health Organization states that "health is a state of complete physical, mental and social well-being and not merely the absence of disease or infirmity."[23] In order to promote optimal health in the child or adolescent, the practitioner needs to understand the community in which the child functions and understand how community systems and community resources can support successful occupational functioning.

The definition of **clients** by the Occupational Therapy Practice Framework: Domain and Process, 2nd edition, includes not only individuals but also organizations and populations within a community.[1] Thus, when the client is a child referred for treatment, the context and environment must be considered as part of the domain of OT. Specifically, the social environment includes the community organizations and groups that are a part of and that affect the child's occupational performance, and the context in which the child interacts with these community systems must be considered in order to provide effective treatment.[1]

Herzberg emphasizes the declining trend of health care provided in traditional inpatient and outpatient medical model settings and the growing trend of health care services offered in a community environment or through a community agency.[10] A variety of perspectives on community interventions are therefore presented here, and the need for OT practitioners to develop the skills for working in communities to enhance full inclusion and social participation for the individual is also discussed. The OT practitioner is required to have certain community service skills, including consultation, policy-making, and program development skills. Defining who the client is may result in the community agency being the client; it may be necessary to broaden the definition of *client* to include the community at large that is supporting the client in order to provide the most effective OT services to the individual client. The distinction between community-based practice and community-built practice is discussed in the context of how the role of the OT practitioner will differ depending on the focus of the community organization. Here, the focus of community-based practice is considered to be the delivery of skilled services and addressing the client's deficits by direct intervention in a community setting. Likewise, community-built practice involves the delivery of skilled services in collaboration with and with support from the appropriate community resources and the building of a sense of client empowerment to resolve client-defined issues. The need for both types of community practice is strongly emphasized, and the two approaches are viewed as existing on a continuum. OT practitioners are encouraged to expand their services to include roles on this continuum and roles that are focused in community environments.[10]

THERAPEUTIC USE OF SELF

While the move toward greater awareness and involvement in community systems is generally perceived as a positive trend in health care, the OT practitioner should be mindful of the possible negative perceptions of the recipients of these types of services. Silverstein, Lamberto, DePeau, and Grossman unexpectedly found that low-income parents of children receiving multiple community and social services had negative experiences and perceptions of the community resources they utilized.[16] Qualitative analysis of 41 interviews revealed parental perceptions of the need to make important decisions based on choices that were often less than satisfactory. A lack of control was experienced by parents when they had to accept community services that were sometimes seen as being ineffective due to lack of individualization. Employees of community agencies were sometimes perceived as being judgmental or too personal; these parents also felt sometimes that they had to compromise on their value systems.

It is essential for occupational therapists and OTAs to practice effective therapeutic use of self when engaging with clients, their families, and individuals within the client's community health care system. **Therapeutic use of self** has been defined as the therapist's "planned use of his or her personality, insights, perceptions, and judgments as part of the therapeutic process"[15] and *conscious use of self* in therapy as "the use of oneself in such a way that one becomes an effective tool in the evaluation and intervention process."[13] Effective therapeutic use of self requires the practitioner to have a thorough self-understanding of personal values and expectations as well as an understanding of the client's values and cultural needs. Understanding how to negotiate a relationship most effectively by using personal skills to an advantage, while respecting the client's values and beliefs, is a skill that one must develop in order to be an effective practitioner. When working with children, the relationship between the practitioner and the child's caretaker(s) must also be considered. In community settings, other individuals such as teachers or community resource providers may be involved in the child's care, too. It therefore becomes a multilayer network of relationships that must be nurtured and developed to ensure the best outcomes for the child or adolescent. The relationships between the practitioner and these individuals need to be taken into account to ensure the most effective treatment for the child. Therefore, OT practitioners working with children in community settings need to have excellent communication and negotiation skills as well as the ability to network with others to establish effective resources for each child. Furthermore, all of this requires a thorough understanding of the mission of the community system in which the child is engaged and how this mission relates to the services being provided by OT.

Therapeutic relationship has been defined as "a trusting connection and rapport established between practitioner and client through collaboration, communication, therapist empathy, and mutual respect.[8] The *intentional relationship model* is a conceptual practice model that thoroughly explains the relationship between the practitioner and the client.[18] This model is specific to the field of OT and explores in detail how the therapeutic use of self promotes occupational engagement that facilitates a positive therapeutic relationship and thus successful therapy outcomes. One aspect of the model is an understanding of one's therapeutic modes. In all, there are six therapeutic modes that a practitioner may utilize. A *therapeutic mode* is defined as an interacting style that a practitioner employs when working with a client. A practitioner may employ more than one mode, and the use of these modes is a function of the individual's innate personality traits and natural communication style. The modes identified in this model include advocating, collaborating, empathizing, encouraging, instructing, and problem-solving. Ideally, a practitioner strives to acquire the ability to use all of the modes and to recognize which mode is the most appropriate to use in a given situation.[18]

Effective therapeutic use of self allows for the development of a therapeutic relationship. As described above, the therapeutic relationship embodies collaboration. It is through this collaboration that client empowerment evolves. When working with children, it is necessary to establish a therapeutic relationship with the child, the caregiver(s), and appropriate individuals within the community system(s) involved in the child's healthcare. This requires the OT practitioner to be acutely aware of the many different relationships that must be nurtured and maintained to promote the most successful outcomes for the child. Not only must the child be empowered, but the significant figures in the child's life must be empowered as well. This requires striving to maintain multiple therapeutic relationships, which necessitates employing different approaches and strategies with the different individuals involved in the child's care. This may

be in contrast to a traditional medical model, where the practitioner may be minimally involved and only have contact with the person transporting the child to therapy sessions.

CLINICAL *Pearl*

The therapeutic use of self is a very important tool used by practitioners in working with the child and communicating with the individuals within the community setting. OT practitioners should constantly engage in self-evaluation of communication and interpersonal skills and strive to increase their ability to work well with others. The practitioner must be able to communicate, empower, and motivate the child and those involved in achieving the child's therapy goals. Treating the child alone is not enough for successful outcomes; it takes the whole community working together.

PUBLIC HEALTH INFLUENCE

The influence of public health on the community practice of many health care disciplines cannot be underestimated. In considering community systems from a very broad perspective, the field of public health employs community-based and community-built approaches for many of its initiatives. Most of the interventions implemented by public health educators are done within community settings and organizations.[12] Understandably, a larger number of people can receive OT interventions when they are provided to groups of people versus individuals or are provided through organizations that include people with similar needs. Traditionally, many OT services have been provided individually, and this is still necessary for specific types of treatment. However, as medical costs rise and health care services continue to move more to community settings, the need and opportunity to broaden the service delivery of OT are expanding.

Developing an appreciation for public health approaches is useful to OT practitioners in understanding community-based and community-built services. For both types of service delivery models, thorough knowledge and awareness of the community is needed to provide effective treatment. Community-based services may be individual services provided in a community setting but still functioning like the medical model;, community-built services, however, can be considered individual or group approaches that embrace and empower the client and the community service providers and may be provided in community settings or through community organizations. The approach used will depend on the needs of the individual or group of clients being served.

Many of the initiatives addressed by the public health discipline are addressed in the objectives of Healthy People 2010.[21] Traditionally, health care in the United States has not been focused on preventive care. In recent years, this trend has changed. The Healthy People initiative was established in 1979 through the Centers for Disease Control (CDC) as a mechanism for identifying objectives and strategies to prevent illness and premature death. Every 10 years, national health priorities are identified, and objectives for prevention are established. Healthy People 2010, the third revision of this initiative, provides a framework for prevention of illnesses in Americans. The two overarching goals of the Healthy People initiative are (1) to increase life quality and lifespan, and (2) to end health disparities.[21]

Healthy People 2010 consists of 10 leading health indicators, 28 focus areas, and 467 objectives. The leading health indicators are used to measure the health of Americans. Several of the leading health indicators—physical activity, overweight and obesity, substance abuse, and mental health—are health concerns that OT practitioners have addressed directly or indirectly through OT interventions. In addition, several of the focus areas and corresponding objectives identified in Healthy People 2010 are areas of interest to OT. The relevant focus areas include educational and community-based programs, mental health and mental disorders, nutrition and overweight, physical activity and fitness, and substance abuse (Figure 5-3).[21] As health care delivery continues to evolve and health care practitioners are challenged to provide services in a variety of settings, numerous opportunities have become available to OT practitioners. By being aware of the objectives set forth in the Healthy People initiative, OT practitioners can partner with other health care providers in the community to meet the health needs and improve the quality of life of clients.

One example of a public health concern in children that OT practitioners can be effective in addressing is childhood obesity. During the past 20 years, the number of Americans considered to be overweight or obese has grown significantly; 32.7% of adults are overweight, 34.3% are obese, and 5.9% are extremely obese.[7] Childhood overweight and obesity are also growing concerns. When categorized by age, 13.9% of children 2 to 5 years of age, 19% of children 6 to 11 years of age, and 17% of adolescents 12 to 19 years of age are considered to be overweight, according to the National Health and Nutrition Examination Survey (NHANES) 2003–2004. Twice as many children are considered to be at risk of becoming overweight.[14]

Campbell and Crawford present a review of data that suggest that eating behaviors are likely to be established early in life and may be maintained into adulthood.[5] Steinbeck suggests that it is important to focus on intervention and prevention in children to establish lifelong healthy eating patterns and regular engagement in physical activity, as it has been documented that treating established adult obesity and overweight is difficult and has poor outcomes overall.[17] Community interventions designed to promote physical activity and nutrition in children present an excellent opportunity to OT practitioners. Programs can be designed for schools, daycare centers, or afterschool settings to address a variety of influences that affect the child's weight; collaboration with caregivers and teachers is essential for effective outcomes. OT practitioners have the necessary skills to provide such programs, and because of the public recognition of childhood obesity as a national concern, the need for these programs is substantial. Refer to Chapter 14 of this text for more on childhood obesity.

In planning a community intervention program, it is necessary to have a well-devised model to follow. A widely used model for planning, implementing, and evaluating community interventions in public health is the Precede-Proceed Model.[9] This model consists of eight phases that provide a framework for intervention. It is an educational and ecologic model that incorporates planning for evidence-based best practices, interventions, and integration of evaluation methods for improvement of quality. It involves careful and thorough assessments of community systems and their influences on the health behavior being addressed. This model provides one example of an appropriate framework; however, the OT practitioner should develop a complete understanding on the use of the model in planning and implementing community interventions.

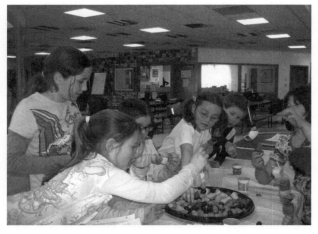

FIGURE 5-3 OT students provide an after school program to children to promote healthy nutritional habits and reduce childhood obesity.

COMMUNITY MENTAL HEALTH MOVEMENT

Possibly the most significant example of the shift from hospital-based care to community care has occurred in the mental health system. During the 1960s, there were many changes in American society. Political, social, and cultural changes resulted from the civil rights movement and activities of the time. Prolonged institutionalization of individuals with disabilities was viewed negatively, which resulted in increasing political support for deinstitutionalization. As a result, the Community Mental Health Center Act of 1963 was signed by President Kennedy, and funds were approved to build comprehensive community mental health centers that would provide a range of mental health services.[4] In some states, OT practitioners were integrated into community mental health services, while in some other states, their roles were replaced by other health care providers. This occurred for a variety of reasons, including lack of awareness with regard to OT, unavailability of OT practitioners with an interest in mental health treatment, higher cost of adding OT practitioners on the staff, and other health care professionals providing services deemed to be similar to OT. OT practitioners wanting to work in mental health need to advocate for the profession and be able to demonstrate the benefit of OT to the mental health directors and administrators to create a role in the community mental health setting. Thinking outside the box and looking at a variety of settings in which to provide services can open up new opportunities. With increased emphasis on the mental well-being of children, there are opportunities to provide community-built OT services to children with mental illnesses.

In a review of community-based mental health OT interventions, Ikiugu presented a model for the design and implementation of community programs. The steps in this model include the following:

1. Educating clients, case managers, other professionals, and the public at large about the role and scope of OT in community mental health
2. Establishing a client referral system
3. Identifying appropriate assessment instruments and completing client evaluation
4. Integrating family caregivers and other key persons controlling community resources into the therapeutic process
5. Implementing individualized interventions as much as possible within the client's natural environment
6. Supporting the client as he or she attempts to reintegrate into the community, for instance by introducing him or her to key individuals within the community.[11]

This model provides another effective framework for approaching OT provided in the community setting.

COMMUNITY OCCUPATIONAL THERAPY INTERVENTIONS

The school system is the largest community system in which occupational therapists and OTAs are employed. According to the 2006 AOTA Workforce Study, which included data from over 3000 OT clinicians, 29.6% of OT practitioners work in school systems and 35% of OT practitioners work with children ages 3 to 21 years.[2,3] In many schools, OT practitioners primarily deal with handwriting skills, fine motor skills, attention to task, and sensory integration. However, the school system provides the opportunity for OT practitioners to address a variety of other health care concerns such as mental health issues, poor social skills, overweight and obesity, and physical inactivity. With so many OT practitioners working in the school systems, this is an opportunity to embrace the school as a community system and provide services beyond the individualized one-on-one treatment in which the OT practitioner may only be interacting with the child's class teacher. The opportunity to address a health concern shared by a large group of students and to work within a community system to create effective outcomes is possible in the school community. However, it requires the practitioner use an effective model or framework for implementing a health intervention program that is occupationally based and addresses the social, political, and environmental demands of the community system. The practitioner must also be willing and able to communicate effectively with administrators, teachers, parents, and children. Excellent communication and negotiation skills are therefore needed. A variety of service delivery methods, such as mentoring, training, educating, and consultation, may be employed as well. An OT practitioner may present the idea for a service or program that benefits the school system and serve as an organizer or leader in its initiation but not in its implementation. Preschools, afterschool programs, and daycare centers can provide similar opportunities as well.

A number of other community systems can also offer the opportunity for OT practitioners to provide services that are community-built interventions. This may include faith-based programs, community recreational programs, community health clinics, camps, group homes and residential care facilities, and shelters for the homeless. With the increase in medical diagnoses such as autism, attention deficit disorder, and a variety of developmental disorders, and with growing health concerns such as obesity, school violence, and behavioral problems, the need for pediatric services is constantly expanding. Treatment and interventions to address these medical issues and concerns must be provided in community settings, as most of these issues require long-term attention.

CLINICAL *Pearl*

> Volunteering is a good way to introduce yourself to a community setting that does not currently employ OT practitioners. Providing in-services regarding the potential role of OT in the community setting can increase awareness and facilitate productive relationships with other team members.

CHALLENGES IN PRACTICE IN COMMUNITY SYSTEMS

A variety of challenges are encountered by OT practitioners when working within a community system. The biggest challenge may be funding. While OT services are required under the Individual With Disabilities Education Act for defined disabilities,[20] these services may not be comprehensive in scope to meet the child's needs, or the child may have health-related concerns that do not meet the criteria for defined disabilities. OT practitioners wishing to expand services in the school system may face funding as well as time constraints. OT practitioners working with children in settings other than the school systems may face difficulties receiving reimbursement for services from insurance or self-pay mechanisms. Grants and donations may be one source; another possibility may be partnering with community organizations that can absorb the costs of the intervention and provide compensation for the practitioner's time. Use of these options requires investment of time and energy upfront to network and establish working relationships with the community organizations. It is therefore important to develop the ability to determine the need for OT services and to establish positive working relationships. The use of evidence-based practices and the ability to communicate the need for this to the appropriate individuals within the community systems as well as to consumers are also necessary to work effectively in a variety of community systems and with a variety of community organizations.

Another challenge for the OT practitioner working within community systems is maintaining good communication with the child's guardians, caregivers, teachers, other health care providers, and administrative or other support persons within the community system. With multiple people involved in the system at different levels, it can be difficult to maintain effective lines of communication regarding the child's care. Support is generally needed to follow through on the child's plan of care or to reinforce certain behaviors and skills. It can be difficult to achieve effective outcomes without a plan for establishing and maintaining open lines of communication. Fragmentation of community services can also affect communication and outcomes by making it more difficult to interact with individuals involved in the child's care.

The cultural competence of the OT practitioner is another area of challenge when working within a community system. The U. S. Census Bureau has projected that by 2050, the non-Hispanic white population will decrease from 69.4% of the population to 50.1% of the population.[19] Minority populations will continue to increase in the United States, which will result in an increasing need for culturally competent health care practitioners. **Cultural competence** is defined in the nursing literature as a process that requires the health care professional to address five constructs: (1) cultural awareness, (2) cultural knowledge, (3) cultural encounters, (4) cultural skill, and (5) cultural desire.[6] *Cultural awareness* means being respectful and sensitive to the values and beliefs of a client's culture and requires one to be aware of one's own personal prejudices and biases about other cultures. *Cultural knowledge* involves understanding the client's worldview. A *cultural encounter* is the experience of interacting with clients from culturally diverse backgrounds. *Cultural skill* is the ability to identify significant cultural data relevant to the client's health status and therapy goals. *Cultural desire* is the health care practitioner's motivation to be culturally competent and to work through the process.[6] OT practitioners who are not culturally competent and OT practitioners who are unwilling to work through the process to develop cultural competence will be challenged to provide effective community services as most communities are becoming increasingly diverse culturally.

CASE *Study*

Mary is an OT assistant working in the school system. She is primarily interested in working with children with psychiatric diagnoses. A K-12 school in the district provides services for 125 children with psychiatric and emotional disorders and works with the community mental health center to address these problems. The community mental health center provides psychiatric evaluations and therapy but does not employ an occupational therapist. Currently no OT services are being provided to these students.

Mary discusses her interest in working with children in this community school setting with her supervisor. At first her supervisor does not support her idea because of Mary's current full-time schedule at other schools within the district. Mary does not receive support to meet with the school principal, teachers, and mental health counselors to discuss the possible need for OT services either. Mary reviews the data on the student population, including diagnoses, academic performance, socioeconomic status, family situation, home environment, and current mental health services provided to these students. To provide current and evidenced-based data regarding the role and efficacy of OT in this setting, she also conducts a literature review of services currently provided in other school districts and networks with other OT practitioners who work with this population. She develops a plan for integrating OT services into the school setting by offering individualized occupation-based treatment following assessment by one of the district OT practitioners. She requests input from the staff for referrals and screens these children. The school is supportive of OT involvement and requests for these services. Mary negotiates with her supervisor to begin with one student at the school and to continue to expand services if successful. Her supervisor agrees with her plan on the basis of the support and request from the school. In order to expand services within the school district, Mary has successfully promoted OT and built relationships within the community of the school system in which she is employed.

SUMMARY

The future of OT is exciting as health care continues to evolve into more diverse settings within the community. OT practitioners are well-suited for community practice. OT's focus on treating the whole person by addressing the occupational needs of the child and its consideration of environmental influences that affect the child's functioning provides for the ability to practice in a variety of settings. OT practitioners have the necessary skills to address the physical, sensory, behavioral, and psychosocial concerns of the child in the community as health care moves more into this context of service provision.

The need to carefully evaluate the community systems in which the child lives, goes to school, and plays, as well as those that provide other services or care to the child, continues to be of utmost importance. Community systems and services are constantly changing, and opportunities for providing health care services in different types of community settings are increasing. These settings may include schools, preschools, after-school programs, daycare centers, faith-based programs, community recreational programs, community mental health centers, community health clinics, camps, group homes, residential care facilities, shelters for the homeless, and home health agencies.

The need for the OT practitioner to continually evaluate and refine interpersonal skills, therapeutic use of self, cultural competence, and other skills such as pro-gram development and consultation is important for successful community practice. The challenges of community practice include funding and reimbursement issues, the challenge of interacting with multiple individuals involved in the child's care, awareness of the different community systems affecting the child's treatment, and addressing cultural influences. As health care opportunities continue to increase in the community environment and more emphasis is placed on evidence-based outcomes and preventive care, OT will continue to be a vital service for children. Occupational therapy practitioners need to be aware of developing opportunities and be at the forefront of providing services to children and adolescents in a multitude of community settings.

References

1. American Occupational Therapy Association: Occupational therapy practice framework: domain and process, ed 2. *Am J Occup Ther* 62:625–683, 2008.
2. American Occupational Therapy Association: *Occupational therapy salaries and job opportunities continue to improve: 2006 AOTA workplace and compensation survey.* Available at: http://www.aota.org/Students/Prospective/Outlook/38230.aspx. Accessed October 12, 2009.
3. American Occupational Therapy Association: *Your career in occupational therapy: workforce trends in occupational therapy,* 2006. Available at: http://www.aota.org/Students/Prospective/Outlook/38231.aspx. Accessed October 12, 2009.
4. Bruce BA, Borg B: *Psychosocial frames of reference: core of occupation-based practice,* ed 3, Thorofare, NJ, 2002, Slack, Inc.
5. Campbell K, Crawford D: Family food environments as determinants of preschool-aged children's eating behaviors: implications for obesity prevention policy—a review. *Aust J Nutr Dietetics* 58(1):19–25, 2001.
6. Campinha-Bacote J: A model of practice to address cultural competence in rehabilitation nursing. *Rehabil Nurs* 26(1):8–11, 2001.
7. Centers for Disease Control and Prevention: *Overweight and obesity: data and statistics.* Available at: http://www.cdc.gov/obesity/data/index.html. Accessed December 15, 2009.
8. Cole MB, Mclean V: Therapeutic relationships re-defined. *Occup Ther Mental Health* 19(2):33–56, 2003.
9. Green LW, Kreuter MW: *Health program planning: an educational and ecological approach,* New York, 2005, McGraw-Hill.
10. Herzberg GL: Preparing ourselves for working with communities. *Home Community Health Special Interest Section Quarterly* 11:2–4, 2004.
11. Ikiugu MN: *Psychosocial conceptual practice models in occupational therapy: building adaptive capability,* St. Louis, 2007, Mosby.

12. McKenzie J, Neiger B, Smeltzer J: *Planning, implementing, and evaluating health promotion program: a primer*, ed 4, San Francisco, 2005, Benjamin Cummings.

13. Mosey AC: *Psychosocial components of occupational therapy*, New York, 1996, Lippincott Williams & Wilkins.

14. National Center for Health Statistics: *Prevalence of overweight among children and adolescents: United States, 2003-2004*. Available at: http://www.cdc.gov/nchs/data/hestat/overweight/overwght_child_03.htm. Accessed December 15, 2009.

15. Punwar J, Peloquin M: *Occupational therapy: principles and practice*, Philadelphia, 2000, Lippincott.

16. Silverstein M et al: "You get what you get": unexpected findings about low-income parents' negative experiences with community resources. *Pediatrics* 122(6):1141–1147, 2008.

17. Steinbeck KS: The importance of physical activity in the prevention of overweight and obesity in childhood: a review and an opinion. *Obes Rev* 2:117–130, 2001.

18. Taylor RR: *The intentional relationship: occupational therapy and use of self*, Philadelphia, 2008, FA Davis.

19. U.S. Census Bureau: *Newsroom*. Available at: http://www.census.gov/Press-Release/www/releases/archives/population/001720.html. Accessed February 1, 2010.

20. U.S. Department of Education: *Building the legacy: idea 2004*. Available at: http://idea.ed.gov/. Accessed January 10, 2010.

21. U.S. Department of Health and Human Services: *Healthy people 2010*. Available at: http://www.healthypeople.gov/. Accessed December 15, 2009.

22. Wittman PP, Velde BP: Occupational therapy in the community: what, why, and how, *Occup Ther Health Care* 13(3–4):1–5, 2001.

23. World Health Organization: Preamble to the Constitution of the World Health Organization as adopted by the International Health Conference, New York, 19-22 June, 1946; signed on 22 July 1946. by the representatives of 61 States and entered into force on 7 April 1948. *Official Records of the World Health Organization* 2:100, 1948.

REVIEW *Questions*

1. What is the definition of community systems?
2. How do OT services in a community differ from traditional OT intervention?
3. What is the difference between community-based practice and community-built practice?
4. How is therapeutic use of self important in providing services in the community and in building community partnerships?
5. How does public health influence community interventions?
6. What are some challenges to providing services in the community?

SUGGESTED *Activities*

1. Develop a community resource notebook describing services available to clients. Share with classmates. Include such things as: address, population served, fees for services, personnel qualifications, special programs.
2. Observe children in a variety of settings in the community. Describe how these settings could be more accessible to children who have special needs.
3. Develop a program to provide community services to children.
4. Volunteer time to a community agency that helps people in need. While at the site, be mindful of the modes of interaction you use and reflect on how successful your interactions with others were. Provide an inservice to serve the needs of the agency and clients.
5. Explore the Healthy People 2010 document to better understand public health policies. Discuss the influence of this policy on health.

## 6

Principles of Normal Development

DIANNE KOONTZ LOWMAN

JEAN W. SOLOMON

CHAPTER *Objectives*

After studying this chapter, the reader will be able to accomplish the following:

- Explain the importance of knowing and understanding the characteristics of typical development while working in the pediatric occupational therapy arena.
- Discuss the relationship among typical development, areas of performance, and contexts.
- Define and briefly describe the periods of development.
- Describe the general principles of development.
- Apply the general principles of development and justify a developmental sequence of skill acquisition in performance and areas of occupation.

KEY TERMS | **CHAPTER OUTLINE**

Development
Typical
Normal
Principles of development
Context
Growth
Periods of development

General Considerations
DEFINITIONS OF TERMS
PREDICTABLE SEQUENCE OF SKILL ACQUISITION
RELATIONSHIP BETWEEN TYPICAL DEVELOPMENT AND CONTEXT

Periods of Development
GESTATION AND BIRTH
INFANCY
EARLY CHILDHOOD
MIDDLE CHILDHOOD
ADOLESCENCE

Principles of Normal Development

Summary

Sally is an occupational therapy assistant (OTA) who is employed by the local public school system. She has been assigned a new client, a 3-year-old girl named Amy. The supervising occupational therapist has begun the occupational therapy (OT) evaluation and has requested that Sally schedule a visit to assess the child's self-care and play skills in order to determine whether the child is functioning at the appropriate age level in these areas. Sally realizes that to accurately assess Amy's skills relative to her chronologic age, she needs to review normal development definitions and principles.

The OT practitioner must understand **development** and the process of **typical** development. The sequence of acquisition in relation to occupational performance skills and areas is the foundation for OT assessment of and intervention with children who have special needs. The sequence of skill acquisition is predictable in the typically developing child.[1] The OT practitioner's knowledge of **normal** development guides the order of expectations and choice of activities for children who are not developing typically. In atypical development, delays in performance skills may make it difficult or impossible for a child to perform activities of daily living (ADLs), engage successfully in play activities, or acquire functional work and productive skills. The OT practitioner identifies deficits in the occupational performance skills (e.g., motor and process skills) that interfere with a child's occupational performance. The practitioner relies on knowledge of typical development to assist the child in developing useful, functional skills.

GENERAL CONSIDERATIONS

An OT practitioner who is attempting to grasp the basics of normal development must consider general pediatric terms, the predictable sequence of skill acquisition in normal development, the **principles of development**, and the relationship between development and **context**. An understanding of the general terms used by pediatric therapists is necessary for effective communication. The pediatric therapist also needs to know the predictable sequence of skill acquisition in a typically developing child. The OT practitioner must understand the relationship between typical development and the occupational performance contexts as delineated in the American Occupational Therapy Association's (AOTA's) Occupational Therapy Practice Framework: Domain and Process (2nd edition).[3]

Definitions of Terms

A basic understanding of the terms used by OT clinicians who work in pediatrics helps practitioners and other individuals working in the area of pediatrics to communicate effectively. Normal is defined as that which occurs habitually or naturally.[2] In this chapter, "normal" is used interchangeably with "typical" in the discussions on development. Development is the act or process of maturing or acquiring skills ranging from simple to more complex.[2] **Growth** is the maturation of a person.[2] Because the concepts of development and growth are analogous, these terms are used interchangeably in this chapter (Box 6-1).

Predictable Sequence of Skill Acquisition

The normal development of skills in terms of performance and areas of occupation occurs in a predictable sequence.[1,4,5,7] The OT practitioner uses knowledge of typical development while working with children who have special needs in order to identify the areas in which there are deficits and develop a plan to improve their ADLs, play, and academic skills. Although developmental checklists and other tools may help a practitioner identify the presence or absence of certain skills, understanding the process of how and why children are able to develop these skills is more useful in the clinical setting. For example, an OT practitioner may use an observational checklist to determine whether a child can independently finger-feed himself or herself. A practitioner who has knowledge of normal development and its predictable sequence of events understands that children usually learn to eat with their fingers before learning to eat with a spoon. Therefore, if a child is not yet finger-feeding, the practitioner would not introduce spoon-feeding (depending on the circumstances). Knowledge and understanding of normal development guide the OT practitioner in the intervention planning process.

Relationship Between Typical Development and Context

OT practitioners need to understand the relationship between typical development and context. Because the events of normal development are sequential and predictable, the chronological age of the child (i.e., how old the child is) has an impact on the child's level of skill development in performance and areas of occupation.[1,4,5,7] Although practitioners obviously cannot change the age

---

BOX 6-1

Definition of Typical Development

Typical development is defined as the natural process of acquiring skills ranging from simple to complex.

of a child, they can offer age-appropriate activities during intervention sessions. Being familiar with age-appropriate activities helps OT practitioners choose tasks for therapy sessions with children. For example, a practitioner may use colored blocks while performing fine motor and sorting activities with a 3-year-old child, but the use of blocks would not be suitable in a session with a 14-year-old adolescent. It would be more appropriate to have the adolescent use objects like coins for fine motor and sorting activities.

Although normal development is predictable and sequential, the rate of skill acquisition varies among children. This variability greatly depends on the context and environment (Box 6-2). These contexts include cultural, personal, temporal, virtual, physical, and social factors.[3]

The *cultural* environment, which comprises customs, beliefs, activity patterns, and behavior standards, also influences the rate of skill development and performance in areas of occupation.[3] Anticipation of behaviors refers to an individual's expectation of repetition of a daily schedule (e.g., waking up, eating, bathing, and dressing—in that order) or consistency of cause and effect behaviors (e.g., washing the dishes and cleaning the room, which cause the mother to be pleased with the child). An adolescent whose parents believe that only adults should be employed may develop work skills later in life than one whose parents believe that summer and after-school jobs are appropriate and should be encouraged. In certain cultures, using eating utensils is not the adult norm. Children in this type of cultural environment may never learn to use a fork or spoon.

The *personal* context includes the child's age, gender, socioeconomic status, and educational level.[3] For example, a 2-year-old boy from a rural community will have different goals and enjoy different activities than would a 10-year-old girl from an inner city.

It is important for OT practitioners working with children to understand the *temporal* context, which refers to the stage of life, time of year, and length of occupation.[3] Adolescents and toddlers have very different goals and experiences. Toddlers experience the "terrible twos" for a short period (it varies for each child). However, a 5-year-old child should be well past this phase, so the observation of this behavior past the expected duration indicates a cause for concern.

The *virtual* context includes communication by means of computers and airways.[3] Children use computers, cell phones, and other electronic means to communicate. These virtual environments provide opportunities for children but also must be monitored.

The *physical*, or *nonhuman*, aspects of the environment have an impact on the rate of skill acquisition in both performance and areas of occupation.[3] For example, if a child lives in a climate that requires warm clothing, he or she will learn to don and doff a sweater or a coat more quickly than one who lives in a temperate climate. A child who lives in a two-story house will more likely learn to ascend and descend stairs before one who lives in a single-story house.

The *social* context refers to the availability and anticipation of behaviors by significant others, which influences the rate of skill acquisition in occupations.[3] An infant who is breastfed will not acquire the ability to drink from a bottle or cup as quickly as one who is bottle-fed. An infant who is carried frequently may not develop gross motor and mobility skills as quickly as one who is allowed to move around on the floor or in a playpen.

Studying the process of normal development allows practitioners to learn about its predictable sequences and contextual variability. Although this knowledge is important, having the skills to solve problems related to the developmental process is more useful than memorizing the sequences of skill acquisition in performance and areas of occupation. Carefully studying this chapter as well as the next two and participating in the suggested activities will give OT practitioners an excellent basis for using the problem-solving approach in the developmental process. One framework to use when studying development is based on the generally accepted periods of development. Another framework

---

BOX 6-2

Contexts

CULTURAL CONTEXT
Customs, beliefs/values, standards, and expectations

PERSONAL CONTEXT
Features of the person such as age, gender, socioeconomic status, and educational level

TEMPORAL CONTEXT
Stage of life, time of day, and time of year

VIRTUAL CONTEXT
Computer or airways, simulators, chat rooms, and radio

PHYSICAL CONTEXT
Nonhuman aspects of the environment

SOCIAL CONTEXT
Significant others and the larger social group

Adapted from the American Occupational Therapy Association: Occupational therapy practice framework: Domain and process, 2nd edition, *Am J Occup Ther* 62, 2008.

involves understanding the general principles of development. Each will be described in the following sections.

PERIODS OF DEVELOPMENT

Periods of development are intervals of time during which a child increases in size and acquires specific skills.[2] Pediatric OT practitioners work with children of varying chronologic ages. The following normal developmental periods are used as the basis for comparison in subsequent chapters dealing with normal development (Box 6-3).

Gestation and Birth

Gestation refers to the developmental period of the fetus, or unborn child, in the mother's uterus. This period begins with conception and ends with birth.[2] The gestational period is also referred to as the *prenatal* (before-birth) *period*.[2] Gestation typically lasts 40 weeks.[2] The birthing process is also known as the *perinatal* (around-birth) *period*. This period varies greatly in duration for a variety of reasons, the discussion of which is beyond the scope of this book. The perinatal period ends when the infant is able to independently sustain life without placental nutrients from the mother. The *postnatal* (after-birth) *period* is the immediate interval of time following birth. During the postnatal period, the infant is known as a *neonate*, or *new baby*.[2]

BOX 6-3

Periods of Development

GESTATION AND BIRTH
From conception to the moment at which the neonate can survive on its own without placental nutrients

INFANCY
From birth through 18 months of age

EARLY CHILDHOOD
From 18 months through 5 years of age

MIDDLE CHILDHOOD
From 6 years of age until the onset of puberty (12 years of age for females and 14 years of age for males)

ADOLESCENCE
From puberty until the onset of adulthood (usually 21 years of age)

Infancy

Infancy is the period from birth through approximately 18 months of age.[9] It is characterized by significant physical and emotional growth.[9] Typically developing infants grow considerably in height and weight during the first 18 months of life.[9] They develop sensory and motor skills, and by 18 months of age they are walking, talking, and performing simple self-care tasks such as eating with a spoon, drinking from a cup, and undressing.

Early Childhood

Toddlers and preschool children represent the period of early childhood, which begins at 18 months of age and lasts through 5 years of age.[2,9] During the early childhood period, children become increasingly independent and establish more of a sense of individuality.

Middle Childhood

Middle childhood begins at 6 years of age and lasts until puberty, which begins at approximately 12 years of age in females and 14 years of age in males.[9] Children in this developmental period spend the majority of their time in educational settings; therefore, the major influence on the child shifts from parents to peers.

Adolescence

Adolescence is the period of physical and psychological development that accompanies the onset of puberty. Puberty is a stage of maturation in which a person becomes physiologically capable of reproduction. This period is marked by hormonal changes and their resulting challenges.[2] Adolescence ends with the onset of adulthood (usually 21 years of age), when individuals begin to function independent of their parents.[2]

OT practitioners use the periods of development as reference points while working with children who have special needs. Knowledge of the sequence of development within each period is used as a guide for the OT process. Practitioners need to know the general principles of development in order to understand the reasons children gain skills predictably and sequentially.

PRINCIPLES OF NORMAL DEVELOPMENT

The general principles of development are widely accepted in the various pediatric disciplines (Box 6-4). The following principles are tools used by OT practitioners to solve problems related to the acquisition of skills.

- Normal development is sequential and predictable. The rate (speed) and direction (vertical or horizontal) of development vary among children, but the sequence remains the same.[1,4,5,7,8] For example, infants who are typically developing acquire head control before trunk control (an example of vertical development). Head and trunk control are necessary for them to sit independently. Infants learn to roll, then sit, then creep, and finally walk. Although most developmental theorists agree that the sequence is the same for all children, recent research in motor control theory demonstrates that motor development does not always follow a set sequence.[1] In either case, each child acquires these skills at a unique rate.

- Maturation and experience affect a child's development.[4-8] Maturation and experience influence the rate and direction of normal development. Maturation is the innate (natural) process of growth and development, and experience is the result of interactions with the environment.[2] In addition, current research on motor control introduces the concepts of arousal states and motivation as additional factors that have an impact on motor learning. The child must be aroused in order to be motivated to move and interact with the environment.[1] Although most developmental theorists agree that maturation, experience, arousal state, and motivation have an impact on a child's development, their opinions vary about which one is the more significant.

- Throughout the course of normal development, changes occur in the biologic, psychological, and social systems.[5] Therefore, development is a dynamic and continuously changing process. Changes in the biologic system include those related to the functions

and processes of internal structures.[6,9] Changes in the psychological system affect the emotional and behavioral characteristics of the individual.[9] Changes in the social system include those that affect individuals in their immediate environment and society as a whole.[5,6,9] These changes occur in all three systems throughout the course of typical development. A change in one system influences the other two.

- Development progresses in two directions: vertical and horizontal.[5,8] As children progress through the various developmental levels related to the specific performance skills or areas of occupation, they are progressing vertically. For example, in the occupational area of ADLs, children learn to eat with their fingers before they learn to eat with a spoon. As children learn to roll, then crawl, and finally walk, they are progressing vertically in gross motor performance skills. In both examples, development is occurring in a vertical direction within a specific performance skill or area of occupation. Development that involves different performance skills and areas of occupation indicates horizontal progression. A child who is simultaneously learning to finger-feed, use a pincer grasp, and creep is progressing horizontally because several different performance skills and areas (i.e., ADLs, fine motor skills, and gross motor skills) are involved.

- Motor development follows three basic rules.
    1. Development progresses cephalad to caudal, or head to tail.[5] For example, a baby is first able to control head and neck movements (beginning at around 2 months), then the arms and hands (grasping begins at about 3 months), then the trunk (most babies sit well by 8 months), and finally the legs and feet (most children walk by 14 to 15 months).
    2. Development progresses in a proximal to distal direction, which means that children develop control of structures close to their body (such as the shoulder) before they develop those farther away from their body (such as the hand).[4] For example, a baby can swat at an object by 3 to 4 months but cannot reach straight ahead and grasp an object in the fingers until around 8 months.
    3. Development progresses from gross control to fine control, which means that children gain control of large body movements before they can perform more refined movements.[4] For example, children are able to catch a large ball using both arms and the body before they learn to catch a tennis ball with one hand. They use the larger arm muscles to catch a large 8-inch ball and the smaller wrist and hand muscles to catch a tennis ball.

These general principles of development provide a framework for OT practitioners to use while solving developmental problems. The principles can be used to guide the intervention planning process while working with children who have special needs.

SUMMARY

Normal development is sequential and predictable. OT practitioners rely on their knowledge and understanding of typical development while working with children who have special needs. Practitioners must also consider the relationship between normal development and contexts.

The periods and general principles of development help provide a framework for organizing and understanding information related to typical development. The periods include gestation and birth, infancy, early childhood, middle childhood, and adolescence. The general principles of development, which are widely used in the various pediatric disciplines, help OT practitioners plan evaluations and interventions while working with children who have special needs.

References

1. Alexander R, Boehme R, Cupps B: *Normal development of functional motor skills*, Tucson, 1993, Therapy Skill Builders.
2. *American heritage dictionary of the English language*, ed 4, Boston, 2000, Houghton Mifflin.
3. American Occupational Therapy Association: Occupational therapy practice framework: domain and process, ed 2. *Am J Occup Ther* 62:625–683, 2008.
4. Boehme R: *Improving upper body control: an approach to assessment and treatment of tonal dysfunction*, Tucson, 1988, Therapy Skill Builders.
5. Case-Smith J, O'Brien J: *Occupational therapy for children*, ed 6, St. Louis, 2010, Mosby.
6. Kielhofner G: *Conceptual foundations of occupational therapy*, Philadelphia, 1997, FA Davis.
7. Kramer P, Hinojosa J: *Frames of reference for pediatric occupational therapy*, ed 3, Philadelphia, 2009, Lippincott Williams & Wilkins.
8. Llorens LA: *Application of a developmental theory for health and rehabilitation*, Rockville, MD, 1976, American Occupational Therapy Association.
9. Meyer WJ: Infancy, *Microsoft Encarta 98 encyclopedia*, Redmond, WA, 1997, Microsoft.

Recommended Reading

Bly L: *Motor skills acquisition in the first year: an illustrated guide to normal development*, Tucson, 1994, Therapy Skill Builders.

Green M, Palfrey JS, editors: *Bright futures: guidelines for health supervision of infants, children, and adolescents*, ed 2, Arlington, VA, 2002, National Center for Education in Maternal and Child Health. Available at: http://www.brightfutures.org. Accessed June 30, 2004.

Gilfoyle ZM, Grady AP, Moore JC: *Children adapt*, ed 2, Thorofare, NJ, 1990, Slack.

Zero to Three: *Brain wonders: helping babies and toddlers grow and develop*, Washington, DC, 2004, Zero to Three. Available at: http://www.zerotothree.org/brainwonders/. Accessed June 30, 2004.

REVIEW *Questions*

1. Explain the following terms: *normal, typical, development, growth.*
2. List and describe the periods of development.
3. List and describe the general principles of development.
4. Define *context.*
5. Describe how contexts have an impact on intervention.

SUGGESTED *Activities*

1. Visit a daycare center or playground to observe children playing. Note the variety of approaches that are used by different children to accomplish the same task.
2. In small study groups, discuss the general principles of development, and then describe these principles in your own words. Give examples of these principles in relation to your own development.
3. In small study groups, describe your cultural background and how it influences your goals and the occupations which you perform. How would it influence the treatment of a child?
4. Provide examples of how contexts (cultural, physical, personal, social, spiritual, temporal, and virtual) influence development. Discuss the techniques practitioners could use to address each context.

## 7

Development of Occupational Performance Skills

DIANNE KOONTZ LOWMAN*

CHAPTER *Objectives*

After studying this chapter, the reader will be able to accomplish the following:

- Describe significant physiological changes that occur at each stage of development.
- Identify the sequences of motor skill development (gross and fine motor).
- Outline the stages of process development (cognitive) as defined by Piaget's theory.
- Describe the issues in each phase of communication and interaction development (psychosocial development) using the theories of Erikson and Greenspan.

* I would like to thank the occupational therapy students at Virginia Commonwealth University's Department of Occupational Therapy for researching the material in this chapter and field-testing the review questions and suggested activities.

KEY TERMS

Performance skills

Motor skills

Gross motor skills

Fine motor skills

Process skills

Communication/interaction skills

Primitive reflexes

Righting reactions

Equilibrium reactions

Psychosocial development

CHAPTER OUTLINE

Infancy

PHYSIOLOGICAL DEVELOPMENT

MOTOR DEVELOPMENT

PROCESS/COGNITION DEVELOPMENT

COMMUNICATION AND INTERACTION/PSYCHOSOCIAL DEVELOPMENT

Early Childhood

PHYSIOLOGICAL DEVELOPMENT

MOTOR DEVELOPMENT

PROCESS/COGNITION DEVELOPMENT

COMMUNICATION AND INTERACTION/PSYCHOSOCIAL DEVELOPMENT

Middle Childhood

PHYSIOLOGICAL DEVELOPMENT

MOTOR DEVELOPMENT

PROCESS/COGNITION DEVELOPMENT

COMMUNICATION AND INTERACTION/PSYCHOSOCIAL DEVELOPMENT

Adolescence

PHYSIOLOGICAL DEVELOPMENT

MOTOR DEVELOPMENT

PROCESS/COGNITION DEVELOPMENT

COMMUNICATION AND INTERACTION/PSYCHOSOCIAL DEVELOPMENT

Summary

Three generations of family members have gathered for a family reunion. While looking at the grandmother's photograph album, conversation centers around how much the 2-year-old grandson looks like his father and grandfather did at the same age. The family is amazed to see how their bodies, sizes, proportions, and postures look similar, even though their clothing and environments are significantly different!

From birth through adolescence, the child progresses through periods of development. Development that occurs within each period is described in the literature in terms of physiologic, motor, cognitive, language, and psychosocial domains. In the Occupational Therapy Practice Framework, the occupational **performance skills** are **motor skills (gross** and **fine motor skills), process skills** (cognition), and **communication/interaction skills** (language and psychosocial) (Box 7-1).[2] Deficits in any of these skills may interfere with the child's performance in the areas of self-care, play, education, and social participation. The normal developmental sequences are presented in this chapter to assist occupational therapy (OT) practitioners in identifying potential deficits or delays. Sequences may vary, and the physical, temporal,

---

BOX 7-1

Occupational Performance Skills

MOTOR SKILLS (Gross and Fine)
Motor skills are those involved in moving and interacting with objects or the environment and include posture, mobility, coordination, strength, effort, and energy. Examples of motor skills include stabilizing the body and manipulating objects.

PROCESS SKILLS (Cognition)
Process skills are those used in completing daily tasks and include energy, knowledge, temporal organization, organizing space and objects, and adaptation. Examples of process skills include maintaining attention to a task, choosing appropriate tools and materials for the task, and accommodating the method of task completion in response to a problem.

COMMUNICATION/INTERACTION SKILLS (LANGUAGE AND PSYCHOSOCIAL DEVELOPMENT)
Communication and interaction skills refer to those needed to interact with other people and include physicality, information exchange, and relations. Examples of communication and interaction skills include gesturing to indicate intention, expressing affect, and relating in a manner that establishes rapport with others.

From the American Occupational Therapy Association: Occupational therapy practice framework: Domain and process, 2nd edition, *Am J Occup Ther* 62:625–683, 2008.

---

social, and cultural aspects of the environment may affect developmental progression.

As children follow a developmental sequence within an individual performance skill, they are also developing other performance skills. For example, an 18-month-old toddler travels and explores independently, has a precise grasp, is beginning to use tools to solve problems, and demonstrates an understanding of the function of objects in play.

INFANCY

Phillip is an active and happy 1-year-old boy. It is his first birthday party, and he is busy experimenting with his new toys. As family and friends watch, he attempts to sit on his push toy and make it move across the kitchen floor. When his older siblings offer help, he pushes them away because he wants to play alone.

Physiologic Development

The newborn's average weight at birth is 7 lb, 2 oz and the average length between 19 and 22 inches. The appearance of the newborn may be characterized by a covering comprising a layer of fluid called *vernix caseosa*; a large, bumpy head; a flat, "board" nose; reddish skin; puffy eyes; external breasts; and fine hair called *lanugo* covering the body.[13] At 1 minute after birth, the newborn's physiological status is tested using the Apgar scoring system, which rates each of the following five areas on a scale of 0 to 2: (1) color, (2) heart rate, (3) reflex irritability, (4) muscle tone, and (5) respiratory effort. The scores are computed at 1 and 5 minutes after birth. The closer the total score (sum of scores for the five areas) is to 10, the better is the condition of the newborn; scores of 6 or less indicate the need for intervention.[12]

The infant's first 3 months of life are characterized by constant physiologic adaptations. Structural changes in the newborn's circulatory system include the expansion of the lungs and increased efficiency of blood flow to the heart. The developing central nervous system (CNS) participates in the body's regulation of sleep, digestion, and temperature.[10]

Physical growth is dramatic—from birth to 6 months of age, infants experience a more rapid rate of growth than at any other time, except during gestation.[19] During the first year, infants triple their body weight, and their height increases by 10 to 12 inches. Their body shape changes, and by 4 months the sizes of their heads and bodies are more proportionate. By 12 months, average infants weigh 21 to 22 lb and are 29 to 30 inches tall. During the second year of life, physical growth slows. By 24 months, an average toddler weighs about 27 lb and is 34 inches tall. The posture of toddlers is characterized by *lordosis* (forward curvature of the spine) and a protruding abdomen, which toddlers retain well into the third year.[33]

At 4 months, sleep patterns begin to be regulated, and some infants may sleep through the night. By 8 months, the average infant sleeps 12 to 13 hours per day, but the range can vary from 9 to 18 hours per day. By 6 to 7 months, the average infant acquires the first tooth, a lower incisor. As a result, saliva production increases, which leads to drooling. At approximately 8 months, the upper central incisor teeth begin to surface, at 9 months the upper lateral incisors appear, and at 12 months the first lower molars are seen.[28]

Motor Development

Brazelton identified six behavioral states observed in the newborn: (1) deep sleep; (2) light sleep; (3) drowsy or semidozing; (4) alert, actively awake; (5) fussy; and (6) crying.[9] The infant's state should be noted when observing the way he or she responds to stimulation.[13]

Sensory Skills

Newborns have vision at birth and can see objects best from about 8 inches away, which is the typical distance between the caregiver's face and the infant's.[29] By the first month of life, an infant shows a preference for patterns and can distinguish between colors. By 3 months, visual acuity develops enough to allow distinction between a picture of a face and a real face.[10] By 12 months, the infant's visual acuity is about 20/100 to 20/50.[24]

Hearing is well developed in newborns and continues to improve as they grow. They tend to respond strongly to the mother's voice.[25] During the first 2 months, infants respond to sound with random body movements. At 3 months, they move their eyes in the direction of sound.[10] At 6 months, they localize sounds to the left and right.[5]

At birth, newborns are able to taste sweet, sour, and bitter substances. Between birth and 3 months, infants are able to differentiate between pleasant and noxious odors. They are very sensitive to touch, cold and heat, pain, and pressure; one of the most important stimuli for infants from birth to 3 months is skin contact and warmth.[27] Holding and swaddling the infant provide skin contact and maintain the infant's body temperature.[13]

Gross Motor Skills

The newborn's body is characterized by physiologic flexion, a position of extremity and trunk flexion.[8] This flexion tends to keep the infant in a compact position and provides a base of stability for random movements to occur. These movements are characterized by a motion called *random burst*, in which everything moves as a

unit.[1] The newborn has numerous **primitive reflexes,** which are genetically transmitted survival mechanisms. These automatic responses to stimuli help the newborn adapt to the environment. Primitive reflexes are controlled by lower levels of the CNS. As higher levels of the CNS mature, higher systems inhibit the expression of primitive reflexes. As infants learn about the environment, primitive reflexes are integrated into their overall postural mechanism, with the more mature righting and equilibrium responses that dominate their movements.[34] Under stress, these reflexes may be partially present, but they are never obligatory in normal development. Some primitive reflexes are present at birth, whereas others emerge later in the infant's development (Table 7-1).

As shown in Table 7-2, infants' gross motor skills become gradually more complex as they develop.[1,8,13] Infants begin to combine basic reflexive movements with higher cognitive and physiologic functioning to control these movements in the environment (Box 7-2). Between birth and 2 months, infants can turn their heads from side to side while in prone and supine positions. As physiologic flexion diminishes, they appear more hypotonic (have less muscular and postural tone), and the movements of each side of their body appear asymmetrical. The asymmetrical tonic neck reflex (ATNR) holds infants' heads to one side. By 4 months, they can raise and rotate their heads to look at their surroundings. In the supine position (on the back), 4-month-old infants begin to bring their hands to their knees and can deliberately roll from the supine position to the side. The increased head and trunk control observed at this age is the result of emerging **righting reactions** and better postural control (see Box 7-2). At 5 months, when pulled to a sitting position, infants can bring their heads forward without lagging. By 6 months, they can shift their weight to free extremities to reach for objects while in the prone position (on the stomach). In the supine position, 6-month-old infants can bring their feet to their mouths and are able to sit by themselves for short periods. At 7 to 8 months, they are able to push themselves from the prone position to the sitting position, roll over at will, and crawl on their stomachs. Between 6 and 9 months, infants develop upper extremity protective extension reactions that allow them to catch themselves when pushed off balance (Figure 7-1). From 7 to 21 months, they develop **equilibrium reactions** that allow them to maintain their center of gravity over their base of support; these reactions are critical for transitional movements patterns (i.e., movements from one position to another) and ambulation (see Box 7-2; Figure 7-2). At 10 to 11 months, infants are practicing and enjoying creeping. By 12 months, they are learning to shift their weight and step to one side by cruising around furniture. At

TABLE 7-1

Reflexes and Reactions

NAME OF REFLEX OR REACTION	POSITION (P) STIMULUS (S)	POSITIVE RESPONSE	AGE SPAN: AGE OF ONSET OR INTEGRATION	LACK OF INTEGRATION OR ONSET
Rooting	P: Supine S: Light touch on side of face near mouth	Opens mouth and turns head in direction of touch.	Birth to 3 mo	Interferes with exploration of objects and head control
Sucking/ swallowing	P: Supine S: Light touch on oral cavity	Closes mouth, sucks, and swallows.	Birth to 2–5 mo	Interferes with development of coordination of sucking, swallowing, and breathing
Moro's	P: Supine, head at midline S: Dropping head, more than 30 degrees extended	Arms extend and hands open; then arms flex and hands close; infant usually cries.	Birth to 4–6 mo	Interferes with head control, sitting equilibrium, and protective reactions
Palmar grasp	P: Supine S: Pressure on ulnar surface of palm	Fingers flex.	Birth to 4–6 mo	Interferes with releasing objects
Plantar grasp	P: Supine S: Firm pressure on ball of foot	Toes grasp (flexion).	Birth to 4–9 mo	Interferes with putting on shoes because of toe clawing, gait, and standing and walking problems (e.g., walking on toes)
Neonatal positive support— primary standing	P: Upright S: Being bounced several times on soles of feet (proprioceptive stimulus)	LE extensor tone increases, and plantar flexion is present. Some hip and knee flexion or genu recurvatum (hyperextension of the knee) may occur.	Birth to 1–2 mo	Interferes with walking patterns and leads to walking on toes
ATNR	P: Supine, arms and legs extended, head in midposition S: Head turned to one side	Arm and leg on face side extend; arm and leg on skull side flex (or experience increased flexor tone)	Birth to 4–6 mo	Interferes with reaching and grasping, bilateral hand use, and rolling
STNR	P: Quadruped position or over tester's knees S: 1. Flexed head 2. Extended head	1. Arms flex and legs extend (tone increases). 2. Arms extend and legs flex (tone increases).	Birth to 4–6 mo	Interferes with reciprocal crawling (children "bunny hop" or move arms and then legs in quadruped position) and walking
TLR	P: 1. Supine, head in midposition, arms and legs extended 2. Prone S: Position (laying on floor); being moved into flexion or extension	1. Extensor tone of neck UE, and LE increases when moved into flexion. 2. Flexor tone of neck UE, and LE increases when moved into extension.	Birth to 4–6 mo	Interferes with turning on side, rolling over, going from lying to sitting position, and crawling; in older children, interferes with ability to "hold in supine flexion" or assume a pivot prone position

Continued

TABLE 7-1

Reflexes and Reactions—cont'd

NAME OF REFLEX OR REACTION	POSITION (P) STIMULUS (S)	POSITIVE RESPONSE	AGE SPAN: AGE OF ONSET OR INTEGRATION	LACK OF INTEGRATION OR ONSET
Landau	P: Prone, held in space (suspension) supporting thorax S: Suspension (usually), also active or passive dorsiflexion of head	Hips and legs extend; UE extends and abducts. Elbows can flex. (Typically used to determine overall development)	3–4 mo to 12–24 mo	Slows development of prone extension, sitting, and standing Early onset (1 mo); may indicate excessive tone or spasticity
Protective extension UE—Parachute, downward forward, sideways, backward	P: Prone, head in midposition, arms extend above S: Suspension by ankles and pelvis and sudden movement of head toward floor P: Seated S: Child pushed: 1. Forward 2. Left, right 3. Backward	Shoulders flex and elbow and wrist extend (arms extend forward) to protect head; infant catches self in directions pushed: 1. Shoulder flexes and abducts; elbow and wrist extend (arms extend forward). 2. Shoulder abducts, elbow and wrist extend (arms extend to side). 3. Shoulders, elbows, and wrists extend (arms extend backward) to protect head.	6-9 mo continues through life	Interferes with head protection when center of gravity displaced
Stagger LE—Forward, backward, sideways	P: Standing upright S: Displacement of body by pushing on shoulders and upper trunk: 1. Forward 2. Backward 3. Sideways	Infant takes one or more steps in direction of displacement. UEs often also have a protective reaction, with elbow, wrist, and fingers extending: 1. Shoulder flexes. 2. Shoulder abducts and extends. 3. Shoulder abducts.	15–18 mo, continues throughout life	Interferes with ability to catch self when center of gravity displaced, causes trips and falls
Equilibrium—sitting	P: Seated, extremities relaxed S: Hand pulled to one side or shoulder pushed	*Head righting: non–weight-bearing side—* trunk flexes; UE and LE abduct and internally rotate; and elbow, wrist, and fingers extend *Head righting: weight-bearing side—* trunk elongates; UE and LE externally rotate; and elbow, wrist, and fingers abduct and extend.	7–8 mo, continues throughout life	Interferes with ability to sit or maintain balance when reaching for objects or displacing center of gravity

TABLE 7-1

Reflexes and Reactions—cont'd

NAME OF REFLEX OR REACTION	POSITION (P) STIMULUS (S)	POSITIVE RESPONSE	AGE SPAN: AGE OF ONSET OR INTEGRATION	LACK OF INTEGRATION OR ONSET
Standing	P: Standing upright, extremities relaxed S: Body displaced by holding UE and pulling to side	*Head righting: non–weight-bearing side*—trunk flexes; UE and LE abduct and internally rotate; and elbow, wrist, and fingers extend. *Head righting: weight-bearing side*—trunk elongates; UE and LE eternally rotate; and elbow, wrist, and fingers extend and abduct.	12–21 mo, continues throughout life	Interferes with ability to stand and walk and make transitional movements
Equilibrium or tilting—prone, su-pine	P: Prone or supine on a tilt board, extremities extended S: Board tilted to left or right	*Head righting: non–weight-bearing side*—trunk flexes; UE and LE abduct; and elbow, wrist, hip, and knee externally rotate and extend. *Head righting: weight-bearing side*—UE and LE internally rotate and abduct and elbow, wrist, fingers, knee, and hip extend.	5–6 mo, continues throughout life	Interferes with ability to make transitional movements, sit, and creep

LE, lower extremity; *UE*, upper extremity; *ATNR*, asymmetrical tonic neck reflex; *STNR*, symmetrical tonic neck reflex; *TLR*, tonic labyrinthine reflex.
Adapted from Alexander R, Boehme R, Cupps B: Normal development of functional motor skills, Tucson, AR, 1993, Therapy Skill Builders; Bly L: *Motor skills acquisition in the first year: An illustrated guide to normal development*, Tucson, AR, 1994, Therapy Skill Builders; Fiorentino MR: *Reflex testing methods for evaluating CNS development*, ed 2, Springfield, IL, 1981, Charles C Thomas; Simon CJ, Daub MM: Human development across the life span. In Hopkins JL, Smith HD, editors: *Willard and Spackman's occupational therapy*, ed 8, Philadelphia, 1993, Lippincott.

13 or 14 months most infants take their first steps, and between 12 and 18 months they spend much of their time practicing motor skills by walking, jumping, running, and kicking. Mobility changes infants' perceptions of their environment. A chair is a one-dimensional object in the eyes of a 6 month old; it is only when the infant can finally climb over, under, and around the chair that he or she discovers what a chair really is.[18]

Fine Motor Skills

Between birth and 3 months, most interactions with the environment are through visual inspection. The grasp reflex allows the infant to have contact with objects placed in the hand. At 4 months, he or she demonstrates visually directed reaching skills. At 5 months, the infant can use a palmar grasp and an ulnar palmar grasp. The

child's fingers are placed on the top surface of an object. The fingers then press the object into the center of the palm toward the little finger (*Figure 7-3, A*). At 5 to 6 months, transferring objects from one hand to another is a two-step process (the taking hand grabs the objects deposited by the releasing hand before the releasing hand lets go). By 6 months, the infant is coordinated enough to reach for an object while in the sitting or prone position. A 6-month-old infant uses a radial palmar grasp (in which the object is held between the thumb and the radial side of the palm) (Figure 7-3, B) to transfer objects from hand to hand in a one-stage process (with the taking hand and releasing hand executing the transfer simultaneously). Grasping skills change significantly between 7 and 12 months. At 7 months, the infant uses a radial digital grasp (in which objects are held between the

TABLE 7-2

Normal Development of Sensorimotor Skills

AGE	GROSS MOTOR COORDINATION	FINE MOTOR COORDINATION
BIRTH OR 37-40 WK OF GESTATION	Is dominated by physiologic flexion Moves entire body into extension Turns head side to side (protective response) Keeps head mostly to side while in supine position	Visually regards objects and people Tends to fist and flex hands across chest during feeding Displays strong grasp reflex but has no voluntary grasping abilities Has no voluntary release abilities
1–2 MO	Appears hypertonic as physiologicalal flexion Practices extension and flexion Continues to gain control of head Moves elbows forward toward shoulders while in prone position Has ATNR with head to side while in supine position When held in standing position, bears some weight on legs	Displays diminishing grasp reflex Involuntarily releases after holding them briefly has no voluntary release abilities
3–5 MO	Experiences fading of ATNR and grasp reflex Has more balance between extension and flexion positions Has good head control (centered and upright) Supports self on extended arms while in prone position props self on forearms Brings hand to feet and feet to mouth while in supine position Props on arms with little support while seated Rolls from supine to prone position Bears some weight on legs when held proximally	Constantly brings hands to mouth Develops tactile awareness in hands Reaches more accurately usually with both hands Palmar grasp Begins transferring objects from hand to hand Does not have control of releasing objects may use mouth to assist
6 MO	Has complete head control Possesses equilibrium reactions Begins assuming quadruped position Rolls from prone to supine position Bounces while standing	Transfers objects from hand to hand while in supine position Shifts weight and reaches with one hand while in prone position Reaches with one hand and supports self with other while seated Reaches to be picked up Uses radial palmar grasp; begins to use thumb while grasping Shows visual interest in small objects rakes small objects Begins to hold objects in one hand
7–9 MO	Shifts weight and reaches while in quadruped position Creeps Develops extension, flexion, and rotation movements, and increases number of activities that can be accomplished while seated May pull to standing position while holding on to support	Reaches with supination Uses index finger to poke objects Uses inferior scissors grasp to pick up small objects Use radial digital grasp to pick up cube Displays voluntary releases abilities
10–12 MO	Displays good coordination while creeping Pulls to standing position using legs only Cruises holding on to support with one hand Stands independently Begins to walk independently Displays equilibrium reactions while standing	Uses superior pincer grasp with fingertip and thumb Use 3-jaw chuck grasp Displays controlled release into large containers

TABLE 7-2

Normal Development of Sensorimotor Skills—cont'd

AGE	GROSS MOTOR COORDINATION	FINE MOTOR COORDINATION
13–18 MO	Walks alone Seldom falls Begins to go up and down stairs	Displays more precise grasping abilities Precisely releases objects into small containers
19–24 MO	Displays equilibrium reactions while walking Runs using a more narrow base support	Uses finger to palm translation of small objects
24–36 MO	Jumps in place*	Uses palm to finger and finger to palm translation of small objects Displays complex rotation of small objects Shifts small objects using palmar stabilization Scribbles Snips with scissors

*From this point on, skills learned during the first 24 months are further refined.
ATNR, asymmetrical tonic neck reflex.
Adapted from Alexander R, Boehme R, Cupps B: *Normal development of functional motor skills,* Tucson, AR, 1993, Therapy Skill Builders; Case-Smith J, Shortridge SD: The developmental process: Prenatal to adolescence. In Case-Smith J, Allen AS, Pratt PN, editors: *Occupational therapy for children,* ed 3, St Louis, 1996, Mosby; Clark GF: Oral-motor and feeding issues. In Royeen CB, editor: *AOTA self-study series: Classroom applications for school-based practice,* Rockville, MD, 1993, American Occupational Therapy Association; Erhardt RP: *Developmental hand dysfunction: Theory, assessment, and treatment,* ed 2, Tucson, AR, 1994 Therapy Skill Builders.

BOX 7-2

Development of Coordinated Movement in Infancy

EXTENSION → FLEXION → LATERAL FLEXION → ROTATION

PRIMITIVE REFLEXES

Primitive reflexes are automatic movements that are usually stimulated by sensory factors and performed without conscious volition. Primitive reflexes cause the first involuntary movements to occur and allow for extension movements to emerge. Primitive reflexes are controlled at the lower levels of the central nervous system. As the higher levels (cerebral hemispheres) mature, the expression of primitive reflexes is inhibited by these higher levels (i.e., they seem to disappear).

RIGHTING REACTIONS

Righting reactions are postural responses to changes of head and body positions. Righting reactions bring the head and trunk back into an upright position. These reactions involve movements called *extension, flexion, abduction, adduction,* and *lateral flexion.*

EQUILIBRIUM REACTIONS

Equilibrium reactions are automatic, compensatory movements of the body parts that are used to maintain the center of gravity over the base of support when either the center of gravity or the supporting surface is displaced. These complex postural responses combine righting reactions with movements known as rotational and diagonal patterns. Essential for volitional movement and mobility, the use of righting reactions begins at 6 months and continues throughout life.

PROTECTIVE EXTENSION RESPONSES

Protective extension responses are postural reactions that are used to stop a fall or to prevent injury when equilibrium reactions fail to do so. These responses involve straightening of the arms or legs toward a supporting surface. Essential for mobility, the use of protective extension reactions begins between 6 and 9 months and continues throughout life.

Adapted from Alexander R, Boehme R, Cupps B: Normal development of functional motor skills, Tucson, AR, 1993, Therapy Skill Builders; Bly L: *Motor skills acquisition in the first year: An illustrated guide to normal development,* Tucson, AR, 1994, Therapy Skills Builders: Florentino MR: *Reflex testing methods for evaluating CNS development,* ed 2, Springfield, IL, 1981, Charles C Thomas; Simon CJ, Daub MM: Human development across the life span. In Hopkins JL, Smith HD, editors: *Willard and Spackman's occupational therapy,* ed 8, Philadelphia, 1993, Lippincott.

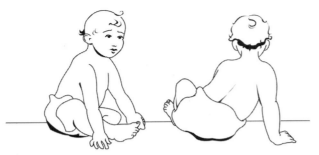

FIGURE 7-1 Equilibrium reactions allow infants to protect themselves by automatically moving forward and sideways after losing balance in the sitting position or when moving from one position to a different one.

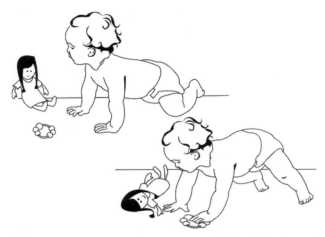

FIGURE 7-2 Infant transition from quadruped (hands and knees) position to vaulting position.

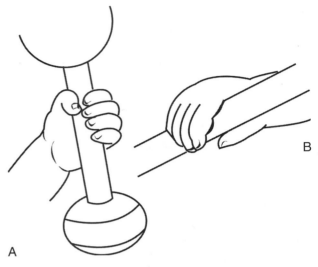

FIGURE 7-3 A, When using the ulnar palmar grasp, the infant places his or her fingers on the top surface of the object, pressing it into the center of the palm toward the little finger. **B,** When using the radial palmar grasp, the infant holds the object between the thumb and the radial side of the palm.

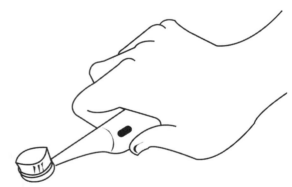

FIGURE 7-4 When using the superior pincer grasp, the infant holds a small object between the tips of the index finger and thumb. The wrist is slightly extended, with the ring and little fingers curled into the palm.

thumb and fingertips), and the ability to voluntarily release an object begins to emerge. At about 9 months, the infant learns to use an inferior pincer grasp (the pad of the thumb is pressed to the pad of the index finger) to pick up a small object. By 10 months, the infant can release an object into a container. By 12 months, he or she uses a superior pincer grasp (the tip of the thumb is pressed to the tip of the index finger) (Figure 7-4) and consistently puts objects into containers. By 12 months, the fine motor skills are developed enough to allow the infant to combine objects and explore their functional uses. These fine motor skills facilitate the development of functional and symbolic play skills.[6,13,16]

Interrelatedness of Development Skills

It is important to note how the interrelatedness of skills affects development. When the newborn is placed in the prone position during periods of alertness, the position of physiologic flexion raises the pelvis off the surface, transferring much of the infant's weight to the head and shoulders. In addition, this position places the hands beside the cheeks. As the infant turns, the head, the mouth, and cheeks rub against the surface, providing the sensory input necessary to elicit the rooting reflex. When the infant turns the head and opens the mouth to root, he or she is able to suck on the hands.[1] This input to the cheeks also helps develop oral motor skills, such as sucking and chewing. As the infant grows, time in the prone position (or "tummy time") will afford the opportunity to raise the head and provide deep-pressure input to the ulnar side and the palm of the hands. This input to the hands facilitates the development of ulnar and palmar grasps. By 6 months, as the infant shifts weight in the prone position, this position provides deep-pressure input to the radial side of the hand, facilitating the radial digital grasp. It is important for the OT practitioner to emphasize the importance of "tummy time" to facilitate the development of oral motor and fine motor skills.

Process/Cognition Development

The infant's cognitive development can be described using Piaget's theory, which states that individuals pass through a series of stages of thought as they progress from infancy to adolescence. These stages are a result of the biologic pressure to adapt to the changing environment and organize structures of thinking. According to Piaget, cognitive development is divided into four stages: (1) sensorimotor, (2) preoperational, (3) concrete operational, and (4) formal operational. During the sensorimotor stage, the infant develops the ability to organize and coordinate sensations with physical movements and actions. As shown in Table 7-3, the sensorimotor period has six substages.[19,27,30]

During the first stage, known as the *reflexive stage*, behavior is dominated by reflexes such as sucking and the palmar grasp. A rattle placed in an infant's hand is retained by the grasp reflex. Random motor movement causes the infant to accidentally shake the rattle. In the second stage, referred to as *primary circular reactions*, the infant repeats the reflexive movements and patterns simply for pleasure. During this stage, he or she may accidentally get the fingers to the mouth and begin to suck on them. The infant then searches for the fingers again but has trouble getting them to the mouth because the coordination to do so has not been mastered yet. The infant repeats this action until the fingers get to the mouth. In the third stage, called *secondary circular reactions*, the infant begins to use voluntary movements to repeat actions that accidentally produced a desirable result. At this age, an infant who accidentally hits a rattle with the foot while kicking would repeat the same kicking movement to reproduce the sound, thus creating a learned scheme, or mental plan, that can be used to reproduce the sound. During the fourth stage, referred to as *coordination of secondary schemata*, several significant changes take place. The infant readily combines previously learned schemes and generalizes them for use in new situations. For example, the infant may visually inspect and touch a toy simultaneously. The major advancement during this period is the emergence of object permanence. The infant searches for an object that seems to have disappeared. In addition, he or she uses existing schemes to obtain a desired object. For example, the infant may pull a string to get an attached toy or object. During the stage called *tertiary circular reactions*, he or she repeatedly attempts a task and modifies the behavior to achieve the desired consequences. The repetition helps the infant understand the concept of cause–effect relationships. Another important hallmark of this stage is the use of tools, such as using a cup to drink something. During the last stage of the sensorimotor period, known as *inventions of new means through mental combinations*, the toddler begins using trial and error to solve problems. For example, he or she learns that pulling on a tablecloth will bring down a plate of cookies to the floor. During the last stage, the child also uses "pretend" play to create new roles for various objects. For example, stuffed animals that were previously used while teething or to hit other objects are now considered playmates (see Table 7-3).[19,27,30]

Communication and Interaction/Psychosocial Development

Language Development

The development of language is closely related to both cognitive and **psychosocial development**.[13] Undifferentiated crying characterizes the newborns' "language." By 3 months, their vocalizations are called *cooing* and usually consist of pleasant vowel sounds. Around 4 months, they begin to *babble*, or repeat a string of vowel and consonant sounds. From birth to 4 months, infants are "universal linguists"—they are capable of distinguishing among the 150 sounds that constitute all human speech. By 6 months, they recognize only the speech sounds of their native language.[23] By the age of 8 months, infants develop a sense of the existence of others, recognizing and imitating the actions of caregivers. They repeat sounds, which is referred to as *lallation* when the repetition is accidental and *echolalia* when the repetition is conscious. By 12 months, infants know between two and eight words and babble short sentences. Their vocabulary increases significantly during the second year. By 24 months, toddlers may have 50 to 200 words in their spoken vocabulary.[13]

Psychosocial Development

The psychosocial development of newborns begins with the earliest emotional connections and interactions with their caregivers. The development of this emotional connection, or feeling of love, between newborns and their caregivers was first examined in the context of attachment, or the development of affectionate ties to the mother by the infant. Ainsworth outlined four stages in the development of infants' attachment to their caregivers.[3]

1. *Initial attachment*: At 2 to 3 months, infants exhibit nondiscriminating social responses.
2. *Attachment in the making*: By 4 to 6 months, infants begin to distinguish between familiar and unfamiliar persons.

TABLE 7-3

Normal Development of Cognitive Skills

AGE	PIAGET'S SENSORIMOTOR PERIOD (BIRTH–2 YR)	COGNITIVE MILESTONES
BIRTH OR 37–40 WK OF GESTATION	REFLEXIVE STAGE	Uses entire body during vocalizations Primarily uses abdomen to breathe Becomes quiet in response to a voice Slowly follows moving objects visually (tracks)
1–2 MO	REFLEXIVE STAGE (1 mo)	Still closely associates all sounds with movement Begins displaying primitive reflexes Does not differentiate between self and objects or between sensation and action Still primarily uses abdomen to breathe, displays rhythmic breathing patterns while at rest Begins to explore environment by putting objects into mouth Stops all activity and experiences a change in breathing patterns while focusing on an object or person Has smoother visual tracking skills
3–5 MO	PRIMARY CIRCULAR REACTIONS (2–4 mo)	Begins to put hand on bottle and find mouth Repeats reflexive sensory motor patterns for pleasure Experiences transition from watching own hands to putting own hands in mouth Increases variety of sounds; exhibits less nasal crying Understands conception of object permanence Experiences transition from searching for only dropped objects to searching for partially hidden objects Pats bottle during feeding
6 MO	SECONDARY CIRCULAR REACTIONS (5–8 mo)	Calls out to get attention Repeats own sounds Uses increasingly varied sounds Increasingly dissociates sounds from movement Understands concept of cause and effect; repeats certain patterns of actions involving objects or people to achieve a particular result Begins to show true voluntary movement patterns Repeats actions that create pleasurable sensations Has a primitive awareness of cause and effect
7–9 MO	CIRCULAR REACTIONS (2–4 mo)	Puts objects in containers Copies movements such as banging objects together Begins to search for objects in containers Responds to word "no" Explores spatial concepts such as in/out and off/on by experimenting with different movements while playing
10–12 MO	COORDINATON OF SECONDARY SCHEMATA (9–12 mo)	Shows a desire for independence in motor development and skills Follows simple directions Uses objects to reach goal in independent problem-solving activities Begins to participate in object permanence problem-solving activities Begins to be capable of decentralized thought (i.e. realization that objects exist apart from self, in different contexts and when out of sight)
13–18 MO	TERTIARY CIRCULAR REACTIONS (12–18 mo)	Solves problems by trial and error Uses objects conventionally and begins to group Uses speech to name, refuse, call, greet, protest, and express feelings Begins to use tools Searches for new schemes

TABLE 7-3

Normal Development of Cognitive Skills—cont'd

AGE	PIAGET'S SENSORIMOTOR PERIOD (BIRTH–2 YR)	COGNITIVE MILESTONES
19–24 MO	INVENTIONS OF NEW MEANS THROUGH MENTAL COMBINATIONS (18–24 mo)	Follows two-step directions Understands object permanence and engages in systematic searching Uses speech as a significant means of communication Begins to show insight Begins to purposefully use tools Mental representation is the hallmark of this stage Develops stability to use mental representation (i.e. label and symbolically use mental schemes to present concepts)

Adapted from Case-Smith J, Shortridge SD: The developmental process: Prenatal to adolescence. In Case-Smith J, Allen AS, Pratt PN, editors: *Occupational therapy for children*, ed 3, St Louis, 1996, Mosby; Maier HW: *Three theories of child development*, rev ed, New York, 1965, Harper & Row.

3. *Clear-cut, or active, attachment*: By 6 to 7 months, infants become more attached to one primary caregiver, seeking proximity to and contact with that person.
4. *Multiple attachments*: After 12 months, infants become attached to persons other than their primary caregivers.

Another facet of the infant–caregiver relationship is called *bonding*, which is characterized by behaviors such as stroking, kissing, cuddling, and prolonged gazing. These behaviors serve two functions: (1) expressing affection and (2) sustaining an interaction between caregivers and infants. By the time infants are 1 month of age, most parents are attuned to them and are able to interpret their cries and comfort them; in other words, a goodness of fit, or a match between infants' temperaments and their environments, exists between their needs and their caregivers' reactions. Caregivers also begin to recognize the early indicators of changes in their infants' temperaments and know ways to calm them or prevent overstimulation.[3,9,27]

Two theories of psychosocial and emotional development in infancy are highlighted in Table 7-4. According to Greenspan, the first stage is called *self-regulation and interest in the world*.[22] During the first few months after birth, the infant is focused on organizing the internal and external worlds, and the job of the primary caregiver(s) is to help him or her regulate these influences. Around the second or third month, the infant moves into the "falling-in-love" stage, in which he or she forms strong a attachment to the primary caregiver(s). He or she responds to the facial expressions and vocalizations of the caregivers with smiles and coos. From 3 to 10 months, the infant begins to learn the art

of purposeful communication. At this stage, smiling is purposeful; he or she has learned that smiling causes adults to smile back. Around 9 or 10 months, the infant develops an organized sense of self and begins to realize how behaviors can be used to get different reactions from others.[22]

EARLY CHILDHOOD

Four-year-old Phillip spends time practicing his fine motor skills. He enjoys drawing pictures and telling long, sometimes exaggerated stories to go with his pictures. When playing with other children in the neighborhood, Phillip tends to play with boys. The boys tend to play rougher games than the girls.

Physiological Development

The beginning of the early childhood period is "marked by the development of autonomy, the beginning of expressive language, and sphincter control."[13] The rapid growth of infancy slows as children enter their second and third years. Their limbs begin to grow faster than do their heads, making their bodies seem less top-heavy. By 6 years, the legs make up almost 45% of the body length, and the children are about seven times their birth weight. The brain of a 5-year-old child is 75% of its adult weight.[14,33,34] Changes in physiological pathways give children the sphincter control necessary for toilet training.[13]

The physiological differences between children in the early childhood stage and adults are significant. The eustachian tube is shorter and positioned more horizontally than that of adults, making children more susceptible to middle ear infections. The digestive tract is not fully mature, and the shape of the stomach is straight, resulting

TABLE 7-4

Psychosocial and Emotional Development

PERIOD	AGE (YR)	ERIKSON	GREENSPAN	TYPICAL BEHAVIORS

INFANCY	0–1	TRUST VERSUS MISTRUST
		Has needs gratified
		Gives to others in return
		Develops drive and hope
			SELF-REGULATION (0–3 mo)
			Calms self
			Regulates sleep
			Notices sights and sounds
			Enjoys touch and movement
				Has fussy periods to
				  relieve stress
				Smiles
				Imitates gestures
				Uses special smiles for
				  different people and
				  events
				May experience joy and
				  anger

			FALLING IN LOVE (2–7 mo)
			Is wooed by significant others
			Responds to facial expressions
			  and vocalizations
			Attachment
			PURPOSEFUL COMMUNICA-
			  TION (3–10 mo)
			Displays reciprocal interactions
			  when initiated by adult
			Initiates interactions
				Fears strangers (8 mo)
				Gives affection
				Learns about cause and
				  effect
				Understands concept of
				  object permanence

EARLY
  CHILDHOOD
	1–3	AUTONOMY VERSUS
		  SHAME AND DOUBT
		Considers self separate
		  from parents
		Develops self-control and
		  willpower
		Struggles with a conflict
		  between holding on and
		  letting go
			EMERGENCE OF
			  ORGANIZED SENSE
			  OF SELF (9–18 mo)
			Knows ways to get different
			  types of reactions
			Is focused and organized while
			  playing
			Initiates complex behaviors
			Is capable of feeling embarrass-
			  ment, pride, shame, joy,
			  empathy, anger
				Early:
				Attaches to transitional
				  object (such as
				  blanket)
				Imitates others
				Understands function of
				  objects and means of
				  behaviors
				May experience joy and
				  anger
				Late:
				Is egocentric
				Experiences separation
				  anxiety (2 yr)

			CREATING EMOTIONAL
			  IDEAS (18–36 mo)
			Uses words and gestures
			Participates in pretend play with
			  others
			Learns to recover from anger
			  or temper tantrums
			Starts associating particular
			  functions with certain people
				Loves an audience and
				  attention
				Often says phrases like
				  "me do it" and "no"
				Has difficulty sharing
				Begins to become
				  independent and
				  spend time alone

TABLE 7-4

Normal Development of Cognitive Skills—cont'd

PERIOD	AGE (YR)	ERIKSON	GREENSPAN	TYPICAL BEHAVIORS
		INITIATIVE AND IMAGI-NATION VERSUS GUILT Displays purpose in actions Has a lively imagination Tests reality Imitates parental actions and roles Seeks new experiences that if successful lead to sense of initiative, needs balance between initiative and responsibility for own actions Accepts consequences of actions Makes choices and plans	EMOTIONAL THINKING (30–48 mo) Differentiates between real and unreal Follows rules Understands relationships among behaviors, feelings, and consequences (is capable of feeling guilty) Interacts in socially appropriate ways with adults and peers	Seems optimistic and confident Asks why Is spontaneous Seeks other playmates Fears monsters, spiders, and so on, has bad dreams (4–5 yr) Plays with imaginary playmates Tells exaggerated stories
MIDDLE CHILDHOOD	5–11	INDUSTRY VERSUS INFERIORITY Sees work as pleasurable Develops sense of responsibility and competence Learns work habits Learns to use tools Likes recognition for accomplishments Is sensitive to performance in comparison with others Tries new activities Becomes scholastically and socially competent	THE WORLD IS MY OYSTER (5–7 yr) Carries out self-care and self-regulatory functions with minimum assistance Enjoys relationship with parents Takes simultaneous interest in wants and needs of parents, peers, and "me first" Forms relationships with peers Struggles to assert own will with peers Better handles not getting own way Better understands reasons for reality limits THE WORLD IS OTHER KIDS (8–10 yr) Cares about role in peer group Has best friends and regular friends Maintains nurturing relationship with parents Continues to enjoy fantasy Follows rules Orders emotions and groups them into categories Experiences competition without becoming aggressive or compliant	**Early (5-7):** Acts assertive and bossy: acts like a "know-it-all" Is critical of self Experiences night-terrors Shares and takes turns May experience joy and anger **Late (9-11):** Desires privacy Acts with impulsivity and more control Looks up to and focuses on being like a certain person a "hero" ("hero worship") Becomes more competitive Expects perfection from others (1 yr)

Continued

TABLE 7-4

Normal Development of Cognitive Skills—cont'd

PERIOD	AGE (YR)	ERIKSON	GREENSPAN	TYPICAL BEHAVIORS
ADOLESCENCE		SELF-IDENTITY VERSUS ROLE CONFUSION Has a temporal perspective Experiments with roles (parents, friends, various groups) Enters sexual relationship Shares self with others Develops ideological commitments	THE WORLD IS INSIDE ME (11-12 yr) Has a developing internal sense of right and wrong Enjoys one or a few intimate friends Takes interest in adults as role models Uses rules flexibly by understanding context Takes interest in opposite sex Has feelings of privacy about own body Has concerns about body and personality related to puberty	Acts as if *right now* is most important thing in life Accepts and adjusts to changing body Plays to imaginary audience Believes in personal fable (of infallibility) and characterized by the phrase "It won't happen to me" Begins working Achieves emotional independence

Courtesy Jayne Shepherd. Adapted from Erikson EH: *Childhood and society*, ed 2, New York, 1963, WW Norton; Greenspan SI: *Playground politics: Understanding the emotional life of your school-aged child*, Reading, MA, 1993, Addison-Wesley; Greenspan S, Greenspan N: *First feelings: Milestones in the emotional development of your baby and child*, New York, 1985, Viking Penguin.

in frequent upset stomachs. Because of the immaturity of the retina, young children are farsighted.[13]

Motor Development

All of the basic components of motor development such as vision, touch, gross motor skills, and fine motor skills exist physiologically during the second and third years. These components are developed as skills and refined through interactions with the environment. Balance and strength increase during the early childhood period. At 2 years of age, toddlers walk with an increased stride length, and by 4 years, their walking pattern more closely resembles that of an adult. The ability to run develops around 3 to 4 years; by 5 or 6 years, a mature running pattern develops. Two-year-old children can climb stairs without holding on to a support; by 3½ years, children are able to walk up and down the stairs independently and with alternating feet.[13]

Like gross motor skills, the coordination and precision of hand and finger movements are refined with maturation and practice, especially when children enter preschool and school. At 2 years, one of the major accomplishments of children is learning to draw. The first type of grasp they learn is the palmar grasp; however, during the second year, they develop the ability to hold a pencil in the hand rather than in the fist. As thumb, finger, and hand precision improves enough to allow children to use the tripod grasp, their drawings progress from scribbles to deliberate

lines and shapes. Mature, dynamic tripod grasp develops by 5 years (Figure 7-5). Three-year-old children are able to snip paper with scissors, and more mature skills with scissors develop around 5 to 6 years.[11,13]

Process/Cognition Development

Piaget's second phase of development, the preoperational period, occurs between the ages of 2 and 7 years; 2- to 4-year-old children are in the preconceptual substage of preoperational thought. The beginning of symbolic thought and strong egocentrism and the emergence of animism characterize this substage. The ability to use symbolism means that the child is able to mentally consider objects that are not present around them. *Egocentrism* is the inability of individuals to realize that others have thoughts and feelings that may not be the same as their own. *Animism* is the mental act of giving inanimate objects lifelike qualities; this characteristic develops around age 3.[34] Children between the ages of 5 and 7 years are in a substage of preoperational thought called *intuitive thought*.

Communication and Interaction/ Psychosocial Development
Language Development

During this phase, cognitive and language development is characterized by the use of symbolism. At this time, children begin to engage in symbolic, or pretend, play

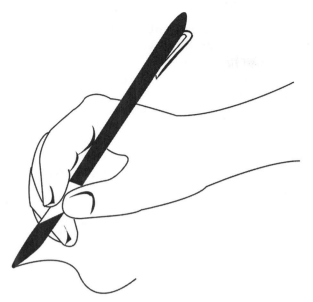

FIGURE 7-5 When using the dynamic tripod grasp, the child holds a pencil with the thumb and index and middle fingers. The fingers move, while other joints of the arm remain stable.

and tend to think more logically. They are able to use words and gestures to represent real objects or events.[13] Their vocabulary expands rapidly, increasing from a repertoire of 200 words at 2 years to 1500 words at 3 years. Two-year-old children label items and ask simple questions, whereas 3-year-old children can express their thoughts and feelings in simple sentences. By age 4, children can narrate long stories, which are sometimes exaggerated. Children 5 or 6 years old are able to enunciate clearly and use their advanced language skills as a tool for learning. For example, they commonly ask questions such as "What is this for?" "How does this work?" and "What does it mean?"[11]

Psychosocial Development

According to Erikson, the 2-to 4-year-old period of early childhood is referred to as the *stage of autonomy versus shame and doubt*. During this stage, a need to be autonomous dominates children's psychosocial development; they are determined to make their own decisions and be independent. Central to this stage is the period known as the *terrible two's*, in which 2-year-olds try to establish their independence. According to Erikson's theories, children begin to doubt themselves and feel ashamed if they are not given adequate opportunities for self-regulation.[10,13,17] Those between the ages of 4 and 6 years are in the stage Erikson calls *initiative and imagination versus guilt*. On the one hand, children show initiative in activities in which their behavior produces successful, effective results and meets with parental approval. On the other hand, guilt results when children assume a sense of responsibility for their own behavior. By imitating others, they learn to take responsibility for their own actions and develop a sense of purpose. Gender role development also occurs during this stage.[11,13,36]

The early childhood years comprise two of Greenspan's stages, which are called *creating emotional ideas* and *emotional thinking*. In the stage of creating emotional ideas, 2-year-olds express them by using words and gestures, engaging in pretend play, and starting to associate certain functions with certain people. In the stage of emotional thinking, 3- and 4-year-olds are able to differentiate between what is real and what is not, follow rules, and understand the relationships between behaviors and feelings.[22]

MIDDLE CHILDHOOD

Ten-year-old Phillip is very concerned about being accepted in his peer group—he insists on wearing the same tennis shoes as the other boys. He and his friends spend hours playing seemingly endless baseball games. They follow the rules but do not really keep scores.

Physiological Development

Between early childhood and adolescence, the growth rate slows down. Although wide variations in growth occur in both sexes during middle childhood, girls and boys typically grow an average of 2 to 3 inches per year, with their legs becoming longer and trunks slimmer.[34] Girls typically grow taller than do boys during this period. Facial features become more distinct and unique, partly because baby teeth have been replaced by permanent teeth. The digestive system matures, so children retain food in the digestive system longer; they eat less frequently but have increased appetites and eat greater quantities.[13] By the age of 10, head and brain growth is 95% complete. Hearing acuity increases, and changes in the position of the eustachian tube decrease the risk of middle ear infections.[12,34]

Motor Development

Because the rate of physical development slows down during middle childhood, children have the opportunity to refine their gross motor skills and become generally more adept at handling their bodies. Children tend to focus on the refinement of previously learned skills. Hours of repetition leads to mastery of these skills, which creates higher self-esteem and greater acceptance from peers.[7] Increased muscle strength and endurance allow children to become more physical; their favorite activities often include running, climbing, throwing, riding a bicycle, swimming, and skating.[34] Refined fine motor skills allow children to improve their performance of tasks such as sewing, using garden tools, and writing. The task of writing is a combination of refined grasping skills and coordinated movements that result in smooth writing strokes and smaller letters. By the age of 10 years, most children have converted from writing in printed letters to writing in cursive letters.[13]

Process/Cognition Development

The middle childhood years, 7 to 11 years, include the Piaget stage of concrete operations. This stage marks the beginning of the ability to think abstractly, or to mentally manipulate actions. For example, children are able to envision what might happen if they threw a rock across the room, without actually throwing a rock. Other characteristics of the concrete operational period include the following:[34]

- Being less self-centered
- Being able to recognize that others may have viewpoints that differ from their own
- Being able to identify similarities and differences among objects
- Being able to use simple logic to arrive at a conclusion
- Being able to simultaneously consider many aspects of a situation rather than just one
- Realizing that a substance's quantity does not change when its form does
- Being able to order objects by size, indicating an understanding of the relationships among objects
- Being able to imagine objects or pieces as parts of a whole

Using Piaget's ideas as a basis, Kohlberg formulated schemes of moral development. During the early elementary years (between the ages of 4 and 10 years), children are in what he calls the *preconventional level of moral development*. They make moral judgments solely on the basis of anticipated punishment or reward (i.e., a "right" or "good" action is one that feels good and is rewarded, and a "wrong" or "bad" action is one that results in punishment[34]). Between 10 and 13 years, children enter a stage called the *morality of conventional role conformity*. They are eager to please others and therefore tend to internalize rules (by applying them to themselves) and judge their actions according to set standards. Ten- and 11-year-olds are concerned about meeting the expectations and following the rules of their peer group. This stage is characterized by conforming, following the "Golden Rule" ("Do unto others as you would have them do unto you"), and showing respect for authority and rules.[31]

Communication and Interaction/Psychosocial Development

Language Development

During middle childhood, the vocabulary of children expands, partly as a result of their focus on reading. Puns and figures of speech become meaningful, and children's jokes are based on the dual meaning of words, slang, curse words, colloquialisms, and secret languages.[19] Communication among children during the middle childhood years has been described as *socialized communication*—conversations center around school activities, personal experiences, families and pets, sports, clothes, movies, television, comics, and "taboo" subjects such as sex, cursing, and drinking.[31]

Psychosocial Development

When children begin attending elementary school, their families are no longer the sole source of security and relationships. During this period, significant social relationships are developed outside the family in the neighborhood and school. In middle childhood, the feeling of belonging is very important to children, so they become increasingly concerned about their status among peers. They seem to have their own personal societies, separate from the adult world, that include rituals, heroes, and peer groups.[7,13,31] Peer groups usually comprise children of the same sex. Girls and boys tend to engage in their own activities, with little communication between the two groups. During this period, children experience more pressure to conform than during any other period of development. Children struggle to simultaneously participate in group activities while balancing the group's identity with their own and establishing their roles within the group.[19]

The middle childhood years include the stage Erikson named *industry versus inferiority*. He believed that children must learn new skills to survive in their culture; if unsuccessful, they develop a sense of inferiority.[19] During this stage, the source of children's feelings of security switches from family to peer group as they try to master the activities of their friends. Greenspan described the 8- to 10-year-old developmental stage as *the world is other kids*.[21] Children develop a mental picture of themselves that is based on interactions with friends, family members, and teachers. The stage called *the world inside me* is representative of an 11-year-old's definition of self, which is based on personal characteristics rather than the peer group's perceptions. At this age, children are able to empathize and understand the feelings of others. They realize that relationships require constant mutual adjustments, so they are able to disagree with a friend but still maintain the friendship.[21]

ADOLESCENCE

Fifteen-year-old Phillip wants to get a job in the music store at the mall. He thinks he would be good at the job because of his extensive knowledge of popular bands and musicians. An additional benefit is that all his friends hang out at the mall.

Physiological Development

Adolescence is a period characterized by many dramatic physiological changes, some of which are related to the adolescent growth spurt and some to the onset of puberty. Preadolescence, characterized by little physical growth, is followed by a period of rapid growth, indicating the onset of puberty.[40] The growth spurt is triggered by neural and hormonal signals to the hypothalamus, resulting in the increased production of and sensitivity to certain hormones. The onset of puberty in boys occurs between 10½ and 16 years, with the average age being 12½ years. The onset in girls occurs between 9½ and 15 years, with the average age being 10½ years. Although boys begin their growth spurt later than do girls, their growth spurt tends to be greater, with height increasing by 8.3 inches, compared with girls' height increasing by 7.7 inches.[15,26,40]

The onset of puberty is usually associated with the first signs of sexual development. The first visible sign of puberty in girls is breast growth, which begins around 10½ years. The average age of menarche is 12.8 years.[33] The onset of puberty in boys is signified by enlargement of the testes, which occurs between the ages of 10 and 13½ years.[15] As the age of the onset of puberty is quite variable, only a range of ages is given here.

Boys who mature earlier than others are described more positively by peers, teachers, and themselves. They tend to be the most popular, are better at sports, and begin dating with more ease than those who mature later. Boys who mature later are described as less attractive, more childish, and less masculine.[15,32,37] In the case of girls, the scenario is reversed. Those who mature the earliest sometimes have a poor body image and low self-esteem. They tend to confide in and share their experiences with older adolescents. Girls who mature later develop at the same age as do their male peers and are likely to develop a better self-concept than do those who mature earlier.[15,32,37] These differences in the rates of development greatly affect adolescents' self-concept and self-esteem. To help ease the transition, adults can educate adolescents about the following:

- Health and preparation for puberty
- Nutrition
- Issues such as smoking prevention, automobile safety, and contraception
- Developing autonomy and independence[39]

Motor Development

The development of gross motor skills in adolescents is directly related to the physical changes that are occurring. Increased muscle mass provides increased dynamic strength, as evidenced by better running, jumping, and throwing skills.[4] Because boys have a greater percentage of muscle mass than do girls, their strength is greater.[7] In addition, motor coordination stops improving in girls around 15 years but keeps improving in boys beyond this age. Fine motor abilities also tend to differ between the sexes. Girls show greater rates of improvement in hand-eye coordination, but overall they still do not perform as well as boys do when it comes to motor skills.[4,36,40]

Process/Cognition Development

The development of formal operational thought is the hallmark of adolescence.[13] Adolescents have the ability to think about possibilities as well as realities. They can formulate hypotheses about the outcome of a certain situation, and after imagining all the possible results, they can test each hypothesis to determine which one is true.[15] This process is called *hypothetical deductive reasoning.*

Adolescents develop their moral thought in the period known as the *conventional level* of Kohlberg's stages. During this stage, adolescents approach moral problems in a social context; they want to please others by being good members of society. Adolescents follow the standards of others, conform to social conventions, support the status quo, and generally try to please others and obey the law.[32]

Communication and Interaction/ Psychosocial Development
Language Development

In high school, adolescents manipulate language; for example, they use codes, slang, and sarcasm. The use of slang during adolescence is important for establishing group membership and being accepted by peers. They also have the cognitive ability to use language for more than simple communication. For example, they can participate in debates or class discussions and argue against a position that they do not agree with; this abstract use of language is not understood by children at younger ages.[7]

Egocentrism

Adolescents tend to believe that if something is of great concern to them, then it is also of great concern to others. Because they believe that others have thoughts similar to their own, they tend to be self-conscious, or *egocentric*. This egocentrism manifests itself in adolescents as having an imaginary audience, or a perception that everyone is watching them. Another way egocentrism manifests itself is through the *personal fable*, or the idea that they are special, have completely unique experiences, and are not subject to the natural rules governing the rest of the world. Egocentrism is the cause of much of the self-destructive behavior of many adolescents who think that they are magically protected from all harm.[32]

Identity

Erikson referred to the adolescent stage of development as *identity versus identity confusion*. During this stage, the main goal for adolescents is to find or understand their identities. They work to form a new sense of self by combining past experiences with future expectations. This process allows adolescents to understand themselves in terms of who they have been and who they hope to become.[17]

The establishment of an occupational identity is one part of the establishment of ego identity. A number of theories about occupational development exist. Ginzberg outlined three periods that apply to this stage: (1) a fantasy period, (2) a tentative period, and (3) a realistic period.[20] Two of Super's stages also apply to adolescents: (1) the growth stage and (2) the exploration stage.[38] Adolescents explore various occupations, identify with workers in a specific occupation, discover which occupations they enjoy, and develop basic habits of work and an identity as a worker.

Peers

Peer groups support adolescents as they experience the transition from childhood to adulthood.[13] Involvement in peer groups provides opportunities to accomplish the following:

- Sharing responsibilities for their own affairs
- Experimenting with new ways of handling new situations
- Learning from each other's mistakes
- Trying out new roles[26]

Early adolescence (ages 12 to 14 years) is the time when children are most concerned about conforming to the values and practices of their peer groups. Older adolescents are less likely to conform to a group and more likely to rely on their own independent thinking and judgment.[26]

Parents

Even though adolescents spend more time with friends, parents still have considerable effects on them. Although adolescents seek the advice of peers on matters such as social activities, dress, and hobbies, they seek the advice of their parents on issues such as occupations, college, and money.[35]

SUMMARY

From birth through adolescence, infants and children progress through a series of stages of development. The sequences of physiological, sensorimotor, cognitive and language, and psychosocial development outlined in this chapter are typical; however, it should be noted that each individual child progresses through these sequences at a different rate. The OT practitioner should consider any physical, social, and cultural factors in the environment that may affect a client's developmental sequence.

References

1. Alexander R, Boehme R, Cupps B: *Normal development of functional motor skills*, Tucson, 1993, Therapy Skill Builders.
2. American Occupational Therapy Association: Occupational therapy practice framework: domain and process, ed 2. *Am J Occup Ther* 62:625–683, 2008.
3. Ainsworth M: Attachment retrospect and prospect. In Parkes CM, Stevenson-Hind M, editors: *The place of attachment in human behavior*, New York, 1982, Basic Books.
4. Ausubel DP: *Theories and problems of adolescent development*, ed 3, 2002, Writers Club Press, iUniverse, Inc.
5. Bax M, Hart H, Jenkins SM: *Child development and child health: the preschool years*, Oxford, 1989, Blackwell Scientific.
6. Benbow M: *Neurokinesthetic approach to hand function and handwriting*, Albuquerque, 1995, Clinician's View.
7. Berger KS: *The developing person through childhood and adolescence*, ed 8, New York, 2009, Worth Publishers.
8. Bly L: *Motor skills acquisition in the first year: an illustrated guide to normal development*, Tucson, 1998, Therapy Skill Builders.
9. Brazelton TB, Nugent JK: *Neonatal behavioral assessment scale*, ed 3, Philadelphia, 1995, Lippincott.
10. Caplan T, Caplan F: *The first twelve months of life*, New York, 1995, Bantam Books.
11. Caplan T, Caplan F: *The early childhood years: the 2 to 6 year old*, New York, 1984, Bantam Books.
12. Bazyk S, Case-Smith J: School-based occupational therapy. In Case-Smith J, O'Brien J, editors: *Occupational therapy for children*, ed 6, St. Louis, 2010, Mosby.
13. Case-Smith J: Development of childhood occupations. In Case-Smith J, O'Brien J, editors: *Occupational therapy for children*, ed 6, St. Louis, 2010, Mosby.
14. Dacey JS, Travers JF: *Human development across the lifespan*, ed 7, New York, 2008, McGraw-Hill.
15. Dusek JB: *Adolescent development and behavior*, ed 3, Englewood Cliffs, NJ, 1995, Prentice Hall.

16. Erhardt RP: *Developmental hand dysfunction: theory, assessment, and treatment*, ed 2, Tucson, 1999, Therapy Skill Builders.

17. Erikson EH: *Childhood and society*, ed 2, New York, 1963, WW Norton.

18. Fraiberg SH: *The magic years: understanding and handling the problems of early childhood*, New York, 1959, Scribner.

19. Freiberg K: *Human development*, 99/00, Guilford, CT, 1999, McGraw-Hill/Dushin.

20. Ginzberg E: Toward a theory of occupational choice: a restatement. *Voc Guide Quart* 20:169, 1972.

21. Greenspan S: *Playground politics: understanding the emotional life of your school-aged child*, Reading, MA, 1994, Addison-Wesley.

22. Greenspan S, Greenspan N: *First feelings: milestones in the emotional development of your baby and child*, New York, 1994, Viking Penguin.

23. Grunwald L: The amazing minds of infants. In Junn EN, Boyatzis CJ, editors: *Annual editions: child growth and development*, Guilford, CT, 1995, Dushkin.

24. Haywood KM, Getchell N: *Life span motor development*, ed 5, Champaign, IL, 2008, Human Kinetics.

25. Hetherington EM et al: *Child psychology: a contemporary viewpoint*, ed 6, New York, 2005, McGraw-Hill.

26. Kimmel DC, Weiner IB: *Adolescence: a developmental transition*, ed 2, New York, 1995, John Wiley & Sons.

27. Lamb ME, Bornstein M: *Development in infancy: an introduction*, ed 4, Mahwah, NJ, 2002, Lawrence Erlbaum Associates.

28. Leach P: *Your baby and child: from birth to age five*, rev ed, New York, 1997, Knopf.

29. Lief NR, Fahs ME, Thomas RM: *The first three years of life*, New York, 1997, Smithmark.

30. Maier HW: *Three theories of child development*, rev ed, New York, 1965, Harper & Row.

31. Minuchin P: *The middle years of childhood*, Pacific Grove, CA, 1977, Brooks/Cole.

32. Papaplia DE, Olds SW, Feldman R: *Human development*, ed 11, New York, 2008, McGraw-Hill.

33. Payne VG, Isaacs LD: *Human motor development: a lifespan approach*, ed 7, London, 2007, Mayfield.

34. Santrock JW: *Life span development*, ed 12, New York, 2008, McGraw-Hill Humanities.

35. Sigelman CK, Rider EA: *Life span human development*, ed 6, Pacific Grove, CA, 2008, Brooks/Cole.

36. Simon CJ, Daub MM: Human development across the life span. In Crepeau EB, Cohn ES, Boyt Schell BA, editors: *Willard and Spackman's occupational therapy*, ed 11, Philadelphia, 2008, Lippincott.

37. Steinberg L: *Adolescence*, ed 8, New York, 2007, McGraw-Hill.

38. Super DE: *The psychology of careers*, New York, 1957, Harper & Row.

39. Vaughan VC, Litt IF: *Child and adolescent development: clinical implications*, Philadelphia, 1989, WB Saunders.

40. Watson RI, Lindgren HC: *Psychology of the child and the adolescent*, ed 4, New York, 1979, Macmillan.

Recommended Reading

Bee HL, Boyd DR: *The developing child*, ed 12, Needham Heights, MA, 2009, Allyn & Bacon.

Berk LE: *Infants, children, and adolescents*, ed 6, Boston, 2007, Allyn & Bacon.

Dixon SD, Stein MT: *Encounters with children: pediatric behavior and development*, ed 4, St. Louis, 2005, Mosby.

REVIEW *Questions*

1. What are primitive reflexes, righting reactions, equilibrium reactions, and protective extension?
2. Briefly describe the gross and fine motor skills of children at the following ages: 1 month, 6 months, 12 months, and 18 months.
3. What are four sequences of Piaget's stages of cognitive development? Give an example of a behavior that might be observed during each stage of cognitive development.
4. Why is Greenspan's stage for 2- to 7-month-olds called *falling in love*? Why is Greenspan's stage for 5- to 7-year-olds called *the world is my oyster*?
5. What are Erikson's five stages of development? Briefly describe each.

SUGGESTED *Activities*

1. Visit a nursery or a child care center that serves infants and toddlers. What postural reactions do you observe? Which ones can you elicit while playing with the infants?
2. Go to a nearby playground and watch normally developing children at play. Using the American Occupational Therapy Association's Occupational Therapy Practice Framework as a guide, record your observations. Develop a chart like the following one to summarize development throughout childhood.

	NEWBORN	I YEAR	4 YEARS	I0 YEARS	I5 YEARS
Physiological development					
Motor skills: gross					
Motor skills: fine					
Process/cognition					
Communication and interaction/psychosocial development					

8

Development of Occupations

DIANNE KOONTZ LOWMAN

JANE CLIFFORD O'BRIEN

JEAN W. SOLOMON

CHAPTER *Objectives*

After studying this chapter, the reader will be able to accomplish the following:

- Describe the developmental sequence of oral motor control.
- Identify the sequences of feeding and eating, dressing and undressing, and grooming and hygiene development.
- Identify the types of food and utensils that are appropriate for infants and young children of different ages.
- Identify the variables affecting a child's development of self-care skills.
- Describe age-appropriate home management activities.
- Discuss care of others as it relates to humans and animals.
- Describe developmentally appropriate activities considered as work or productive in the context of the Occupational Therapy Practice Framework.
- Explain the difference between formal and informal educational activities.
- Identify age-appropriate vocational activities.
- Define play and leisure skills.
- Describe the progression of play skills.
- Explain the relevance of play to occupational therapy practice.
- Identify occupational therapy professionals who have made significant contributions to the study of play.

KEY TERMS | CHAPTER OUTLINE

Area of occupation

Activities of daily living

Feeding

Eating

Dressing and undressing

Oral motor development

Personal hygiene and
grooming skills

Oral hygiene

Bathing and showering

Toilet hygiene

Instrumental activities of daily
living

Readiness skills

Home management activities

Community mobility

Care of others

Educational activities

Work

Vocational activities

Play

Leisure activities

Social participation

Activities of Daily Living
DEFINITION AND RATIONALE

FEEDING AND EATING SKILLS

Oral Motor Development

Infancy

Early Childhood

DRESSING AND UNDRESSING SKILLS

Infancy

Early Childhood

PERSONAL HYGIENE AND GROOMING

BATHING AND SHOWERING

TOILET HYGIENE

Instrumental Activities of Daily Living
READINESS SKILLS

HOME MANAGEMENT ACTIVITIES

COMMUNITY MOBILITY

CARE OF OTHERS

SUMMARY

Education
READINESS SKILLS

Preschool Readiness Skills

Kindergarten Readiness Skills

Elementary School Readiness Skills

Middle Childhood and Adolescent Readiness Skills

EDUCATIONAL ACTIVITIES

Work/Vocational Activities
SUMMARY

Play/Leisure Activities
DEFINITION OF PLAY

OCCUPATIONAL THERAPY THEORISTS AND THEIR CONTRIBUTIONS TO PLAY

Reilly

Takata

Knox

Bundy

PLAY SKILL ACQUISITION

Infancy

Early Childhood

Middle Childhood

Adolescence

DEVELOPMENTAL RELEVANCE OF PLAY AND LEISURE

SUMMARY

Social Participation

Chapter Summary

Occupational therapy (OT) practitioners focus on improving a child's ability to perform daily living, education, work, play and leisure, and social activities. These activities occur in cultural, physical, social, personal, and temporal contexts. The OT practitioner evaluates a child's ability to perform in these areas by examining the performance skills of each area. Knowledge of each **area of occupation** is therefore important to pediatric OT practice. This chapter provides a description of the areas of occupation within the framework of normal development.

Activities of Daily Living

DEFINITION AND RATIONALE

Activities of daily living (ADLs) constitute one of the areas of occupation described in the American Occupational Therapy Association's (AOTA's) Occupational Therapy Practice Framework.[2] The ADLs listed in Box 8-1 are the most basic tasks that children learn as they grow and mature.[34] Basic self-care skills include **feeding** and **eating, dressing and undressing,** and grooming and hygiene.[2] Because eating is a critical daily living skill essential to the child's survival, growth, health, and well-being, it falls within the OT practitioner's domain of concern.[3] A child with sufficient eating skills is able to actively bring food to the mouth without assistance. A child who requires feeding must receive assistance in the activity of eating.[3] Oral motor control relates to the child's ability to use the lips, cheeks, jaw, tongue, and palate.[36] **Oral motor development** refers to feeding, sound play, and oral exploration.[28] Feeding is an oral motor skill, but some

BOX 8-1

Activities of Daily Living

Bathing and showering
Bowel and bladder management
Toileting hygiene
Dressing and undressing
Eating and feeding
Functional mobility
Personal device care
Personal hygiene and grooming
Communicative device use
Community mobility
Health management/medication routine
Meal preparation and cleanup

From the American Occupational Therapy Association: Occupational therapy practice framework: Domain and process, (2nd ed), *Am J Occup Ther* 62:625–683, 2008.

oral motor skills, such as oral motor awareness and exploration, do not involve food at all.[14]

The normal development of oral motor skills related to eating and feeding involves sucking from a nipple, coordinating the suck–swallow–breathe sequence, drinking from a cup, and munching and chewing solid foods.[12,24,25] The maturation of these skills is closely tied to the physical maturation of the infant.

FEEDING AND EATING SKILLS
Oral Motor Development

The infant's oral mechanisms differ anatomically from those of the adult; the oral cavity of the infant appears to be filled by the tongue. The small oral cavity, coupled with sucking fat pads that stabilize the infant's cheeks, allows the infant to compress and suck on a nipple placed in the mouth. The limited mobility of the tongue results in the back and forth movement of the tongue known as *suckling*.[24,28,29] As the size ratios in the mouth change with the infant's growth, a more mature oral motor pattern emerges. By 4 to 6 months of age, the area inside the infant's mouth increases as the jaw grows and the sucking fat pads decrease. These changes allow increased movement of the infant's cheeks and lips. A "true sucking" pattern develops, as the infant's tongue can move up and down as well as forward and backward. Increased control of the jaw, lips, cheeks, and tongue allows the infant to move food and liquid toward the back of the mouth and prepares the infant to accept and control strained baby food.[28,30]

Full-term infants are born with reflexes that allow them to locate the source of food, suck, and then swallow. The following describes these reflexes in relation to oral motor development.[30]

- *Rooting reflex:* When the infant's cheeks or lips are stroked, he or she turns toward the stimulus. This reflex, which allows the infant to search for food, is maintained for a longer period in breast-fed infants.
- *Suck–swallow reflex:* When the infant's lips are touched, the mouth opens, and sucking movements begin.
- *Gag reflex:* The gag reflex protects the infant from swallowing anything that may block the airway.[28] At birth, the gag reflex is highly sensitive and elicited by stimulation to the back three fourths of the tongue. This reflex gradually moves to the back one fourth of the tongue as the infant matures and engages in oral play.
- *Phasic bite–release reflex:* When the infant's gums are stimulated, he or she responds with a rhythmic up-and-down movement of the jaw. This reflex forms the basis for munching and chewing.

- *Grasp reflex:* When a finger is pressed into the infant's palm, he or she grasps the finger. As the infant sucks, the grasp tightens, indicating a connection between sucking and the grasp reflex. Most of these early reflexive patterns begin to change or disappear between 4 and 6 months of age, when the cortex develops.[28,30]

Infancy

Oral skills develop concurrently and are closely related to the overall development of sensorimotor skills. Table 8-1 presents a brief overview of the development of normal sensorimotor, oral motor, and feeding skills during the first 3 years of life. Feeding initially requires that the adult provide head support and head–trunk alignment to enable the infant to coordinate the suck–swallow–breathe sequence. The infant's first suckling pattern predominates for the first 3 to 4 months of life.[12] Beginning at 4 months, a "true sucking" pattern—an up-and-down tongue movement—develops as head and jaw stability appears.

At 6 months, the infant has complete head control and more jaw stability, allowing for better control of tongue movements. This stability allows the infant to effectively suck from a bottle and take in soft food from a spoon.[24] At 4 to 5 months, the infant demonstrates a reflexive phasic bite–release pattern when given a soft cracker. With practice, the rhythm progresses into a munching pattern, which involves an up-and-down jaw movement. The munching pattern is effective for eating baby food or other dissolvable foods.[12,24] By 7 to 8 months, some diagonal jaw movements are added to the munching pattern. Infants use their fingers to eat soft crackers and cookies.[12,24]

Around 12 months, infants enjoy and prefer eating with their fingers. Rotary chewing movements and a well-graded bite are observed. At this time, many infants transition from drinking from a bottle to drinking from a cup. While learning to drink from a cup, the infant's jaw initially continues to move in the up-and-down sucking pattern. In addition, the infant bites the rim of the cup to stabilize the jaw. By 15 months, the infant demonstrates some diagonal rotary movements of the tongue and jaw while chewing food. Between 15 and 18 months, the infant begins to independently eat with a spoon.[12]

Early Childhood

By 24 months of age, the foundation has been established for all adult eating patterns.[27] At age 2, children eat independently, consuming most meats and raw vegetables (Figure 8-1). Circular rotary chewing develops between the second and third year of life and allows toddlers to eat almost all adult foods.[24,30]

By 24 months, children can hold a spoon and bring it to the mouth with the wrist supinated into the palm-up position.[28] At 30 to 36 months, children experiment with forks to stab at food. A variety of spoons are available for children learning to use utensils.[21] The size of the spoon's bowl should match the size of the child's mouth. Children learning to use spoons typically use ones with shallow bowls; they have to work harder to eat food from spoons with deeper bowls. Child-size spoons and forks are easier for children to hold and manipulate, and bowls and plates with raised edges also make it easier for children to scoop the food.[21,28]

By 24 months, toddlers can also efficiently drink from cups. Children may begin drinking through straws between 2 and 3 years of age, especially if they have been exposed early to the use of straws. Given the variety of playful long, short, and decorated straws that are available on the market, children are happy to independently use their own straws.[21] By 30 to 36 months, children try to serve themselves liquids and family-style servings of food.[28]

DRESSING AND UNDRESSING SKILLS

Dressing and undressing are also essential, basic self-care skills learned in infancy and early childhood.[2] Dressing includes selecting clothing and accessories appropriate for the weather and occasion, putting clothes on sequentially, and fastening and adjusting clothing and shoes.[2] Young children develop independent dressing skills at various ages according to the family's cultural expectations for self-dressing and the types of clothing worn, opportunities for practice, and the child's motivation for independence.[10] Dressing skills require coordinated movements of almost every body part.[31] The development of independent dressing skills typically occurs at age 4 to 5 years.[10,19,35] Table 8-2 lists the general sequence of dressing and undressing skills.

Infancy

During the first year of development, the infant establishes the daily routine and begins to cooperate in dressing activities.[16] He or she learns to remove loose-fitting clothing such as hats, mittens, and socks. By age 1, most infants have achieved many of the motor skills needed for the development of dressing skills. They can separate movements so that the arms or legs can move separate from the trunk, have begun to stabilize with one hand the action of the other, and can adjust their posture during reaching.[20] Infants have the necessary control to push arms and legs through sleeves and pants or play at pulling off a hat.[20]

TABLE 8-1

Normal Development of Sensorimotor, Oral Motor, and Feeding Skills

AGE	SENSORIMOTOR SKILLS	ORAL-MOTOR SKILLS	FEEDING SKILLS
BIRTH/37–40 WK GESTATION	Is dominated by physiologic flexion Moves total body into extension or flexion Turns head side to side in prone position (a protective response) Keeps head mostly on side in supine position Tends to keep hands fisted and flexed across chest during feeding Has strong grasp reflex	Possesses strong gag reflex Possesses rooting reflex Possesses automatic phasic bite–release pattern Sucks and suckles when hand or object comes into contact with mouth Shows minimal drooling in supine position and increased drooling in other positions	Begins bottle- or breast-feeding with total sucking pattern Uses mixture of suckling and sucking on bottle (dependent on head position) Possesses incomplete lip closure Is unable to release nipple
1–2 MO	Appears hypotonic as physiologic flexion diminishes Practices extension and flexion Continues to gain control of head Moves elbows forward toward shoulders in prone position Possesses ATNR, with head to side in supine position Experiences weakening grasp reflex Does not possess voluntary release skills	Continues to show strong gag reflex Continues to show rooting reflex Continues to show automatic phasic bite–release pattern Continues to suck and suckle when hand or object comes in contact with mouth Drools more as jaw and tongue move in wider excursions	May lose coordination of sucking–swallowing–breathing pattern with increased head movements Opens mouth and waits for food Has better lip closure Uses active lip movement when sucking
3–5 MO	Experiences diminishing ATNR and grasp reflex Possesses more balance between extension and flexion Has good head control (centered and upright) Brings hands to mouth constantly Supports on extended arms and props on forearms in prone position Brings hand to feet and feet to mouth in supine position Props on arms, with little support in sitting position Develops tactile awareness in hands Reaches more accurately, usually with both hands Begins transfer of objects from hand to hand Does not possess controlled release skills; may use mouth to assist	Experiences diminished rooting reflex and automatic phasic bite–release pattern Experiences diminished strong gag reflex at 5 months Drools less in positions with greater postural stability Uses mouth to explore objects Begins to show new oral movements in association with increased head and body control	Anticipates feeding; recognizes bottle and readies mouth for nipple Demonstrates voluntary control of mouth during bottle-feeding or breast-feeding Loses liquid from lip corners Is able to receive solid food from a spoon at 5 months Uses suckling during spoon feeding; gags on new textures Shows tongue reversal after spoon is removed; ejects food involuntarily

Continued

TABLE 8-1

Normal Development of Sensorimotor, Oral Motor, and Feeding Skills—cont'd

AGE	SENSORIMOTOR SKILLS	ORAL-MOTOR SKILLS	FEEDING SKILLS
6 MO	Has total head control Shifts weight and reaches with one hand in prone position Begins shifting weight in quadruped position Transfers objects from hand to hand in supine position Reaches with one hand while supporting with other in sitting position Reaches to be picked up Begins to use thumb in grasp Begins to hold objects in one hand Shows visual interest in small things	No longer has rooting reflex or autonomic phasic bite–release pattern Experiences decrease in strength of gag reflex Maintains lip closure longer in supine, prone, and sitting positions Drools when babbling, reaching, and teething; drools less during feeding	Sucks from bottle or breast with no liquid loss and long sequences of coordinated sucking–swallowing–breathing Suckles liquid from a cup with liquid loss Coughs and chokes when drinking too much liquid from cup Moves upper lip down to scrape food from spoon and uses suckling with some sucking to move food back Gags on new textures Opens mouth when spoon approaches Uses phasic up-and-down jaw movements, suckling, or sucking when presented with solids Moves tongue laterally when solids placed on side biting surfaces Begins finger feeding Plays with spoon
7–9 MO	Shifts weight and reaches in quadruped position Creeps Develops extension, flexion, and rotation; expands movement options in sitting position May pull to stand and hold on to support Reaches with supination Uses index finger to poke Develops voluntary release skills	Experiences diminishing gag reflex; becomes more similar to an adult protective gag reflex Uses facial expressions to convey likes and dislikes Uses mouth in combination with visual examination and hand manipulation to investigate new objects Bites on fingers and objects to reduce teething discomfort Produces more coordinated jaw, tongue, and lip movements in supine, prone, sitting, and standing positions; rarely drools except when teething	Suckles liquid in cup; loses liquid when cup is removed Takes fewer sucks and suckles before pulling away from cup to breathe Independently holds bottle Feeds self cracker using fingers Holds jaw closed on soft solids to break off pieces Uses variable up-and-down movement while chewing; moves tongue laterally and jaw diagonally when solids placed on biting surfaces Assists with cup and spoon feeding

Age	Gross and fine motor skills	Oral motor development	Feeding/eating skills
10–12 MO	Creeps with good coordination Cruises holding on to support with one hand Stands independently Learns to walk independently Uses superior pincer grasp with finger tip and thumb Smoothly releases large objects	Produces more coordinated jaw, tongue, and lip movements when sitting, standing, and creeping on hands and knees; rarely drools except when teething	Easily closes lips on spoon; uses upper and lower lips to remove food from spoon Uses controlled, sustained biting motion on soft cookies or crackers Chews with mixture of up-and-down and diagonal rotary movements Feeds self independently using fingers Likes to feed self but needs assistance with using spoon; inverts spoon before putting in mouth
13–18 MO	Walks alone Learns to go up and down stairs Has more precise grasp and release	Moves upper and lower lips By 15 to 18 months, has excellent coordination of sucking, swallowing, and breathing	Uses an up-and-down sucking pattern to obtain liquid from a cup Shows well-coordinated rotary chewing movements by 18 months Has well controlled and sustained biting movements Practices self-feeding; becomes neater Holds cup and puts cup down without spilling liquid
19–24 MO	Demonstrates equilibrium reactions while standing and walking Runs with more narrow base of support	Uses up-and-down tongue movements and tip elevation Develops internal jaw stabilization Swallows with easy lip closure	Efficiently drinks from cup Has well graded and sustained bite
24-36 MO	Jumps in place* Pedals tricycle* Scribbles* Snips with scissors*	Uses tongue humping rather than tongue protrusion to initiate swallow	Possesses circular rotary jaw movements* Closes lips while chewing* Holds cup in one hand* Handles spoon more accurately* Uses fingers to fill spoon* Begins to drink from straws*

ATNR, asymmetrical tonic neck reflex.

*From this point on, skills learned during the first 24 months are further refined.

Adapted from Alexander R, Boehme R, Cupps B: Normal development of functional motor skills, Tucson, AR, 1993, Therapy Skill Builders; Bly L: Motor skills acquisition in the first year: An illustrated guide to normal development, Tucson, AR, 1994, Therapy Skill Builders; Case-Smith J, Humphrey R: Feeding and oral motor skills. In Case-Smith J, Allen AS, Pratt PN, editors: Occupational therapy for children, ed 2, St Louis, 1995, Mosby; Clark GF: Oral-motor and feeding issues. In Royeen CB, editor: AOTA self-study series: Classroom applications for school-based practice, Rockville, MD, 1993, American Occupational Therapy Association; Glass RP, Wolf LS: Feeding and oral-motor skills. In Case-Smith J, editor: Pediatric occupational therapy and early intervention, Boston, MA, 1993, Andover Medical; Lowman DK, Murphy SM: The educator's guide to feeding children with disabilities, Baltimore, MD, 1999, Paul H Brookes; Lowman DK, Lane SJ: Children with feeding and nutritional problems. In Porr S, Rainville, EB, editors: Pediatric therapy: A systems approach, Philadelphia, 1999, FA Davis; Morris SE, Klein MD: Pre-feeding skills: A comprehensive resource for feeding development, Tucson, AR, 1987, Therapy Skill Builders.

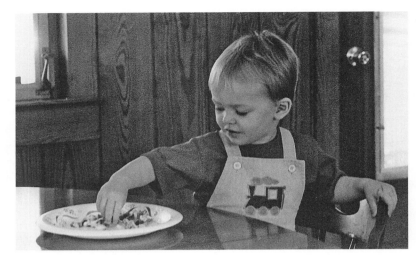

FIGURE 8-1   At age 2, children are able to sit up at the table, feed themselves, and eat almost all adult foods.

TABLE 8-2

Developmental Sequence for Self-Care Skills

AGE (YR)	DRESSING AND UNDRESSING SKILLS	GROOMING AND HYGIENE
1	Cooperates in dressing (e.g., holds foot up for shoe or sock, holds arm out for sleeve) Pushes arms through sleeves and legs through pants	Cooperates during hand washing and drying Has regular bowel movements
1½	Takes off loose clothing (such as mittens, hat, socks, and shoes) Partially pulls shirt over head Unties shoes or takes off hat as an act of undressing Unfastens clothing zippers with large pull tabs Puts on hat	Allows teeth to be brushed Pays attention to acts of eliminating Indicates discomfort from soiled points Begins to sit on potty when placed there and supervised (for a short time)
2	Removes unfastened coat Purposefully removes shoes (if laces are untied) Helps pull down pants Finds armholes in over-the-head shirt	Attempts to brush teeth in imitation of adults Washes own hands with assistance Shows interest in washing self in bathtub Urinates regularly
2½	Removes pull-down pants or shorts with elastic waist Removes simple clothing (such as open shirt or jacket) Assists in putting on socks Puts on front-button-type coat or shirt Unbuttons large buttons	Dries hands Wipes nose if given a tissue and prompted to do so Has daytime control of bowel and bladder; experiences occasional accidents Usually indicates need to go to toilet; rarely has bowel accidents
3	Puts on over-the-head shirt with some assistance Puts on shoes without fastening (may be on wrong feet) Puts on socks with some difficulty positioning heel Independently pulls down pants or shorts Zips and unzips coat zipper without separating or inserting zipper Needs assistance to remove over-the-head shirt Buttons large front buttons	Washes own hands Uses toothbrush with assistance Gets drink from fountain or faucet with no assistance Uses toilet independently but needs help wiping after bowel movements

TABLE 8-2

Developmental Sequence for Self-Care Skills—cont'd

AGE (YR)	DRESSING AND UNDRESSING SKILLS	GROOMING AND HYGIENE
3½	Usually finds front of clothing Snaps or hooks clothing in front Unzips front zipper on coat or jacket, separating zipper Puts on mittens Buttons series of three or four buttons Unbuckles belt or shoe Puts on boots Dresses with supervision (needs help with front and back)	Pours well from small pitcher Spreads soft butter with knife Seldom has toileting accidents; may need help with difficult clothing
4	Removes pullover garment independently Buckles belt or shoe Zips coat zipper, inserting zipper Puts on pull-down pants or shorts Puts on socks with appropriate heel placement Puts on shoes with assistance in tying laces Consistently knows front and back of clothing	Washes and dries hands and face without assistance Brushes teeth with supervision Washes and dries self after bath with supervision Cares for self at toilet (may need help with wiping after bowel movement)
4½	Puts belt in loops	Runs brush or comb through hair Tears toilet tissue and flushes toilet after use
5	Puts on pullover shirt correctly each time Ties and unties knots Laces shoes Dresses unsupervised	Scrubs fingernails with brush with coaching Brushes and combs hair with supervision Cuts soft foods with knife Blows nose independently when prompted Wipes self after bowel movements
5½	Closes back zipper	Performs toileting activities, including flushing toilet, independently
6	Ties bow knot Ties hood strings Buttons back buttons Snaps back snaps Selects clothing that is appropriate for weather conditions and specific activities	Brushes and rinses teeth independently

Adapted from Case-Smith J: Self-care strategies for children with developmental deficits. In Christiansen C, editor: *Ways of living: Self-care strategies for special needs*, Bethesda, MD, 1994, AOTA; Coley IL: *Pediatric assessment of self-care activities*, St Louis, 1978, Mosby; Cook RE, Tessier A, Klein MD: *Adapting early childhood curricula for children in inclusive settings*, Columbus, OH, 1996, Merrill; Johnson-Martin NM: *The Carolina curriculum for preschoolers with special needs*, ed 2, Baltimore, MD, 2004, Paul H Brookes; Johnson-Martin NM: *The Carolina curriculum for infants and toddlers with special needs*, ed 3, Baltimore, MD, 1990, Paul H Brookes; Klein MD: *Pre-dressing skills: Skill starters for self-help development*, rev ed, Tucson, AR, 1983, Communication Skill Builders; Orelove, FP, Sobsey, D: *Educating children with multiple disabilities: A transdisciplinary approach*, ed 3, Baltimore, MD, 1996, Paul H Brookes; Shepherd J, Procter SA, Coley IL: Self-care and adaptations for independent living. In Case-Smith J, Allen JA, Pratt PN, editors: *Occupational therapy for children*, ed 2, St Louis, 1996, Mosby.

Early Childhood

By age 2, refined balance and equilibrium reactions provide children with the necessary motor skills to raise their arms to pull shirts over their heads. They can move their hands behind them to attempt to put their arms into the sleeves of a button-front shirt. By 3 years, children are more aware of details and can find arm and leg holes easily. By 4 years, they recognize correct and incorrect sides; as fine motor skills progress, they can also use buckles, zippers, and laces. By 5 years, all skills of balance, equilibrium, and fine motor coordination are refined enough to allow children to dress themselves unsupervised.[16,20] Figure 8-2 shows some children putting on their boots before going outdoors.

PERSONAL HYGIENE AND GROOMING

Grooming and hygiene are important self-care skills that tend to develop after the development of eating and dressing skills. (See Table 8-2 for the general sequence of

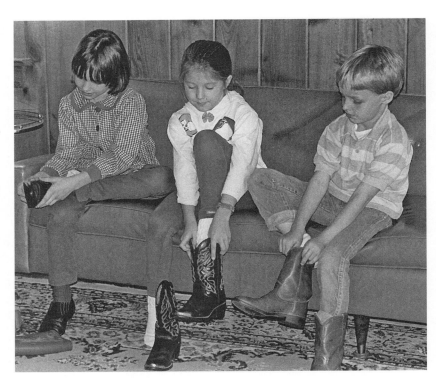

FIGURE 8-2 By age 5, children are able to dress themselves without adult supervision. They show adequate strength, balance, equilibrium, and fine motor coordination.

personal hygiene and grooming.) The cultural expectations and social routines of the family determine when independence in grooming and hygiene is achieved.[35] Face washing, hand washing, and hair care are typical **personal hygiene and grooming skills** learned in early childhood. The infant cooperates in hand washing. By age 2, children can wash their hands but need assistance turning on water and getting soap. By age 4, children can perform hand and face washing unsupervised. With supervision and coaching, 5-year-olds can scrub fingernails with a brush and comb hair.[16]

In early childhood, **oral hygiene** involves brushing teeth.[2] Before age 2, infants allow their parents to brush their teeth. Two-year-olds imitate parents brushing their teeth. Children continue to brush their own teeth with supervision until the age of 5 or 6 years.[35] At that time, refinement of skill in the use of tools enables children to independently complete all steps of dental care, including making the necessary preparations and then brushing the teeth and rinsing the mouth.[12]

BATHING AND SHOWERING

Bathing and showering involve soaping, rinsing, and drying the body. Around age 2, children begin to show interest in bathing by assisting in washing while in the bathtub. Because bathing is a pleasurable activity for most children and parents, learning to wash oneself begins in the context of play.[12] Typically, most children are able to wash and dry themselves with supervision by age 4. It is not until age 8 that most children can independently prepare the bath or shower water, wash, and dry themselves.[35]

TOILET HYGIENE

Toilet hygiene involves clothing management, maintaining toileting position, transferring to and from toileting, and cleaning the body. Physiologically, voluntary control of urination does not usually occur until between 2 and 3 years of age. Independent toileting is a developmental milestone, which varies widely among children. During infancy, regularity in bowel movement and urination develops gradually. The infant may also indicate when diapers are wet or soiled and even sit on the toilet when placed there. Toilet training is not typically introduced until the child remains dry for 1 or more hours at a time, shows signs of a full bladder or the need to toilet, and is at least 2½ years old.[31] Daytime bowel and bladder control is usually attained between 2½ and 3 years of age, although the child may still need assistance with difficult clothing or fasteners.[16] Night-time bladder control may not be attained until age 5 or 6. During the day, 5-year-olds can anticipate immediate toilet needs and completely care for themselves while toileting, including wiping themselves and flushing the toilet.[16]

Instrumental Activities of Daily Living

Instrumental activities of daily living (IADL) are the complex activities of daily living that are necessary to function independently in the home, school, or community.[2] During childhood, children learn home management tasks that help them participate in family routines and community mobility skills that help them to be active outside the home. As they get older, they are given the responsibility of caring for others.[35]

READINESS SKILLS

Readiness skills are necessary for successful participation in home management, community mobility, and care of others' activities. Specific readiness skills are related to particular tasks. Activity analysis (breaking an activity into steps) can determine the readiness skills needed to perform a specific task. For example, making a bed requires the coordination of both sides of the body, sequencing skills, and a pad-to-pad pinch. Setting the dinner table requires sequencing, balance, and dexterity while carrying and placing plates and silverware. The different readiness skills necessary to care for others can be illustrated by comparing the requirements for caring for a pet with those for babysitting a sibling. These two tasks obviously require different abilities. Readiness skills acquired by children and adolescents are determined by the contexts and environments in which they engage on a daily basis.

HOME MANAGEMENT ACTIVITIES

Home management activities are tasks that are necessary to obtain and maintain one's personal and household possessions.[2] The context significantly influences a child's or adolescent's participation in home management tasks. Children's ages and their physical, social, and cultural environments determine their roles in this domain. Children and adolescents may have chores that they are expected to complete on a regular schedule. Examples of chores include making the bed, setting the dinner table, and cutting the grass. Some children and adolescents have the incentive of a monetary allowance to complete the assigned chores, whereas others do not have a monetary incentive but are still expected to assist in the maintenance of their households.

COMMUNITY MOBILITY

Mobility in the community outside the home is critical to the child's development. During the preschool years, **community mobility** may mean accompanying parents; during adolescence, it may be driving to run errands. Environmental factors that have an impact on mobility might be crowds, street crossings, public transportation, and architectural barriers.[35] Family and cultural expectations also determine the age and independence of community mobility skills.

CARE OF OTHERS

Care of others refers to the physical upkeep and nurturing of pets or other human beings.[2] As with household management, the care of others is also significantly influenced by performance contexts. In large families, older siblings may be required to assist their parents in the care of younger siblings. A child living on a farm may assist with feeding and caring for the farm animals. A child living in an urban area may walk the family dog several times a day in the park or around the neighborhood.

SUMMARY

The ADLs of feeding and eating, dressing and undressing, personal hygiene and grooming, and toilet hygiene are the most basic tasks learned by children as they grow and mature. The IADLs of home management, community mobility, and caring for others are critical to the child's development and ability to be active outside the home. The specific age at which young children develop independent ADL and IADL skills varies according to the family's cultural expectations, opportunities for practice, and the child's motivation for independence. OT practitioners are in an excellent position to teach parents and teachers ways to facilitate the development of self-care skills in children.

Education

READINESS SKILLS

Readiness skills are those performance abilities that are necessary to effectively engage in educational and vocational activities. Readiness is a stage of preparedness for "what comes next."[35] Different readiness skills are necessary for different tasks. Readiness skills must be considered within the temporal and environmental contexts of the Occupational Therapy Practice Framework. The chronologic age of the child or adolescent is directly related to the necessary readiness skills. For example, readiness skills expected of a kindergarten student are different from those expected of a high school student. Social, cultural, and physical environments also influence expectations of readiness.

The readiness skills necessary for successful participation in formal educational activities vary according to performance contexts. This section discusses educational readiness skills for children enrolled in preschool programs, kindergarten, and elementary school.

Preschool Readiness Skills

Children entering preschool programs need certain readiness skills, which include independence in toileting with a minimum of assistance for handling fasteners, independence in self-feeding, and cooperative play behavior. Children attending a preschool program are also expected to understand rules and schedules. They need to exhibit the beginning of behavioral and emotional maturity (i.e., controlling tempers and mood swings).

Kindergarten Readiness Skills

The child attending kindergarten is expected to have the readiness skills of a typical preschooler with additional preacademic and academic skills. He or she must be able to sit quietly while listening to a story and should have adequate fine motor skills for coloring and for manipulating small objects.[11] The child must possess gross motor skills such as running, hopping, and jumping and is expected to recognize letters and numbers.

Elementary School Readiness Skills

Children attending elementary school are expected to have greater independence as well as skills in the occupational performance areas than younger children. Independence in the bathroom and cafeteria is necessary. In addition to independence in eating, children in elementary school are expected to carry their lunch trays and assist in cleaning the table at the end of a meal. They must remain in their classroom chairs for extended periods. The ability to remain "on task" and attend to work while seated is termed *in-seat behavior*.

Expectations of reading, writing, spelling, and math skills increase with grade level. The child attending elementary school should have adequate perceptual and motor skills to participate in games and organized sports.

Middle Childhood and Adolescent Readiness Skills

Educational readiness skills for middle childhood and adolescence build on the competencies gained during the preceding periods. Appropriate social skills and manners are expected, and increased skill in creative

thinking, problem solving, and the development of ideas is required. Expressive writing is learned during this period. During middle childhood, children and adolescents also begin to seek independence. They question authority figures but must learn to work with them effectively in educational settings.

EDUCATIONAL ACTIVITIES

Educational activities are the opportunities that facilitate learning for children and adolescents.[35] These activities can be formal or informal. Formal educational activities are structured and may be mandated by public law for specific age groups. These activities are provided in settings such as preschool programs, daycare centers, public schools, and Sunday school classes. Informal educational activities are less structured and occur in a variety of settings. Examples of activities in which younger children engage include playing school with an older sibling and playing a shopping game with peers. Figure 8-3 shows children engaged in "playing school," a typical informal educational activity. Adolescents frequently study together, creating opportunities for informal learning.

Work/Vocational Activities

In preparation for entering the world of **work** as adults, adolescents engage in a variety of **vocational activities**. These activities are work related and typically have a monetary incentive or salary.[1] Like educational activities, vocational activities can be formal or informal. An example of a formal vocational activity is having a job. Public laws determine the age at which a person may hold a job. Informal vocational activities include neighborhood lemonade stands and cutting a neighbor's grass for a fee. Figure 8-4 shows a child "selling" cookies to a friend. Like home management and the care of others, vocational activities in which a child or adolescent might participate are significantly influenced by performance contexts for that individual.

Readiness skills for formal and informal vocational activities are as varied as and depend greatly on performance contexts. To successfully engage in formal vocational activities, skills such as promptness, appropriate dressing, and effective communication with peers and supervisors are important. Activity analysis is beneficial when considering appropriate formal and informal vocational activities.

SUMMARY

Education and work are two of the areas of occupation described in the Occupational Therapy Practice Framework. Readiness skills also develop during childhood

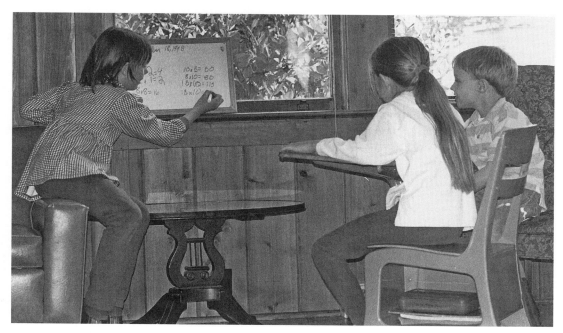

FIGURE 8-3   Children enjoy "playing school," a typical informal educational activity. Note the students attending to the "teacher."

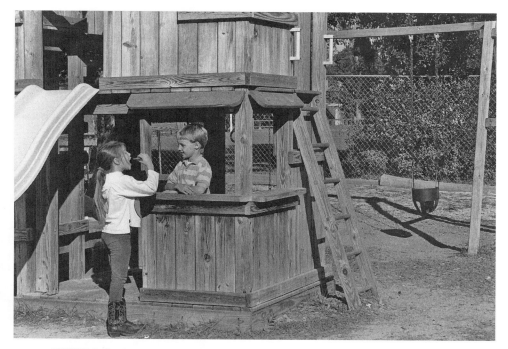

FIGURE 8-4   A young boy sells cookies (an informal vocational activity) to his friend.

and can differ according to each child's age and the task being performed. Although all children and adolescents participate in educational tasks, great variability exists in the ways they participate in home management activities, the care of others, and vocational activities.

Play/Leisure Activities

Play is the occupation of childhood. Through play, children learn cognitive, social–emotional, motor, and language skills.[4,5,15,32,34] In adulthood, play often takes the form of **leisure activities**, which are not associated with time-consuming duties and responsibilities.[2] During play and leisure activities children, adolescents, and adults refine skills, relax, reflect, and engage in creativity. Children develop problem-solving skills and flexibility as well as motor skills during play. Importantly, children need a variety of skills to engage in play, such as motor skills (e.g., coordination, strength, balance, timing, sequencing), social (e.g., sharing, negotiating, communicating), and cognitive skills (e.g., problem solving, creativity, planning). OT practitioners evaluate the play of children to determine ways to facilitate play and enable children to play at their highest potential. In this way, OT practitioners assist children in gaining skills for adulthood.

DEFINITION OF PLAY

Scholars have struggled for centuries to define play.[6,7,13,15,18,19,32-34] Play has been viewed as (1) a method to release surplus energy, (2) a link in the evolutionary change from animal to human being (recapitulation theory), (3) a method to practice survival skills, and (4) an attitude or mood.[26,31] More recent theories have asserted that play provides the stimulation needed to satisfy a physiologic need for optimal arousal.[32] Theorists describe play in terms of the development of cognitive, emotional, social, language, and motor skills.[4,5,15,32,34] These theorists propose that play develops as children learn necessary skills. For example, Piaget proposed that children's play developed from sensorimotor (practice) play to symbolic play to games with rules as the child acquires cognitive skills.[34] Table 8-3 describes Piaget's stages of play. McCune-Nicolich proposed that children engage in more make-believe play as their language skills develop.[34] See Table 8-4 for a description of the progression of symbolic or make-believe play. Figure 8-5 shows an 18-month-old toddler playing "dress-up" with her mother's shoes. Early theorists such as Erikson and Freud

TABLE 8-3

Piaget's Stages of Play

AGE (YEARS)	STAGE
0–2	*Sensorimotor:* Practices games, exploratory behaviors, reflexive behaviors, repetition
2–6	*Symbolic:* Uses imaginary objects, pretend play
6–10	*Games with rules:* Participates in team sports, activities with flexible rules, goals

TABLE 8-4

Symbolic Play

AGE (MONTHS)	PLAY CHARACTERISTICS
12	Play directed towards self Imitation of pat-a-cake and other movements Simple pretend play directed toward self (eating, sleeping) Imitation of familiar actions
18–24	Role-playing with objects (such as feeding a doll) Use of nonrealistic objects in pretend
24–36	Engagement in multistep scenarios (such as giving doll a bath, dressing the doll, and putting the doll to bed)
36–48	Use of language in play Advance plans and development of stories Acting out sequences with miniatures
48	Imaginary play Role-playing entire scenarios Creation of stories with "pretend" characters

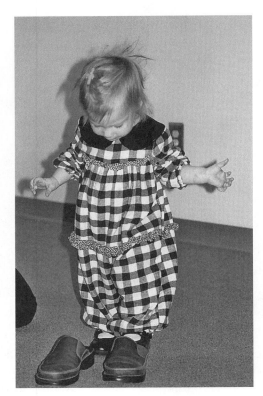

FIGURE 8-5 A toddler enjoys playing "dress-up" wearing her mother's shoes, a typical activity for an 18-month- old.

believed that children work out emotional conflicts during play.[35]

Psychoanalysts also theorized that play could be used to evaluate conflicts. Developmental theorists described the changes in play in terms of motor skill progression.[5,22,32] In doing so, they divided play into the categories of functional (sensorimotor), constructive (manipulative), dramatic ("pretend"), and formal (rule governed).[32] Parham identified the social aspects of play as progressing from solitary to parallel to group play.[32] Figure 8-6 shows two children engaged in cooperative play. Play encompasses a variety of skills and occupies much of the child's day. Thus, OT practitioners must have a firm understanding of its complexities. The Occupational Therapy Practice Framework defines play or leisure activities as "any spontaneous or organized activity that provides enjoyment, entertainment, amusement, or diversion."[2]

OT practitioners view play as an area of performance in addition to ADLs and work and productive activities. As such, OT practitioners work with children to facilitate and remediate play skills. The following section discusses OT theorists who made significant contributions to the study of play in OT practice.

OCCUPATIONAL THERAPY THEORISTS AND THEIR CONTRIBUTIONS TO PLAY

Reilly

Mary Reilly, a noted occupational therapist and researcher, described play as a progression through three stages: (1) exploratory behaviors, (2) competency, and (3) achievement.[33] Exploratory behaviors are intrinsically motivated and are engaged in for their own sake.[33] Infants engage in exploratory behaviors that focus on sensory experiences.[33] The second stage of development, competency, occurs when children search for challenges, novelty, and experimentation. In this stage, they often want to do everything alone and "their way."[33] This stage is observed in early and middle childhood. The achievement stage of play emphasizes performance standards (such as winning) and competition. Children at this stage of development take more risks in their play.

Takata

Occupational therapist Nancy Takata developed Play History, a format that helps OT practitioners obtain information about a child's play.[33] The interview format helps describe a child's play skills. OT practitioners with a solid knowledge of typical play patterns can use this information to design intervention plans.

Knox

The Knox Preschool Play Scale (PPS) was constructed by occupational therapist Susan Knox and is based on Piagetian cognitive stages and Parham's social stages.[32] The revised Knox PPS divides play into four domains: (1) space management, (2) material management, (3) imitation, and (4) participation. The scale provides age equivalents for each domain and an overall play age. This scale is easy to administer and provides information on the motor skill requirements for play.

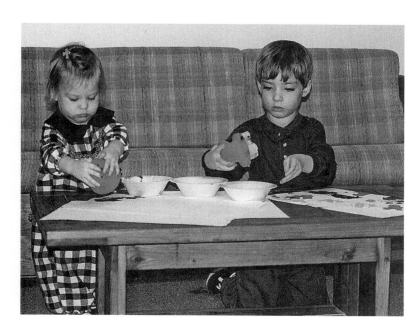

FIGURE 8-6 Children share their paints as they create pictures. They are absorbed in the play process.

Bundy

Professor and occupational therapist Anita Bundy designed the Test of Playfulness (ToP) to objectively measure playfulness.[7,8] Bundy found that a child's attitude about and approach to activities (i.e., playfulness) provide valuable information to OT practitioners. Some children who do not possess the skills for play may still be playful. Others have the skills but do not appear to be having fun. The ToP examines the context in which children perform play activities.[7,8] For example, two 4-year-old boys playing "Godzilla" may engage in rough and tumble "fighting." Because the context of the fighting is play, the children are not being mean spirited or hurtful. They are clearly playing and not fighting.

PLAY SKILL ACQUISITION

Children acquire play skills as they mature and develop, and play affords opportunities for development. For example, a child needs balance and coordination to ride a bike. At the same time, riding the bike improves the child's balance and coordination. Table 8-5 provides an outline of toys and play activities suitable for different age groups.

Infancy

Infants explore the environment and learn through their senses.[5,23] They enjoy visual, tactile, auditory, and movement sensations.[6] Toys with bells and noise encourage infants to explore the environment.[22] Play should focus on enhancing their capabilities while furnishing new opportunities for exploration. OT practitioners and caregivers must allow children to repeat activities until they have mastered them.[5,33] Infant play encourages body awareness. They typically explore their hands and feet spontaneously. Playing games such as pat-a-cake helps them understand that their bodies are fun, as does face-to-face play with an adult.[4,5,14] Peek-a-boo is a favorite game at this age. Enjoyable toys encourage mobility, elicit actions, increase motor skills, and facilitate natural creativity.

Parents and caregivers establish bonds with infants by playing comfortably with them. Adults must respond to the infants' cues. Cues that indicate stress include crying, hiccups, gaze aversion, yawning, finger splaying, and tantrums.[6,26] If infants cry or show signs of stress, they should be comforted and the type of play changed. OT practitioners should remember that play is fun.

Early Childhood

Continued exploration and the development of friendships accentuate childhood play.[6,23] Play provides children with opportunities to learn negotiation, problem-solving, and communication skills. Figure 8-7 shows children challenging their skills in play. Play in early childhood helps children develop and refine motor skills.[6,15,23] Consequently, adults should be cautious about intervening too quickly during play. Children need opportunities to work out differences among themselves.

TABLE 8-5

Toys and Play Activities for Various Ages

AGE (YEARS)	TOYS AND ACTIVITIES
0–1	*Manipulative, sensory:* rattles, musical sounds, bells, swings, soft toys, boxes, pots and pans, wooden spoons, books
1–2	*Movement, manipulative, sensory:* push-pull toys, balls, pop-beads, pop-up toys, toy phones, musical books, noisy toys, ride-on toys, trucks, cause and effect toys
2–4	*Pretend play, movement, manipulative, sensory:* dolls, trucks, action figures, play-doh, markers, water play, balls, blocks, Lego, books, dress-up toys, hats, shoes, clothes, tricycles
4–6	*Pretend play, craft activities, movement:* swings, gyms, bicycles, scooters, ball games, beads, painting, play-doh, arts and crafts, dolls, cooking, group games (for example, follow-the-leader, tag, red rover)
6–8	*Pretend play, craft activities, movement:* gymnastic play, jumping rope, coordinated games (for example, keep-away with ball), arts and crafts, wood kits, model airplanes, painting, drawing, skating, bike riding, swimming
8–10	*Movement, group games, manipulative:* basketball, baseball, soccer, bike riding, skateboarding, tennis, swimming, volleyball, arts and crafts requiring more skill, cooking, collecting
10	*Movement, games that challenge, skilled manipulative resulting in products:* competitive sports, sewing, knitting, woodworking, bowling, walking, going to the beach, flying kites, boating, camping, reading

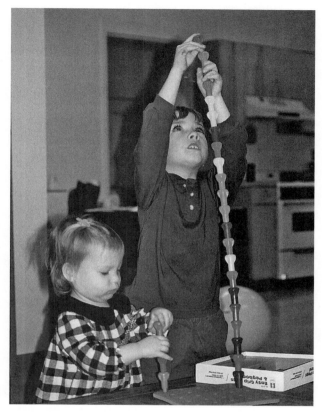

FIGURE 8-7 Children challenge their motor, social, and cognitive skills during play. They must use their fine motor skills to build a tower.

Children enjoy manipulative play, imitation, games, and social play with other children of the same sex.[6] They enjoy dramatic and rough and tumble play.[6,34] Role-playing scenarios that facilitate dramatic play stimulates a child's imagination, creativity, and problem-solving abilities.

Middle Childhood

Middle childhood is a time of refinement of skills, such as speed, dexterity, strength, and endurance. Children become more competent in play activities. They enjoy games with rules and competition. Childhood is a time for them to experiment with many play activities. Some of these activities are easy, whereas others are difficult. Children should be encouraged to play, have fun, and realize that everyone has different talents. This is all part of growing up and finding their identities.

Adolescence

Adolescents are in search of independence.[6,23] Parents need to facilitate socially appropriate play and leisure activities. Adolescents enjoy activities in which they can participate with peers.[6,23] They may wish to participate in school or community clubs. OT practitioners and parents need to listen carefully to adolescents to help them discover their goals and talents. At this stage of development, play is beneficial in the establishment of independence.

DEVELOPMENTAL RELEVANCE OF PLAY AND LEISURE

Play is important in each stage of development. It provides children with opportunities to develop motor, social–emotional, cognitive, and language skills. (The Appendix titled "Play Analysis Guide" at the end of this chapter provides a guide to the observation of play.) Play also allows children to interact with others, challenge themselves, and identify their own strengths and weaknesses; therefore, play contributes to the quality of life. Play and leisure remain important throughout a person's life. People engage in play and leisure activities because they enjoy them and are intrinsically motivated to participate in them.[9]

SUMMARY

Play and leisure activities are crucial components in the development of children and in the acquisition of skills children will use in adulthood. These activities provide the foundation for problem solving, skill development, social interaction, and negotiating.

OT practitioners can play a key role in teaching parents, teachers, and peers ways to play and be playful with children who have special needs. OT practitioners assist children who have disabilities in developing play skills so they may reach their potential.

Social Participation

Social participation includes organized patterns of behavior expected of a child interacting with others within a given social system, such as the family, peer group, or community.[2] Children who have disabilities or special needs are members of a family system. Interventions that have an impact on one member of the family system do so on all members of that system. Therefore, it is important for OT practitioners to understand the family system. Refer to Chapter 2 for a detailed description of the patterns associated with the family system. Likewise, peers can positively or negatively influence a child's willingness to perform a task.[35] For example, if peers ridicule an adaptive device, it will not be used by the child. Consideration of the child's social routines and cultural and physical contexts is critical in determining the appropriate intervention techniques. Understanding the issues faced by children with disabilities or special needs may help OT practitioners better address social participation needs. Children may experience limited access to activities because of a disability. Many parents cite lack of adequate supervision or trained staff as factors that prevent them from allowing their children with special needs to participate in after-school events. As children develop a desire to socialize with peers away from the family, new issues arise. For example, competitive sports and activities become more valued in the middle school and high school years. Children who have special needs may, however, be excluded from these activities. OT practitioners who are aware of leisure and social events that include all children are a great resource for children and families. Other issues interfering with social participation of children with disabilities include lack of transportation, excessive costs, and inaccessibility of the event. For example, children who are in wheelchairs require special transportation which may not be readily available in rural communities. One adolescent remarked when asked about his social life in middle school, "I can go to dances after school; a special bus brings me home. That's cool – I like that." However, he later remarked, "But I can't go to the store with the other kids and my brother on the weekends. My mom won't let me ride my wheelchair on the road. There is no good sidewalk for me, and the cars drive too fast."

CHAPTER SUMMARY

OT practitioners must have a firm knowledge of the occupational areas of daily living, education, work, play and leisure, and social participation to effectively work with children and their families. OT practitioners use their knowledge of the contexts in which activities occur to design appropriate interventions because contexts influence any given activity and the success of the child in performing it. Finally, the ability to analyze each of the areas of occupation through activity analysis is essential to effectively work with children and adolescents.

References

1. *American Heritage Dictionary*, ed 4, Boston, 2000, Houghton Mifflin. 1981.
2. American Occupational Therapy Association: Occupational therapy practice framework: domain and process, ed 2. *Am J Occup Ther* 62:625–683, 2008.
3. American Occupational Therapy Association: Specialized knowledge and skills in feeding, eating, and swallowing for occupational therapy practice. *Am J Occup Ther* 61, 2007.
4. Axline VM: Play therapy procedures and results. In Schaefer C, editor: *The therapeutic use of play*, New York, 1976, Jason Aronson.
5. Bantz DL, Siktberg L: Teaching families to evaluate age-appropriate toys. *J Pediatr Health Care* 7:111, 1993.
6. Berger KS: *The developing person through the lifespan*, ed 8, New York, 2009, Worth Publishers.
7. Bundy AC: Assessment of play and leisure: delineation of the problem. *Am J Occup Ther* 47:217, 1993.
8. Bundy AC: Play and playfulness: what to look for. In Parham LD, Fazio LS, editors: *Play in occupational therapy for children*, ed 2, St. Louis, 2010, Mosby.
9. Bundy AC: Play theory and sensory integration. In Fisher AG, Murray EA, Bundy AC, editors: *Sensory integration: theory and practice*, Philadelphia, 1991, FA Davis.
10. Case-Smith J: Self-care strategies for children with developmental deficits. In Christiansen C, Matuska K, editors: *Ways of living: self-care strategies for special needs*, ed 3, Bethesda, MD, 2004, American Occupational Therapy Association.
11. Case-Smith J, editor: *Occupational therapy for children*, ed 6, St. Louis, 2009, Mosby.
12. Case-Smith J, Humphrey R: Feeding intervention. In Case-Smith J, editor: *Occupational therapy for children*, ed 6, St. Louis, 2009, Mosby.
13. Cass JE: *The significance of children's play*, London, 1971, Batsford.
14. Clark GF: Oral-motor and feeding issues. In Royeen CB, editor: *AOTA self-study series: classroom applications for school-based practice*, Rockville, MD, 1993, American Occupational Therapy Association.
15. Cohen D: *The development of play*, New York, 1987, New York University Press.
16. Coley IL: *Pediatric assessment of self-care activities*, St. Louis, 1978, Mosby.
17. Florey L: Development through play. In Schaefer C, editor: *The therapeutic use of play*, New York, 1976, Jason Aronson.
18. Greenstein DB: It's child's play. In Galvin J, Sherer M, editors: *Evaluating, selecting, and using appropriate assistive technology*, Gaithersburg, MD, 1996, Aspen.
19. Johnson-Martin NM: *The Carolina curriculum for infants and toddlers with special needs*, ed 3, Baltimore, 2004, Paul H. Brookes.
20. Klein MD: *Pre-dressing skills: skill starters for self-help development*, rev ed, Tucson, 1999, Communication Skill Builders.
21. Klein MD, Delaney TA: *Feeding and nutrition for the child with special needs: handouts for parents*, Tucson, 1994, Therapy Skill Builders.
22. Linder TW: *Transdisciplinary play based assessment*, ed 2, Baltimore, MD, 2008, Paul H. Brookes.
23. Llorens LA: *Application of a developmental theory for health and rehabilitation*, Rockville, MD, 1976, American Occupational Therapy Association.
24. Lowman DK, Lane SJ: Children with feeding and nutritional problems. In Porr S, Rainville EB, editors: *Pediatric therapy: a systems approach*, Philadelphia, 1999, FA Davis.
25. Lowman DK, Murphy SM: *The educator's guide to feeding children with disabilities*, Baltimore, 1999, Paul H. Brookes.

26. Marfo K, editor: *Parent-child interaction and developmental disabilities*, New York, 1988, Praeger.
27. Millar S: *The psychology of play*, New York, 1974, Aronson.
28. Morris SE, Klein MD: *Pre-feeding skills: a comprehensive resource for mealtime development*, ed 2, Tucson, 2000, Therapy Skill Builders.
29. Murphy SM, Caretto C: Anatomy of the oral and respiratory structures made easy. In Lowman DK, Murphy SM, editors: *The educator's guide to feeding children with disabilities*, Baltimore, MD, 1999, Paul H. Brookes.
30. Murphy SM, Caretto C: Oral-motor considerations for feeding. In Lowman DK, Murphy SM, editors: *The educator's guide to feeding children with disabilities*, Baltimore, 1999, Paul H. Brookes.
31. Orelove FP, Sobsey D, Silberman R: *Educating children with multiple disabilities: a collaborative approach*, ed 4, Baltimore, 2004, Paul H. Brookes.
32. Parham LD, Primeau L: Play and occupational therapy. In Parham LD, Fazio LS, editors: *Play in occupational therapy for children*, ed 2, St. Louis, 2010, Mosby.
33. Reilly M, editor: *Play as exploratory learning: studies in curiosity behavior*, Beverly Hills, 1974, Sage.
34. Rubin K, Fein GG, Vandenberg B: Play. In Mussen PH, editor: *Handbook of child psychology*, ed 4, New York, 1983, Wiley.
35. Shepherd J: Activities of daily living. In Case-Smith J, O'Brien J, editors: *Occupational therapy for children*, ed 6, St. Louis, 2010, Mosby.
36. Wolf LS, Glass RP: *Feeding and swallowing disorders in infancy: assessment and management*, Tucson, 1992, Therapy Skill Builders.

REVIEW *Questions*

1. Describe the developmental sequence of oral motor control, feeding, and eating skills.
2. Which foods and utensils are appropriate for children at various ages?
3. List the developmental sequences of dressing and undressing, toilet hygiene, grooming, bathing and showering, and oral hygiene.
4. Provide examples describing the progression of play skills.
5. Which terms describe play?
6. Describe the contributions of Reilly, Takata, Knox, and Bundy to the study of play in occupational therapy.
7. What is the difference between formal and informal work and productive activities? Give an example of each.
8. List the readiness skills expected of a child entering kindergarten. Why are these skills important?

SUGGESTED *Activities*

1. In a small group, list and discuss examples of how different cultural expectations might affect the development of self-care skills.
2. Visit a local child care center.
   a. Observe preschool children of different ages eating lunch. What similarities and differences do you notice?
   b. Note all the different ways you see children putting on their coats.
   c. Visit a daycare class of 2-year-olds. How many children are in diapers? How many are toilet trained?
3. Participate in play with an infant, child, and adolescent. Describe the way their play differed.
4. Watch a child playing for 15 minutes. Describe the way Reilly, Knox, Takata, and Bundy would describe the child's play.
5. Describe your favorite play activities as a child, adolescent, and adult. Record the setting, materials, group members, and feelings. Share your activities with classmates. How are the activities similar? Different?
6. In a small group, discuss your recollections of your formal education. In what ways do your stories differ and at what age?
7. Make a log of home management, the care of others, and vocational activities that you remember engaging in as a child and adolescent. Compare logs with classmates.

Play Analysis Guide

NAME OF CHILD: **DATE OF EVALUATION:**

DATE OF BIRTH:

CHILD'S AGE:

I. Describe the physical setting.
   Who was present?
II. Describe the activities performed by the child.
   A. Gross Motor
      Balance:
      Coordination:
      Motor Planning:
      Sequencing:
      Endurance:
      Mobility:
      Quality of Movement:
      Overall Skill:
   B. Fine Motor
      Manipulation of Objects:
      Grip:
      Strength:
      Overall Effectiveness:
   C. Social
      Participation:
      Negotiating:
      Peer Interactions:
      Sharing:
   D. Imitative
      Creativity:
      Novelty:
      Use of Toys:
   E. Language
      Expression:
      Communication:
      Imagination:
   F. Attitude
      Approach:
      Affect:
      Spontaneity:
      Teasing:
      Mischief:
III. Describe the adult supervision. Did it facilitate or inhibit play?
IV. Other

9

Adolescent Development: Becoming an Adult

KERRYELLEN G. VROMAN

CHAPTER *Objectives*

After studying this chapter, the reader will be able to accomplish the following:

- Describe the physical, cognitive, and psychosocial development of adolescents.
- Recognize the interrelationship between health and adolescent development.
- Identify the role and responsibilities of the occupational therapy assistant in facilitating the adolescent client's healthy transition to young adulthood.
- Apply developmental stage to the choice of therapeutic activities, interventions, and strategies used with adolescent clients.

KEY TERMS | **CHAPTER OUTLINE**

Working with adolescents is both rewarding and frustrating. Flexibility, a sense of humor, the capacity to see strengths before weaknesses, to validate positively, and to constructively establish boundaries are the attributes of an occupational therapy (OT) practitioner who works successfully with adolescents. Equally important is an OT practitioner's ability to identify and integrate the adolescent's developmental needs into OT evaluations and interventions.

This chapter describes adolescent development and the occupations and performance that are vital to an adolescent's transition from childhood to early adulthood. Case studies illustrate the role of cognitive, physical, and psychosocial development in the choice and delivery of OT services (Table 9-1). The practitioner integrates all these areas of development to view adolescence as a dynamic interrelated process of growth. The practice guidelines included in this chapter assist the reader to apply the principles of adolescent development. It is essential to consider the unique work setting and individually apply this information to each adolescent (Box 9-1).

ADOLESCENCE

Most definitions of adolescence attempt to capture the distinct physical, emotional, and social changes that characterize this turbulent, stage of human development. Writing in her diary, young Anne Frank voiced her experience of adolescent angst.

TABLE 9-1

Summary of Adolescent Development

TYPE OF DEVELOPMENT	DESCRIPTION
Physical	Skeletal growth spurt
	Growth in muscle mass and strength
	Growth and maturation of reproductive organs
	Growth of secondary sex characteristics; pubic and body hair
	Advanced motor and coordination skills
	Boys:
	Significant increased muscle mass
	Onset of sperm production and ejaculation
	Girls:
	Development of female body shape, including breast development
	Menarche
Cognitive	Increased capacity for abstract thinking—logical thinking
	Advanced reasoning— hypothetical deductive reasoning
	Development of impulse control—emotional self-regulation
	Increased ability to assess risk and consequence versus reward
	Increased problem-solving skills
	Improved use and manipulation of working memory
	Improved language skills, especially in girls
	Future-oriented planning and goal setting
	Increased capacity to cognitively regulate emotional states
	Emergence of moral reasoning—conventional level of morality
	Greater ability to perceive others' perspectives
	Focus on role obligations and how one is perceived by others
	Questioning of values of parents and institutions
Psychosocial	Emotional separation from parents
	Exploration of interests, ideas, and roles
	Experimentation related to interests and preferences
	Formation of personal identity
	Identification with a peer group
	Exploration of romantic relationships
	Development of a sense of one's sexuality
	Developing sexual orientation
	Establishing occupational identity for future worker role

Adapted from Hazen E, Schlozman S, Beresin E: Adolescent psychological development: A review, *Pediatr Rev* 29:161, 2008.

"They mustn't know my despair, I can't let them see the wounds which they have caused, I couldn't bear their sympathy and their kind-hearted jokes, it would only make me want to scream all the more. If I talk, everyone thinks I'm showing off; when I'm silent they think I'm ridiculous; rude if I answer, sly if I get a good idea, lazy if I'm tired, selfish if I eat a mouthful more than I should, stupid, cowardly, crafty, etc. etc."

Adolescents experience a full spectrum of emotions: elation and joy, overwhelming loneliness, laughter and fun, seemingly unbearable emotional pain, anger, and frustration and embarrassment. Supreme confidence and a sense of immortality contrasts with moments of hopelessness, which they perceive are an eternity. They experience the closeness of friendships and discover the pleasure of intimacy. They have intense passions, often reinforced and heightened by the mass media, for music, video games, sports, or other interests, which for a week, a month, or a year are all-absorbing.

Adolescents also have remarkable creativity, energy, compassion, and potential. The teenage years are a time of exploration, idealism, and cynicism. They will make some of the most important decisions of their lives. Ideally, they will plan and prepare for their futures, develop positive attitudes and make healthy, safe, behavioral choices.

STAGES OF ADOLESCENT DEVELOPMENT

The term *adolescence* defines the psychosocial development that occurs during puberty. However, there is little agreement about the ages at which adolescence begins and ends. This chapter uses the most commonly agreed-upon period of adolescence, 10 to19 years. By age 19, most young people have completed high school; they are experiencing living outside the family home; and they are pursuing divergent paths (e.g., work, college, parenting, or military service) to adulthood. However, the transition to adulthood often continues through the ages of 20 to 24 years, and these years of young adult life are often included as part of a continuum of adolescence. Therefore, the chapter also includes some data related to this age group.

Physical maturation and psychosocial development shape an adolescent's capacities to think, relate, and act as a future adult. This development affects and is influenced by adolescents' choices of occupations and the quality of their occupational performance. The end of adolescence is marked by the legal status of adulthood with all its rights and responsibilities. As OT practitioners, we understand development as a maturational process, which we observe in the age-related tasks and occupational performance challenges that adolescents undertake. These developmental tasks include seeking independence from parents, learning and adopting the norms and lifestyles of peer groups, accepting the physical and sexual development of one's body, and establishing sexual, personal, moral, and occupational identities. If successfully achieved, these developmental tasks result in a sense of well-being, whereas failure leads to further life difficulties.[27] However, developmental tasks do not stand alone, and they are best understood when viewed in the context of adolescents' sociocultural and economic environments.

PHYSICAL DEVELOPMENT AND PUBERTY

Physical development is the result of significant biological changes. Adolescents gain approximately 50% of their adult weight and 20% of their adult height during this rapid period of physical growth. This dramatic increase in height, weight, and changes in body proportions occur as the result of a complex regulatory process, involving pituitary gland initiation of the release of growth and sex-related hormones from the thyroid, adrenal glands, and ovaries and testes.[11]

Due to individual differences, growth varies in onset and duration. The average growth period lasts about 4 years. It can begin as early as when the child is 9 years old, and in some adolescents, it may continue to around age 17. In the United States, the average peak of growth for girls occurs around age 11, and they usually reach their full height 2 years after they begin menstruating. In boys, age 13 is typically the time of peak growth. Skeletal growth and muscle development result in an overall increase in strength and endurance for physical activities. Bones grow; increase in length, width, strength; and change in composition. This skeletal growth is not consistent; head, hands, and feet reach their adult size earliest. Bones calcify, replacing the cartilaginous composition of bones making them denser and stronger.

During this period of bone growth, muscles also increase in size and strength. Strength is greatest around 12 months after an adolescent's height and weight have reached his or her peak. The related development in coordination and endurance results in an overall improvement in skilled motor performance.[11] These gains in muscle mass and increased capacity in heart and lung functions are greatest in males, and their performance peaks around 17 to 18 years of age.[9] The difference between the sexes in strength and gross motor performance continues throughout adulthood.

Girls show an increase in motor performance earlier, around the age of 14 years. It also includes enhanced speed, accuracy, and endurance. However, motor performance changes in girls' are highly variable. A complex interaction of physical and social factors such as their musculoskeletal development and menses as well as their interest, motivation, participation, and attitude toward physical activities influence their motor performance and response to their physical abilities.[9]

Many adolescents find social confidence in fitting within the "typical" pattern of physical development. They derive comfort in being similar to their peers, but there are also advantages in physical competence in sport activities that build **self-esteem** and enhance social status. In particular, early-maturing boys are more likely to be described as being popular, well adjusted, and leaders at school and in social groups. These adolescents are often more concerned about being liked and adhering to rules and routines than later-developing males. However, there is a downside to early physical development; it brings about the expectations of coaches, parents, and peers to excel in physical activities. This unwelcome pressure can lead to anxiety. In contrast, late-maturing boys are reported to feel self-conscious about their lack of physical development.[50] A comparable pattern of early physical competence and increased social status is not observed in girls.

Puberty

Puberty, the biological process of sexual reproductive maturity that occurs with the rapid physical growth of adolescence, is controlled by a complex interactive feedback loop involving the pituitary gland, hypothalamus, and the gonads (ovaries in females and testes in males). Similar to physical growth, the age of puberty varies by as much as 3 years.[45,50]

In puberty, specific changes occur in the sex organs. Menstruation begins in girls; the penis and testicles increase in size in males. Race, socioeconomic status, heredity, and nutrition influence menarche in girls. Ovulation typically starts 12 to 18 months after menarche and at the peak period of physical growth.[50,53] In boys, in addition to primary sexual growth changes such as increase in the size of the penis, spermarche (first ejaculations) generally occurs between 12 and 13 years of age. At the same time that secondary sex characteristics develop, boys experience the development of facial hair and a lower voice, and girls experience the development of breasts and areolar size changes; pubic hair develops over a 3- to 4-year period in both sexes. Many adolescents will also experience acne, but it is more common in males (70% to 90%) due to the effect of testosterone.[21,45]

Only minimal research has been conducted on puberty in adolescents with developmental and physical disabilities. Therefore, little specific information exists to assist these adolescents, their caregivers, or their health professionals in understanding how puberty may differ for them.[49] Some research suggests that in girls with moderate-to-severe cerebral palsy, sexual maturation begins earlier or that it ends much later than in the general population.[62] Another retrospective study involving women with autism spectrum conditions reported that menstruation begins 8 months earlier (i.e., around the age of 13 years) or ends later than is typical.[32]

OT practitioners who work with adolescents, including those with disabilities and chronic conditions, need to be receptive to teen-initiated discussions and be willing to talk to them and their parents on topics ranging from physical development, sexual expression, and contraception. Information about sex education as it relates to people with disabilities can be found at sites such as www.sexualhealth.com and the National Information Center for Children and Youth with Disabilities (NICHCY). Referral to counselors and health care providers who offer counseling or are specialists in women's or men's reproductive health can be beneficial. In addition, OT practitioners need to recognize the signs of sexual abuse (see Box 13-2 in Chapter 13).

Implications of Physical Growth and Sexual Maturation for Adolescents

An adolescent's adjustment to his or her physical and sexual development influences global self-esteem.[53] Family, friends, and available information are important factors that contribute to a healthy adjustment. Some adolescents accept their physical development easily, with a degree of pride, considering it a welcomed sign of their transition to adulthood. For other adolescents, these changes can be a source of confusion, anxiety, or emotional turmoil.[66]

Psychosocial development accompanies puberty, integrating physical and physiologic changes into a positive **body image**. The perception of one's own image affects a person's emotions, thoughts, and attitudes towards self and others. It influences choice of behaviors and relationships, especially intimate relationships.[9] Helping adolescents learn about their bodies, understand their feelings, express their thoughts about their bodies, and recognize that many of their peers share their experiences can contribute significantly to reducing anxiety.

Adolescents compare their bodies and appearances with "ideal masculine and feminine" images (Box 9-2). This social comparison is a significant dimension of body image perception and attitude toward one's body. It is pervasive in the media and manipulated by marketing (e.g., advertisements, teen magazines, TV shows, music videos, and the fashion industry). These images bear little relationship to the ethnic or physical appearance of the diverse population of American teens or their lifestyles. Therefore, it is not surprising that many adolescents struggle with their physical images and are critical of their bodies.[8,12]

CASE *Study*

Alisha is an attractive 14-year-old girl, 5 ft 3 in tall. Her outward appearance to her friends, family, and teachers is that of a successful adolescent. She achieves good grades, plays in the high school band, and is a member of the dance team. However, in the past 6 months she has become increasingly self-conscious, especially about her developing body and about the fact that she does not have a boyfriend like her friends do. To her delight, Alisha quickly

---

BOX 9-2

Healthy Development of Body Image

The practitioner may observe the following behaviors in the early and middle years of adolescence. These behaviors are typical of an adolescent concerned with developing a positive body image.

EARLY ADOLESCENTS
- Evaluate physical attractiveness and explore self-identity with single mindedness.
- Make comparisons between their bodies/appearances with those of others', especially those portrayed in the media.
- Have interest in and anxiety about their sexual development.

MIDDLE ADOLESCENTS
- Have achieved most of the physical changes associated with puberty and are developing an acceptance of their bodies.
- Are less preoccupied with their physical changes, and their interest now is oriented toward developing their appearance, grooming, and "trying to be attractive."
- Eating and other body image–related disorders develop and are established.

Adapted from Radizik M, Sherer S, Neinstein L: Psychosocial development in the normal adolescent. In Neinstein LS, editor: *Adolescent health: A practical guide*, Philadelphia, 2002, Lippincott Williams & Wilkins.

---

loses weight on a diet program. However, her dramatic weight loss does not change Alisha's belief that she is overweight and unattractive. She withdraws from her friends and increases her exercise routine. When her mother finds Alisha purging after eating, she becomes concerned and takes her to a psychiatrist. The psychiatrist diagnoses Alisha's condition as anorexia nervosa, a disorder characterized by a distorted self-image and a dysfunctional pattern of restricting food intake, purging, or both.

Negative body image, such as Alisha's view of herself, reflects low self-esteem. Both are often associated with mental health problems. Depression, anxiety, and body image disorders (e.g., dysphoria and anorexia nervosa) are common among adolescents. It is estimated that between 40% and 70% of girls, especially in early adolescence, are dissatisfied with two or more aspects of their physical appearance.[22] When listening to conversations among teenage girls, one is likely to hear comments such as "Do you think my backside is too big in these jeans?" or "I'm too fat, I need to lose weight." Studies of body image report that body dissatisfaction is universal and that most girls, regardless of ethnicity, express a desire to be thin.[39] Boys also experience dissatisfaction with their bodies. Their internalized perception of how they "should" be in relation to the images of masculinity involves greater muscle definition and muscle mass, typically in the upper body (i.e., shoulders, arms, and chest).[65]

Adjusting to these physical changes and developing a healthy body image contribute to a positive **self-concept**. This is a process of self-evaluation related to other abilities and competencies in physical activities (e.g., competitive sports). It also involves experimenting with changing one's physical appearance to express individuality. This can be simple and temporary, such as dying or cutting one's hair, or a more permanent statement such as body piercing and tattoos.

Adolescents with disabilities do not always have opportunities to make choices about their appearance and to experiment with change as part of their adolescence experience. Exploring self and body image is more difficult for them, since these adolescents may depend on others for their self-care, may not have their own money, and often lack independence in community mobility. Maintaining their child-like status, rather than adjusting to the emotional and psychological changes and demands of adolescence, may be more comfortable for their parents. Within the framework of therapy, OT practitioners can facilitate experimentation and also support parents in their attempts to encourage typical adolescent activities.

Another dimension of physical maturation is sexual identity. Adolescents explore their sexuality and learn to form intimate relationships. Similar to physical development in strength and motor performance, early sexual maturity has social consequences. An outward appearance of sexual maturity can make adolescents seem older than their actual age, resulting in demands and expectations from peers and adults that they are not psychologically prepared to handle. As mentioned earlier, physically mature adolescents are more likely to have concerns about being liked than later-maturing peers. Despite these concerns, they are often popular and are successful in heterosexual relationships, whereas late-maturing boys are more likely to develop inappropriate dependence, feel insecure, exhibit disruptive behaviors, and abuse substances.[21,65] Some late-maturing boys find validation in academic pursuits and nonphysical competitive activities, especially those from middle and upper socioeconomic families that value such achievement.[24] However, studies report that early-maturing girls do not fare as well as do their male counterparts. They have lower self-esteem, have poorer body image, and are more likely to experience psychological difficulties such as eating disorders and depression than do their average maturing peers.[66] Like late-maturing boys, they are also are more likely to have lower grades, engage in substance abuse (alcohol, drugs), and exhibit behavioral problems.

With sexual maturation of the body, adolescents also develop further awareness of their gender and sexual orientation. *Gender identity* refers to a person's perception of and identification with being either masculine or feminine, which is not the same as being biologically female or male. Gender identity is subjective and internal to the individual; it is expressed through personality and how a person presents himself or herself to others.

Sexual orientation refers to a person's preference pattern of physical and emotional arousal, and sexual attraction toward others of either the opposite sex or the same sex/gender.[19] Adolescence is a time of sexual exploration, dating, and romance, and this period heightens awareness of one's sexual orientation.

Most adolescents identify their sexual orientation as heterosexual, whereas about 15% of teens in mid-adolescence experience an emotional and/or sexual attraction to their same sex. Approximately 5 percent of teens will identify themselves as gay or lesbian, but they often delay openly identifying their sexual orientation until late adolescence or early adulthood.[51] This postponement of identification as gay or lesbian is attributed to lack of support and acceptance among peers, prejudicial attitudes, and experiences of verbal and physical harassment in high school.[19]

Openness as well as willingness to discuss emerging sexuality and sexual and gender orientation is important in all OT practitioners. This openness includes using gender-neutral language (e.g., *partner* rather than *boyfriend* or *girlfriend*; *protection* rather than *birth control*), inquiring if they suspect violence in intimate relations, and providing nonjudgmental support.

COGNITIVE DEVELOPMENT

The quality of thinking evolves in adolescence. Cognitive development is the evolution of mental processes: higher-level thinking, construction, the acquisition and use of knowledge, as well as perception, memory, and the use of symbolism and language.[48] Piaget, the most notable theorist of cognitive development, referred to this phase as *formal operations*, the development of logical thinking.

The development of formal operation varies among adolescents. Their ability to think becomes more creative, complex, and efficient (speed and adeptness). It is more thorough, organized, and systematic than it was in late childhood.[11] Adolescents' ability to problem-solve and reason becomes increasingly sophisticated, and they develop the capacity to think abstractly (i.e., they do not require concrete examples). Initially, they are less likely to apply this more sophisticated thinking to new situations.[31,65]

The distinction between preadolescent thinking, which is characterized by consideration of possibilities as generalizations of real events, and logical thinking is the realization that the world is one of possibilities, imagined as well as real.[48] This process of thinking about possibilities without the use of concrete examples is referred to as *hypothetical–deductive reasoning* and is essential for problem-solving and arguing. This type of reasoning makes it possible for a person to identify, imagine, and theoretically explore potential outcomes to determine the most likely or best one. With this newly acquired abstract thinking, adolescents develop the ability to make decisions about their behaviors that integrates values and weighs options. For the first time in their lives, adolescents begin to develop a perspective of time that is future oriented. They see the relationship between their present actions and the future consequences of these actions.

Some gender differences are present in cognitive development. On average, girls exceed boys in verbal abilities, possibly because they acquire language skills earlier. In contrast, boys tend to outperform girls in tasks that use visual–spatial skills, especially manipulating images (e.g., mental rotation). In the area of math performance, boys demonstrate skills in geometry and word problems, whereas girls excel in computational tasks.[50]

As advanced cognitive abilities become established, adolescents achieve independence in thought and action.[10] The quality of performance in academic learning activities (i.e., educational achievement) improves, and adolescents begin to consider and develop occupational skills that will translate into career and work. Personal, social, moral, and political values that denote membership in adult society also evolve. Kohlberg, an important moral development theorist, describes this level of thinking as *postconventional*.[26] It refers to the ability to base one's moral judgment on one's own values and moral standards. Adolescents comprehend the bases of laws, the principles that underpin right and wrong, and the implications of violating these principles. This development of moral and social reasoning enables them to deal with concepts such as integrity, justice, truth, reciprocity, and ambiguity.[26]

Cognition informs occupational performance. One dimension of cognition in the American Occupational Therapy Association (AOTA's) Practice Framework is self-regulation, the ability to control and monitor one's behavior and emotions relative to the situation and social cues.[1] Impulsive ill-conceived behaviors with little or no consideration of the consequences are more characteristic of junior high school or early high school students.[30] Adolescents with mild-to-moderate cognitive impairments associated with head injuries, severe mental health disorders, and mild intellectual disabilities also exhibit impulsive and poor self-monitoring of their behaviors. They sometimes fail to comprehend the consequences of their actions or to recognize the subtle social cues used as feedback to modify our responses.

BOX 9-3

Strategies for Working With Adolescents With Cognitive Impairments

- Identify how each teen learns best. Ask the teen, family, or teachers.
- Identify strengths and build from existing skills.
- Offer specific choices (*Which of these three things would you like to do?*) rather than an open-ended choice (*What would you like to do?*).
- Select activities that match the teen's abilities, needs, and interests. Offer activities that are age related but within the performance level of the teen (e.g., themes that deal with developmental needs such as relationships, appearance, grooming, and self-identity).
- Break down activities into simple steps that are achievable, but provide a challenge.
- Keep instructions simple.
- Present only one instruction or step at a time.
- Increase instructions only if the client consistently follows current directions.
- Present directions systematically.
- Use many methods of instruction (e.g., verbal instructions, demonstrations, visual cues such as pictures, step-by-step diagrams, and the hand-over-hand technique).
- Help the client develop and learn a new skill in a familiar setting before using the skill in novel settings (e.g., the community).
- Give specific feedback with concrete examples. Describe the correct or incorrect skill or behavior demonstrated. "Good" is an example of encouragement; it does not give clear feedback on performance.
- Be consistent, and use repetition.
- Do not introduce variety without a reason. Change can mean new cognitive demands for the teen and can increase the stress of learning. Flexibility and behavioral and cognitive adaptations are difficult for adolescents with cognitive impairments.

Difficulty in processing social cues (nonverbal body language and facial expressions) adversely influences the quality of their social interactions and ability to maintain relationships.[55] Their cognitive impairment may also result in limited problem-solving skills and poor insight as to the implications of behaviors and decisions. Box 9-3 lists some strategies for working with adolescents with cognitive impairments.

PSYCHOSOCIAL DEVELOPMENT

Psychosocial development is the essence of adolescence. There are three characteristic phases of psychosocial development. Phase 1 is *early adolescence* during the middle school years between the ages of 10 and 13; phase 2 is *middle adolescence* during the high school years between the ages of 14 and 17; and phase 3 is *late adolescence* between the ages of 17 and 21 in the first years of work or college.[2,50] Table 9-2 outlines common behaviors seen in each of these phases.

The critical task of adolescence is achieving a stable, multidimensional self-identity. It involves reflection to identify and integrate one's values, beliefs, and perceptions into a view of one's self as an autonomous and valued member of society. This *egocentric* process of self-absorption has cognitive and psychosocial dimensions. A cognitive component is adolescents' belief that others are just as concerned about and interested in their appearances, behaviors, and activities as they are themselves. It involves thinking one is special and invulnerable. The risks and poor decisions with regard to personal safety taken by adolescents are a reflection of this egocentric thinking.

The middle years comprise the most intense period of psychosocial development during adolescence. Family activities are less interesting to adolescents, whereas peer relationships become all-important. Peers become increasingly influential in the adolescent's life, which makes acceptance into peer groups highly desirable and conformity to the opinions of friends and peers likely.[50]

Late adolescence is a period of consolidation. In this phase, adolescents ideally become responsible young adults who are able to make viable decisions, have a stable and consistent value system, and can successfully take on adult roles such as worker or even parent. It is the stable, positive sense of self and awareness of one's own abilities that enables late adolescents and young adults to establish healthy relationships. In this transition from emotional and physical dependency upon parents, familial relationships are reframed to reflect the adult status.

An increased vulnerability to most mental health disorders is present in adolescence. Difficulty or failure in successfully navigating psychological and social developmental tasks can have far-reaching health and social consequences. The problems an OT practitioner might observe include deterioration in school performance, dropping out of school, suicide attempts, withdrawing from social participation, self-critical comments, and self-harm. Early recognition and effective intervention are crucial.

Theoretical Stages of Identity

The hallmark of psychosocial development is the quest for self-identity. From birth, infants begin this process by establishing themselves as separate entities from their mothers. Throughout childhood and across adult life, a person's sense of self continues to evolve, but the process is most intense in adolescence.[11]

Self-identity has two components: (1) an individual component—*who am I as a person*; and (2) a contextual component—*where and how do I fit into my world*. The contextual component is one's understanding of one's relationship to others and the world.[34] The individual component is the persona from which a person relates to others and his or her environment.[40] Outwardly, a person's **identity** is visible in his or her values, beliefs, interests, and commitments to work, and the social role he or she assumes, such as daughter or parent.[40] When people believe that others value the qualities and characteristics that define them, they are more likely to experience emotional well-being.

Identity Formation: "Who am I?"

Erik Erikson was the first developmental theorist to propose that acquiring a sense of identity (*identity formation*) was the foremost psychosocial task of adolescent development.[40] He theorized that one's self-identity develops through the recognition of one's abilities, interests, strengths, and weaknesses and continues to dictate how identity formation is viewed in research and clinical practice.[40] He described identity formation as crisis resolution and commitment to an identity through a complex process. The outcome, self-identity, is a composite of spiritual and religious beliefs, intellectual, social, and political interests, and a vocational or occupational commitment. It also includes gender orientation, identification with culture and ethnicity, and perceptions of one's personality traits (e.g., introverted, extroverted, open, conscientious).

Adolescents' quest for self-identity is a frequent theme in films and literature and is the angst expressed in the lyrics of popular music. Daydreams and fantasies about real and imagined selves energize and motivate adolescents as they attempt to make sense of their world. To achieve this, they experiment; they try different roles, express a variety of opinions and preferences, and make choices. They try out different activities and lifestyles before eventually settling upon a set of values, moral perspectives, and life goals. Adolescents engage in introspection (internalized thinking about the self and making social comparisons between themselves and peers) and self-evaluation. They also evaluate how their family and friends view them. They set goals, take action, and resolve conflicts and problems.[34] All of these behaviors help them identify what makes them individuals.

Promoting psychosocial development is implicit in all adolescent OT services. Meeting an adolescent's psychosocial needs requires recognition of the dimensions of identity and the activities that encourage identity formation. This recognition assists OT practitioners in planning therapy interventions that encourage exploration and

TABLE 9-2

Typical Characteristics of Psychosocial Development

PHASE	CHARACTERISTICS
Early adolescence	Being engrossed with self (e.g., interested in personal appearance)
	Emotional separation from parents (e.g., reduced participation in family activities); less overt display of affection toward parents
	Decrease in compliance with parents' rules or limits, as well as challenging of other authority figures (e.g., teachers, coaches)
	Questioning of adults' opinions (e.g., critical of and challenging their parents' opinions, advice, and expectations); seeing parents as having faults
	Changing moods and behavior
	Mostly same-sex friendships, with strong feelings toward these peers
	Demonstration of abstract thinking
	Idealistic fantasizing about careers; thinking about possible future self and role(s)
	Importance of privacy (e.g., having own bedroom with doors closed, writing diaries, having private telephone conversations)
	Interest in experiences related to personal sexual development and exploring sexual feelings (e.g., masturbation)
	Self-consciousness, display of modesty, blushing, awkwardness about self and body
	Ability to self-regulate emotional expression; limited behavior (e.g., not thinking beyond immediate wants or needs, therefore being susceptible to peer pressure)
	Experimenting with drugs (cigarettes, alcohol, and marijuana)
Middle adolescence	Continuation of movement toward psychological and social independence from parents
	Increased involvement in peer group culture, displayed in adopting peer value system, codes of behavior, style of dress and appearance, demonstrating individualism and separation from family in an overt way
	Involvement in formal and informal peer groups such as sports teams, clubs, or gangs
	Acceptance of developing body; sexual expression and experimentation (e.g., dating, sexual activity with partner)
	Exploring and reflecting on the expressions of own feelings and those of other people
	Increased realism in career/vocational aspirations
	Increased creative and intellectual ability; growing interest in intellectual activities and capacity to do work (e.g., mentally and emotionally)
	Risk-taking behaviors underscored by feelings of omnipotence (sense of being powerful) and immortality; engaging in risky behaviors, including reckless driving, unprotected sex, high alcohol consumption, and drug use
	Experimenting with drugs (cigarettes, alcohol, marijuana, and other illicit drugs)
Late adolescence	More stable sense of self (e.g., interests and consistency in opinions, values, and beliefs)
	Strengthened relationships with parents (e.g., parental advice and assistance valued)
	Increased independence in decision making and ability to express ideas and opinions
	Increased interest in the future; consideration of the consequences of current actions and decisions on the future; this behavior leads to delayed gratification, setting personal limits, ability to monitor own behavior, and reach compromises
	Resolution of earlier angst at puberty about physical appearance and attractiveness
	Diminished peer influence; increased confidence in personal values and sense of self
	Preference for one-to-one relationships; starting to select an intimate partner
	Becoming realistic in vocational choice or employment, establishing worker role, and working toward financial independence
	Definition of an increasingly stable value system (e.g., regarding morality, belief, religious affiliation, and sexuality)

Data from Radizik M, Sherer S, Neinstein LS: Psychosocial development in normal adolescent. In Neinstein LS, editor: *Adolescent health care: A practical guide*, ed 4, Philadelphia, 2002, Lippincott Williams & Wilkins; American Academy of Child and Adolescent Psychiatry: http://www.aacap.org/publications: Accessed September 7, 2004.

resolution of identity-related challenges appropriate to an adolescent's developmental state.

Adolescents' behaviors, thoughts, and emotions may seem contradictory, particularly in those between the ages of 13 and 15. Adolescents may choose healthy behaviors, become a vegetarian, or participate in sports, but they may also experiment with alcohol, tobacco, street drugs, or junk food. They may explore different belief systems and argue passionately against their parent's ideological views. They may express disinterest in relationships with the opposite sex and then hang out exclusively with a girlfriend or boyfriend.

CASE *Study*

Sam has body piercings and recently got a tattoo. He frequently breaks his parents' curfew rules and is increasingly argumentative. Lately, he has been skipping classes and is talking about dropping out of his high school basketball team. At the same time, Sam has a job at his uncle's car dealership; he dresses appropriately for work and is reliable. He gets along well with his uncle, takes directions, and shows initiative.

Today's permissive and tolerant society permits adolescents a period of experimentation and exploration. To cite an example, when a teen's parents commented on her recent behavior, she retorted indignantly, "I don't have to be responsible. I am an adolescent." However, adolescents are expected to become young adults whose thinking, emotions, and behaviors are congruent with and reflect the prevailing social norms and values of their communities.

Building on Erickson's theory, developmental theorists describe identity as a series of states. They pose it as an ongoing process of negotiation, adaptation, and decision making. Marcia illustrates this perspective by describing four states of identity—(1) identity diffusion, (2) identity moratorium, (3) identity foreclosure, and (4) identity achievement—whose characteristics are different dimensions of exploration of or commitment to stable future goals.[40]

Identity diffusion, common in early adolescence, is the least defined sense of personal identity. In this identity state, an adolescent avoids or ignores the task of exploring his or her identity and has little interest in exploring options. These adolescents have yet to make a commitment to choices, interests, or values. The question "who am I" is not a significant issue. They tend to avoid or have difficulties meeting the day-to-day demands of life, such as completing school work or participating in sports or extracurricular activities.[10] In a state of identity diffusion, adolescents seldom anticipate or think about the future. Those who continue to experience identity diffusion well

into their middle and late adolescent years may demonstrate impulsivity, disorganized thinking, and immature moral reasoning.[11] Identity diffusion is associated with lower self-esteem, a negative attitude, and dissatisfaction with one's life, parents' lifestyle, and school.[11] Because they have not explored their interests or considered their strengths in relation to work, they sometimes have problems finding employment.

Identity moratorium in early and middle adolescence is emotionally healthy. It can continue into late adolescence, particularly for college students. Adolescents in this state openly explore alternatives, strive for autonomy, try out different interests, and pursue a sense of individuality. Adolescents experiencing a prolonged state of identity moratorium are likely to be undecided about the major course of study and their goals for the future and to still be actively exploring options. When the uncertainty of the moratorium state continues for too long, it is associated with anxiety, self-consciousness, impulsiveness, and depression.[12]

Adolescents who choose to avoid experiencing an identity crisis by prematurely committing to an identity, experience *identity foreclosure*. These adolescents do not engage in the process of self-exploration and experimentation. Without considering other possibilities, they typically accept their parents' values and beliefs and follow family expectations regarding career choices. Foreclosure is associated with approval-seeking behaviors and a high respect for authority. Compared with their peers, these adolescents are more conforming and less autonomous.[11] They prefer a structured environment, are less self-reflective, have few intimate relationships, and are less open to new experiences.[11] However, foreclosure on an identity makes them less anxious than many of their peers, who struggle with identity issues throughout adolescence.

Identity achievement following identity moratorium is an exploration of possibilities and the healthy resolution of the quest. It is reached in the final years of high school, in college, or in the first years of work. It is characterized by a commitment to interests, values, gender and sexual orientation, political views, career or job, and a moral stance. This relatively stable sense of self enhances self-esteem. Adolescents and young adults who attain identity achievement are autonomous, exhibit mature moral reasoning, and are independent. In resolving their identity issues, they are able to change and adapt in response to personal and social demands without undue anxiety, since they are less self-absorbed, self-conscious, and less vulnerable to pressure from peers. They are open and creative in their thinking.[11] A sense of identity also gives a person greater capacity for intimacy and self-regulation. Identity achievement represents congruency between a person's sense of identity, self-expression, and behavior (Box 9-4).[45]

BOX 9-4

Behavioral Indicators of Self-Esteem

POSITIVE SELF-ESTEEM
- Expresses opinions
- Mixes with other teens (e.g., interacts with social group of teens)
- Initiates friendly interactions with others
- Makes eye contact easily while speaking
- Faces others when speaking with them
- Maintains comfortable, socially determined space between self and others
- Speaks fluently in first language without pauses or visible discomfort
- Participates in group activities
- Works collaboratively with others
- Gives directions or instructions to others
- Volunteers for tasks and activities

NEGATIVE SELF-ESTEEM
- Avoids eye contact
- Is overly confident; for example, brags about achievements or skills
- Acts as class clown; seldom contributes to class constructively
- Is verbally self-critical; makes fun of self as a form of humor; puts self down
- Speaks loudly or dogmatically to avoid listening to others' responses
- Is submissive and overly agreeable to others' requests or demands
- Is reluctant to give opinions or views, especially if it will draw attention to himself or herself
- Monitors behaviors; for example, hypervigilant of surroundings and other people
- Makes excuses for performance; seldom evaluates personal performance as satisfactory
- Engages in putting others down, name calling, gossiping, and, at worst, bullying

Adapted from Santrock JW: *Adolescence*, New York, 2003, McGraw-Hill.

In late adolescence, the inability to achieve a stable positive identity is associated with lack of confidence and with low self-esteem. As adults, adolescents with this issue tend to have difficulties in many areas of their lives, such as work and intimate relationships. They are challenged by the countless responsibilities and stresses of adult life.

Social Roles

A person's roles are closely associated with self-identity. Social roles have characteristics and expectations assigned to them, and are universal to a particular cohort (i.e., a group of people with similar attributes, such as age and cultural affiliations). Therefore, the roles of adolescents place demands and constraints on their behaviors and define the occupational performance skills needed to successfully fulfill them. The relative importance of roles varies with age. Some roles provide social status, while others need to be assumed in order to transition to early adulthood; therefore, these roles influence social development, self-esteem, and identity. Examples of adolescent specific roles that are associated with identity are sport related, (e.g., jock, hockey player, cheerleader); some are academic (e.g., geek, nerd); and others have negative connotations (e.g., dork) or are associated with sexual or racial slurs. All of these roles have inferences to various sets of common behaviors, characteristics, and expectations, and they assign group membership.

Adolescents receiving OT services may have disabilities or disorders that marginalize or stereotype them. To some degree, these disabilities or disorders are roles, implying identities, and become barriers to others in recognizing adolescents' characteristics and qualities. An example is the characteristics that are stereotypical of "being disabled." Therefore, a goal associated with OT is to assist adolescents with disabilities to avoid internalizing these labels as integral to their identities and to help them define themselves by their interests, values, and competencies in social and occupational roles. This is achieved by providing adolescents with choices, building skills through individualized interventions and strategies that support inclusion, and advocating for community support.[42]

Adolescents with physical disabilities deal with the paradox of striving to achieve the typical adolescent independence while remaining physically dependent on their parents or caregivers. However, an identity as a self-determining autonomous person is subjective and does not require an adolescent to be physically independent. An adolescent with a physical disability may attain emotional and psychological independence by employing an attendant caregiver, taking on the responsibility to provide instructions about meeting needs, and determining the organization of his or her own daily routine. It may involve moving out of the family home and driving a modified vehicle.

OCCUPATIONAL PERFORMANCE IN ADOLESCENCE

In this section, we discuss four areas of occupation: (1) work, (2) instrumental activities of daily living (IADLs), (3) leisure, and (4) social participation.[1] Through their participation in occupations, adolescents explore activities that capture their curiosity and reflect their values, interests, and needs. They will take on the values associated with these activities while learning new skills or improving performance skills.[17] The competence they achieve enhances their peer acceptance, social status, and self-esteem.

Work

Work that includes paid employment and volunteer activities contributes to adolescents' developing interests and values.[33] It is a setting in which adolescents interact with adults on a more equal level, have opportunities to assume responsibilities, learn work behaviors and values, and develop preferences for future areas of work/careers. Work also develops other life and social skills such as managing money, organizing time, developing a routine, working collaboratively with other people, and communicating with social groups outside family and school. The earned disposable income gives some adolescents discretionary spending and a sense of economic independence. Other adolescents assume the responsibility for contributing to family income. In late adolescence, work is a recognized societal indicator of adulthood.

Studies of work patterns report that approximately 70% of adolescents work and attend school.[2] However, regulations state that they cannot work more than 4 hours on a school day and that the evening hours of work are restricted. Although some part-time work is beneficial, excessive hours of work (i.e., more than 20 hours a week) can be detrimental. It takes time away from academics, recreation and social activities, and participation in sports, and it increases the risk of work-related injuries.[52] It is also associated with emotional distress, sexual activity, and substance abuse at an early age.[4,63] Despite the adverse consequences, approximately 18% of high school students work 20 hours or more per week.[44] In addition to their paid employment, the 2000 edition of *America's Children: Key National Indicators of Well-Being* reported that 55% of high school students participated in volunteer activities. Studies have shown that adolescents who volunteer do better in school, feel more positive about themselves, and avoid risky behaviors such as substance abuse.[29]

OT programs can help adolescents effectively deal with the transition from school to work through prevocational assessment, establishment and maintenance of routines, work site coaching, managing community mobility, and building social skills. This takes care of one aspect of the transition. Adolescents also engage in a process of developing an **occupational identity**, which combines their interests, values, and abilities in the pursuit of a realistic choice of a job or a career path. This process optimally results in a work choice that integrates psychosocial identity and matches skills, values, and interests with job requirements.

Occupational identity begins to develop in early adolescence. As abstract thinking and the capacity to think about the future develops, adolescents start to fantasize about their future work. Initially, these fantasies are idealistic and combine aspirations and dreams about a possible adult self. By middle adolescence, the aspirations are more realistic, and by late adolescence, their work goals combine their interests and values with a realistic match between their performance abilities and actual job demands. Attending college or university can defer the determination of an occupational identity as it delays the transition to work.

Instrumental Activities of Daily Living

To gain competency in the instrumental activities of daily living (IADLs), adolescents gradually take on more responsibilities. It starts with personal or simple family chores, for example, cleaning one's room or emptying the dishwasher, and develops into tasks that contribute to the management of the household (e.g., mowing the lawn, doing laundry, cleaning the car, and cooking). As adolescents become more independent in these routines, they prepare meals for themselves and learn to drive or use public transport so that they can move about the community independently. Still with some parental oversight, they take on their own *health management*, such as taking medications, learning about health risks, and making decisions about health behaviors (e.g., smoking, having protected sex, nutrition, and personal hygiene routines).[1] They develop money management skills, beginning with activities such as shopping, and progressing to planning how and when to spend money, paying bills, or managing a credit card.

By middle adolescence, some adolescents will take on responsibilities of caring for children by babysitting and assisting with coaching or life guard work. With these tasks, they develop knowledge and awareness of *safety and emergency procedures*.[1] These roles and associated responsibilities extend their skill repertoire.

Cognitively able adolescents with physical disabilities, who are physically dependent, face unique challenges in the area of IADLs. If they are to live independently, their IADL learning involves decision making and problem solving to enable them to manage their health and finances and to acquire skills to instruct and oversee attendant caregivers who maintain their physical care and their environment. OT practitioners, along with parents, can assist these adolescents to take on these responsibilities.

Another dimension of IADL development includes the use and maintenance of a wide variety of communication technologies. A study of Canadian adolescents recommended that their use of technologies be seen as a continuum of personal communication (telephone and cell phone), social communication (e-mail, instant messaging, chat, and bulletin boards), interactive environments (Web sites, search engines, and computers), and unidirectional sources (television, radio, and print).[56]

Eighty-seven percent of adolescents between the ages of 12 and 17 years interact through online social networks such as MySpace or Facebook.[37] They are constantly connected to friends through text messaging, cell phones, instant messaging, and Twitter. They have contact with adults such as teachers and coaches via e-mail and social network sites. Girls dominate most of the content created online by adolescents; 35% of girls blog, whereas only 20% of boys do; 54% of girls post photos on the Internet, compared with 40% of boys; but boys post video content more than girls do.[38]

Adolescents have access to a vast amount of information and are connected to people beyond their immediate social network and geographic location. The benefits of the enjoyment of social networking and the use of the Internet have to be weighed against the risks involved in these activities. The use of technology integrates cognitive skills, values, and interests. Adolescents make moral decisions about the information they will access or share and who they interact with. It is important that they protect their personal identities and maintain privacy. However, they are of an age when risk taking is more likely, anticipation of consequences is underdeveloped, and problem-solving skills are inconsistent.

Leisure and Play

American adolescents spend more than half their waking hours in free time and **leisure** activities, and the choices they make in these situations are important to their development.[35] Adolescents can use leisure activities to explore and try out new behaviors and roles, establish likes and dislikes, socialize, and express themselves within peer groups. Outside the structured school and work settings, adolescents can assess their strengths, values, interests, and positions in the social context differently through leisure activities.[61] Often, in these activities, adolescents experience more personal choice, more scope for creativity, and fewer performance expectations from parents. An OT study of teens' views of leisure reported that they engage in leisure for enjoyment and describe it as "freedom of choice" and "time out."[50]

Not all leisure activities are equal. Some provide a constructive use of time and participation in organized leisure activities and promote the development of physical, intellectual, and social skills.[17] Structured leisure activities that are part of extracurricular school programs (e.g., sports teams, school band or orchestra, drama club, and cheerleading) or community-based activities such as scouts and music and dance classes involve goal-directed challenges but are also fun. These programs promote healthy development and teach skills that are associated with higher academic performance and occupational achievement.[17,25] Other outcomes for adolescents involved in extracurricular activities include an increased likelihood of attending college, better interpersonal skills, greater community involvement, and lower alcohol and drug use and antisocial behavior.[17,25] For

example, boys from low socioeconomic backgrounds who exhibit low-to-moderate academic performance but play sports are more likely to finish high school.

Participation in physical leisure activities have long-term health advantages and are predictive of adult physical activity levels.[61] The increase in obesity and chronic health conditions in the American population highlights the importance of adolescent physical activity.[32] Many high school, college, and community programs actively promote participation in physical activity as a public health objective. Despite these initiatives, the number of adolescents who engage in sports and physical activities has declined overall. While a number of studies have identified the many factors (parents, teachers, peers) that influence an adolescent's physical activity level, friends are one of the most influential.[61] Boys are more likely to participate in and have a positive attitude toward physical activities than are girls because of the relationship between masculine identities, sports, and competition (Figure 9-1).[61]

> **CLINICAL *Pearl***
>
> Physical activity is important for all children, including adolescents with disabilities. The recommended amount of physical activity for children and adolescents is 1 hour or more per day, ideally including both aerobic and strength activities. Even if the children do not achieve this level of intensity or duration of physical activity, benefits from moderate levels of physical activity, 20 to 30 minutes of activity three or more times a week, can be significant. The level and type of physical activity can be adapted for adolescents with disabilities and integrated into their individualized education program (IEP). Physical activities for adolescents with physical disabilities reduce their risk of acquiring secondary disabilities in adulthood. Many of the secondary disabilities are associated with poor lifestyle habits and are preventable.[58]

Adolescents spend much of their unstructured time watching television and playing computer games, and these passive leisure activities have little benefit. The main criticism is that they contribute to boredom, which is associated with a greater risk of dropping out of school, drug use, and antisocial or delinquent activities.[61] Another risk factor is the development of a lifelong pattern of sedentary leisure activities, which is associated with obesity and increased incidence of chronic health problems.

Leisure activities are a valuable therapeutic area of OT practice. Enhancing leisure and related skills, especially those related to social behavior, has other beneficial outcomes. For example, an improvement in skills

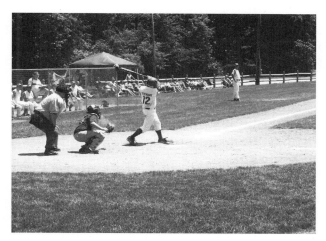

FIGURE 9-1   Baseball games and other team sports provide a peer group and competition.

related to a leisure activity may enable an adolescent to join and succeed in extracurricular school activities. Successful participation in these popular age-related groups can transfer beyond the context of therapy by building **self-efficacy** and autonomy. Furthermore, as mentioned previously, extracurricular activities are positively associated with healthy life choices.

CLINICAL *Pearl*

Adolescents with disabilities have the challenge of achieving a sense of identity that constructively integrates their differences into a coherent and healthy self-concept. Labeling adolescents by using their disorder to describe them (e.g., "disabled teens") is not acceptable. Client-centered occupational therapy (OT) identifies adolescents by their abilities. Like most of their peers, self-conscious and acutely aware of themselves, adolescents with disabilities or chronic health problems want to be "like everyone else," namely, other teenagers in their social groups. The OT practitioner's role is to assist adolescents with disabilities develop personal identities that do not make their disabilities a central or defining characteristic of how they view themselves. For example, labeling Jane "the cerebral palsy student" or Doug "the disruptive student" or "the clumsy student" can encourage adolescents to shape their identities around the labels they hear. As a consequence of this behavior of others, they will set limits upon themselves rather than focus on their abilities and characteristics that make them more like other adolescents. Identifying and developing performance skills enhance self-efficacy and self-esteem, which, in turn, promotes a positive sense of self.

Social Participation

Social participation, which involves patterns of behavior and activities expected of an individual, is an important area of occupational performance. Social integration, a sense of belonging, acceptance, and friendships, all play a significant role in an adolescent's emotional adjustment.[65] By engaging in a spectrum of social activities, adolescents explore and develop social roles and relationships.[60,61] These roles and relationships provide adolescents with social status and a social identity separate from that which is associated with their roles within their families and expands their sources of emotional and social support to include friends and nonfamily adults.[5,10]

Being part of *cliques* is one form of social participation. Cliques are small, cohesive groups of adolescents and have a somewhat flexible membership. They meet the personal needs of their members, who share a broad range of activities and modes of communication. They provide a normative reference for comparison with peers and significantly influence the development of social attitudes and behaviors.[5] The transition from junior high school to high school is easier with membership in supportive and peer-recognized cliques.

In early and middle adolescence, the membership of cliques initially develops spontaneously around common interests, school activities, and neighborhood affiliations. The cliques in junior high school are usually same sex groups; in middle to late adolescence, the cliques expand to include the opposite sex. In late adolescence, cliques weaken, and loose associations among couples replace this social structure.[10]

Exclusion from social cliques has a cost. Adolescents experience the exclusion as rejection, social isolation, lack of social status, and loss of opportunities to participate in the array of identity-developing activities. An adolescent who does not find his or her niche in a clique or social group is more likely to be depressed, be lonely, and have psychological problems.[10] One explanation for some adolescents joining less constructive peer groups, such as gangs or groups who engage in illegal or antisocial activities, is their exclusion from desired social cliques or the lack of alternatives for peer group experiences (Box 9-5).

Marginalized adolescents excluded from social groups may experience bullying. While the occurrence of verbal abuse is consistent across grades, physical bullying peaks in middle school and declines during high school.[28] Newer trends in bullying involve social networking sites like MySpace and other computer-mediated communication modes such as texting, and e-mail. Signs of bullying are loneliness, deterioration in performance (grades), and avoiding school or even dropping out.[14]

In 2000, the U.S. Department of Education issued an official statement regarding disability harassment in

BOX 9-5

Quick Facts: Health and Health Risks Behaviors Among American Teenagers

- Child and adolescent obesity in the United States is a significant health problem. Eighteen percent of adolescents, 12 -19 years, are overweight (Data: 2003-2006). Seventy percent of overweight adolescents are likely to be obese or overweight as adults unless they adopt and maintain healthier patterns of eating and exercise.
- Depression is a significant health concern among adolescents. In 2005, 20% of male and 37% of female students reported being so sad or hopeless almost every day for two or more consecutive weeks in the past 12 months that they stopped doing some activities.
- Adolescent death rates due to injury in 2005 were:
  - Unintentional injury death rate was 31.4 deaths per 100,000; 73 percent of the unintentional injuries were motor-vehicle traffic related.
  - Adolescent homicide rate was 9.9 deaths per 100,000; 84 percent of the homicides were firearm-related.
  - The adolescent suicide rate was 7.7 deaths per 100,000; 46 percent of the suicides were firearm-related and 40 percent of the suicides were by hanging. About 25% of female and 15% of male high school students stated that they had attempted or seriously considered suicide. Suicide is the third leading cause of death among adolescents.
- For every adolescent suicide death, it is estimated another 10 adolescents make a suicide attempt. Statistics for 2008 show that 8.8 percent of drug-related emergency department visits made by adolescents aged 12 to 17 involved suicide attempts. Seventy-two percent (almost three out of four) of these visits for drug-related suicide attempts were adolescent girls.
- Alcohol is the most widely used drug by adolescents. It is the typical first drug used by boys. The percentage of adolescents (12-19 years) who reported drinking alcohol in the past month was 17% (Center for Disease Control [CDC] 2006). Nineteen percent reported binge drinking; 26 percent report episodic heavy drinking and a further 6 percent reported heavy alcohol use. Overall 44.7 percent of high school students report current use of alcohol.
- Typically, the first drug used by girls is nicotine (cigarettes). Approximately 25.7% of students reported current cigarette use, current smokeless tobacco use, or current cigar use. Forty five percent of American adolescents have tried cigarettes by 12th grade, and one out of five (20%) 12th graders report being current smokers. Even in 8th grade, one in five (21%) have tried cigarettes, and 1 in 15 (7%) has already become a current smoker (Monitoring the Future Study [MFS], 2008; Youth Risk Behavior Surveillance [YRBSS], 2007 data).
- Thirty-eight percent (almost 1 in 4) of high school high school students reported having used marijuana in their lifetime. It is the most common illicit drug used by high school adolescents (YRBSS 2007 data).
- The National Survey of Drug Use and Health found that 8.2% of 12- to 17-year-olds depended on/abused alcohol or illicit drugs; this behavior was slightly higher among female adolescents than male peers (8.4% vs. 7.9%). The use of ecstasy is more prevalent than that of cocaine. Other illicit drugs that have increased in use by teenagers are anabolic steroids and heroin (MFS, 2006, 2008).
- Approximately 47.8% of high school students have had sexual intercourse and the prevalence is highest among female students. Nationally, 35.0% of high students had had sexual intercourse with at least one person during the proceding 3 months i.e., currently sexually active when surveyed in 2007 (YRBSS 2007 data).
- National CDC in the YRBSS survey data 2008 reports that 7.8% of students had ever been forced physically to have sexual intercourse when they did not want to. The overall prevalence of having been forced to have sexual intercourse was higher among female (11.3%) than male (4.5%) students.
- The teenage birth rate declined for a 14 year period, but rose in 2005-2006 by 3 percent to 41.9 births per 1,000. This increase was greatest for non-Hispanic black teens, whose overall rate rose 5 percent in 2006 and the lowest increase was for Hispanic teens (2 percent).

This information was compiled from the following resources retrieved in June 2010:

National Institute on Drug Abuse National Institutes of Health (2008).

Monitoring the Future, National results on adolescent drug use - Overview of Key Findings. http://www.monitoringthefuture.org/pubs/monographs/overview2008.pdf

1.1 **The DAWN Report May 13, 2010: Emergency Department Visits for Drug-related Suicide Attempts by Adolescents: 2008 retrieved from the SAMHSA National Clearinghouse for Alcohol and Drug Information.** http://ncadi.samhsa.gov/

1.2 **Center for Disease Control and Prevention:**

Adolescent Health in the United States, 2007 http://www.cdc.gov/nchs/fastats/adolescent_health.htm

Summary Health Statistics for U.S. Children: National Health Interview Survey, 2008. http://www.cdc.gov/nchs/data/series/sr_10/sr10_244.pdf

Morbidity and Mortality Weekly Report YRBSS Summaries, June 8 2008, Vol. 57, SS-4. http://www.cdc.gov/mmwr/PDF/ss/ss5704.pdf

Knopf, D., Park, M. J., & Mulye, T. (2008). The Mental Health of Adolescents:

A National Profile, NAHIC http://nahic.ucsf.edu/downloads/MentalHealthBrief.pdf

school.[28] That same year, the National Center on Secondary Education and Transition provided strategies for school interventions and educational programs to address and deter bullying (http://www.ncset.org). Improving an adolescent's social skills and facilitating participation in social and extracurricular activities can reduce his or her vulnerability to bullying.

Friendships are different from peer groups or clique relationships. Friendships involve openness and honesty and are equally important in an adolescent's development. Adolescents with friends are more emotionally intense and are less concerned about social acceptance.[11] Friends share common characteristics: ethnicity, interests, age, sex, and behavioral tendencies. Girls generally have more friends and their friendships have more closeness; they perceive greater support and intimacy (sharing) than do boys (Figure 9-2).[10] The friendships of boys are congenial relationships established around shared interests such as sports, music, or other common activities (see Figure 9-1).

The friendships of adolescence evolve over time and reflect cognitive and psychosocial development.[10] Initially, adolescent friendships are between individuals of the same sex and develop around shared activities and possessions and from a closeness of mutual understanding. In middle adolescence, friendships develop around shared loyalty and an exchange of ideas. During these years, emotional intensity and sharing of confidences heighten the vulnerability in peer relationships.[11] By the latter years of adolescence, friendships evolve to incorporate both autonomy and interdependence; dependence on friends diminishes, and sharing of *all* activities is no longer an essential aspect of the relationship. This is partly because the focus of late adolescents shifts to developing meaningful, intimate relationships.

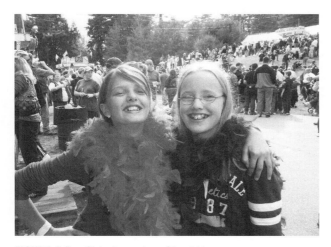

FIGURE 9-2   Girls share close friendship.

Close friendships are important for self-esteem and are associated with less anxiety and depression in adolescence.[11] The social participation and closeness provide intimacy and social and emotional adjustments, which contribute to adult interpersonal skills. Adolescents talk to their friends, share concerns and fears, and learn from each other. This is important because this is a time of emotional separation from parents for most adolescents when they are apt to claim, "My parents don't understand me."

Contrary to popular opinion, major conflicts between parents and adolescents are *not* a normal part of the adolescent–parent relationship.[36] Stability and security provided by parents or significant adults are critical in adolescence, and for the most part, they continue to maintain a loving and respectful relationship with their parents, provided it existed even before adolescence. The physical and emotional separation from parents and the questioning of parents' values and beliefs are healthy, especially if the family context includes parental positive regard, constructive limit setting, and emotional stability. While peer influence is mostly around tastes, interests, and lifestyle, parents' influence continues to inform goals, personal values, and morals. When child–parent conflicts exist, they occur mostly in early adolescence and are about autonomy or control. Therefore, it is not surprising that adolescents in families with an authoritative parenting style exhibit competitive behaviors.

Quality relationships with adults who are not family members are beneficial to healthy adolescent development. Structured out-of-school activities, such as nonacademic extracurricular and leisure activities, provide the venue for relationships with nonfamilial adults. Adults often reflect on those positive influential experiences with coaches, adult leaders, and teachers who gave them attention during their adolescence. These activities and interactions facilitate problem solving, provide social support outside the family, increase self-esteem, and promote skill acquisition.[17] Research shows that high-risk adolescents benefit from nonfamilial relationships and that they participate less in risky behaviors (e.g., carrying a firearm or using illegal drugs.[6] A number of studies have demonstrated the value of mentoring programs such as Big Brothers and Little Sisters and participation in extracurricular activities.

THE CONTEXT OF ADOLESCENT DEVELOPMENT

This chapter, as does the OT literature, uses the terms *context* and *environment* interchangeably. These terms refer to the settings and the characteristics of the settings in which adolescents live, work, and play. The relationship between an adolescent and his or her context is reciprocal; it has an impact on what is done and how it is done. Salient contexts influence occupational performance by encouraging or supporting development. Others may compromise adolescents' development by being unsafe or by not offering the necessary resources for learning healthy behaviors and acquiring skills.

Social context comprises friends, team members, other students, parents, siblings, extended family, coaches, and teachers, who have expectations, provide support and resources, and are positive or negative role models. *Physical context* involves the adolescent's school, home, and community, including the socioeconomic factors and the resources that are available. Culture and ethnicity also shape the social and physical contexts.[48] Culture represents the beliefs, perceptions, values, and norms of the group. The dominant culture (mainstream American) can sometimes conflict with family culture, particularly for adolescents who belong to minority groups or immigrant families that have their own cultural, ethnic, or religious beliefs. The values of both the dominant culture and the minority culture have an internalized component related to identity and an externalized component that takes the form of expectations. Adolescents can feel torn between the desire to belong to a peer group within the dominant culture and the desire to identify with and respect the family's culture.[47]

An OT practitioner working in a diverse setting needs to understand the social and cultural norms and expectations of adolescents' ethnic and sociocultural backgrounds. Cultural factors may influence their choices of activities and interests, self-esteem, and the expectations of their families.[47] Cultural perceptions of a disability or a disorder may also influence the family's and adolescent's therapy goals. The expectations of the adolescent's social peer context and family cultural context will together shape his or her "adaptive social and emotional development."[5]

The influence of activities on development varies, since contexts may determine the relative importance and value of the activities.[25] For example, in low-income communities, success in high school sports defines a "good student," whereas in higher-income communities that value academic achievement, other types of extracurricular activities will also define a "good student."[25]

Social contexts, for example, a low-income or disorganized family, increase the likelihood of deviant or high-risk behaviors.[41] Similarly, adolescents from disadvantaged or marginalized groups may have limited access to resources and fewer positive and healthy opportunities to develop self-esteem and complex cognitive skills.[41] Therefore, school, therapy, and extracurricular activities may play a significant role in meeting their needs and alleviating the harmful effects of their social and home contexts. Client-centered OT can facilitate development by providing a variety of choices and opportunities for decision making; this will foster a sense of personal control and provide constructive feedback. Likewise, a therapeutic milieu can offer adolescents opportunities for self-directed exploration in a safe, stable, and supportive environment. Acceptance, positive regard, and opportunities to make mistakes and self-correct without negative consequences (e.g., emotional or physical abuse) are all important contextual characteristics for healthy development. Table 9-3 lists some of the contextual characteristics that foster adolescent self-development and skill acquisition.

TABLE 9-3

Contextual Factors That Contribute to Healthy Adolescent Development

CONTEXTUAL FACTOR	CHARACTERISTICS
Support	Family support, including positive parent–adolescent communication Parental involvement in school activities and schoolwork Constructive relationships with other adults Caring neighborhood and school environment
Empowerment	Community valuing the youth Adolescents given useful and valued roles in the community Community involving adolescents in community service activities and valuing their contributions Safe home and community environments
Boundaries and expectations of adolescents	Family boundaries that include rules and consequences School and neighborhood boundaries that include rules, consequences, and community monitoring of behavior Adult role models Positive peer influences High expectations—family, friends, and school expect adolescent to do well

From the Search Institute, 2004: http://www.search-institute.org.

NAVIGATING ADOLESCENCE WITH A DISABILITY

The estimated 23% to 35% of American adolescents with chronic health conditions or special care needs experience the same development as adolescents without disabilities.[18,46] They will make the same adjustments to physical growth, puberty, psychological independence from parents or caregivers, and social relationships with same and opposite sexes and seek to acquire a sense of identity. However, their chronic health conditions, disabilities, and physical dependence upon others create additional challenges for them and their families. Undertaking these developmental tasks such as the prerequisite of choosing a job, being out of school, working and living outside the family home are more complicated.[13,23] Parents also can find the transition challenging. Many have been the primary supports and caregivers for their adolescents and have advocated vigorously for their children's needs. However, the time has come for them to let go of the role that has dominated their lives.

Adolescents with disabilities have fewer opportunities to engage in typical adolescent experiences, to make their own choices, to engage in social relationships, or explore the world of ideas, values, and cultures different from those of their families.[7,59,64] Yet, they need opportunities to experience and learn from successes and failures they initiate in order to develop a sense of self-efficacy and determine realistic goals for themselves.[58,64]

Adolescents with disabilities or chronic illnesses (e.g., cancer, diabetes) deal with additional issues: negative self-perceptions, lower expectations, and social isolation. Some confront stigma associated with their disabilities, discrimination, and environmental barriers such as lack of resources, and community accessibility.[15]

Adolescents with physical disabilities report experiencing more loneliness and feeling more isolated than their peers without disabilities. They struggle with social acceptance from peers in and out of the school setting.[16,59] Adolescents without disabilities consider their peers with physical disabilities less socially attractive and report that they are less likely to interact with them socially.[20] Even adolescents with disabilities who have good social relationships in school have less contact with friends outside the school setting than their peers without disabilities.[20]

While most adolescents strive to be included in peer groups, those with physical disabilities may experience role marginalization. Since they are unable to perform the tasks of many typical age-related roles, they sometimes lack clear roles among their peers.[43]

For example, in early and middle adolescence, the basis of social interaction is often physical play and leisure activities, which excludes adolescents with disabilities.[3] However, success in academic activities can promote better social acceptance for adolescents with disabilities.[43] Another factor is how teens with disabilities view themselves. Self-perceptions of social attractiveness and value can be a self-imposed barrier to seeking friendships or group participation. Doubt and McColl shared this account of one student whose positive self-perception promoted his inclusion in a team.[16]

"I approached the [hockey team] about being a statistician because I really wanted to get involved in the team. This is probably the closest without playing...that I could.... plus I'm doing work for them too, so I am useful and that's a good way to get involved...and it really gives me a chance to be one of the guys finally; a secondary guy, but one of the guys, nonetheless" (p. 149).

Social status among adolescents often is acquired through personal characteristics such as excelling in sports and physical attractiveness. For adolescents with disabilities, the typical access points for social inclusion and status are limited. Additionally, the personal challenge of self-evaluation based on social comparison, which is typical of all adolescents, is also present. For example, body image includes comparison with the "ideal," which is characterized by physical perfection in appearance and athletic performance. This is unrealistic for many adolescents, but especially so for adolescents with obvious physical disabilities or motor disorders. Accepting their bodies is an important step in feeling competent in social and eventually intimate relationships. One strategy to "fit in" employed by adolescents with disabilities is an attempt to mask their disabilities, to make fun of them or themselves, or to self-exclude themselves from social groups. Their underlying motive is to make their peers without disabilities more comfortable with them in spite of their disabilities.

Adolescents with emotional and behavioral problems or disabilities and those from socially and economically lower backgrounds can also lack supportive environments for healthy development. Violence, poverty, school failure, sexual and emotional abuse, and discrimination negate healthy adolescent development.[64] For example, at-risk teens can have pseudo-independence (i.e., a false sense of independence). Their circumstances lead them to be prematurely independent from the support and nurturing of adults and to be without a safe and stable environment. They assume responsibility for themselves without the skills or the cognitive and psychological maturity to competently meet the demands associated with independence.

OCCUPATIONAL THERAPY PRACTITIONER'S ROLE AND RESPONSIBILITIES

All adolescents from the ages of 3 to 21 with special needs are eligible for OT services under the 1975 Public Law 94-142, Education of All Handicapped Children's Act; Part B. Under the 1997 Public Law 105-17, Individuals with Disabilities Education Act (IDEA), every adolescent receiving special education services when he or she reaches age 14 requires an individualized transition plan in his or her individualized education program (IEP); by age 16, it should include a statement of the needed transition services, objectives, and activities. Furthermore, an amendment to the IDEA (PL105-17) expanded the scope of alternative education programs for at-risk students to include all those with disabilities and behavioral issues that need be addressed outside the mainstream educational system. Lastly, the 2004 Individuals with Disabilities Improvement Education Act sought to ensure that schools and parents have the resources they need to promote academic achievements and life skills in students with disabilities.

The mainstream as well as the alternative school systems have identified the need for OT services for adolescents with cognitive deficits; sensory impairments; and physical, communicative, and behavioral disabilities who attend high schools.[14,59] Specific areas of occupations that have been identified are students' decreased participation in leisure activities and hobbies, poor time management, and poor coping skills such as self-regulation of anger and stress and unhealthy lifestyle behaviors.[14] However, the current role of the OT practitioner in the high school system is often one of consultation or periodic review and monitoring. The transition from high school provides an excellent opportunity to advocate the need for OT reassessment and collaborative interdisciplinary program planning in life and prevocational skills. The OT practitioner working in the school system or a health care setting has an important role in assisting adolescents to participate fully in the social and academic opportunities provided by the school and the community. They work collaboratively with students, their families, and teachers to establish students' strengths and therapy needs in order to assist them to develop the life and coping skills they will need in the future.

CASE *Study*

Tom is a 15-year-old African American youth with Down syndrome. Psychological test scores place him in the mildly intellectually disabled group under the guidelines of the fourth edition of the *Diagnostic and Statistical Manual (DSM-IV)*. Until he started high school, Tom used to participate well in mainstream school activities, with some accommodations. However, as the cognitive demands of education have increased, he spends most of his day in a special class setting. The prioritized goals of Tom's recent individualized education program (IEP) facilitate his transition from high school to the community and to work.

Tom and adolescents like him who have special needs require assistance to achieve most developmental milestones. OT programs within the comprehensive education plan help these adolescents acquire the performance skills needed to transition from an educational setting to the community and to a work environment. The objective is independence appropriate to their abilities. Programming would involve understanding their physical challenges and adapting their self-care routines appropriately, and training them in the IADLs. Training in social skills is particularly important, since these skills are the basis for forming friendships and maintaining appropriate work relationships.[53]

In working with adolescents with cognitive impairments, an OT practitioner needs to identify the cognitive functional level of each adolescent and how this affects his or her ability to perform everyday activities. For example, in the case above, Tom's cognition affects his understanding of basic information and his ability to learn new information, which determines the number and the complexity of instructions he can follow. An adolescent's cognitive ability influences how well he or she is able to recall information, and it will determine the strategies the OT practitioner should use for teaching new skills. The goal of the OT practitioner is to optimize each adolescent's functioning at his or her full capacity. Therefore, the skilled OT practitioner develops expectations, goals, and treatments that include just the "right" amount of challenge while still ensuring success. Targeting tasks appropriately to an adolescent's level includes modifying the demands of the environment to help him or her function effectively. Examples of modifications to improve function include a list of the steps to complete an activity or the use of a color coding system for medication.

SUMMARY

Although growing up and making the transition from childhood to young adulthood is challenging, most American adolescents do become healthy young adults.[54]

Fundamental to an adolescent's growth and well-being is the formation of social relationships and the development of a sense of competency through participation in all areas of occupational performance. OT practitioners have the expertise and responsibility to promote the healthy development of the adolescent in the school system as well as in the health care setting. However, it will be only through the active recruitment of OT practitioners who specialize in the high school setting that adequate OT services will be provided to meet the unique needs of adolescents with special needs or disabilities.[42,57]

References

1. American Occupational Therapy Association: Occupational therapy practice framework: domain and process, ed 2. *Am J Occup Ther* 62:625–683, 2008.

2. Arnett JJ: Emerging adulthood: a theory of development from the late teens through the twenties. *Am Psychol* 55:469, 2000.

3. Arnold P, Chapman M: Self-esteem, aspirations and expectations of adolescents with physical disability. *Devt Med Child Neurol* 34:97, 1992.

4. Bachman JG, Schulenberg J: How part-time work intensity relates to drug use, behavior, time use and satisfaction among school seniors: are these consequences or merely correlates? *Dev Psychol* 29:220, 1993.

5. Bagwell CL et al: Peer clique participation and social status in preadolescence. *Merrill-Palmer Quart* 46:280, 2000.

6. Beier SR et al: The potential role of an adult mentor in influencing high-risk behaviors in adolescents. *Arch Pediatr Adolesc Med* 15:32, 2000.

7. Brollier C, Shepherd J, Markey KF: Transition from school to community living. *Am J Occup Ther* 48:346, 1994.

8. Cash TF, Putzinsky T: *Body image*, New York, 2002, Guilford.

9. Cech DJ, Martin S: *Functional movement development across the life span*, ed 2, Philadelphia, 2002, Saunders.

10. Coleman JC, Hendry L: *The nature of adolescence*, ed 2, New York, 1990, Routledge.

11. Conger JJ, Galambos NL: *Adolescence and youth: psychological development in a changing world*, ed 5, New York, 1997, Longman.

12. Croll J: Body image and adolescents. In Strang J, Story M, editors: *Guidelines for adolescent nutrition services*, Center for Leadership, Education, and Training in Maternal and Child Nutrition, Division of Epidemiology and Community Health, School of Public Health, University of Minnesota, 2005. Available at: www.epi.umn.edu/let/pubs/adol_book.htm. Accessed November 10, 2008.

13. Davis SE: Developmental tasks and transitions of adolescents with chronic illness and disabilities. *Rehabil Counseling Bull* 29:69, 1985.

14. Deshler D et al: *High schools and adolescents with disabilities: challenges at every turn*, 2005. Available at: http://www.corwinpress.com/upm-data/10858_Chapter_1.pdf. Accessed June 2008

15. Dirette D, Kolak L: Occupational performance needs of adolescents in alternative education programs. *Am J Occup Ther* 58:337, 2004.

16. Doubt L, McColl MA: A secondary guy: physically disabled teenagers in secondary schools. *Can J Occup Ther* 70:139, 2003.

17. Eccles JS et al: Extracurricular activities and adolescent development. *J Soc Issues* 59:865, 2003.

18. Foundation for Accountability: *A portrait of adolescents in America 2001: a report from the Robert Wood Johnson Foundation national strategic indicator surveys*, Portland, 2001, The Foundation for Accountability.

19. Frankowski BL, Committee on Adolescence: Sexual orientation and adolescents. *Pediatrics* 113:1827, 2004.

20. Frederickson N, Turner J: Utilizing the classroom peer group to address children's social needs: an evaluation of the circle of friends intervention approach. *J Special Educ* 36:234, 2002.

21. Ge X, Conger R, Elder, G: The relation between puberty and psychological distress in adolescent boys. *J Res Adolesc* 11:70, 2000.

22. Gilligan C, Lyons NP, Hanmer TJ: *Making connections: the relational worlds of adolescent girls at Emma Willard School*, Cambridge, 1990, Harvard University Press.

23. Goldberg RT: Towards an understanding of the rehabilitation of the disabled adolescent. *Rehab Lit* 42:66, 1981.

24. Graber J et al: Is pubertal timing associated with psychopathology in young adulthood? *J Am Acad Child Adolesc Psychiatr* 43:718, 2004.

25. Guest A, Schneider B: Adolescents' extracurricular participation in context: the mediating effects of schools, communities, and identity. *Sociol Educ* 76:89, 2003.

26. Hazen E, Schlozman S, Beresin E: Adolescent psychological development: a review. *Pediatr Rev* 29:161, 2008.

27. Hooker K: Developmental tasks. In Lerner RM, Petersen AC, Brooks-Gunn T, editors: *Encyclopedia of adolescence*, vol 1, London, 1991, Garland Publishing.

28. Hoover J, Stenhjem P: *Bullying and teasing of youth with disabilities: creating positive school environments for effective inclusion*, 2003. Available at: http://www.ncset.org/publications/issue/NCSETIssueBrief_2.3.pdf. Accessed August 20, 2008.

29. Johnson MK et al: Volunteerism in adolescence: a process perspective. *J Res Adolesc* 8:309, 1998.

30. Keating DP: Cognition, adolescents. In Lerner RM, Petersen AC, Brooks-Gunn T, editors: *Encyclopedia of adolescence*, vol 1, London, 1991, Garland Publishing, p 987.

31. Kemper HCG: The importance of physical activity in childhood and adolescence. In Haynan L, Mahon MM, Turner JR, editors: *Health behavior in childhood and adolescence*, New York, 2002, Springer Publishing.

32. Knickmeyer RC et al: Age of menarche in females with autism spectrum conditions. *Development Med Child Neurol* 48:1007, 2006.

33. Kirkpatrick JM: Social origins, adolescents' experiences and work value trajectories during the transition to adulthood. *Soc Forces* 80:32, 2002.

34. Kunnen ES, Bosma HA, VanGeert PLC: A dynamic systems approach to identity formation: theoretical

background and methodological possibilities. In Nurmi JE, editor: *Navigating through adolescence: European perspectives*, New York, 2001, Routledge Falmer.

35. Larson R, Verma S: How children and adolescents spend time across the world: work, play and developmental opportunities. *Psychol Bull* 125:701, 1999.

36. Laursen B, Coy KC, Collins WA: Reconsidering changes in parent-child conflict across adolescence: a meta-analysis. *Child Dev* 69:817, 1998.

37. Lenhart M, Madden M: *Teens and technology: youth are leading the transition to a fully wired and mobile nation*, 2005. Available at: http://www.pewinternet.org/report_display.asp?r=162. Accessed November 2, 2008.

38. Lenhart M et al: *Teens and social media: the use of social media gains a greater foothold in teen life as they embrace the conversational nature of interactive online media*, 2007. Available at: http://www.pewinternet.org/PPF/r/230/report_display.asp. Accessed November 2, 2008.

39. Levine MP, Smolak L: Body image development in adolescence. In Cash TF, Putzinsky T, editors: *Body image*, New York, 2002, Guilford.

40. Marcia JE: Identity and self-development. In Lerner RM, Petersen AC, Brooks-Gunn T, editors: *Encyclopedia of adolescence*, vol 1, London, 1991, Garland Publishing.

41. Mechanic D: Adolescents at risk: new directions. *J Adolesc Health* 12:638, 1991.

42. Michaels CA, Orentlicher ML: The role of occupational therapy in providing person-centred transition services: implications for school-based practice. *Occup Ther Int* 11:209, 2004.

43. Mpofu E: Enhancing social acceptance of early adolescents with physical disabilities: effect of role salience, peer interaction, and academic support interventions. *Int J Disabil Dev Educ* 50:435, 2003.

44. National Institute of Occupational Safety and Health: *Child labor research needs* (NIOSH Publication No 97-143), Cincinnati, 1997, NIOSH—Publications 84.

45. Neinstein LS, Kaufman FR: Normal physical growth and development. In Neinstein LS, editor: *Adolescent health care: a practical guide*, ed 4, Philadelphia, 2002, Lippincott Williams & Wilkins.

46. Newacheck PW, Halfon N: Prevalence and impact of disabling chronic conditions in childhood. *Am J Public Health* 88:610, 1998.

47. Oetting ER, Beauvais F: Orthogonal cultural identification theory: the cultural identification of minority adolescents. *Subst Use Misuse* 25:655, 1991.

48. Overton WF, Byrnes JP: Cognitive development. In Lerner RM, Petersen AC, Brooks-Gunn T, editors: *Encyclopedia of adolescence*, vol 1, London, 1991, Garland Publishing.

49. Quint E: Menstrual Issues in adolescents with physical and developmental disabilities. *Ann NY Acad Sci* 1135:230, 2008

50. Rathus S: *Childhood and adolescence voyages in development*, ed 3, Belmont, CA, US, 2008, Thomson Wadsworth.

51. Rotherman-Borus MJ, Langabeer KA: Developmental trajectories of gay, lesbian, and bisexual youth. In D'Augelli AR, Patterson C, editors: *Lesbian, gay, and bisexual identities among youth: psychological perspectives*, New York, 200, Oxford University Press.

52. Rubenstein H, Sternabach MR, Pollock SH: Protecting the health and safety of working teenagers. *Am Fam Physician* 60:575, 1999.

53. Santrock JW: *Adolescence*, ed 9, New York, 2003, McGraw-Hill Higher Education.

54. Scales PC, Leffert N: *Developmental assets: a synthesis of the scientific research on adolescent development*, ed 2, Minneapolis, 2004, Search Institute.

55. Simmons CD, Griswold L: Evaluation of social interaction in a community based program for persons with traumatic brain injury. *Scand J Occup Ther* 17:49–56, 2010.

56. Skinner H et al: Adolescents use technology for health information: implications for health professionals from focus group studies. *J Med Internet Res* 5. Available at: http://www.jmir.org/2003/4/e25/HTML. Accessed October 10, 2008.

57. Spencer JE, Emery LJ, Schneck CM: Occupational therapy in transitioning adolescents to post-secondary activities. *Am J Occup Ther* 57:435, 2003.

58. Steele CA et al: Lifestyle health behaviours of 11- to 16-year-old youth with physical disabilities. *Health Ed Res Theory Pract* 11:173, 1996.

59. Stewart DA et al: A qualitative study of the transition to adulthood for youth with physical disabilities. *Phys Occup Ther Pediatr* 21:3, 2001.

60. Vilhjalmsson R, Krisjansdottir G: Gender difference in physical activity in older children and adolescents: the central role of organized sport. *Soc Sci Med* 56:363, 2003.

61. Widmer MA, Ellis GD, Trunnell ER: Measurement of ethical behavior in leisure among high and low risk adolescents. *Adolescence* 31:397, 1996.

62. Worley G et al: Secondary sexual characteristics in children with cerebral palsy and moderate to severe motor impairment: a cross-sectional survey. *Pediatrics* 110:897, 2002.

63. Wynn JR: High school after school: creating pathways to the future for adolescents. *New Dir Youth Dev* 97:59, 2003.

64. Zajicek-Faber ML: Promoting good health in adolescents with disabilities. *Health Social Work* 23:203, 1998.

65. Zastrow CH, Kirst-Ashman KK: *Understanding human behavior*, ed 6, Belmont, CA, 2004, Brooks/Cole, Thomson Learning.

66. Zehr JL et al: Early puberty is associated with disordered eating and anxiety in young adults. *Front Neuroendocrinol* 27:139, 2006.

REVIEW *Questions*

1. What physical changes occur in adolescence?
2. What cognitive changes occur in adolescents? Give examples of how these developments are seen in an adolescent's occupational performance.
3. With the maturation of the reproductive systems, what changes occur in body image?
4. What are some of the psychosocial issues for each stage: early, middle, and late adolescence?
5. What are some behavioral indicators of positive and negative self-esteem?
6. What are the characteristics of play/leisure and social participation in adolescence?
7. What are some of the issues that children with special needs may face in adolescence?

SUGGESTED *Activities*

1. Interview a teen to learn about interests, hobbies, concerns, and occupations that are important to him or her.
2. Read some teen magazines, and discuss how the themes and images in them might influence an adolescent reader.
3. Make presentations to each other on current teen trends, such as music, dress, styles, and social behaviors. Discuss cultural differences.
4. Develop a list of activities that teens enjoy that might be used in occupational therapy, and identify the relevant developmental learning of task associated with each activity.
5. Spend time alone with a teenager for a few hours, in a group and at home. How does he or she show individuality? How does his or her behavior change with context? How does he or she "fit in" in each setting?
6. View "*Breakfast Club*" or a similar movie that explores adolescence. Examples of other movies are *16 Candles*, *Angus*, *Can't Buy Me Love*, *Juno*, *Can't Hardly Wait*, *Dead Poet's Society*, *Fast Times at Ridgemont High*, *Pretty in Pink*, *Say Anything*, *St. Elmo's Fire*, and *The Outsiders*. Identify the roles, developmental stages, and tasks identified in the chosen movie. How does this movie exemplify adolescent development?
7. Compare adolescent or teen culture in America with that in another part of the world.

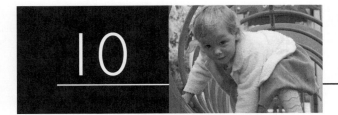

10

The Occupational Therapy Process

JEAN W. SOLOMON

JANE CLIFFORD O'BRIEN

CHAPTER *Objectives*

After studying this chapter, the reader will be able to accomplish the following:

- Describe different pediatric frames of reference and practice models.
- Explain the way in which assessment relates to program planning and intervention.
- Differentiate among long-term goals, short-term objectives, and mini-objectives.
- Apply activity analysis to intervention(s) with children and adolescents.
- Define and describe therapeutic use of self.
- Be aware of the importance of family-centered intervention and cultural diversity.
- Discuss the preparation for and process of discharge planning or discontinuation of occupational therapy services.
- Understand the top-down approach to intervention.
- Identify and describe the tools of practice for working with children and adolescents.

This chapter describes the occupational therapy (OT) process by first presenting the role of the OT practitioner and then the pediatric practice models. The authors describe considerations during the provision of OT services. The OT process begins with referral, screening, and evaluation and moves to intervention planning, goal setting, and treatment implementation and then to re-evaluation and discharge planning. A discussion of specific frames of reference used in pediatric practice is also presented.

ROLES OF OCCUPATIONAL THERAPIST AND OCCUPATIONAL THERAPY ASSISTANT IN THE OCCUPATIONAL THERAPY PROCESS

The roles of the occupational therapist and occupational therapy assistant (OTA) in the OT process differ. The occupational therapist is responsible for the selection of assessments used during evaluation, interpretation of results, and development of the intervention plan. The OTA may gather evaluative data under the supervision of the occupational therapist using an approved structured format but is not responsible for the interpretation of assessment results; he or she may contribute to the process by sharing knowledge of the client gained during the assessment process.

MODELS OF PRACTICE

A model of practice (MOP) helps OT practitioners organize their thinking.[13] For example, practitioners using the Model of Human Occupation (MOHO) know that they will gather information about volition (e.g., the child's or parents' goals and priorities or occupational choices), habituation or routines (e.g., how the child spends the day), performance (e.g., the physical skills and abilities of the child), and environment (e.g., the physical layout of the home). Practitioners using the Person–Environment–Occupational-Performance model will organize their thinking into information about the child (e.g., the child's physical abilities), the environment (e.g., where the child attends school) and occupational performance (e.g., how the child is performing his or her daily occupations). Other commonly used pediatric MOPs include Occupational Adaptation and the Canadian Occupational Performance Model.

MOPs provide practitioners with a framework for thinking about and arranging their materials. They help practitioners focus on factors that influence functioning. MOPs are developed from OT theory and philosophy. As such, they fit with the Occupational Therapy Practice Framework (OTPF) in their emphasis on occupation. See Table 10-1 for an overview of selected MOPs.

TABLE 10-1

Models of Practice

MODEL	AUTHOR(S)	COMPONENTS	PREMISES
Model of Human Occupation (MOHO)	Kielhofner	Volition Habituation Performance Environment	The human is an open system. Volition drives the system. The clinician's role is to understand the client in terms of these systems (and subsystems) and intervene to facilitate engagement in occupations.
Canadian Occupational Performance Model	Occupational Therapy Association Townsend, et al.	Spirituality Occupation Context (institutional included)	The worth of the individual is central to this model. Spirituality is the core of a person. Thus, occupational therapy practitioners must understand the client's spirituality to facilitate engagement in occupations. Performance of occupations takes place within social, physical, and cultural environments.
Person–Environment–Occupation Model	Law, et al.	Person Environment Occupation	Looks at the person in terms of physical, social, and emotional factors. The environment (context) influences the person and occupations. The environment includes culture. Occupations are the everyday things people do.

Data from Kielhofner G: *A model of human occupation: Theory and application*, ed 4, Baltimore, MD, 2008, Lippincott, Williams & Wilkins; Law M, Cooper B, Stewart D, et al: The person-environment-occupation model: A transactive approach to occupational performance, *Can J Occup Ther* 63:9, 1996; Townsend E, Brintnell S, Staisey N: Developing guidelines for client-centered occupational therapy practice, *Can J Occup Ther* 57:69, 1990.

REFERRAL, SCREENING, AND EVALUATION

The referral, screening, and evaluation aspects of the OT process are concomitantly referred to as the *evaluation period*. During this period, the OT practitioner meets the child, the family, or other referral sources (e.g., teacher, early interventionist) to collect information that will assist in setting goals and developing an activity configuration for the child.

Referral

Children are usually introduced to OT by means of a **referral**. The reason for a referral depends on the individual state licensure law or regulations within the area of practice. It is the responsibility of the OT practitioner to know the laws and regulations that govern his or her area of practice setting. Some states require a referral before an OT practitioner can see a client. Other states require a referral only for the intervention process. A physician or a nurse practitioner generally gives the referral, depending on the state's laws; it is called *physician's referral* or *doctor's orders*.

According to the *Standards of Practice for Occupational Therapy* published by the American Occupational Therapy Association (AOTA), only occupational therapists may accept a referral for assessment.[1] The OTA, if given a referral, is responsible for forwarding it to a supervising occupational therapist and educating "current and potential referral sources about the scope of occupational therapy services and the process of initiating occupational therapy referrals."[1] OTAs may acknowledge requests for services from any source. However, they do not accept and begin working on cases at their own professional discretion without the supervision and collaboration of the occupational therapist.

Screening

Clients may first be introduced to OT through a **screening**. Screenings provide a general overview of a child's functioning to determine if the child requires further evaluation. Both occupational therapists and OTAs can conduct such screenings. For example, an OTA may be hired to screen children in a well-baby clinic or an incoming kindergarten class to determine the need for additional evaluation before entering school. Once the OTA has identified the need for a more complete evaluation, the occupational therapist determines the specific evaluation or format to be used. The data gathered by the OTA are interpreted by the occupational therapist. An OTA "may contribute to this process under the supervision of a registered occupational therapist."[1]

Evaluation

The **evaluation** is a critical part of the OT process. The occupational therapist is responsible for determining the type and scope of evaluation. An evaluation includes assessments of an individual's areas of performance (e.g., activities of daily living [ADLs], instrumental ADLs [IADLs], work, education, play/leisure, social participation), client factors (e.g., neuromusculoskeletal, specific and global mental functions, body system), performance skills, performance patterns, contexts, and activity demands.[2] According to AOTA, an entry-level OTA "assists with data collection and evaluation under the supervision of the occupational therapist."[3] An intermediate- or advanced-level OTA "administers standardized tests under the supervision of an occupational therapist after service competency has been established."[3] Although the OTA may participate in the evaluation process, the occupational therapist is responsible for interpreting the results and developing the **intervention plan**.

Levels of Performance

The evaluation provides the OT practitioner with a picture of the child's occupational needs as well as the child's strengths and weaknesses. This occupational profile consists of a description of the level of performance at which the child functions. A child's level of function may differ in relation to task, pattern, and context (Box 10-1). For example, a child may feed himself or herself independently at home after setup but be unable to do so at school in the time provided while sitting at the table because of the loud noises and confusion of the lunch room.

Functional independence refers to the completion of age-appropriate activities with or without the use of assistive devices and without human assistance (e.g., eating independently with an offset spoon).

BOX 10-1

Components of the Occupational Profile

Who is the client?

Why is the client seeking services?

What occupations and activities are successful or are causing problems?

What contexts and environments support or hinder desired outcomes?

What is the client's occupational history?

What are the client's priorities and targeted outcomes?

From American Occupational Therapy Association: Occupational therapy practice framework: Domain and process, 2nd edition, *Am J Occup Ther* 62:625–683, 2008.

Assisted performance refers to a child's participation in a specific age-appropriate task with some assistance from the caregiver (e.g., putting on a shirt and receiving assistance with buttoning).

Dependent performance occurs when a child is unable to perform an age-appropriate task. A caregiver is required to perform the task for the child (e.g., holding a cup for a child with cerebral palsy).

INTERVENTION PLANNING, GOAL SETTING, AND TREATMENT IMPLEMENTATION

Intervention Planning

The occupational therapist develops an intervention plan after the evaluation has been completed. The evaluation includes parental concerns, the client's strengths and weaknesses, a statement of the client's rehabilitation potential, long-term goals, and short-term objectives. The plan describes the type of media (i.e., specific types of materials) and modalities (i.e., intervention tools) that will be used and the frequency and duration of treatment. The plans for re-evaluation and discharge as well as the level of personnel providing the intervention are also included.[1]

The intervention plan is based on a selected MOP or a frame of reference (FOR). The FOR provides guidelines and intervention strategies. The OTA utilizes knowledge of the selected frames of reference, the activity analysis, and the selection, gradation, and adaptation of activities to carry out the intervention plan.

Frames of Reference

Once practitioners have gained information by using an MOP, they must decide how to intervene. FORs are used to direct OT intervention. They inform practitioners on what to do and are based on theory, research, and clinical experience.[13] FORs define the populations for which they are suitable, describe the continuum of function and dysfunction, provide assessment tools, describe treatment modalities and intervention techniques, define the role of the practitioner, and suggest outcome measures. FOR helps the OT practitioner identify problems and develop solutions. Common pediatric FORs in OT are MOHO, developmental, sensory integration, biomechanical, sensorimotor, motor control, and rehabilitation FORs. See Table 10-2 for an overview of FORs. MOHO is both a MOP and a FOR, since this model has numerous assessment tools and intervention strategies. As such, it provides an overall way of thinking and also meets the criteria for a FOR. See Chapter 25 for a description of MOHO.

Practitioners may choose a variety of FORs. However, they should be careful to choose an appropriate one and be clear about the theories and methodologies used with the given FOR. In cases when intervention does not progress as planned, practitioners adhering to one FOR may explore other suggested intervention techniques or change to another FOR. Intervention techniques are based on evidence from research. Given the need for evidence-based intervention, clinicians adhering to an FOR are using techniques investigated through research. Therefore, practitioners must keep themselves informed by reading and critically analyzing current research literature.

The following sections provide an overview and examples of specific FORs used with children.

Developmental Approach

CASE *Study*

Corey is a 2-year-old boy diagnosed with global developmental delays. Corey attends an early intervention center twice weekly for 2 hours of "group" time and 1 hour weekly for direct OT services. Roanna, the OTA, works with Corey and provides activities that can be continued at home with the family. The OT evaluation, which was based on the Hawaii Early Learning Profile (HELP), had revealed that Corey functions at a level between 16 and 20 months for most skills, with gross motor skills being his strength and fine motor and language skills his weak areas. Cognitively, Corey recognizes and points to four animal pictures (16–21 months), identifies himself in a mirror (15–16), identifies one body part (15–19), and searches for a hidden object (17–18). Expressive language skills include saying no meaningfully (13–15), naming one or two familiar objects (13–18), and using 10 to 15 words spontaneously (15–17). Gross motor skills are solid to 20 months: Corey picks up a toy from the floor without falling (19–24), runs fairly well (18–24), and squats when playing (20–21). He does not walk upstairs independently (22–24) or jump in place (22–30). Fine motor skills are scattered to 18 months. Corey builds a tower with two cubes (12–16) and scribbles spontaneously (13–18). He uses both hands at midline (16–18) but has difficulty pointing with his index finger (12–16) and placing one round peg in a pegboard (12–15). Social-emotional skills include enjoying rough-and-tumble play (18–24), expressing affection (18–24), and showing toy preferences (12–18). Corey has developed self-help skills to 12 months. He holds a spoon and finger-feeds himself (9–12), naps once or twice each day (9–12), cooperates with dressing (10–12), and removes a hat (15–16).

The OTA designed an intervention plan based on this developmental picture of Corey and the parents' concern that Corey is not "playing like his 30-month-old cousin." The overall goal of the intervention based on the developmental FOR is to facilitate the child's ability to perform

TABLE 10-2

Pediatric Frames of Reference

FRAME OF REFERENCE	REFERENCE(S)	PRINCIPLES	SAMPLE POPULATIONS	TREATMENT MODALITIES
Developmental	Llorens	Development occurs over time and between skills (e.g., gross and fine motor). Some children experience a gap in their development due to physical, emotional, and/or social trauma. The role of occupational therapy is to bridge this gap.	Down syndrome Intellectual disability Failure to thrive Cerebral palsy Pervasive developmental disorder	Identify current level of functioning. Work on the next step to achieve the skill. Intervention includes practice, repetition, education, and modeling of skills.
Biomechanical	Pedretti and Paszuinielli	Improve strength, endurance, range of motion.	Children with cardiac concerns Brachial plexus Cerebral palsy Juvenile rheumatoid arthritis Down syndrome	*Strength*: Increase weight of toys or repetitive use of objects. *Endurance*: Increase time engaged in occupation. *Range of motion*: Repetitively provide slow, sustained stretch to increase end range.
Sensory integration	Ayres	Children with sensory integration dysfunction have difficulty processing sensory information (vestibular, proprioceptive, tactile). Improvements in sensory processing lead to improved engagement in occupations.	Sensory integrative dysfunction Developmental coordination disorder Sensory modulation disorder Pervasive developmental disorder	Provide controlled sensory input to improve the child's ability to process sensory stimuli. Use suspension equipment and the "just-right challenge." Provide activities that are child directed.
Motor control	Shumway-Cook	Acquisition of motor skills is based on dynamic systems theory. (All systems, including sensory, motor, and cognitive, work on each other for movement to occur.)	Cerebral palsy Developmental coordination disorder Down syndrome	*Task-oriented approach*: Children learn motor skills best by repeating the occupations in the most natural settings, varying the requirements. They learn from their motor mistakes.
Neuro-developmental	Bobath, Schoen, and Anderson	Children learn motor patterns when they "feel" normal.	Cerebral palsy Traumatic brain injury movement patterns	Clinician uses handling techniques and key points of control to inhibit abnormal muscle tone and facilitate normal movement patterns. Children learn through "feeling" normal patterns and thus should not make motor mistakes.

Continued

TABLE 10-2

Pediatric Frames of Reference—cont'd

FRAME OF REFERENCE	REFERENCE(S)	PRINCIPLES	SAMPLE POPULATIONS	TREATMENT MODALITIES
Model of Human Occupation	Kielhofner	Volition Habituation Performance Environment	All diagnoses	The human is an open system. Volition drives the system. The clinician's role is to understand the client in terms of these systems (and subsystems) and intervene to facilitate engagement in occupations.
Rehabilitation	Early, Pendleton & Schultz-Krohn	Children relearn skills lost; develop compensatory strategies; and develop adaptive techniques.	Acquired brain injury trauma Stroke	Help children regain function for independence in occupations Help children to practice; improve strength, ROM, and endurance.

Data from Ayres AJ: *Sensory integration for the child,* Los Angeles, 1979, Western Psychological Services; Bobath B: Sensorimotor development, *NDT Newsletter* 7:1, 1975; Early MB: *Physical dysfunction practice skills for the occupational therapy assistant,* ed 2, St. Louis, 2006, Mosby; Llorens LA: *Application of a developmental theory for health and rehabilitation,* Rockville, MD, 1976, American Occupational Therapy Association; Shultz-Krohn W, Pendleton H: Application of the occupational therapy framework to physical dysfunction. In Pendleton, H. & Shultz-Krohn, editors: *Pedretti's occupational therapy: Practice skills for physical dysfunction,* ed 6, St Louis, 2006, Mosby; Schoen S, Anderson J: Neurodevelopmental treatment frame of reference. In Kramer P, Hinojosa J, editors: *Frames of reference for pediatric occupational therapy,* Baltimore, MD, 2009, Lippincott, Williams & Wilkins; Shumway-Cook A, Woolacott M: Motor control: Issues and theories. In Shumway-Cook A, Woolacott M, editors: *Motor control: Theory an practical applications,* ed 2, Baltimore, MD, 2002, Lippincott, Williams & Wilkins.

age-appropriate tasks in the areas of self-care, play/leisure, education, and social participation. The developmental FOR targets intervention at the level at which the child is currently functioning and requires that the clinician provide a slightly advanced challenge. Clinicians using the developmental FOR need a clear understanding of the logical progression of skills. A typical therapy session is illustrated by the following SOAP (subjective, objective, assessment, and plan) note.

S

His mother stated that Corey draws a line now.

O

Corey scribbled spontaneously, holding the crayon in a palmar grasp. He imitated a vertical stroke (18–24) consistently and a circular stroke 1 out of 5 times (20–24). Corey built a tower of 4 cubes (18–22). He pointed with his index finger on command (two out of five times). Corey had difficulty isolating his index finger for finger games. Corey removed his socks (15–18), placed a hat on his head (16–18), and held a cup handle (12–15). He showed difficulty scooping food with a spoon (15–24) and continued to drink from a bottle (18–24).

A

Corey exhibits fine motor and self-care skills consistently to 18 months. He shows many emerging self-care skills.

Corey is making progress in achieving age-appropriate skills for play, self-care, and academics.

P

Corey will continue to participate in group sessions, which are designed to facilitate social-emotional and play skills.

Corey will continue to receive weekly individual OT services to improve fine motor and self-care skills for play, self-care, and academics. The parents have been provided with developmental activities for Corey to engage in at home.

Roanna used the developmental FOR to treat Corey. She focused on fine motor and self-care skills because Corey was participating in group sessions to develop social-emotional and play skills. Roanna designed the intervention to be fun and playful and began at the level at which Corey was functioning. She gradually increased the level of difficulty and provided developmentally appropriate activities for the parents to use at home.

Sensory Integration Approach

CASE *Study*

Jamar is a 13-year-old boy with sensory integration dysfunction. His movements are awkward, and he has poor balance and coordination; associated reactions with effort are noted (such as both hands moving when he writes). Jamar shows poor eye–hand coordination, poor rhythmic skills, and poor body awareness. He also shows signs of poor tactile, vestibular, and proprioceptive processing. The occupational therapist classified Jamar's dysfunction as poor motor planning and body awareness due to inadequate processing of vestibular input (vestibular-based somatodyspraxia).

Jamar is an intelligent child who has expressed the desire to "be smoother, learn to dance, and not be the last one in every sport in gym." He also reports handwriting difficulties leading to lower grades in school.

Jamar receives OT services from Jackie, an OTA with 10 years of experience in a community-based sports injury clinic. The following SOAP note describes an intervention session. The goal of Jamar's intervention sessions is to improve body awareness, vestibular processing, and overall quality of movement so that he will be more confident in his body. Sensory integration theory postulates that by improving the ability to process sensory information, the body's ability to plan and execute movements will improve. Ayres emphasized movement-related activities with the use of suspended equipment (to get the intensity needed) and the "just-right challenge."[9]

S

Jamar states that a dance is taking place at school in 2 weeks.

O

Jamar reluctantly participated in a fast-moving tire-swing activity. He quickly became dizzy with the spinning and enjoyed bouncing into objects. Jamar had difficulty getting on new pieces of equipment. He "talked" his way through a difficult five-step obstacle course. Jamar showed difficulty clapping to the rhythm (five beats before an error) while on the trampoline but was able to clap to the rhythm (20 beats without an error) when sitting on the platform swing. On hearing a noise, he jumped into hoops placed randomly on the floor, showing some difficulty in sequencing and planning. Jamar was able to sequence and plan a

difficult three-step obstacle course that involved crawling, swinging, and throwing a ball at a target. He completed 10 minutes of the Mavis typing program with a 70% success rate and was able to imitate simple dance moves (from song 1 of the Twister Moves game). Jamar was not able to successfully complete the dance moves and could not stay with the music after song 1.

A

Jamar exhibits difficulty with motor planning, sequencing, and timing of movements, which interferes with his leisure activities (dancing) and academics (writing).

P

Jamar will continue with sensory integration therapy twice weekly (1 hour sessions) for 3 months to improve his processing of vestibular, proprioceptive, and tactile information for quality of movements and educational and leisure activities. Jamar was provided with a homework assignment to select one song from Twister Moves and complete the dance steps from the game. Jamar will complete a Mavis typing program at the eighth-grade level and use a laptop computer for writing assignments. He will discuss these activities with his parents and teacher.

Jackie, the OTA, used a sensory integration frame of reference to improve the motor planning, sequencing, and timing of movements. Jamar chose the activities, and the session was tailored to address his concern about looking "awkward or weird" (i.e., not dancing to the beat of the music) at the school dance. Using goals that children pick themselves empowers and gratifies them. Furthermore, the child will work very hard to achieve these goals, making the likelihood of success greater. In this example, Jackie used suspended equipment to provide the intensity of input needed for a 13-year-old. She also challenged Jamar to participate in a slightly uncomfortable activity. Children gain confidence when they succeed in activities they deem to be slightly "tougher." In this way, Jackie worked on Jamar's self-concept as well. Recommending the use of a laptop is not necessarily a sensory integration technique. However, Jamar is 13 years old and needs to be able to communicate in writing for success in school. Therefore, Jackie decided that it was time to move away from teaching writing skills and help Jamar perform his educational occupation.

Biomechanical Approach

CASE *Study*

Abigail is a 14-month-old infant who suffered a left brachial plexus injury (i.e., damage to the nerves that control arm movement) during birth. She is treated by an occupational therapist once every 2 weeks. Teresa, an OTA, visits Abigail twice a week to work on the goals that have been established by the occupational therapist in collaboration with the child's family. Abigail's long-term OT goals include (1) increasing active range of motion (AROM) in her left arm, (2) increasing the functional strength in her left arm, and (3) increasing her ability to use her left arm during age-appropriate activities such as playing with a toy and self-feeding. Abigail's treatment sessions with Teresa last 30 minutes. A typical therapy session is shown in the following daily progress note. The goals of therapy sessions using a biomechanical FOR are to increase strength, endurance, and ROM for successful engagement in chosen occupations (e.g., play and self-care).

S

Abigail's mother stated that Abigail enjoys the ROM exercises she performs each day. She especially enjoys singing "Row, row, row your boat" during the stretching exercises.

O

Abigail received a 30-minute therapy session in her home. Her mother and older brother were present for the entire session. Stretching and AROM left-arm exercises were performed. Left-shoulder AROM was 0 to 105° and passive ROM (PROM) 0 to 180°. Activities included weight bearing on her extended (straightened) left arm for 1 minute while reaching for toys with her right arm. Abigail also reached for toys with her left arm while bearing weight on her right arm. Abigail spontaneously used her left arm as an assist while playing with a shape sorter.

A

Abigail actively participates in the activities throughout the session. Her ability to sustain weight on her left arm with minimum physical assistance has improved from 20-second to 1-minute intervals. Left shoulder AROM from 0 to 105° has shown an increase of 5° since last month.

P

Abigail will participate in OT twice weekly to work on improving left upper extremity functioning for play, self-care, and academic work. Her goals include (1) achieving full AROM for the left upper extremity, (2) strengthening her left arm to lift objects, and (3) spontaneously using the left upper extremity as an assist.

Teresa used the biomechanical frame of reference to treat Abigail. It is used with children who have orthopedic (i.e., bone, joint, or muscle) problems such as hand injuries or lower motor neuron disorders (affecting the nerve

connections outside the central nervous system [CNS]) such as brachial plexus injuries. The goals of the biomechanical approach are to (1) assess physical limitations on the client's ROM, muscle strength, and endurance; (2) improve ROM, strength, and endurance; and (3) prevent or reduce contracture and deformities.[10] This approach focuses on the physical limitations that interfere with the client's ability to engage in the occupational performance areas of ADLs, play and leisure activities, and work and productive activities. Teresa will work on the overall goal of improving Abigail's ability to use both arms for play, self-care, and academics.

Neurodevelopmental Approach

CASE *Study*

Raja is a 4-year-old child who has been diagnosed with spastic right hemiplegia cerebral palsy. A brain lesion caused abnormal muscle tone on the right side of his body, which prevents him from properly using the right arm and leg. He is receiving outpatient OT services at the local hospital; his mother usually brings him to the clinic. Raja recently had a phenol alcohol nerve block—an injection into the nerves that innervate the arm—to help reduce the increased flexor tone in his right arm. Because of the recent changes in Raja's right arm, Alejandro, the occupational therapist, is currently providing all of the direct OT services. His sessions with Raja typically last 45 minutes. An example of a therapy session is described in the following SOAP note.

The goal of therapy sessions with a neurodevelopmental FOR is to normalize muscle tone and to improve movement patterns for occupations (e.g., academics, self-care, and play).

S

Raja's mother stated that Raja's right arm is easier to wash and the elbow is straighter since the nerve block.

O

Raja arrived this morning eager to work on the therapy ball. He performed activities on the therapy ball while lying on his stomach and bearing weight on his elbows, followed by bearing weight on his extended arms. Tapping—using fingertips to deliver successive light blows to the belly muscle—over the triceps to facilitate full extension (straightening) of Raja's elbow was performed. (The triceps muscle is primarily responsible for elbow extension.) Raja participated in bilateral hand activities, such as fastening large buttons and creating pictures using finger paint. When necessary, the wrist extensor muscles were stroked to encourage maintenance of a functional wrist position (e.g., wrist extension while grasping) during the bilateral tasks. Gentle cueing at the shoulder was used to promote weight shifting on the right. Raja did not spontaneously weight-bear on the right during movements. Raja fastened five large buttons in 2 minutes.

A

Raja's ability to use his right arm has improved, as shown by his ability to fasten five large buttons while his wrist is extended.

P

Raja will receive OT weekly to work on increasing right arm functioning for self-care, academics, and play.

Alejandro is using a neurodevelopmental (NDT) frame of reference to treat Raja. This type of approach involves the use of sensory input to change muscle tone and movement patterns in infants, children, and adolescents who have central nervous system (CNS) damage.[10] Because using an NDT approach requires skill and experience, entry-level occupational therapists and OTAs should be closely supervised while using it.

Motor Control Approach

CASE *Study*

Talasi is a 6-year-old child who shows a slight intention tremor in her right arm and walks with a wide-based gait. She performs the skills expected of her age, yet the quality of the movement is poor and she falls frequently. She is unable to keep up with her peers on the playground, is slow in getting dressed or undressed, frequently has her clothes on backwards, and spills food and drink during mealtimes. Her parents are concerned that she is "falling behind" in school because she is forgetful and disorganized. Brian is the OTA responsible for treating Talasi at school. The following SOAP note describes a therapy session with a motor control FOR to improve Talasi's quality of movement for play, academics, and self-care.

S

Talasi stated that she was having a bad day. She forgot to bring her "show and tell" book from her Grammy.

O

Talasi participated in a game of "dress-up." She put on a sweater and pants, buttoned them, and then removed them. Talasi dressed her doll and played a timed game of

dress-up. She played eye–hand games using beanbags, targets, and catching a ball. The placement of the targets, the speed, and her position in relation to the target varied. Talasi balanced herself for 45 seconds on the right foot with eyes open and for only 5 seconds with eyes closed. She drank her juice without spilling it but did spill apple sauce from a spoon. An intention tremor was noted in her right arm during spoon feeding. Talasi was instructed to hold the spoon closer to the bowl. A weighted spoon eased some of the tremor and resulted in less spilling.

A

Talasi demonstrates poor quality of movement, an intention tremor in her right arm, and slow movements interfering with her functioning in school, at play, and during self-care.

P

Talasi will receive OT weekly to work on increasing the quality of movement for self-care, academics, and play.

Brian used the motor control FOR to improve Talasi's quality of movement. This FOR follows a task-oriented approach that encourages the repetition of desired movements in a variety of settings and circumstances. For example, Talasi practiced dressing herself with large clothing and dressing a small doll. Both these tasks involve dressing and undressing skills. Motor control theory promotes a practice approach. The clinician provides verbal feedback but allows the child to perform the task and learn from his or her mistakes. For example, Brian allowed Talasi to feed herself; then he instructed her on a different technique, which she practiced. Finally, Brian used a weighted spoon to see if this would decrease the tremor and thus the spilling.

Motor control theories support using activities that motivate the child and have as close a resemblance to the actual task as possible. Imagery and practice are intervention techniques used in the motor control approach.

Rehabilitative Approach

CASE *Study*

Dewayne is a 6-year-old child whose left arm was amputated below the elbow following a car accident 2 years ago. Dewayne goes to Shriner's Hospital in another town for the fitting of his prosthesis, an artificial limb, and for training in its use. He has outgrown his old prosthesis and is meeting with Missy, an OTA, to work on using and caring for his new artificial arm and learn activities that will improve his ability to use it functionally. A typical therapy session is shown in the following daily SOAP note.

S

Dewayne said that his new arm felt good.

O

Dewayne was treated in the OT department for prosthetic training and home/family instruction on its care. The department's Prosthetic Checklist was completed during the session. No red areas were noted. Dewayne's father was shown how to don and doff the stump sock and the new artificial arm. Dewayne dressed and undressed himself using the artificial arm. He stabilized a paper with the prosthetic arm and wrote with his right hand.

A

The new artificial arm fits well. Dewayne and his father demonstrated knowledge of proper care, donning and doffing, and using the prosthesis. Dewayne is able to engage in age-appropriate self-care and writing activities while using his prosthesis.

P

Dewayne is discharged from Shriner's Hospital. He will be monitored by an occupational therapist at school.

Missy used the rehabilitative frame of reference to treat Dewayne. This FOR is used after an injury or illness to return a person to the highest possible level of functional independence as well as teach any compensatory methods that may be needed to perform certain activities.[10]

Because many children are born with disabilities, OT practitioners are required in some cases to teach new skills (habilitate) instead of teaching previously known skills (rehabilitate). However, for cases in which a child acquires a disability after birth, a rehabilitative approach is appropriate. The methods used during rehabilitation and habilitation include the following:

- Self-care evaluation and training
- Acquisition and training in the use of assistive devices
- Prosthetic use training
- Wheelchair management training
- Architectural and environmental adaptation training
- Acquisition and training in the use of augmentative communication devices and assistive technology
- Play assessment and intervention

An OT practitioner who is using a rehabilitative approach or a habilitative approach focuses on skill acquisition in the occupational performance areas of ADLs, play and leisure skills, and work and productive activities.

Model of Human Occupation

CASE *Study*

Peter is an 8-year-old boy with asthma, food allergies, and attention deficit disorder (ADD). Peter has difficulty following rules at school and frequently gets into trouble. He does not do well academically and has few friends. On the playground, Peter tends to play hard and often is "rough" with his friends. His parents are concerned that Peter is not succeeding in school and struggles socially. Peter is on a strict diet and receives medication for his ADD.

S

Peter stated, "I'm fine, I just want to run."

O

Volition: Peter smiled and was easily invested in outdoor active games such as tag, relay races, and swinging. He became agitated while performing reading and writing tasks indoor. However, he enjoyed drawing a picture of outdoor games.

Habits: Peter participated in active games outside at the end of the school day. He followed multistep directions outside and made eye contact with the clinician. Peter was resistant when it was time to come inside. He completed writing tasks reluctantly.

Performance: Peter was able to climb, pump himself on the swing, and played outside for 30 minutes with no evidence of fatigue. Inside, Peter struggled with writing assignments and became frustrated easily. Peter enjoyed drawing a picture of his outside play.

Environment: The playground was equipped with a variety of swings and tires, and many children were playing. At home, Peter has a swing and a trampoline and also plays in the woods. His parents are supportive of his outdoor play.

A

Peter shows strengths in gross motor skills; he has interests in outdoor activities with friends. Peter shows weaknesses in indoor fine motor activities and displays poor attention to details.

P

Peter's enjoyment of gross motor outdoor activity may be used to help him develop academic skills. He would benefit from activities emphasizing outdoor activities.

Consultation with teachers and parents on how to use outdoor activities for school work may prove motivating for Peter and help him succeed in school. Peter will receive occupational therapy for 1 hour weekly during the school year.

The OT practitioner used MOHO to guide clinical reasoning. Upon finding out that Peter was volitionally motivated toward active outdoor activities, the clinician planned the intervention around ways to support Peter while working on his poor fine motor skills and his decreased attention to details. Targeting activities that motivate Peter may help him improve his academics. (See Chapter 25 for more information on MOHO in practice).

Legitimate Tools

Legitimate tools are the instruments or tools that a profession uses to bring about change. Legitimate tools change over time based on the growing knowledge of the profession, technological advances, and the needs and values of both the profession and society.[12] OT practitioners use occupations, purposeful activities, activity analysis, activity synthesis, and therapeutic use of self as tools to help children in their care.

Occupation

The goal of OT is to help children participate in their desired occupations. These occupations include social participation, self-care tasks (e.g., feeding, dressing, bathing), educational activities, and play. Intervention is designed to help them actively participate to the fullest in these occupations. Therefore, OT practitioners analyze occupations to determine why a child is not performing well and use the tools of practice to assist them. Intervention is then designed to remediate the underlying skill deficits that are causing the child's difficulty, to compensate for problem areas, or to adapt the requirements of the skills so that the child may be successful at performing them in a different way.

OT practitioners provide occupation-based interventions.[2,8] The intervention involves having the child actively participate in the actual occupation with which he or she struggles. For example, an intervention to improve a child's ability to play with others may consist of inviting another child to the therapy session(s) to facilitate playing.

Purposeful Activities

Purposeful activities are defined as goal-directed behaviors or tasks that constitute occupations.[9] An activity is purposeful if the individual is a voluntary, active participant and the activity is directed toward a goal that the individual considers meaningful. OT practitioners use purposeful activities to evaluate, facilitate, restore,

or maintain individuals' abilities to function in their daily occupations.

Purposeful activities provide opportunities for individuals to achieve mastery, and successful performance promotes feelings of personal competence. Those involved in purposeful activities focus on the processes required for achievement rather than on the goals. Purposeful activities occur within the contexts of personal, cultural, physical, and other environmental conditions and require a variety of client factors (e.g., neuromusculoskeletal, global, and specific mental functions, and body systems).[2] Purposeful activities are unique to the individual; therefore, the OT practitioner grades or adapts a chosen activity for the individual.[9]

Activity Analysis

Activity analysis is the process of analyzing an activity to determine how and when it should be used with a particular client.[3] It involves the identification of the components or client factors necessary to perform an activity.[3] Several methods are used to analyze activities, two of which are discussed in this chapter.

The first method is **task-focused activity analysis**. This method of analyzing activity identifies the physical, social, and mental factors involved in a specific task. The OT practitioner uses an activity analysis to describe the materials needed for the activity, the sequential steps of the activity, and safety concerns.[4] Task-focused activity analysis identifies the most and least important performance components needed to complete the activity. The physical, personal, social, and cultural conditions and influences are described. Using this analysis, the OT practitioner identifies how the activity may be graded and adapted for the client. Task-focused activity analysis is used to understand the activity in terms of skills and personal and cultural meanings to help the OT practitioner understand how the activity can be used therapeutically. This type of analysis enables him or her to quickly identify the demand of an activity (Figure 10-1).[6]

The second method comprises both **child- and family-focused activity analyses** (Figure 10-2). The OT practitioner analyzes the actual intervention and identifies the child's and family's strengths and weaknesses. The practitioner then identifies the objectives and plans activities that are specifically designed to meet those objectives. The practitioner describes the types of materials, supplies, and equipment that will be needed; identifies the position of the child and the OT practitioner during intervention; and documents the expected results or recommendations. Several activities may meet the requirements of the plan.

There is a degree of overlap between the two types of activity analysis. Although each one emphasizes distinct aspects of activity, both require that the practitioner

TASK-FOCUSED ACTIVITY ANALYSIS

CHILD'S NAME: _____ *Kellie Peralta* _____ DATE: _____ *12/30/05* _____

ACTIVITY DESCRIPTION: *Closing Velcro tabs on shoes* _____

SUPPLIES/EQUIPMENT: *Socks, shoes, chair* _____

STEPS OF ACTIVITY:

1) *Prepare work area with chair, socks and shoes.*

2) *Position child on chair.*

3) *Put socks and shoes on.*

4) *Demonstrate how to close tabs.*

5) *Allow the child to practice closing tabs with hand-over-hand assistance.*

6) *Allow child to begin practicing closing tabs.*

LIST THE MOST IMPORTANT PERFORMANCE COMPONENTS REQUIRED FOR THIS ACTIVITY:

Sensorimotor	Cognitive	Psychosocial/Psychological
1) *Sensory awareness*	1) *Level of arousal*	1) *Values*
2) *Tactile*	2) *Attention span*	2) *Interests*
3) *Proprioception*	3) *Sequencing*	3) *Role performance*
4) *Kinesthesia*	4) *Learning*	4) *Self-expression*
5) *Fine coordination / dexterity*	5) *Concept formation*	5) *Coping skills*

LIST THE LEAST IMPORTANT PERFORMANCE COMPONENTS REQUIRED FOR THIS ACTIVITY:

Sensorimotor	Cognitive	Psychosocial/Psychological
1) *Oral-motor control*	1) *Orientation*	1) *Self-concept*
2) *Reflexes*	2) *Recognition*	2) *Social conduct*
3) *Pain response*	3) *Categorization*	3) *Interpersonal skills*
4) *Olfactory*	4) *Spatial operations*	4) *Time management skills*
5) *Gustatory*	5) *Problem-solving skills*	5) *Self-control*

ENVIRONMENTAL CONTEXTS:

1. Physical	2. Social	3. Cultural
Activity can be done in the child's room or another room in the home. *Area should be well lighted.* *Child can sit on chair or floor.*	*Practitioner and child will work together until task is learned.* *Mother will practice with child.*	*In own culture, people are expected to wear shoes.*

Gradation	Adaptation	Safety Hazards
Method of instruction can vary to accommodate child's learning needs. *Task can be taught using hand-over-hand method.*	*D rings can be placed on tip of tabs to facilitate grasping the tabs.*	*None*

FIGURE 10-1 Task-focused activity analysis form for Kellie Penalta.

CHILD- AND FAMILY-FOCUSED ACTIVITY ANALYSIS

DATE: ___*12/30/05*___

CHILD'S NAME: ___*Kellie Peralta*___   AGE: ___*2 years, 7 months*___

DIAGNOSIS: ___*Pervasive Development Disorder-Austism*___

SETTING: ___*Home Based*___   FREQUENCY OF OT: ___*5 times per week*___

DURATION: ___*1 hour per session*___

Strengths	Limitations
Strong family support system	*Decreased eye contact*
Enjoys proprioceptive activities	*Delays in fine motor skills*
Enjoys vestibular activities	*Delays in gross motor skills*
	Delay with self-care skills

OBJECTIVE: ___*Kellie will be able to engage in at least three activities without tantrums within 6 months*___

Planned Activities	Materials	Supplies and Equipment
1) Hair brushing *2) Vestibular activities* *3) Dressing activities*		*1) Hair brush* *2) Therapy ball* *3) Clothing, shoes*

Position of Child and Practitioner	Performance Results	Recommendations
1) Child sits on floor in front of therapist.	*1) Child had difficulty tolerating hairbrushing.*	*1) Continue with deep pressure hairbrushing with corn brush. Allow child to initiate hairbrushing activity.*
2) Child initially sits on a 9-inch ball. Practitioner is positioned behind child and supports child at hips.	*2) Child was able to tolerate sitting on ball. She was able to carry out a task while sitting on a ball.*	*2) Introduce a 12-inch ball during next session.*
3) Child sits on floor in front of practitioners. Practitioner also sits on floor.	*3) Child was receptive and able to follow directions. Hand-over-hand assistance was required.*	*3) Mother should practice activity with child everyday. Discrete trial teaching will be used during therapy sessions.*

FIGURE 10-2   Child- and family-focused activity analysis form for Kellie Penalta.

understand the needs of the child, a variety of theoretical approaches, and the context of intervention.

Activity Synthesis
Activity synthesis includes adapting, grading, and reconfiguring activities and is considered a legitimate tool used in OT practice.

Adaptation refers to the process of changing steps during an activity so that the client is able to engage in it. An activity is adapted by modifying or changing the sequence of its steps, the way in which the materials are presented, or the way in which the child is positioned, or by presenting the activity in such a way that the child is expected to perform only certain aspects of it. Activities can also be adapted by changing the characteristics of the materials that are used, such as their size, shape, texture, or weight.[12] For example, in the case of a child who is fearful of movement and needs to improve or develop righting reactions, the practitioner may have him or her sit on a therapy ball to elicit righting reactions. However, because of the child's fear of movement, the practitioner might begin the intervention with a smaller ball that allows the feet to stay on the ground and provides slow, controlled movements. The practitioner can make the activity easier or more difficult to find the right challenge for the child.

Gradation refers to the process of arranging the steps of an activity in a sequential series to change or progress, allowing for gradual improvement by increasing the demand for a higher level of performance as the child's abilities increase. For example, the practitioner provides a frame that limits the movement of the ball to help the child feel more comfortable sitting on the ball. Once the child feels comfortable, the practitioner can take away the stabilizing frame. The OT practitioner determines the type and extent of grading based on clinical reasoning. A client's level of performance changes when he or she participates in activities that are graded for his or her needs. Once the practitioner has adapted and graded an activity, it is presented in its "real" form, thus synthesizing the analysis, adaptation, and grading into the activity itself.[11] For example, finger-feeding is acceptable while a child is learning self-feeding. The activity is then adapted by the introduction of a utensil. It would be acceptable initially for the child to hold the utensil and attempt to use it to scoop or spear food. The practitioner ultimately expects the child to grasp the utensil, spear the food, and bring it to the mouth, thus synthesizing the activity of self-feeding into the child's repertoire of abilities. The goal of adapting and grading activities is participation in occupations in the given context.

Activity Configuration

Activity configuration is the process of selecting, on the basis of a child's age, interests, and abilities, specific activities that will be used during the intervention process. For example, a long-term goal for the child may be the ability to feed himself or herself independently. One short-term objective may be scooping food with a spoon. A session objective may be learning how to control the grasp and release of a spoon.

Therapeutic Use of Self

Therapeutic use of self is the ability of the OT practitioner to communicate with the child and the child's family or caregivers while being aware of his or her own personal feelings. OT practitioners use their individual characteristics to relate to families, interact with children, and help them perform occupations. As such, those OT practitioners who are aware of their own strengths and weaknesses have insight into how one's use of self has an impact on intervention, so they may help children and their families more effectively.

Taylor developed the Intentional Relationship Model (IRM) which describes six modes of interacting with clients for their benefit.[15] These interpersonal modes include advocating, collaborating, emphathizing, encouraging, instructing, and problem solving.[15] OT practitioners may favor one mode over the other, but understanding how one uses these modes with different clients can help OT practitioners develop improved therapeutic use of self. Some clients will respond better to certain modes than to others. Becoming mindful of one's use of self in a therapeutic setting benefits clients and strengthens the therapeutic relationship. Taylor provides reflective exercises and examples to help practitioners develop skill and awareness in therapeutic use of self.[15]

In a therapeutic relationship, the OT practitioner helps the child and the family without any expectation of the help being reciprocated.[10] He or she develops and maintains a good relationship with the child and the family.[5] Therefore, OT practitioners must possess a basic knowledge of family dynamics, cultural and ethnic concepts in the provision of services, and family systems. As Peloquin stated, "concern for the patient as a person remains essential to effective practice."[14]

OT practitioners recognize that a child is treated in the contexts of the child's family, culture, and environment. The OT practitioner's role is to create an atmosphere of freedom and challenge within the structure of the intervention. The intervention should not be so simple that the child becomes bored or so difficult that he or she feels inadequate. The practitioner prepares a setting to meet the child's needs by guiding him or her toward mastery of the skill.[14]

OT practitioners work with the family to guide them as they care for the child. Because families may experience emotional stress associated with the issues of raising a child who has special needs, they may not always be able to participate in the therapeutic process. Clinicians must work with parents where they are and not have unreal expectations or judgments with regard to the parents "getting through" things. Working on goals that are important to a family at a particular time is an effective way to help them. Parents will understand their children's needs better as they work with the OT practitioner to meet the agreed-upon goals.

CASE *Study*

Tyrone is an 18-month-old child with developmental delays; he is unable to walk, speaks very little, and does not manipulate toys. His mother has three other children (ages

9, 7, and 3), lives alone, and receives public assistance. The OT practitioner provides the mother with an extensive home program, which she refuses to carry out. The practitioner documents that the mother is "noncompliant and in denial about her son's diagnosis."

In this scenario, the OT practitioner has failed to examine the context and therefore has too quickly judged Tyrone's mother. The mother may be overwhelmed by this new diagnosis and the demands of caring for four young children by herself on a limited income. She may not be carrying out the home program because she has no time or energy to do it. The OT practitioner has not targeted the goals that support the mother and the family.

Consider the same case with the OT practitioner providing the mother with techniques to include her other children in playing with Tyrone to improve his abilities. This would allow the mother some free time and involve all the children in the activity. The OT practitioner may even provide activities that they could all perform together as "family game time" (e.g., "Simon Says" or finger plays). The OT practitioner may work more closely with the mother in determining how Tyrone's developmental delays are having an impact on the family. After identifying that feeding Tyrone is problematic, the OT practitioner may target feeding issues. Targeting the issues of concern to parents is the best way to involve them in the intervention process. OT practitioners who target parental concerns seldom find parents who are "in denial" or "noncomplaint."

CLINICAL *Pearl*

Examining situations from all angles provides insight that may help OT practitioners working with children.

CLINICAL *Pearl*

The parents may not understand the entirety of the diagnosis, but they generally understand their child. They can learn about their child's strengths and weaknesses during the intervention process. OT practitioners can help the parents understand their child better by involving them in goal setting.

CLINICAL *Pearl*

Parents want the best from their children. OT practitioners help them care for their children and play a role in empowering parents.

CLINICAL *Pearl*

Making eye contact, getting to the child's level, and pointing out his or her strengths to the parents help OT practitioners gain trust from the child and from the family. These abilities are considered part of therapeutic use of self.

One way to help parents understand their child better is through modeling behaviors. Parents report that they learn more easily by observing the practitioner work with the child. Being able to observe and ask questions helps them develop skills and routines to care for their child.[6,9] The OT practitioner models handling techniques, management, and attitudes toward the child. The clinician also models patience, understanding, and acceptance, which, in turn, helps parents show the same. The OT practitioner learns from parents by listening and opening lines of communication; this therapeutic relationship empowers parents. While the OT practitioner comes into contact with many children with special needs, parents may find this new experience overwhelming. Therefore, a clinician who models understanding, caring, and acceptance of the child may teach parents the same, which has an impact on the child and the family in ways that cannot be measured. This is the essence of therapeutic use of self.

Therapeutic use of self requires that OT practitioners be aware of their body language; read parents' verbal and nonverbal cues; and interact in a caring, nonjudgmental manner. Making eye contact, nodding one's head, and using facial expressions to communicate are all aspects of therapeutic use of self that clinicians must understand and use effectively.

Multicultural Implications

CASE *Study*

Maria is a 2-year-old girl diagnosed with spastic quadriplegia. Her parents have recently immigrated to the United States from the Dominican Republic. Maria is evaluated at the early intervention center by an occupational therapist, a physical therapist, and a speech therapist. The team decides that Maria needs all the services. The occupational therapist meets with the parents to decide on goals for sessions. The social worker, who speaks Spanish, is present. Using a family-centered approach (mandated by early intervention laws), the OT practitioner asks the parents what their concerns are and what they would like to work on in therapy sessions. The parents are hesitant to respond throughout the meeting. The OT practitioner feels that the parents are not interested in receiving services for their daughter. The OT practitioner and the social worker meet after the meeting to discuss the events.

This case study illustrates the need to understand cultural expectations. The OT practitioner does not understand why the parents do not quickly express what they desire for Maria. The practitioner interprets this as lack of caring and interest in the child's progress.

The social worker explains to the OT practitioner that while many American parents feel empowered to discuss their concerns and advocate for their child, parents from the Dominican Republic look to the professional to tell them what to do. Maria's parents have not yet been socialized to the American system. They are not uninterested but, rather, somewhat confused as to why a medical health care professional (e.g., the OT practitioner) would ask them what they wanted. They view health care professionals as the experts and, as such, will follow through with any requirements set forth by the team.

Once the OT practitioner understands this cultural difference, he holds the next meeting in a different way, is more directive, and provides the parents with the team's recommendations. However, the team acknowledges that Maria will require OT services when she enters school, and so they will have to help socialize the parents to advocate for their child with professionals. However, the OT practitioner may first have to be more direct than they would need to be with parents already socialized to the American system.

Cultural values have an impact on all areas of family life. OT practitioners need to understand the cultural context of the child in order to meet the child's and the family's needs. Although the OT practitioner may not have direct understanding of each culture, sensitivity and open communication may bridge the gap. Disregard for cultural concerns may interfere with establishing rapport; as a result, the practitioner may find the child or caregiver not investing in the intervention. When this happens, the lack of compliance and satisfaction generally makes the therapy process ineffective.

Goal Setting

The OTA collaborates with the occupational therapist and the family on the development of long-term goals and short-term objectives for any child they are treating. Through this collaborative process, the occupational therapist, the OTA, and the family agree on the needs of the child as well as the appropriate priorities for intervention. This makes the intervention process more efficient and effective and leads to a better understanding of the child. Based on the evaluation and discussion of needs, realistic goals for the child can be established.

Long-Term Goals

Long-term goals are statements that describe the occupational goals the client should achieve after intervention. These goals should be measurable, observable, clear, and written in behavioral terms. Goals need to be very specific and address the problems that have been identified. A practitioner can use the mnemonic device referred to as the **RUMBA criteria** to write up the goal statements (Box 10-2).[7]

Short-Term Goals

Short-term goals are the steps the client needs to achieve in order to meet the long-term goal. They are statements that describe the skills that should be mastered in a relatively short period. For example, consider a client whose long-term goal is independent dressing. The short-term objectives for this client may include developing the pincer grasp for buttoning, learning to button, and developing sequencing skills for dressing.

Treatment Implementation

Treatment implementation (intervention) involves working within the system through which the child is receiving therapy, working with the family, and working

---

BOX 10-2

RUMBA Criteria

R (RELEVANT)
A relevant goal reflects the client's current life situation and future possibilities. Everyone involved in the client's care (client, therapist, family, and members of other disciplines) should agree on the goal.

U (UNDERSTANDABLE)
An understandable goal is stated in clear language. Jargon and very specialized or difficult words should be avoided.

M (MEASURABLE)
A measurable goal contains criteria for success.

B (BEHAVIORAL)
A behavioral goal focuses on the behavior or skill that the client must eventually demonstrate.

A (ACHIEVABLE)
An achievable goal describes a behavior or skill that the client should be able to accomplish in a reasonable period.

Adapted from Early MB: *Mental health concepts and techniques for the occupational therapy assistant,* ed 2, New York, 1993, Raven Press.

directly with the child. Working with the child involves planning each session, developing and analyzing activities, and then grading and adapting those activities as necessary. This process is geared toward reaching the short-term objectives first and then the long-term goals.

Intervention includes the methods used to work toward meeting the goals, the media or activities used during the intervention, and documentation of the child's progress or lack of progress.

Session or Mini-Objectives

Session or mini-objectives are the goals the practitioner has set for an intervention session. They are planned before the session in collaboration with the child and parents. Sometimes mini-objectives will remain for several sessions because it may take more than one intervention to meet them. Once the session objectives are identified, the OT practitioner analyzes the activities that will facilitate meeting the objectives.

RE-EVALUATION AND DISCONTINUATION OF INTERVENTION

Re-evaluation

Although the occupational therapist determines whether a re-evaluation is indicated, the OTA is responsible for reporting any change in the child's condition to the supervisor. Therefore, if the OTA observes changes, the changes are brought to the attention of the occupational therapist, and the OTA may suggest a re-evaluation. The OTA participates in the re-evaluation in collaboration with and under the supervision of the occupational therapist.[3]

Discontinuation of Intervention

In pediatric OT practice, discharge planning or discontinuation of intervention may be mandated by laws that govern the type of system in which the child receives OT services. Regardless of the system, the discontinuation process is the responsibility of the occupational therapist. The OTA collaborates in the discontinuation process under the supervision of the occupational therapist by reporting on the child's progress and making suggestions regarding future needs.

Services are typically discontinued once the child has met the predetermined goals and achieved maximum benefit from OT or when the parents and the child decide that the child no longer wants to receive OT. Services may be discontinued when the child moves away or enters another system. The OTA may recommend discontinuation of services to the

occupational therapist when any of the conditions mentioned above exist. Discontinuation plans should include a plan for follow-up when indicated. Figure 10-3 provides a summary of the OT process from referral to the follow-up plan.

While many systems do not allow for children to be discharged and re-admitted, this may, in fact, be the best method. For example, a child who is no longer receiving OT services may need OT periodically in junior high school to help him or her successfully adjust to physical changes or to advanced requirements.

REFERRAL	
OTR:	Accepts any referral to occupational therapy and determines plan for evaluation
COTA:	Forwards all referrals to OTR

EVALUATION	
OTR:	Determines type and scope of evaluation
COTA:	Administers specific assessments under direction of OTR

INTERVENTION PLAN	
OTR:	Develops intervention plan
COTA:	Collaborates with OTR

INTERVENTION	
OTR:	Carries out intervention plan and supervises COTA
COTA:	Participates in carrying out intervention plan under supervision of and in collaboration with OTR

DISCHARGE PLANNING	
OTR:	Determines when discharge is appropriate and develops discharge plan
COTA:	Contributes knowledge about patient and collaborates in discharge planning

FOLLOW-UP PLAN	
OTR:	Develops plan and scope of plan
COTA:	Collaborates in development process

FIGURE 10-3 Responsibilities of occupational therapist and occupational therapy assistant (OTA) in OT intervention process.

OCCUPATION-CENTERED TOP-DOWN APPROACH

Since OT practitioners are interested in helping children engage in their occupations, evaluation and intervention focusing on occupations are recommended. Fisher proposed a model for OT evaluation and intervention using a client-centered, occupation-based, **top-down approach** called the **Occupational Therapy Intervention Process Model (OTIPM)**.[8]

The following is a case study illustrating how this translates to practice. The focus of this evaluation and intervention plan is on the child's occupations.[8] Later in the process, the OT practitioner will determine the client factors or components that are interfering with performance. However, goals for intervention can be developed on the basis of overall performance. As highlighted in this case study, OT practitioners are encouraged to address the concerns of parents, caregivers, and teachers when designing an intervention that focuses on occupational performance. OT practitioners are encouraged to read Fisher's work for additional information.[8]

The following case illustrates the top-down approach to OT intervention.

CASE *Study*

Hannah is a 2-year and 7-month-old girl with a diagnosis of pervasive developmental disorder. She was referred to an early intervention program for evaluation by the pediatrician.

Parental Concerns

Her parents express concern that Hannah does not talk as clearly as her cousin does and never has; becomes agitated very easily and screams, especially during bath time; and does not play with her cousins and sisters. Furthermore, her mother is concerned about the lack of variety in her diet. Hannah's parents are concerned that she is not developing like her sisters (ages 5 and 1), and they are unsure about how to manage her behaviors. Her mother is "worried about Hannah's lack of interest in her mother, father, or siblings."

Areas of Performance
Activities of Daily Living

- *Feeding.* Hannah is currently able to drink from a bottle but does not like to drink from a cup. She is very particular about the food she eats and likes only very soft, almost liquid types of food. Her food preferences currently include Cheerios with milk, pasta soup, and bland mashed potatoes. Hannah sometimes eats very ripe bananas.

- *Dressing.* Hannah does not yet dress or undress independently. Her mother reports that she likes to wear only long-sleeved shirts and leggings and refuses to walk around barefoot. Hannah is able to remove her socks. She is able to remove mittens, hats, and coats after they are unzipped. She is unable to remove slip-on shoes or unlace or unbuckle other shoes. She is unable to put on or take off pants, skirts, or shirts.

- *Bathing.* Hannah often hides and becomes tearful when her mother announces that it is bath time. She cries, has tantrums, and hits others when placed in the tub. She hates having her face washed; however, her mother reports that sometimes Hannah will rub her face with a washcloth on her own.

- *Toileting.* Hannah does not indicate when she is wet or soiled and shows no discomfort.

- *Sleep.* Hannah sleeps through the night. She goes to bed around 9:00 p.m. and wakes up around 7:00 a.m. She takes a 2-hour nap during the day.

Play

Hannah does not interact with others while playing but plays alone quietly. She likes balls and stares at them for long periods of time. Hannah sometimes enjoys going to the playground, especially when there are few or no other children around. She goes up and down the slide, sometimes as often as 30 times in an hour. She is terrified of the swing and refuses to go in the sandbox. Hannah enjoys roughhousing with her father.

Social Participation

Her mother reports that Hannah prefers to sit in front of the television watching children's programs and does not play with toys. She does not respond to her name when called despite having had a normal audiologic examination. Hannah's eye contact is limited; she does not look at her mother when asking for things. She does not verbalize her needs but, instead, takes her mother's hand to guide her to whatever she wants. Hannah does not initiate conversation with her sisters or parents.

Habits/Routines

Hannah stays at home with her mother and younger sister; her older sister attends morning kindergarten. Hannah's family lives in a two-story house in the country. Hannah has a swing and sandbox in the yard. She has a variety of toys. Hannah eats breakfast around 8:00 a.m., lunch at noon, and dinner at 6:00 p.m. She takes a 2-hour nap after lunch. Hannah bathes once a week, although her mother would like her to do it more often. The family enjoys taking hikes and spending time together. The children go to gymnastics classes once a week. Hannah frequently does not participate in classes.

Each Sunday the family gets together at the grandmother's house for dinner and socializing. Many children are playing there. Hannah finds it difficult to be around them and frequently goes to a quiet room in the house. The family leaves early on many occasions when she has tantrums.

Assessment

Hannah's family has established routines in which she is able to participate. She experiences some difficulty at family gatherings but has also demonstrated the ability to adapt (e.g., finding a quiet space). Hannah is able to indicate her wants by pulling on her mother's hand, which indicates that she has motivations and desires.

Hannah is demonstrating delays in all areas of self-care, play, and social participation. She shows signs of sensory modulation difficulties that interfere with these occupations.

Plan

Hannah will attend an early intervention program three mornings a week, which will include OT services for improving her ability to play with others, dress and feed herself, and get along with family members.

Abbreviated Intervention Plan

The goals and objectives were designed to meet parental concerns (Box 10-3). The first goal of dressing will help Hannah's parents see that she can participate in daily tasks, and this may empower them to set other goals. Other goals and objectives center around parental concerns that Hannah does not play with other children and shows a lack of interest in her mother, father, and siblings. Since play is so important in a child's life, the OT practitioner decided to start there. Furthermore, her mother has repeatedly expressed concern that Hannah is not interested in the family. Therefore, helping the child become part of the family will benefit everyone.

Because Hannah already gets her mother's attention to show her what she wants, the OT practitioner will build upon this skill. This will help the parent and child feel successful early on, build a trusting relationship between parent and child in order to meet other goals, and reinforce the connections between Hannah and other family members. Children with a diagnosis of pervasive developmental disorder may not express themselves in the same manner as do typically developing children. Therefore, grabbing her mother's hand and expressing her desires by means of pointing at pictures close to her mother may be Hannah's way of staying close to her. This may cause her mother to feel needed and thus connected to her. Once Hannah is accustomed to pointing to pictures, the OT practitioner may give the pictures to the father, sisters, and teachers.

BOX 10-3

Goals and Objectives

1. Hannah will be able to dress herself with verbal prompting within 6 months.
   - Hannah will be able to button a shirt with demonstrative prompts 3 out of 4 times.
   - Hannah will be able to unbutton a shirt independently 3 out of 4 times.
   - Hannah will show improved bilateral coordination by putting together five pop beads independently 4 out of 6 times.
2. Hannah will play with her sisters for 15 minutes, sharing toys at least twice during the session.
   - Hannah will engage in parallel play with her sister and cousin (both 5 years old) for 5 minutes without interfering in the play.
   - Hannah will play "pass the ball" with her sister (5 years old) for 5 minutes without becoming upset.
   - Hannah will dance with her sisters for 3 minutes as part of family game night.
3. Hannah will seek her mother's help at least five times a day.
   - Hannah will indicate her desires to her mother by pointing to the objects she wants 3 out of 5 times.
   - Hannah will hold her mother's hand to lead her to the objects she wants.
   - Hannah will make eye contact with her mother twice while playing peek-a-boo.

When the family has seen some progress and Hannah's behaviors are more under control, the OT sessions may focus on the underlying components, such as fine motor skills. For example, once Hannah is able to play with her sisters at home with a large ball, the practitioner may recommend coloring activities or other activities that are more challenging for her. The OT practitioner knows that targeting family issues has the greatest impact on the child's performance. The goal of the sessions is not that Hannah becomes "normal"; instead, the goal is for her to fit in with the family so that other family members can begin to understand her better and make the necessary accommodations.

Frame of Reference

A sensory integration frame of reference will be used to help Hannah modulate sensory information. The OT practitioner will work with the family to determine her sensory needs and provide home strategies for the parents that will help manage Hannah's behaviors more easily.

A developmental frame of reference will also be used to help Hannah participate in everyday play activities at home. The OT practitioner will provide other family members with simple, easily implemented goals to help them relate to and better understand Hannah. Hannah will learn how to play better through practice and rewards (e.g., sensory or verbal).

Intervention Strategies

Intervention strategies are tailored to meet the child's and family's needs and thus require creativity, analysis, and reflection on how the activities are meeting the goals. Since children change, intervention strategies must also change.

Hannah's OT sessions may focus on sensory modulation activities, including brushing programs and tactile exploration (e.g., playing with sand, water, or rice). Many children with pervasive developmental disorder benefit from a sensory integration approach that includes child-directed experiences on suspended equipment, requiring adaptive responses. See Chapter 24 for more treatment suggestions.

The OT practitioner carefully adapts and grades activities while reading the child's cues so that the child can succeed. Occasionally including the parents and siblings in the sessions helps model how to promote positive behaviors and provides the parents with strategies to use at home. Because the goal of the sessions is to improve play skills, intervention resembles play and may include small play groups with other children. The OT practitioner gives the child a reward for positive behaviors (e.g., sharing), which could be a sticker, positive verbal praise, or an extra turn.

To help the child ask for assistance from her mother, the clinician sets up a picture board with the activities of the day and teaches the child how to point to the next activity. Hannah will eventually learn to pick out the activities by pointing. This same strategy can be implemented at home by placing pictures on the refrigerator, from which she may choose. The clinician may decide to give the mother an apron with pictures on it so that Hannah has to go to her to choose a picture. Each intervention session includes a variety of play activities, strategies for parents, and successful performances from Hannah. The OT practitioner pays close attention to Hannah and her family's needs.

SUMMARY

OT services are provided to children from birth to 21 years of age. Before engaging in pediatric practice, the practitioner must be familiar with the profession's tools, the OT intervention process, and federal and state laws in order to effectively design OT services. OT practitioners in pediatrics work not only with the children but also with the families and caregivers. Specialized training in intervention techniques, family dynamics, and cultural considerations are beneficial. OT practitioners help children participate in everyday occupations. Therefore, a top-down approach focusing on occupations as the means and ends and emphasizing client-centered care is recommended.[8]

References

1. American Occupational Therapy Association: *Standards of practice for occupational therapy*, Bethesda, MD, 1998, American Occupational Therapy Association.
2. American Occupational Therapy Association: Occupational therapy practice framework: domain and process, ed 2. *Am J Occup Ther* 62:625–683, 2008.
3. American Occupational Therapy Association: *Occupational therapy roles*, Bethesda, MD, 1994, American Occupational Therapy Association.
4. Blesedell-Crepeau E: Activity analysis: a way of thinking about occupational performance. In Neistadt ME, Crepeau EB, editors: *Willard and Spackman's occupational therapy*, ed 10, Philadelphia, 2003, Lippincott.
5. Case-Smith J: *Pediatric occupational therapy and early intervention*, ed 2, Boston, 1998, Butterworth-Heinemann.
6. Crowe T et al: Role perceptions of mothers with young children: the impact of a child's disability. *Am J Occup Ther* 49:221, 1997.
7. Early MB: *Mental health concepts and techniques for the occupational therapy assistant*, ed 3, Philadelphia, 1999, Lippincott Williams & Wilkins.
8. Fisher A: *OTIPM: a model for implementing top-down, client-centered, and occupation-based assessment, intervention, and documentation*, Durham, NH, January 12–14, 2005, University of New Hampshire.
9. Hinojosa J, Sabari J, Pedretti LW: Purposeful activities. *Am J Occup Ther* 47:1081, 1993.
10. Humphry R, Link S: Preparation of occupational therapists to work in early intervention programs. *Am J Occup Ther* 44:28, 1990.
11. Kramer P, Hinojosa J: Activity synthesis. In Hinojosa J, Blount M, editors: *The texture of life: purposeful activities*, Bethesda, MD, 2004, American Occupational Therapy Association.
12. Luebben A, Hinojosa J, Kramer P: Legitimate tools of pediatric occupational therapy. In Kramer P, Hinojosa J, editors: *Frames of reference in pediatric occupational therapy*, ed 2, Baltimore, MD, 1999, Lippincott Williams & Wilkins.
13. MacRae N: *Foundations of occupational therapy*. Unpublished lecture notes, 2001, University of New England.
14. Peloquin S: The patient-therapist relationship in occupational therapy: understanding visions and images. *Am J Occup Ther* 44:13, 1990.
15. Taylor R. *The intentional relationship: use of self and occupational therapy*, Philadelphia, 2007, FA Davis.

Recommended Reading

Dunbar S: *Occupational therapy intervention models with children and families*, Thorofare, NJ, 2007, Slack.

Kielhofner G: *Conceptual foundations of occupational therapy*, ed 4, Philadelphia, 2009, FA Davis.

Kramer P, Hinojosa J: *Frames of reference for pediatric occupational therapy*, ed 3, Philadelphia, 2009, Lippincott Williams & Wilkins.

REVIEW *Questions*

1. In what way does assessment of a child guide the OT practitioner in the processes of program planning and treatment implementation?
2. Define and differentiate among long-term goals, short-term objectives, and mini-objectives.
3. What are the components of an activity analysis?
4. In what ways are activity analysis and adaptation used by the OT practitioner during program planning and treatment implementation?
5. What are the levels of performance?
6. Provide examples of using a top-down approach to OT intervention.

SUGGESTED *Activities*

1. Using the task-focused activity analysis form as a guide, analyze the specific daily routines that you personally perform, such as brushing your teeth, getting dressed, and preparing lunch.
2. Visit a daycare center or observe a neighbor's child performing specific tasks. Analyze what you observe using the task-focused activity analysis.
3. Choose an activity in which you typically engage and experiment by changing your position and the materials used for the activity. For example, eat a bowl of ice cream while sitting at the table and then do the same thing on your stomach in front of the television. Try different sizes of bowls and spoons. Write down how the change in position or in the bowl and spoon made a difference in your performance.
4. Identify at least one long-term personal goal. Write short-term objectives about the way you plan on reaching your goal(s). Consider what methods you will use in attaining the objectives and ultimately your goal(s). The goal(s) should be attainable within 12 months. Use the RUMBA criteria when writing up your goal(s).
5. Ask some parents what they would like for their children in the near future. Write these as measurable goals. Describe the trends you observed and what you have learned that may help you in practice.

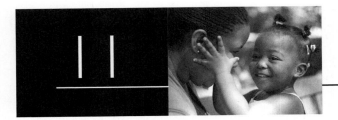

Anatomy and Physiology for the Pediatric Practitioner

JEAN W. SOLOMON*

CHAPTER *Objectives*

After studying this chapter, the reader will be able to accomplish the following:

- Distinguish between two branches of biology: anatomy and physiology.
- Understand and describe the hierarchy of organization of the human body.
- Describe the anatomic position.
- Understand and define the descriptive and movement terminology.
- Understand the cardinal planes and axes.
- Describe the structures and functions of the organ systems of the human body.
- Provide examples of pediatric health conditions or disorders of the organ systems of the human body.
- Understand and describe the relationship among body structures, the function of body structures, and one's successful engagement in daily occupations.

* I would like to thank Robert (Bob) Hunter for his review of this chapter as a content expert in anatomy and physiology.

CHAPTER OUTLINE

Terminology, Planes, and Axes

Skeletal System

Muscular System

Integumentary System

Cardiovascular System

Respiratory System

Nervous System

Endocrine System

Digestive System

Urinary System

Lymphatic System

Immune System

Reproductive System

Relationship Among Body Structures and Functions and Occupational Performance

Summary

The Occupational Therapy Practice Framework (OTPF) describes the domains and processes inherent to the profession of occupational therapy (OT). According to the OTPF, the term *client factors* refers to those components that influence actions or occupations.[1] For example, a child's neuromuscular status is considered a client factor. Client factors include both body structures and functions (Table 11-1). The term *body structures* refers to the parts that make up the human body. For example, the structure of the hand includes bones, muscles, tendons, nerves, and blood vessels. A child with a missing thumb would have a deficient body structure that may interfere with his occupational performance. The term *body functions* refers to how the body part, organ, or organ system works. In the former example, body function would include the child's hand strength or coordination. Deficits in body functions may also result in poor occupational performance. Since body functions and body structures are essential to understanding occupational performance, this chapter provides an overview of the structures in each body system. Lastly, the author provides an overview of how body structures and body functions influence occupational performance.

Successful engagement in daily occupations is dependent upon the interactions of many client factors including one's values, beliefs, and spirituality. However, the focus of this chapter is on the client factors related to body structures and functions.

Anatomy is the branch of biology that studies the structures of the human body. *Physiology* is the branch of biology that studies the functions of the structures of the human body. The human body comprises living matter. A unifying concept in biology is that structure or shape determines function in all living matter. One's successful engagement in chosen daily occupations may be impaired if specific client factors related to body structures and functions are impaired or abnormal.

The organization of the human body is hierarchical. *Atoms* are the smallest unit of matter. By definition, *matter* is anything that takes up space and has mass or weight. Atoms of different elements have unique masses and space requirements. The most abundant elements found in living matter are carbon, hydrogen, oxygen, nitrogen, and phosphorus. Atoms link together (bond) to form *molecules*. For example, two hydrogen atoms bond with one oxygen atom to form one molecule of water (H_2O). Molecules come together to form *cells*. Cells are the smallest units of living matter. The cells found in the human body are eukaryotic cells. Eukaryotic cells have a membrane bound nucleus that contains a person's genetic information, for example, deoxyribonucleic acid (DNA) and genes. Cells come together to form *tissues*. There are four basic types of tissue found in the human body. The four tissue types are epithelial, connective, muscle, and nervous (Table 11-2). Tissues come together to form *organs*. Organs, for example, the heart, are made of two or more types of tissues. Organs come together to form *organ systems*, for example, the cardiovascular system, or the circulatory system, which consists of the heart and associated vessels. Organ systems come together to form organisms. The human body has numerous organ systems that work together to allow one's active participation in chosen daily occupations.

The OT practitioner needs to understand the interrelatedness of various organs and organ systems in the human body. Knowledge of the terminology that is used in the study of the human body's structures and functions also is necessary. The anatomic position is used as a reference point when studying the anatomy and physiology of the human body. By definition, the term *anatomic position* refers to a person standing upright with the arms resting at the side of the body, palms forward, and the head and feet pointing forward. The fingers of both hands are adducted (not spread apart) (Figure 11-1). The human body has bilateral (two-sided) symmetry, that is, the right side of the body is a mirror image of the left side of the body.[3,4] The human body is divided into front (anterior/ventral) and back (posterior/dorsal) cavities. Organ systems are located in specific regions of the ventral and dorsal cavities. The ventral cavity is subdivided into thoracic, abdominal, and pelvic cavities. The dorsal cavity is subdivided into cranial and spinal cavities (Figure 11-2).

TERMINOLOGY, PLANES, AND AXES

In the course of their work, OT practitioners use their knowledge of terminology to examine and understand the structures and functions of the human body. The term *anterior* or *ventral* refers to the front of the body. The eyes are located in the sockets found on the anterior surface of the head. The term *posterior* or *dorsal* refers to the back of the body. The spinous processes of the vertebra are found on the posterior surface of the neck and trunk. The term *superior* or *cephalad* refers to the head, or "above." The nose is superior to the lips. The term *inferior* or *caudal* refers to the tail/foot, or "below." On the face, the lips are inferior to the nose. *Proximal* means "closer to the body," whereas *distal* means "farther away from the body." The shoulder is proximal to the hand, and the hand is distal to the elbow. *Medial* means "closer to the midline" or to the "midsaggittal plane of the body." *Lateral* means "farther away from the midline of the body." With a person standing in the anatomic position, the styloid process of the ulna is medial to the styloid process of the radius.

TABLE 11-1

Client Factors

CLIENT FACTORS	
CATEGORY AND DEFINITION	EXAMPLES
Values: Principles, standards, or qualities considered worthwhile or desirable by the client who holds them.	Honesty with self and with others Personal religious convictions Commitment to family.
Beliefs: Cognitive content held as true.	He or she is powerless to influence others Hard work pays off.
Spirituality: The "personal quest for understanding answers to ultimate questions about life, about meaning, and the sacred" (Moyers & Dale, 2007, p. 28).	Daily search for purpose and meaning in one's life Guiding actions from a sense of value beyond the personal acquisition of wealth or fame.

BODY FUNCTIONS
Categories
Mental Functions (affective, cognitive, perceptual)
Specific Mental Functions

Higher-level cognitive	Judgment, insight
Attention	Awareness, sustained, selective, attention
Memory	Short-term, long-term, and working memory
Perception	Discrimination, spatial, and temporal relationships
Thought	Recognition, categorization, generalization,
Mental functions of sequencing complex movement	Execution of learned movement patterns
Emotional	Coping, adapting
Experience of self and time	Body image, self-concept, self-esteem

Global Mental Functions

Consciousness	Level of arousal, level of consciousness
Orientation	Orientation to person, place, time, self, and others
Temperament and personality	Emotional stability
Energy and drive	Motivation, impulse control, and appetite
Sleep (physiological process)	

Sensory Functions and Pain

Seeing and related functions	Detection/registration, modulation, and integration of sensations from the body and environment
Hearing functions	
Vestibular functions	Visual awareness
Taste functions	Sensation of securely moving against gravity
Smell functions	Association of taste & smell
Proprioceptive functions	Awareness of body position and space
Touch functions	Comfort with the feeling of being touched by others
Pain	Localizing pain
Temperature and pressure	Thermal awareness

Neuromusculoskeletal and Movement-related Functions

Functions of joints and bones	ROM
Joint mobility	Postural alignment
Joint stability	Strength
Muscle power	Degree of muscle tone (e.g., flaccidity, spasticity, fluctuating)
Muscle tone	Endurance
Muscle endurance	Righting and supporting
Motor reflexes	Eye–hand/foot coordination, bilateral integration,
Involuntary movement reactions	Walking patterns and impairments
Control of voluntary movement	
Gait patterns	

Continued

TABLE 11-1

Client Factors—*cont'd*

CLIENT FACTORS	
CATEGORY AND DEFINITION	EXAMPLES
Cardiovascular, Hematologic, Immunologic, and Respiratory System Function Cardiovascular system function Hematological and immunological system function Respiratory system function	Blood pressure functions (hypertension, hypotension, postural hypotension), and heart rate Rate, rhythm, and depth of respiration Physical endurance, aerobic capacity, stamina, and fatigability
Voice and Speech Functions • Voice functions • Fluency and rhythm • Alternative vocalization functions	
Digestive, Metabolic, and Endocrine System Function • Digestive system function • Metabolic system and endocrine system function	
Genitourinary and Reproductive Functions • Urinary functions • Genital and reproductive functions	
Skin and Related-structure Functions • Skin functions • Hair and nail functions	Protective functions of the skin–presence or absence of wounds, cuts, or abrasions Repair function of the skin–wound healing
BODY STRUCTURES **Categories** Structure of the nervous system Eyes, ear, and related structures Structures involved in voice and speech Structures of the cardiovascular, immunologic, and respiratory systems Structures related to the digestive, metabolic, and endocrine systems Structure related to the genitourinary and reproductive systems Structures related to movement Skin and related structures	

Moyers, P. A., & Dale, L. M. (2007). *The guide to occupationaltherapy practice* (2nd ed.). Bethesda, MD: AOTA Press.

Note. Some data adapted from the ICF (WHO, 2001).
World Health Organization. (2001). *International classification of functioning, disability, and health (ICF).* Geneva: Author.
*Adapted from Table 2 from: American Occupational Therapy Association: Occupational therapy practice framework: Domain and process, 2nd edition, *Am J Occup Ther* 62(6):625–703, 2008.

Knowledge of the three cardinal planes and their axes is important to understand the anatomy and physiology of the human body, especially when analyzing the cross-sections of structures and movements at individual joints. (1) The *sagittal plane* divides the body into left and right sides. If the body is divided into equal left and right parts, then the plane is called the *midsaggital plane.* The axis for the sagittal plane is the *frontal axis,* which is perpendicular to the saggital plane. (2) The *frontal plane* divides the human body into anterior and posterior parts. The axis for the frontal plane is the *saggital axis.* (3) The *horizontal or transverse plane* divides the body into upper and lower parts. The axis for the horizontal plane is the *vertical axis.* Specific movements occur in each of the three cardinal planes, and the axes are the points about which a body part rotates. For example, bending of the elbow occurs in the sagittal plane. The elbow joint rotates about the frontal axis. Understanding these

TABLE 11-2

Major Tissues of the Body

TISSUE TYPE	STRUCTURE	FUNCTION	EXAMPLES IN THE BODY
Epithelial	One or more layers of densely arranged cells with very little extracellular matrix May form either sheets or glands	Covers and protects the body surface Lines body cavities Movement of substances (absorption, secretion, excretion) Glandular activity	Outer layer of skin Lining of the respiratory, digestive, urinary, reproductive tracts Glands of the body
Connective	Sparsely arranged cells surrounded by a large proportion of extra-cellular matrix often containing structural fibers (and sometimes mineral crystals)	Supports body structures Transports substances throughout the body	Bones Joint cartilage Tendons and ligaments Blood Fat
Muscle	Long fiberlike cells, sometimes branched, capable of pulling loads; extracellular fibers sometimes hold muscle fiber together	Produces body movements Produces movements of organs such as the stomach, heart Produces heat	Heart muscle Muscles of the head/neck, arms, legs, trunk Muscles in the walls of hollow organs such as the stomach, intestines
Nervous	Mixture of many cell types, including several types of neurons (conducting cells) and neuroglia (support cells)	Communication between body parts Integration/regulation of body functions	Tissue of brain and spinal cord Nerves of the body Sensory organs of the body

From Patton KT: *Anatomy and physiology*, ed 7, St. Louis, 2009, Mosby.

concepts is crucial to the analysis and measurement of the range of motion (ROM) of joints (Figure 11-3).

Knowledge of terms that are used to describe movements is useful while studying the muscular and skeletal systems to analyze the activity demands and client factors necessary for occupational performance. *Flexion* is the bending at a joint, which decreases the angle of the joint. *Extension* is the straightening of a joint, which increases the angle of the joint. Flexion and extension occur in the sagittal plane, with rotation about the frontal axis. *Abduction* is movement *away* from the midline of the body, whereas *adduction* is movement *toward* the midline of the body. Abduction and adduction occur in the frontal plane, with rotation about the sagittal axis. Horizontal abduction and adduction, for example, moving the arm across the chest or toward the back of the body, are movements that occur in the horizontal plane. Internal (medial) and external (lateral) rotations, that is, movements of the head of the humerus in and out of the glenoid fossa, occur in the transverse plane. Forearm supination is turning palms up. Forearm pronation is turning palms down so that the palms of the hands face the floor.

Supination and *pronation* occur in the transverse or horizontal plane, with rotation about the vertical axis. All of these movements are possible only with intact skeletal and muscular organ systems.

CLINICAL *Pearl*

To remember the definition of *supination*, think about how you carry a bowl of soup, palm up; *pronation* is the opposite.

SKELETAL SYSTEM

The **skeletal system** consists of bones, cartilage, ligaments, and joints. The two major subdivisions of the skeletal system are the axial and appendicular systems. The *axial skeletal system* consists of the bones, cartilage, ligaments, and joints of the neck and trunk. The *appendicular skeletal system* consists of the bones, cartilage, ligaments, and joints of the arms and legs (upper and lower extremities) (Figure 11-4).

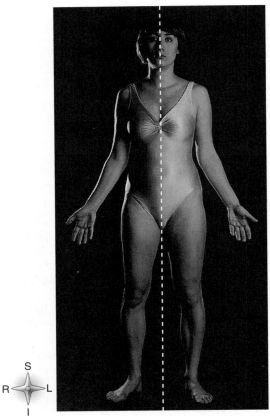

FIGURE 11-1 Anatomic position and bilateral symmetry. (From Thibodeau GA and Patton KT: *Anatomy and physiology,* ed 6, 2006, Mosby.)

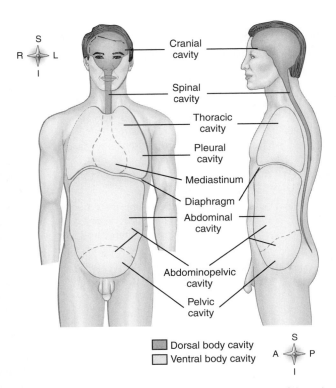

FIGURE 11-2 Major body cavities. (From Thibodeau GA and Patton KT: *Anatomy and physiology,* ed 6, Mosby, 2006.)

CLINICAL *Pearl*

To remember the number of vertebra in the first three regions of the vertebral column, know that breakfast is at seven in the morning, lunch is at noon, and dinner is at five in the afternoon. This translates into 7 cervical vertebrae, 12 thoracic vertebrae, and 5 lumbar vertebrae. The vertebrae of the sacrum and coccyx are fused, and the number of vertebrae can be variable.

The primary functions of the skeletal system are support of the human body and protection of internal vital organs. In concert with the muscular system, the skeletal system allows movement at joints (articulations between two or more bones) or supports movement-related functions in the human body.[1] Different types of joints are found in the human body. Shoulder and hip joints are called *ball and socket joints,* which are freely movable in all three of the cardinal planes. During typical development, bones fully ossify and provide stability. Examples of disorders of the skeletal system include fractures and congenital amputations. Subsequent chapters cover disorders and health conditions of the skeletal system.

MUSCULAR SYSTEM

The three types of muscle in the **muscular system** are cardiac, smooth, and skeletal muscles. *Cardiac muscle* is found in the heart; it contracts to maintain blood circulation throughout the body. Cardiac muscle contracts involuntarily and is controlled by its own pacemaker. *Smooth muscle* is found in the internal organs of the body and is not under conscious control. For example, smooth muscle in the organs of the digestive system contracts to move nutrients through the digestive tract. The third type of muscle is *skeletal* or *striated muscle(s).* The contraction and relaxation of skeletal muscle is under conscious control. Skeletal muscle has at least two attachments to bone—the origin and the insertion, which consist of bands of connective tissue called *tendons.* Between the origin and the insertion is the *muscle bulk* or *muscle belly* (Figure 11-5). Skeletal muscle contracts to create movement at joints. Skeletal muscles have a role in *thermoregulation* (regulating the temperature of the body) and *osmoregulation* (regulating the amount of water in the human body). Skeletal muscles function as agonists or antagonists when contracting to

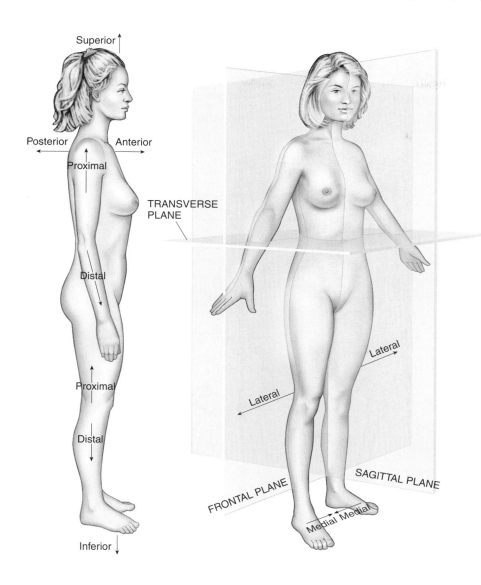

FIGURE 11-3 Directions and planes of the body. (From Thibodeau GA and Patton KT: *Anatomy and physiology*, ed 6, Mosby, 2006.)

create movement at a joint. The *agonist* is the prime mover muscle that shortens, producing movement at a joint. The *antagonist* is the muscle that lengthens to allow movement at a joint (Figure 11-6). An example of a minor disorder of the muscular system is a sprain. Subsequent chapters address health conditions and disorders associated with the muscular system.

CLINICAL *Pearl*

Agonists and antagonists simultaneously shorten and lengthen because of reciprocal innervation that results in the coactivation (simultaneous contraction) of both muscle groups.

CLINICAL *Pearl*

Skeletal muscles are named in a variety of ways that include the location, the action, and the shape of the muscle. Extensor carpi radialis is located on the radial or thumb side of the forearm (radialis) and extends (extensor) the wrist (carpi). Pronator quadratus is shaped like a rectangle with four sides (quadratus) and pronates (pronator) the forearm.

CLINICAL *Pearl*

Co-contraction is a term used to describe agonistic and antagonistic muscle groups contracting simultaneously at a joint to provide stability proximally or distally to support movement. For example, when you brush your hair, the muscles of the shoulder and wrist contract to stabilize these joints, while the elbow straightens and bends moving the brush through your hair.

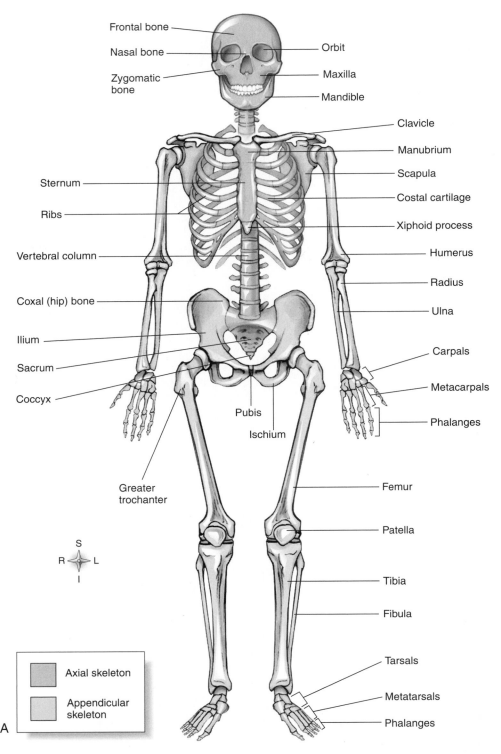

Frontal bone

Nasal bone

Zygomatic bone

Orbit

Maxilla

Mandible

Clavicle

Manubrium

Scapula

Costal cartilage

Xiphoid process

Humerus

Radius

Ulna

Carpals

Metacarpals

Phalanges

Sternum

Ribs

Vertebral column

Coxal (hip) bone

Ilium

Sacrum

Coccyx

Pubis

Ischium

Greater trochanter

Femur

Patella

Tibia

Fibula

Tarsals

Metatarsals

Phalanges

S

R   L

I

Axial skeleton

Appendicular skeleton

A

FIGURE 11-4   Skeleton. **A**, Anterior view. Skeleton. (From Thibodeau GA and Patton KT: *Anatomy and physiology*, ed 6, Mosby, 2006.)

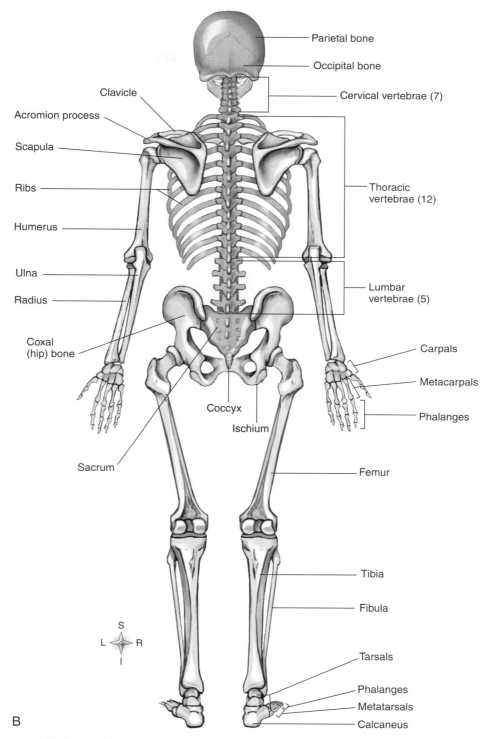

FIGURE 11-4, cont'd B, Posterior view. (From Thibodeau GA and Patton KT: *Anatomy and physiology*, ed 6, Mosby, 2006.)

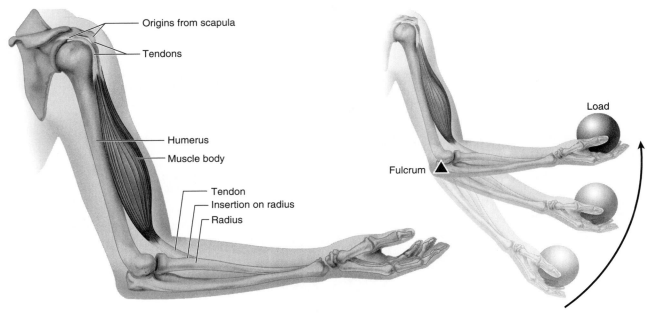

FIGURE 11-5 Attachments of the skeletal muscle. (From Thibodeau GA and Patton KT: *Anatomy and physiology,* ed 6, Mosby, 2006.)

INTEGUMENTARY SYSTEM

The structures of the **integumentary system** are the skin, hair, nails, and sebaceous glands. The skin is the largest organ in the human body. Skin has two primary layers: (1) the epidermis and (2) the dermis. The *epidermis* is the thin outer layer that is composed of epithelial cells. Epithelial tissue or thin skin also lines the internal organs. The *dermis* is the deeper, thicker layer of skin that consists of dense connective tissue. The skin functions as the body's first line of defense against potential invading microbes, acting as an external barrier associated with the immune system (immunologic function within the OTPF). It also functions in *homeostasis,* that is, thermoregulation (relatively stable internal body temperature) and osmoregulation (balance among water and electrolytes). The skin also has a role in sensory functions and pain.[1] Acne, typically seen in adolescents and young adults, is a disorder involving the skin and its associated structures. Decubitis ulcers (pressure sores) can be a serious disorder involving the integumentary system. Decubitus ulcers develop from extended pressure on bony prominences that causes skin cells to die. OT practitioners can help prevent decubitus ulcers by recommending a variety of positioning options. Additional information on positioning can be found in subsequent chapters.

CLINICAL *Pearl*

In the absence of sensation, the child or adolescent can be taught to relieve pressure through weight shifting. Simple adaptations may also be useful. Using a foam doughnut to distribute pressure around the elbow on the olecranon process (funny bone) can prevent skin breakdown while the child lying on the floor props himself or herself on the elbows to read, watch TV, and so on.

CARDIOVASCULAR SYSTEM

The **cardiovascular system** consists of the heart, blood, blood vessels (arteries, veins, and capillaries), and bone marrow (which is the site of blood cell formation). The cardiovascular system functions in the transport and exchange of oxygen, nutrients, and waste products. It also has hematologic (blood) function. Three circuits of blood flow are found in the cardiovascular system: pulmonary, systemic, and coronary paths. (1) The *pulmonary circuit* allows transport and exchange between the heart and lungs. Oxygen-poor blood is pumped from the right atrium to the right ventricle into the left and right pulmonary arteries going to the capillary beds at the alveoli of the lungs. Carbon dioxide diffuses out of the cardiovascular system and oxygen diffuses in. The

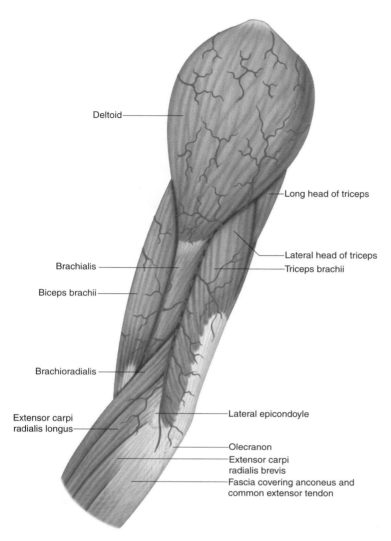

Deltoid

Long head of triceps

Brachialis

Lateral head of triceps
Triceps brachii

Biceps brachii

Brachioradialis

Extensor carpi
radialis longus

Lateral epicondoyle

Olecranon
Extensor carpi
radialis brevis
Fascia covering anconeus and
common extensor tendon

FIGURE 11-6   Muscles of the left upper arm. (From Standring S: Gray's anatomy: *The anatomical basis of clinical practice*, ed 39, Philadelphia, 2004, Churchill Livingstone.)

pulmonary veins return the oxygen-rich blood to the left atrium of the heart. (2) In the *systemic circuit*, blood is pumped into the left ventricle and then into the aorta to the entire body. The blood returns to the heart via the superior and inferior vena cavae (Figure 11-7). (3) The *coronary circuit* transports and exchanges oxygen, nutrients, and waste products between heart cells and the pulmonary system. Common disorders or health conditions associated with the cardiovascular system are presented in subsequent chapters. Table 11-3 lists normal values for vital signs.

CLINICAL *Pearl*

When stabilizing the blood pressure cuff, use the pads of the index and middle fingers on the dial. If the practitioner uses the thumb to stabilize the stethoscope, the practitioner's radial pulse may be heard instead.

CLINICAL *Pearl*

To determine heart rate, locate the radial (volar surface of forearm slightly proximal to the wrist on thumb side) or the coronary (neck region) pulse, and then place your index and middle fingers firmly over the artery. Count the number of beats for 15 seconds, and then multiply by four to determine the beats per minute.

CLINICAL *Pearl*

To determine breaths per minute, watch and count the number of times a person inhales/exhales for 15 seconds. Multiply this number by four to determine the number of breaths per minute. If a person is aware that he or she is being watched, the rate of respiration may change. This is one of the very few instances in which the practitioner does not tell the child or adolescent what is happening. Under most circumstances, the practitioner verbally and physically lets a client know what is happening.

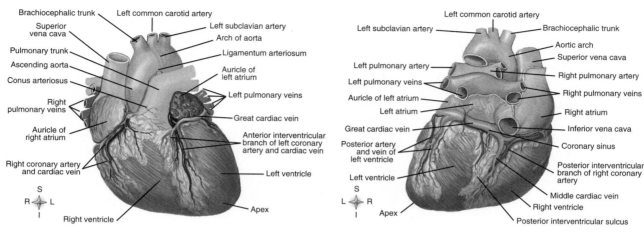

FIGURE 11-7   The heart and great vessels. (From Thibodeau GA and Patton KT: *Anatomy and physiology,* ed 7, Mosby, 2009.)

TABLE 11-3

Normal Values for Vital Signs in Infants, Children, and Adults

PARAMETER	INFANT	CHILD	ADULT
Heart rate	120 bpm (beats per minute)	70–110 bpm	60–80 bpm
Blood pressure	75/50 mm Hg (millimeters of mercury)	95/56 mm Hg	120/80 mm Hg
Respiratory rate	20–40 br/min (breaths per minute)	20–30 br/min	12–18 br/min

RESPIRATORY SYSTEM

The structures of the **respiratory (pulmonary) system** are the nose, mouth, pharynx, larynx, trachea, diaphragm, and lungs. The nose and mouth are the organs of entrance and exit of materials transported and exchanged with the environment by the respiratory system. Breathing, the primary function of the respiratory system, involves ventilation and respiration. *Ventilation* is the movement of gases into and out of the lungs. *Respiration* involves an exchange of gases between the alveoli (plural for alveolus) of the lungs and the capillaries of the cardiovascular system. The diaphragm is the major muscle of ventilation. It is a dome-shaped muscle that sits below the lungs separating the thorax from the abdomen of the body. When the diaphragm contracts, the vertical volume increases, thus allowing air to come in (inspiration). When the diaphragm relaxes, the vertical volume decreases, thus forcing air out of the lungs (exhalation). The two major categories of diseases of the respiratory system are obstructive and restrictive diseases. *Obstructive diseases* cause a decrease in air flow. *Restrictive diseases* cause a decrease in the volume or the amount of air that is able to enter the respiratory system. Asthma and cystic fibrosis are examples of obstructive diseases. Kyphoscoliosis is an example of a restrictive respiratory

disease.[2] *Respiratory distress syndrome (RDS)* is a health condition associated with prematurity. Other pediatric disorders associated with the pulmonary system are presented in subsequent chapters.

NERVOUS SYSTEM

The **nervous system** is one of the two organ systems in the human body that functions in communication and control throughout the body, integrating the functions of all other organ systems. It functions in rapid communication. From the OTPF perspective, the nervous system has the following primary functions: mental, sensory and pain, and neuromuscular as well as movement-related functions. The structures of the nervous system include the brain, spinal cord, cranial nerves, peripheral nerves, and the special sense organs. The two major subdivisions of the nervous system are (1) the central nervous system (CNS) and (2) the peripheral nervous system (PNS). The CNS consists of the brain and the spinal cord. The PNS consists of the network of peripheral nerves, the autonomic nervous system, and the special sense organs such as eyes and ears. The autonomic nervous system consists of the sympathetic (flight or fight) and parasympathetic (rest and digest) nervous systems. The neuron is the basic unit of the nervous system. There are efferent (motor) and afferent (sensory) neurons. Motor nerves carry electrical messages to effectors such as muscles. Sensory nerves carry sensory information from the periphery to the CNS for processing. Most neurons consist of cell body, dendrite, and axon. The capacity of neurons to communicate rapidly is dependent upon the myelin sheath. In certain health conditions, for example, Guillain-Barre syndrome, demyelinization occurs and results in temporary paralysis of the muscles innervated by the affected nerves. The disorders associated with the nervous system are presented in subsequent chapters.

CLINICAL *Pearl*

The nervous system stimulates skeletal muscles to contract in order to create movement at the joints. The agonist shortens while the antagonist lengthens because of reciprocal innervation.

CLINICAL *Pearl*

The lower motor neuron (LMN) system includes the cell bodies of the anterior horn of the spinal cord and the spinal and cranial nerves that effect target muscles. The upper motor neuron (UMN) system includes nerve cells in the spinal cord (excluding the cells located in the anterior horn) and all superior structures. Disorders of the LMN system result in flaccidity, decreased or absent deep tendon reflexes, and muscle atrophy. Disorders of the UMN system result in spasticity, exaggerated deep tendon reflexes, and the emergence of primitive reflexes.

ENDOCRINE SYSTEM

The **endocrine system** is the second organ system that functions in communication and control and integrates the functions of other organ systems throughout the human body. From the OTPF perspective, the endocrine system has the following primary functions: digestive and metabolic. Unlike the nervous system, the endocrine system does not necessarily communicate rapidly with other organ systems. The endocrine system contains glands that secrete hormones, which travel to target cells. The circulatory system is the primary means of transport of hormones throughout the body. The endocrine system has hormones that act as agonists and antagonists. Most agonistic and antagonistic hormones function via negative feedback mechanisms. Negative feedback involves the presence of one synergistic hormone signaling another not to be released. The glands of the endocrine system are widespread throughout the body (Figure 11-8). The nervous and endocrine systems often work in concert with one another. A comparison of the nervous and

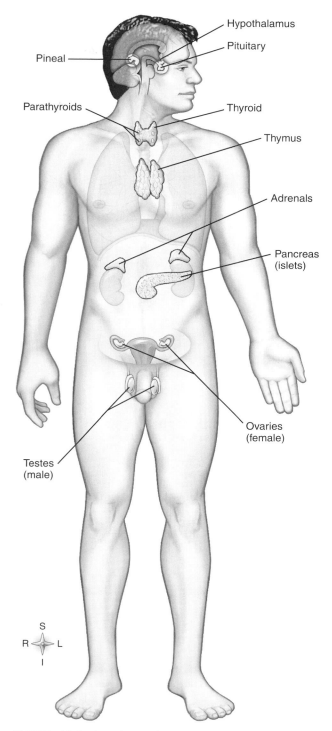

FIGURE 11-8 Locations of some major endocrine glands. (From Thibodeau GA and Patton KT: *Anatomy and physiology,* ed 6, Mosby, 2006.)

TABLE 11-4

Comparison of the Endocrine System and Nervous System

FEATURE	ENDOCRINE SYSTEM	NERVOUS SYSTEM
Overall Function	Regulation of effectors to maintain homeostasis	Regulation of effectors to maintain homeostasis
Control by regulatory feedback loops	Yes (endocrine reflexes)	Yes (nervous reflexes)
Effector tissues	Endocrine effectors: virtually all tissues	Nervous effectors: muscle and glandular tissues only
Effector cells	Target cells (throughout the body)	Postsynaptic cells (in muscle and glandular tissue only)
Chemical Messenger	Hormone	Neurotransmitter
Cells that secrete the chemical messenger	Glandular epithelial cells or neurosecretory cells (modified neurons)	Neurons
Distrance traveled (and method of travel) by chemical messenger	Long (by way of circulating blood)	Short (across a microscopic synapse)
Location of receptor in effector cell	On the plasma membrane or within the cell	On the plasma membrane
Characteristics of regulatory effects	Slow to appear, long lasting	Appear rapidly, short lived

endocrine systems is depicted in Table 11-4. Cushing's syndrome, in which there is redistribution of body fat resulting in a moon face and reddening of the skin, is an example of a disorder of the endocrine system.

DIGESTIVE SYSTEM

The structures of the **digestive system** are the mouth, pharynx, esophagus, stomach, small intestine, large intestine, and accessory organs. The *mouth,* or *oral cavity,* is composed of the teeth, mandible, maxilla, hard and soft palates, and the muscles of the tongue. Certain muscles of facial expression create movement of the lips and the temporomandibular joint (jaw, or the articulation between the maxilla and mandible). The solid, semisolid, or liquid food enters the digestive system through the mouth. Solids are chewed and mixed with saliva to form a bolus in preparation for the food to be digested throughout the digestive system (oral preparation phase of swallow). There are three phases of swallow: (1) oral preparation, (2) oral transit, and (3) pharyngeal phases. The oral transit phase of swallow involves the bolus being actively moved from the front of the mouth to the back. Both the oral preparation and oral transit phases of swallow are voluntary. After the bolus passes into the pharynx, the movement of the bolus is involuntarily controlled by smooth muscles. The movement of food through the digestive system is caused by the involuntary contraction and relaxation of smooth muscle. This movement is known as *peristalsis.* The bolus goes from the pharynx into

the esophagus, into the stomach, into the small intestine, and then into the large intestine. The food continues to be chemically digested by these organs. Most of the nutrient resorption occurs in the small intestine, whereas most of the water resorption occurs in the large intestine. Waste products are eliminated though the anus by defecation. Examples of disorders of the digestive system are dysphagia and gastroesophageal reflux disease (GERD). *Dysphagia* means difficulty swallowing. Some children and adolescents who have special needs have sensory impairment in the structures of the digestive system. Subsequent chapters further explain how the digestive system is associated with secondary impairments in children and adolescents with special needs.

> **CLINICAL** *Pearl*
>
> Children who have low muscle tone often are hyposensitive to tactile and other sensory input. Children who have high muscle tone tend to be hypersensitive to input. Children who are hyposensitive may be unaware of the bumps and bruises. Children who are hypersensitive typically over-respond to input.

URINARY SYSTEM

The **urinary system** is also known as the *genitourinary system.* The structures of the urinary system are the kidneys, ureters, urinary bladder, and urethra. The functional unit of the kidney is the nephron. The ureters connect the kidneys with the urinary bladder. The urinary bladder is the storage organ for urine. Urine is excreted from the body through the urethra. The primary functions of the urinary system are filtering blood plasma and excreting urine. A developmental hallmark is a toddler's gaining control of the urinary bladder. The sphincter muscle that prevents urine from flowing from the urinary bladder into the urethra must be intact for a child to be able to become toilet trained. An example of health conditions involving the urinary system is incontinence. Disorders of this system can have a significant impact on occupational performance and self-esteem. Toilet hygiene is covered in detail in the chapter on activities of daily living (ADL).

LYMPHATIC SYSTEM

The **lymphatic system** is closely associated with the cardiovascular, or circulatory, system. The primary structures of the lymphatic system are the tonsils, spleen, thymus, lymph, lymphatic vessels, and lymph nodes. The lymph, or lymphatic fluid, is a watery substance that is similar to the fluid found in the spaces between cells throughout the human body. The lymph circulates freely through the lymphatic vessels. The lymphatic system is critical in maintaining homeostasis, or the relatively stable internal environment, within the human body. The second primary function of the lymphatic system is fighting microbes disease-causing organisms in concert with the immune system (immunologic function). An example of a disorder of the lymphatic system is tonsillitis.

CLINICAL *Pearl*

If a word ends in "-itis," it means that inflammation is present in the organ whose name mostly forms the word root. For example, *Tonsillitis* means inflammation of the tonsils. *Pericarditis* means inflammation of the pericardium of the heart.

IMMUNE SYSTEM

The **immune system** does not have a distinct structure. Blood cells, skin cells, brain cells, and many other cells support the function of the immune system. The primary function of the immune system is to maintain homeostasis of the body and to fight diseases and disorders. Immunity is either nonspecific or specific. *Nonspecific immunity* mechanisms provide a more general defense. The skin is our body's first line of defense against potentially harmful microbes. *Specific immunity* involves different types of mechanisms that target only certain foreign agents called *antigens*. Examples of specific immunity cells are phagocytes and natural killer cells. An inflammatory response occurs when there is injury. The cardinal signs of an inflammatory response are swelling, redness, pain, decreased movement, and warmth to touch (heat). An allergy is a hypersensitivity to a particular substance that is relatively harmless. Allergens are antigens that cause an allergic response. Juvenile rheumatoid arthritis is an example of a disease of the immune system.

REPRODUCTIVE SYSTEM

The **reproductive system** is necessary for sexual reproduction, but not for other forms of reproduction, for example, mitosis (cell division) or budding (reproduce a new organism from a single parent from a bud). The structures of the human male and female reproductive systems are different. However, both males and females have essential organs known as *gonads*, which produce *gametes* (sex cells that are haploid, i.e., have half the amount of genetic information of the parent cell).

The structures of the male reproductive system include the testes (male gonads), accessory reproductive glands, and supporting organs such as the scrotum and the penis. The function of the male reproductive system is to produce and store gametes. During sexual intercourse, ejaculation of sperm occurs, and subsequently fertilization of the ovum (egg) can occur in the female.

The structures of the female reproductive system include the ovaries, fallopian tubes, uterus, vagina, and accessory reproductive glands. The ovaries are the organs that produce the female gametes, or eggs. The female reproductive system has a cycle between the years of onset of menstruation (menarche) and cessation of menstruation (menopause). The typical menstrual cycle is 28 days, with menstruation lasting approximately 5 days. During menstruation, the outer layer of the uterine wall is shed in preparation for the implanting of a fertilized egg, should it occur.

In the event that an egg is fertilized by a sperm, the resulting embryo will implant itself into the endometrium of the uterine wall within several days after fertilization. The fertilized egg is called a *zygote* (diploid cell), which has the same amount of genetic information as each parent. The embryo goes through cell division, or *mitosis*, for approximately nine months, during which cells, tissues, and organs grow and specialize. The sequence of fetal development is predictable and well documented. During the first trimester, the tactile (touch) system responds to stimuli, the vestibular system begins to develop, and the fetus begins to move inside the womb. During the second trimester, the tactile receptors begin to differentiate and specialize. The fetus begins to process visual and auditory stimuli. The fetus has a wake–sleep cycle. The movement patterns of the fetus are reciprocal and symmetrical. During the third trimester, the muscles of the fetus mature. The fetus has tactile, olfactory, and gustatory discrimination. The fetus exhibits primitive reflexes such as rooting and palmar grasp reflexes. Following 36 to 42 weeks of gestation (the average being 40 weeks), a neonate is born. The development from birth through adolescence was discussed in previous chapters, and genetic disorders are discussed in subsequent chapters.

CLINICAL *Pearl*

Identical twins have identical genetic information but different finger and foot prints. Finger and foot prints develop as a result of the tactile experiences of the fetus in the womb.

RELATIONSHIP BETWEEN BODY STRUCTURES AND FUNCTIONS AND OCCUPATIONAL PERFORMANCE

This chapter provides a discussion of the structures and functions of organ systems from the perspective of a biologist. OT practitioners use this knowledge to better understand how body structures and body functions influence occupational performance and to provide interventions to address areas of deficit. For example, the OT practitioner examines a child's hands to determine whether the structure of the hand (e.g., congenital deformity, edema, or structural anomaly) interferes with the child's performance. The intervention may focus on improving the structure, if possible (e.g., splinting to increase range of motion), or on compensating for the deficit, as might be the case for a child with a congenital anomaly of missing digits.

The OTPF presents body functions with reference to the World Health Organization (WHO) perspective and includes the following categories: mental functions; sensory functions and pain; neuromuscular and movement-related functions; cardiovascular, hematologic, immunologic, and respiratory system functions; digestive, metabolic, and endocrine system functions; genitourinary and reproductive functions; and functions of the skin and related structures.

The OT practitioner also determines how specific body functions are influencing a child's occupational performance. For example, the OT practitioner examines neuromuscular and movement-related functions such as joint mobility (range of motion), muscle

power (strength), and control of voluntary movements (eye–hand coordination and oculomotor control). If the child's structures are intact, their functions may be influencing the ability of the child to engage in his or her occupations. For example, a child with hypertonicity may have adequate body structures in that the muscles, bones, and joints are within normal limits; but the child may be experiencing difficulty with body functions, including range of motion, muscle tone, and control of voluntary movements.

Functions of the cardiovascular and respiratory systems include aerobic capacity and endurance. Again, the OT practitioner uses his or her knowledge of the involved structures to determine the best way to intervene. For example, a child may show decreased endurance secondary to prolonged inactivity, not due to structural dysfunction of the cardiac or respiratory system, such as might be observed when a child has a cardiac abnormality. Thus, the OT practitioner acknowledges that the child is showing difficulty in terms body function of the cardiovascular system and that it is interfering with the child's ability to play with peers on the playground, complete activities of daily living, and perform other occupations.

An immunologic response may be inflammation. Children who have juvenile rheumatoid arthritis may have inflammation in the joints of the wrists and hands that interferes with their occupational performance. OT practitioners observe responses to activities and may provide these children with techniques to lessen the work load, thus reducing inflammation. Subsequent chapters discuss specific joint protection and energy conservation techniques.

Functions of the digestive, endocrine, genitourinary, reproductive, and integumentary systems have been discussed above. *Metabolism* is the term that sums up all chemical reactions that occur in the human body. Metabolism is important to the maintenance of homeostasis.

OT practitioners examine children's performances in the following areas of occupation: activities of daily living (ADLs), instrumental activities of daily living (IADLs), rest and sleep, education, work, play, leisure, and social participation. ADLs may also be referred to as *basic activities of daily living* (BADLs), or *personal activities of daily living* (PADLs). Practitioners analyze children's ability to perform occupations taking into consideration the structures and functions of the associated body systems. For example, eating is an ADL that involves the digestive system and the neuromuscular movement-related system. The OT practitioner considers the body structures by evaluating the child's oral motor structures (e.g., palate, tongue) and consulting with the child's physician to rule out an abnormality in the digestive system function or structure. The OT practitioner analyzes the movement-related functions of the child's oral motor structures and their ability to prepare food to be digested through the digestive tract.

OT practitioners analyze children's ability to perform occupations in light of their body structures and body functions. OT practitioners understand that these occupations occur in a variety of environments (e.g., home, school, community) and contexts (e.g., culture, periods, lifespan) and that many factors influence the child's performance.

SUMMARY

This chapter presents an overview of human anatomy and physiology to help OT practitioners understand how body structures and body functions influence occupational performance. The chapter reviews basic terminology and planes and their associated axes. Following general information about the organs and organ systems of the human body, body functions from an OT perspective was presented. The chapter concludes by describing the relationship between body structures and functions to occupational performance.

References

1. American Occupational Therapy Association: Occupational therapy practice framework: domain and process, ed 2. *Am J Occup Ther* 62:625–703, 2008.
2. Moore A: Respiratory lecture, fall 2009, Trident Technical College, OTA Program, Charleston, SC.
3. Thibodeau P: *Anatomy and physiology*, ed 7, St. Louis, 2010, Mosby.
4. Thibodeau GA and Patton KT: *Mosby's handbook of anatomy and physiology*, St. Louis, 2000, Mosby.

Recommended Reading

Daniels et al: *Body: the complete human*, Washington, DC, 2007, National Geographic Society.
Chamley CA, et al: *Developmental anatomy and physiology of children: a practical approach*, St. Louis, 2005, Mosby.

REVIEW *Questions*

1. What is the difference between anatomy and physiology?
2. Describe the hierarchy of organization of the human body.
3. What is *anatomic position*?
4. What are the structures and functions of the organ systems of the human body?
5. How do body structures and functions impact a child's or adolescent's occupational performance?

SUGGESTED *Activities*

1. Make a table of the organ systems of the human body with three columns for each system: structure, function, and potential impact on occupational performance.
2. Design a three-dimensional model representing planes and axes.
3. Demonstrate the movements of the upper extremity (arm).

12

Pediatric Health Conditions*

GRETCHEN EVANS PARKER

JEAN W. SOLOMON

JANE CLIFFORD O'BRIEN

CHAPTER *Objectives:*

After studying this chapter, the reader will be able to accomplish the following:

- Describe the characteristics of a variety of pediatric conditions.
- Describe the signs and symptoms of pediatric orthopedic, genetic, neurologic, developmental, cardiopulmonary, neoplastic, sensory and environmentally induced conditions.
- Describe the types and classification of burns.
- Describe treatment precautions associated with specific pediatric conditions.
- Summarize the ways in which different conditions affect children's and adolescent's occupational performance.
- Describe general intervention principles and strategies associated with pediatric health conditions or diagnoses.
- Describe the roles of the occupational therapy assistant and the occupational therapist in interventions for children with a variety of diagnoses.
- Use knowledge of pediatric conditions to plan interventions.

* The section on developmental coordination disorder (DCD) was written as part of a doctoral dissertation. Special thanks go to Harriet Williams, PhD; Anita Bundy, ScD; Jim Lyons, PhD; and Bruce McCleneghan, PhD, for their assistance.

KEY TERMS

Adaptive equipment
Joint protection techniques
Prosthesis
Contusion
Crush wound injury
Dislocation
Sprain
Fractures
Closed fracture
Open fracture
Orthotics
Scoliosis
Peripheral nervous system
Central nervous system
Kyphosis
Cortical blindness
Visual perception
American sign language
Partial-thickness burns
Acute medical management
Rehabilitation
Universal precautions

CHAPTER OUTLINE

Orthopedic Conditions
ACHONDROPLASIA
ARTHROGRYPOSIS
JUVENILE RHEUMATOID ARTHRITIS
OSTEOGENESIS IMPERFECTA
CONGENITAL HIP DYSPLASIA
AMPUTATION
ACQUIRED MUSCULOSKELETAL DISORDERS
Soft Tissue Injuries
Fractures
GENERAL INTERVENTIONS

Genetic Disorders
DUCHENNE MUSCULAR DYSTROPHY
DOWN SYNDROME
CRI DU CHAT SYNDROME
FRAGILE X SYNDROME
PRADER-WILLI SYNDROME
GENERAL INTERVENTIONS

Neurologic Disorders
SPINA BIFIDA
TRAUMATIC BRAIN INJURY
SHAKEN BABY SYNDROME
ERB'S PALSY
SEIZURES
GENERAL INTERVENTIONS

Developmental Disorders
AUTISM
ATTENTION DEFICIT HYPERACTIVITY DISORDER
RETT SYNDROME
DEVELOPMENTAL COORDINATION DISORDER
GENERAL INTERVENTIONS

Cardiopulmonary System
CARDIAC DISORDERS
PULMONARY DISORDERS
HEMATOLOGIC DISORDERS
GENERAL INTERVENTIONS

Sensory System Conditions
VISION IMPAIRMENTS
HEARING IMPAIRMENTS
GENERAL SENSORY DISORGANIZATION

CHAPTER OUTLINE—cont'd

FUSSY BABY
LANGUAGE DELAY AND LANGUAGE IMPAIRMENTS
GENERAL INTERVENTIONS

Other Pediatric Health Conditions
BURNS

Neoplastic Disorders
LEUKEMIA
TUMORS OF THE CENTRAL NERVOUS SYSTEM
BONE CANCER AND TUMORS

Immunologic Conditions
CHRONIC FATIGUE SYNDROME
HUMAN IMMUNODEFICIENCY VIRUS
LATEX ALLERGY

Environmentally Induced and Acquired Conditions
FAILURE TO THRIVE
FETAL ALCOHOL SYNDROME
EFFECTS OF COCAINE USE
LEAD POISONING
ALLERGIES TO FOODS AND CHEMICALS
GENERAL INTERVENTIONS

*Role of Occupational Therapy Assistant and Occupational
    Therapist in Assessment and Intervention*

Summary

This chapter describes the major characteristics, signs and symptoms, and intervention strategies of a variety of pediatric conditions encountered by occupational therapy (OT) practitioners. Knowing the course and characteristics of each of these conditions serves as a framework for assessment, evaluation, and intervention planning. This knowledge enables the OT practitioner to be a valuable member of the intervention team. Box 12-1 lists some potential members of the pediatric team.

A brief description of the major characteristics of each condition is presented and is followed by intervention principles that are useful in OT practice. Case examples are provided to describe OT interventions. This chapter presents an overview of orthopedic, genetic, neurologic, developmental, cardiopulmonary, neoplastic, sensory system, and environmentally induced conditions.

ORTHOPEDIC CONDITIONS

Orthopedic or musculoskeletal conditions involve bones, joints, and muscles. The musculoskeletal system consists of the skeletal and muscular systems. The skeletal system consists of bones, joints, cartilage, and ligaments. The muscular system consists of muscles, tendons, and the fascia covering them (Box 12-2). Tendons, which are bands of tough, inelastic fibrous tissue, connect muscles to bones. Muscles are activated by the nervous system and move bone(s) to create movement at a joint.

BOX 12-1

Potential Team Members

- Behavior specialist
- Cardiologist
- Cardiac surgeon
- Emergency medical technician
- Geneticist
- Neonatologist
- Neurologist
- Neuropsychologist
- Neurosurgeon
- Nurse
- Occupational therapist
- Occupational therapy assistant
- Orthopedist
- Orthopedic surgeon
- Orthotist
- Physical therapist
- Physical therapy assistant
- Prosthetist
- Psychologist
- Pulmonologist
- Respiratory therapist

BOX 12-2

Musculoskeletal Disorders: Signs and Symptoms

- Misalignment of joints
- Swelling
- Pain
- Warmth to touch
- Immobility
- Discoloration (redness, blueness, whiteness)

Congenital disorders of the musculoskeletal system include achondroplasia (dwarfism), arthrogryposis, juvenile rheumatoid arthritis, osteogenesis imperfecta (brittle bones), and congenital hip dysplasia. Children may be born with missing digits or limbs (amputations). Acquired orthopedic disorders include fractures and sprains.

CLINICAL *Pearl*

Therapy for an older child who has lost a limb as a result of trauma or surgery is different from therapy for a child with a congenital amputation. A child who loses a limb later in childhood benefits from having a prosthesis fitted as soon as possible for psychological and rehabilitation reasons.

Children with orthopedic conditions may experience difficulties in the performance of daily occupations such as activities of daily living (ADLs), play and leisure, and work and productive skills.

Achondroplasia

Achondroplasia, or dwarfism, is a pathologic condition of arrested or stunted growth that occurs during fetal development. It is a disorder of the growth cartilage. Typical physical features include a large protruding forehead and short, thick arms and legs on a relatively normal trunk.

Due to their physical stature and features, children with achondroplasia may require **adaptive equipment** to perform daily occupations. OT practitioners may provide compensatory strategies to help these children achieve independence despite their small stature and short, yet large, hands. Frequently children with achondroplasia exhibit poor hand coordination and require OT intervention to develop hand skills for occupations. Occasionally, medical intervention might include orthopedic surgery, and the OT practitioner would address range of motion (ROM) and relearning of movements postsurgically.

Arthrogryposis

Arthrogryposis is sometimes genetic but is also attributed to reduced amniotic fluid during gestation or central nervous system (CNS) malformations.[39] In the classic form of arthrogryposis, all the joints of the extremities are stiff, but the spine is not affected. Shoulders are turned in, elbows are straight, and wrists are flexed, with ulnar deviation. Hips may be dislocated, and knees are straight, with the feet turned in. Arm and leg muscles are small, with webbed skin covering some or all of the joints. The condition is worse at birth, so any increases in ROM or joint motion are improvements.[4] In typical cases, all the joints of the arms and legs are fixed in one position, partly due to muscle imbalance or lack of muscle development during gestation (Figure 12-1).

Ongoing occupational and physical therapies help children with arthrogryposis meet educational, self-care, and play needs. Children with arthrogryposis have many physical limitations that interfere with all areas of occupational performance. OT practitioners may help these children maintain or increase ROM and adapt themselves to perform their occupations and daily activities. OT practitioners may elect to use technology to help these children engage in ADLs, play, education, and social participation (see Chapter 26). Due to the multiple issues associated with arthrogryposis, OT practitioners consult with family members and school personnel to provide the best intervention. The following case example illustrates some intervention principles.

CASE *Study*

Courtney is a 4-year-old girl, who has a large vocabulary. Her arms and legs have a tubular shape; the skin between her fingers and in the folds of her knees and elbows is webbed. During the first 2 years of life, Courtney could not sit on the floor to play because she could not bend her hips and knees, and her feet turned in so much that

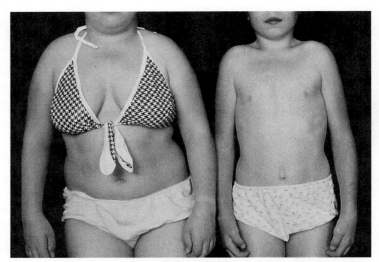
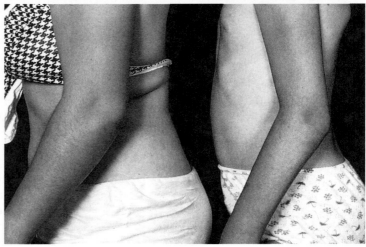

FIGURE 12-1 Child with arthrogryposis. (From Zitelli BJ, Davis HW: *Atlas of pediatric physical diagnosis,* ed 5, St. Louis, 2007, Mosby.)

the soles faced each other (i.e., she had clubbed feet). To get from place to place, she rolled along the floor using the normal movement of her trunk. Her shoulders and forearms turned inward, so the backs of her hands always touched her sides. She currently cannot bend her elbows, and her wrists are permanently bent toward her forearms. She has limited and weak finger movement. The palms of her hands are narrow and almost fold together.

Courtney had surgery at the age of 2 years to repair clubbed feet to enable her to place the soles of her feet on the floor. Before the surgery, she used to stand on the sides of her feet; after the surgery, she can stand for short periods, but she still cannot get to a standing position without help. To keep her legs stable while standing, she wears braces on her knees and ankles. Seated at a table of the right height, Courtney can move toys that are moderately sized and not too heavy. She grasps small things by pressing them between the backs of her wrists.

Courtney has been receiving occupational and physical therapies since birth. OT intervention consists of performing ROM, stretching, and play activities to maintain and improve Courtney's movement for all activities. The OT practitioner has provided Courtney's parents with home programs of fun activities to promote social interaction and play; has integrated stretching activities into the morning dressing routine so as to not overwhelm the parents; and has fabricated wrist extension orthoses to encourage functional wrist and hand positioning. The OT practitioner has also provided soft fabric bands to help Courtney keep her elbows flexed (and not outstretched) for 10 to 15 minutes at a time.

CLINICAL *Pearl*

Parents of a newborn with arthrogryposis have a lot to learn in a short period. Functional gains are made only in the early months of the infant's life. To maintain the gains in joint movement made during therapy, a clearly written home program should be created so that the parents can have easy-to-follow guidelines. The program should include specific exercises, precautions, and a clearly written orthotic-wearing schedule.

CLINICAL *Pearl*

A dynamic elbow flexion orthosis for an infant with arthrogryposis can be made with elastic and orthoplast. The elbow straightens against the pull of the elastic; the elastic then pulls the elbow into flexion, allowing hand-to-mouth movement. The dynamic elbow flexion orthosis allows infants to do activities such as eating finger food or blowing bubbles.

Juvenile Rheumatoid Arthritis

The three types of *juvenile rheumatoid arthritis* (JRA) are (1) Still's disease (20% of JRA cases), (2) pauciarticular arthritis (40% of JRA cases), and (3) polyarticular arthritis (40% of JRA cases) (Table 12-1).[5,10] Children with JRA experience exacerbations and remissions of symptoms. During exacerbations, or flareups, symptoms worsen, and the joints become hot and painful; joint damage can occur. During remissions, or pain-free periods, children with JRA may resume typical activities. **Joint protection techniques** are encouraged at all times so that these strategies become a habit (Box 12-3).

By the time they are adults, 75% of individuals with JRA have permanent remission.[12] However, these children may have functional limitations due to contractures and deformities. The OT practitioner helps educate them on how to protect their joints, compensate for lack of ROM during exacerbations, and complete activities with less stress on the joints (work simplification techniques). Furthermore, the OT practitioner provides these children with stretching and movement activities to maintain the functioning of the joints and prevent contractures. The OT practitioner may prescribe adaptive equipment or technology to help these children engage in everyday activities (Box 12-4).

CASE *Study*

Five-year-old Amber, a cheerful child in the kindergarten, loves riding her bike. Amber has pauciarticular arthritis, a type of JRA, and as a result her joints periodically become painful, hot, and swollen. The OT practitioner provides Amber with a home program of passive and active stretching and strengthening activities and suggests that Amber do these activities right before playing outside or riding her bike. The OT practitioner stresses that stretching will help Amber ride more easily and without getting injured. The OT practitioner has measured all of Amber's joints with a goniometer to ensure that Amber's ROM is not deteriorating and has adapted her bicycle to include built-up handle bars, making it easier for Amber to grasp them without causing damage to her wrist and finger joints.

OT practitioners working with children with JRA frequently provide adaptations to activities to help these children perform activities. This may include providing built-up handles on items such as spoons or hair brushes (adaptive equipment), showing the children how to perform activities more easily (e.g., work simplification), or instructing them in an alternative method to perform an activity (e.g. using a computer instead of writing as a means of written expression).

TABLE 12-1

Three Types of Juvenile Rheumatoid Arthritis

TYPE	LIMB INVOLVEMENT	FUNCTIONAL IMPLICATIONS
PAUCIARTICULAR (FEW JOINTS)		
Affects four or fewer joints Comprises approximately 40% of JRA cases	Only a few unmatched joints are affected. Leg joints are usually affected, but elbows can also be affected. Children often recover in 1–2 yr. Children can develop an eye inflammation called *iritis*, which can lead to blindness unless it is treated early.	Pain and joint stiffness may limit activities. Contractures can develop. Orthoses may be needed. Work simplification may be necessary. Adaptive equipment may be needed. Climbing stairs may be difficult.
POLYARTICULAR (MANY JOINTS)		
Comprises approximately 30% of JRA cases Five or more joints affected Girls more commonly affected than boys	Symmetrical joints of legs, wrists, hands, and sometimes the neck are affected.	Onset is fast. Functional implications are the same as those for pauciarticular arthritis but also include the following: Activities can be limited by fatigue. There is difficulty with fine motor activities.
STILL'S DISEASE		
Affects joints as well as internal organs Comprises approximately 20% of JRA cases	Speed of onset and affected limbs are the same as those for polyarticular arthritis. Other organs, for example, the spleen and lymph system, may also be affected. Bone damage may affect growth.	Functional implications are the same as those for polyarticular arthritis but also include the following: Rash and fever may develop, last for weeks, and require bed confinement.

JRA, juvenile rheumatoid arthritis.
Data from Rogers, S. Common conditions that influence children's participation. In Case-Smith J, O'Brien J: *Occupational therapy for children*, ed 6, St. Louis, 2010, Mosby, pp. 153-154.
Arthritis Foundation: http://www.arthritis.org/disease-center.php?disease_id=38&df=effects : Accessed June 14, 2010. .

Osteogenesis Imperfecta

Osteogenesis imperfecta is a congenital condition in which bones fail to develop and are brittle. Consequently, children are prone to fractures with typical handling and movement. Children who have osteogenesis imperfecta also have secondary osteoporosis.

Osteoporosis may also be caused by a lack of weight-bearing activities such as crawling and standing. The bones are weakened as a result of mineral loss; weight-bearing activities and muscles pulling on bones during movement make bones stronger. Children who develop osteoporosis are usually severely affected by another condition, such as osteogenesis imperfecta or cerebral palsy. These children are usually very inactive and unable to stand; their bones can become so brittle that even simple activities such as dressing could cause a fracture.

OT practitioners who work with children with osteogenesis imperfecta and osteoporosis must be gentle when helping them experience play, ADLs, education, and social participation. The OT practitioner educates family, teachers, and others on how to handle the child and also educates the child on how best to move through any given space and pay attention to body positions. Weight-bearing activities help develop bone growth and should therefore be encouraged. Children with osteogenesis imperfecta may require orthoses to protect bones and prevent contractures.

CLINICAL *Pearl*

With proper joint management, children can be placed in prone or supine standers for weight-bearing activities. Standing is good not only for bone growth and strengthening but also for body functions such as circulation and digestion.

Rules of Joint Protection for Children With Juvenile Rheumatoid Arthritis

- If the joints are warm and swollen, encourage the children to use them carefully during all activities and to continue to do range-of-motion (ROM) exercises as much as they can.
- Because tired muscles cannot protect the joints, teach the children that they should not remain in the same position, such as holding a pencil to write, for long periods without stretching or taking a break.
- Larger muscles are found around the big joints, so teach the children the correct way to use the big joints for heavy work. For example, they can balance a lunch tray on their forearms, wear a backpack on both shoulders, or carry a purse over a shoulder rather than in a hand.
- If the children become tired or are in pain, stop the activity.
- Proper positioning prevents contractures and deformities. Teach the children that they should always use good posture.

Intervention for Juvenile Rheumatoid Arthritis

- Orthoses to prevent development of contractures
- AROM and PROM exercises to maintain ROM
- Careful monitoring of each joint to maintain functional level and to prevent deformity
- Providing exercises to maintain or increase strength
- Teaching the importance of joint protection during all activities to prevent deformities or contractures

AROM, active range of motion; *PROM,* passive range of motion; *ROM,* range of motion

Congenital Hip Dysplasia

Congenital hip dysplasia (or dislocation of the hip) may be caused by genetic or environmental factors. An infant may be genetically prone to instability of one or both of the hip joints, and sudden passive stretching of an unstable hip or prolonged time in a position that makes the hip vulnerable may cause a dislocation.[14,35] Medical intervention at an early age is critical to preventing permanent physical or body structure damage. Surgery may be necessary. Less invasive procedures, such as bracing and casting, may promote proper hip alignment and stability (Figure 12-2).

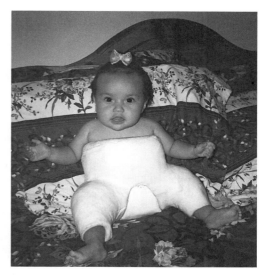

FIGURE 12-2 A spica cast. (From Leifer G: *Introduction to maternity and pediatric nursing,* ed 5, 2006, Philadelphia: Saunders.)

OT practitioners may work with infants and children who have casts to support hip alignment. Helping parents and children with daily living skills during this period involves simplifying activities and providing adaptive equipment to ensure successful engagement in activities. For example, it may be necessary to provide a bath seat in which a child can be positioned for a sponge bath. These children may need seating that is adapted to accommodate the cast. Those children who are in a full body brace will not be able to explore their environments, so the OT practitioner may adapt developmentally appropriate activities to help these children to explore.

Amputation

An infant born missing all or part of a limb has a *congenital amputation*. A *traumatic amputation* is the result of an accident, infection, or cancer. Each year, approximately 26 out of 10,000 children in the United States are born missing all or part of a limb. The types of amputations vary greatly (Table 12-2). Thumb and below-elbow amputations are the most common types of upper extremity congenital amputations.[12]

OT practitioners analyze the activities that the child with an amputation will engage in and determine how to compensate for or adapt the task so that the child can be successful. In some cases, use of technology or a **prosthesis** may be prescribed to help the child engage in daily activities. The OT practitioner considers the child's age and the type of amputation and works with a team of professionals to determine the course of treatment.

TABLE 12-2

Types of Congenital Upper Extremity Amputations

TYPE OF DEFICIENCY	MISSING SKELETAL PARTS
TRANSVERSE AMELIA	
Forequarter amputation	All or most of the arm is missing from the shoulder and below.
TRANSVERSE HEMIMELIA	
Below-elbow amputation	All of the arm is missing from the elbow and below.
LONGITUDINAL HEMIMELIA	
Partial amputation	One of the long bones of the forearm is missing. Fingers or thumb may or may not be missing.
PHOCOMELIA	
	Bones of the upper or lower arm are missing. All or part of the hand remains.

Data adapted from Rothstein JM, Roy HR, Wolf SL: *The rehabilitation specialist's handbook*, ed 2, Philadelphia, 1998, FA Davis.

CASE *Study*

Beth was born with an above-elbow amputation. The occupational therapist completed a developmental evaluation at 3 months and determined that Beth was achieving all her developmental milestones. The attending physician, occupational therapist, physical therapist, and social worker discussed the pros and cons of a prosthesis with Beth's parents. The team explained that most children with congenital upper extremity amputations choose to use a prosthesis as a tool some of the time, but they learn adaptive techniques for performing many activities without it. Very young children often use the sensations in their stumps to learn about their environments. The OT practitioner provided the parents with some informational books as well as the phone numbers of other parents who had children with congenital upper extremity amputations; the OT practitioner suggested that Beth's parents spend some time talking to those with experience raising a child with an upper extremity amputation.

Beth's parents decided to wait to have her fitted with a prosthesis until she was 2 years of age because she could then begin to understand its use as a tool. They also thought that at 2 years her language skills would make it easier for her to learn to use the prosthesis. They felt that Beth would gradually learn when to do things with or without the prosthesis.

Beth's first prosthesis had a rubber mitt and a friction elbow that did not lock. Later, an adept hand, which was made of plastic and had one C-shaped "finger" with an indentation in which the end for the opposing "thumb" could be fit, was added. The adept hand would remain open until Beth chose to close it by pulling on a cable attached to a shoulder harness.

Beth is now 7 years old. She has had two surgeries to the end of the bone in her stump. Every year she has a prosthesis revision, and small details are added or changed. Now that she is older, Beth's parents include her in the decisions for changes. The family has learned that Beth usually knows what works for her better than anyone on her treatment team. Whenever a change is made, the OTA spends a few OT sessions with Beth exploring the new uses and operation of the updated prosthesis. During these sessions, the occupational therapist and the OTA work closely together; Beth's training requires specific understanding of the ways in which the components of the prosthesis work and function.

Fitting a prosthesis on a child with a congenital amputation at a very young age allows the child to reach developmental milestones in a timely manner and for the prosthesis to become a part of the child's body image. A prosthesis is more likely to be rejected when the child is older. In the case of a less severe congenital amputation, a child often does well without a prosthesis. The use of a prosthesis depends on the severity of the amputation and whether one or both arms are involved. See Box 12-5 for stump and prosthesis care.

Acquired Musculoskeletal Disorders

Acquired musculoskeletal disorders are conditions that are not present at birth and involve injury or trauma to the skeletal and/or muscular systems. Soft tissue injuries and fractures require the attention of an orthopedist, a medical doctor who specializes in diseases of the musculoskeletal system.

CLINICAL *Pearl*

To avoid causing fractures, use care when handling and doing range-of-motion (ROM) exercises with severely affected, inactive children. Maintaining good joint mobility with daily careful passive stretching and proper positioning initiated during infancy helps control osteoporosis.

BOX 12-5

Care of the Residual Limb and Prosthesis

- Decreased skin surface may result in overheating.
- Bandages must be dry and must be monitored.
- Examine the stump site for excessive redness, irritation, or swelling when the prosthesis is removed each night.
- Report any discomfort, redness, or pressure areas to the occupational therapist immediately.
- Wash the residual limb daily with soap and water, rinse, and dry carefully. Do not soak it.
- Cleanse the residual limb at night, ensuring enough time for it to dry thoroughly.
- Do not shave or apply lotions or moisturizers to the residual limb.
- Check the correct fitting of the prosthesis, and make sure that there are no pressure areas.
- Change the stump socks daily, and wash them by hand using mild soap and water.
- Keep the leather parts, liners, and webbing of the prosthesis clean and dry. Inspect for wear.
- Check the mechanical parts or components frequently.

NSW Artificial Limb Service: Care of the residual limb and prosthesis. Adapted from http://www.monash.edu.au/rehabtech/pub/reports/CAREOFPR.PDF Retrieved June 14, 2010.

Soft Tissue Injuries

Soft tissue injuries involve damage to muscles, nerves, skin, and/or connective tissue and include contusions, crush injuries, dislocations, and sprains. A **contusion** is an injury that does not disrupt the integrity of the skin and is characterized by swelling, discoloration, and pain. In the absence of any complicating health conditions, contusions heal with time and do not require medical or therapeutic intervention.

A **crush wound or injury** is a break in the external surface of the bone caused by severe force applied against tissues (e.g., a finger caught in a door). This type of injury may require medical or OT intervention if alignment and immobility are necessary for the injury to heal. Untreated crush injuries may result in permanent deformity and pain of the joint(s) involved. The permanent misalignment of a body structure may have functional implications.

A **dislocation** is the displacement of a bone from its normal articulation at a joint. Dislocations of the shoulder and hip joints are frequently seen in infants and young children, since these joints are freely movable. The shallowness of the shoulder joint increases the likelihood of dislocation occurring at this structure.

A **sprain** is a traumatic injury to the tendons, muscles, or ligaments around a joint and is characterized by pain, swelling, and discoloration. Sprains can occur when children or adolescents lose their balance and consequently use a protective response that makes the wrist and ankle the most vulnerable joints for injury. Sprains are most frequently seen in the ankles and wrists. Most do not require emergency medical attention or OT intervention.

CLINICAL *Pearl*

Immediately apply ice to a soft tissue injury for a minimum of 20 minutes or until the area becomes pain free. The application of ice will reduce swelling at the involved site and relieve pain.

Fractures

Fractures are breaks, ruptures, or cracks in bone or cartilage. They may be defined as *closed* or *open*. A **closed fracture** has no open wounds from the broken bone penetrating the skin, whereas an **open fracture** involves an open wound, where complications are more common. Fractures require immediate realignment followed by immobilization to allow the bone(s) to heal. Immobilization requires casts, orthoses, pins, or other external fixations.

General Interventions

Children with orthopedic conditions may exhibit difficulty performing ADLs, instrumental activities of daily living (IADLs), education, play, or social participation because of improper joint alignment. For example, children with achondroplasia often have difficulty grasping and manipulating objects because of their short but large hands. They benefit from practice, modification, and adaptation (Table 12-3). They may need work space modifications (e.g., adapted chairs). Furthermore, their physical stature may interfere with play. Children with JRA may develop contractures that limit their active ROM and interfere with their ability to perform play, leisure, and academic activities and ADLs. They benefit from stretching exercises and work simplification techniques.

OT practitioners help children who have orthopedic conditions engage in play, leisure, and educational activities, ADLs, IADLs, and social activities.

OT interventions for orthopedic conditions frequently involve the following:

- Helping children engage in all areas of occupation (e.g., play, ADLs, education, social participation, IADLs)
- Developing home programs to facilitate engagement in occupations that can easily be integrated into the child's and family's daily activities

TABLE 12-3

Orthopedic Conditions: General Intervention Considerations

CONSIDERATION	DEFINITION AND EXAMPLE(S)
Promotion of proper joint alignment	Through static (nonmovement) and dynamic (movement) orthotic devices, facilitating the typical alignment of muscles and joints. (*Note:* In the absence of soft tissue contracture and/or bony deformities)
Application modalities such as ice or moist heat	Placing a moist heat pack or ice pack on the inflamed area
Immobilization with a cast or orthosis	Keeping the involved area in proper alignment
Instruction in proper positioning to reduce edema or swelling	Elevating the involved/inflamed area to increase flow of body fluids back to the trunk
Compensation	Helping the child engage in occupations through changing the ways or techniques used to participate
Modification/adaptation	Helping the child participate in occupations by changing how the activities are performed
Emotional/psychosocial consideration	Addressing emotional/psychosocial issues associated with disorders. Children may need to work on developing a positive self-concept, body awareness, and sense of control
Social participation	Promoting social participation in children

- Providing passive or active stretching exercises to improve ROM for occupations. This may be accomplished through activities, orthoses, or casting. OT practitioners may design orthoses to help with the alignment of joints. Clinicians frequently consult with orthopedists to explore the functional outcome of the **orthotic**, or procedure
- Providing work simplification/joint protection techniques to rest inflamed joints and to protect joints
- Adapting equipment to compensate for limited ROM or congenital anomalies
- Providing compensatory techniques to allow children to succeed by performing their occupations differently
- Remediation to strengthen muscles and stability around the joints

GENETIC CONDITIONS

Inherited pediatric health conditions occur in response to changes in the genetic makeup of the fetus. Humans have 23 pairs of chromosomes, which are tiny thread-shaped structures found in each cell of the body. Each chromosome is made up of tiny sections called *genes*. Half of the genetic information (genome) comes from the mother through her egg, and the other half of the genome comes from the father through the sperm. The offspring's genome is unique to the individual and determines every aspect of a person's characteristics (phenotype or the physical expression of the genotype). Because so many genes (23 pairs of chromosomes per cell multiplied by 250 to 2000 genes per chromosome) and mutations are possible, genetic disorders occur. Sometimes a gene carrying a specific problem can be passed from one or both parents to the child. Problems develop when genes mix and match improperly or mutate (i.e., a gene that has been damaged or is abnormal in some way). Genetic conditions cause characteristic physical features involving body structures and patterns of involvement in body functions that have an impact on one's successful performance in occupations. An understanding of certain genetic conditions helps OT practitioners design and implement interventions.

Approximately 30% of developmental disabilities are related to genetic conditions; 50% of major hearing and vision problems are caused by genetic syndromes.[12] The descriptions that follow highlight genetic conditions commonly encountered in OT practice. Table 12-4 and Box 12-6 provide an overview of other selected genetic disorders and the signs and symptoms or genetic disorders.

Duchenne Muscular Dystrophy

One of the more common types of muscular dystrophy (MD) is *Duchenne muscular dystrophy*, or pseudohypertrophic (which means "false overgrowth") MD. In children with Duchenne MD, the muscle mass breaks down and is replaced by fat and scar tissue. The buildup of fat and scar tissue can make the muscles, especially those of the calves, look unusually large. Duchenne MD is seen only in boys. About 3 individuals per 100,000 develop the condition.[12] Most children who have Duchenne MD survive until they

TABLE 12-4

Selected Genetic Conditions

CONDITION AND GENETIC CAUSE	INCIDENCE	COMMON SYMPTOMS AND SIGNS	FUNCTIONAL IMPLICATIONS
TUBEROUS SCLEROSIS			
Autosomal dominant gene or mutation	1 in 20,000 births[16]	Very mild to severe symptoms Tumors in brain; can cause seizures, intellectual disability, delayed language skills, and motor problems, which is rare Tumors in heart, kidneys, eyes, or other organs; can (but may not) cause problems	Possible learning disabilities Possible aggressive or hyperactive behavior Possible inability to speak and need for alternative communication Possible severe delays in gross and fine motor skills Mild to severe delays in self-help skill
ANGELMAN SYNDROME			
Deletion of chromosome 15 from mother[10]	1 in 25,000[13]	Tremors and jerky gait Developmental delays Severe language impairment; nonverbal or severe speech delay Very happy mood (happy puppet syndrome) Possible seizure disorder	Microencephaly Gross and fine motor delays, delayed walking skills Severely delayed self-care skills Inability to speak but possible use of alternative communication Sleep disorders (can be very disruptive to family life) Severe sensory processing problems Behavior problems such as biting, hair pulling, stubbornness, and screaming
PRADER-WILLI SYNDROME			
Deletion of chromosome 15 from father[19]	1 in 15,000[19]	Growth failure related to poor suck–swallow reflex in infancy Obsessed with food, possibly causing obesity (parents must lock all kitchen cabinets as a precaution; the child may eat anything) Developmental delays, low intelligence Hypotonia and poor reflexes Speech problems related to hypotonia Laid-back attitude but possible stubbornness and violent tantrums Severe stress on families resulting from behavior problems	Obsession with eating (can be dangerous during treatment) Gross and fine motor delays Delayed development of self-help skills Difficulty walking resulting from obesity or low muscle tone May need alternative communication Possible benefits from prevocational and vocational training

Continued

TABLE 12-4

Selected Genetic Conditions—cont'd

CONDITION AND GENETIC CAUSE	INCIDENCE	COMMON SYMPTOMS AND SIGNS	FUNCTIONAL IMPLICATIONS
RETT SYNDROME			
Genetic but undetermined[14]	Seen only in girls	Normal or nearly normal development during first 6–18 mo of life	Gross and fine motor problems
		Loss of skills and functional use of hands beginning at approximately 18 mo	Lacking or delayed self-help skills
		Loss or severely impaired ability to speak	Difficulty walking or inability to walk
		Development of repetitive, almost constant hand movements such as hand washing and wringing, clapping, and mouthing	Delayed response to requests, possibly taking up to 2 min to respond
		Shakiness in trunk and limbs	Possible need for alternative communication
		Unsteady, wide-based, stiff-legged walking	
FRAGILE X SYNDROME			
Mutation on X chromosome (most common genetic disease in humans)[11]	1 in 2000 males and 1 in 4000 females[1]	Boys more severely affected than girls	Mobility problems; delayed walking skills
		Possible hyperactivity	Gross and fine motor delays
		Low muscle tone	Delayed development of self-help skills
		Sensory processing problems involving touch and sound	Possible learning problems ranging from learning disabilities and ADD to intellectual disability
		Possible autistic behavior	Possible need for alternative communication in boys (unusual for girls)
		Language delays (more common in boys); possible dysfunctional speech	Possible benefits from prevocational and vocational training
		Intelligence problems ranging from learning disabilities to severe intellectual disability	

ADD, attention deficit disorder.

BOX 12-6

Genetic and Chromosomal Disorders: Signs and Symptoms

- Developmental delays
- Microencephaly
- Impaired cognitive development
- Unusual or excessive eating habits or patterns
- Small body structure
- Congenital anomalies
- Facial features characteristic of syndrome
- Simian crease in hands (characteristic of Down syndrome)
- Failure to thrive

are in their 20s, and a few live until they are in their 30s. The cause of death is usually cardiopulmonary system (heart and lung) complications that lead to pneumonia.

Sometimes parents suspect that something is wrong when their infant begins to walk on his toes around 1 year of age (Box 12-7). The diagnosis is usually made by the age of 4 years after a muscle biopsy is performed. By then the child's calves look large and progressive weakness has begun, especially in the joints closest to the body. **Scoliosis** (Figure 12-3) can develop because of muscle weakness, especially during growth spurts. Proper wheelchair positioning and support are important to prevent scoliosis. Older children with Duchenne MD may have to use a ventilator, so good body alignment is important for maintaining chest capacity that is vital for breathing.

BOX 12-7

Progression of Functional Losses in Children with Duchenne Muscular Dystrophy

LEVEL 1

Initially independent but has progressive functional losses over a period of several years; for example, walks independently but then loses stair-climbing ability and needs leg braces to walk and assistance to get up from a chair

LEVEL 2

In wheelchair: sits erect and is able to roll chair and perform ADLs such as upper extremity dressing, eating, and brushing the teeth in bed or chair

LEVEL 3

In wheelchair: sits erect but is unable to perform ADLs in bed or chair, such as placing equipment conveniently or rolling over without assistance

LEVEL 4

In wheelchair: sits erect with support and can do minimum ADLs such as brushing teeth or eating with adapted equipment

LEVEL 5

In bed: can do no ADLs without assistance

ADLs, activities of daily living.
Adapted from Rothstein JM, Roy HR, Wolf SL: *The rehabilitation specialist's handbook,* ed 2, Philadelphia, 1998, FA Davis.

CASE *Study*

Kevin has Duchenne MD. He is in Grade 2 in a regular class. When seated at his desk, he looks like the rest of the students in the class, even though his arms and legs look chubby. He is bright, but he has trouble keeping up with his classmates. He struggles to write, and his handwriting is hard to read. Of late, when he needs to get his pencil, he walks his fingers across the desk. It is hard for him to raise his hand to get the teacher's attention or to get his books out of his desk. When the class goes to other parts of the school for gym or music, Kevin can easily be spotted by his waddling gait. He has lordosis (see Figure 12-3); to keep from falling forward, he carries his shoulders and head back. His gait looks like a slow march because he has to pick his feet up high so that his toes do not drag. He falls a lot. To rise from the sitting position, he "walks" his hands up his legs (Gowers' sign).

The OT practitioner works with Kevin at school on a weekly basis and provides his teacher with suggestions to help meet Kevin's classroom needs. For example, the OT practitioner has suggested that Kevin start using a computer for his written work, sit at a larger table, and have all his books within easy reach. The OT practitioner monitors Kevin's needs for adaptive equipment. Because Kevin's ability to move has decreased, the practitioner has provided Kevin's family with some ROM exercises that will help him keep his joints loose, which, in turn,

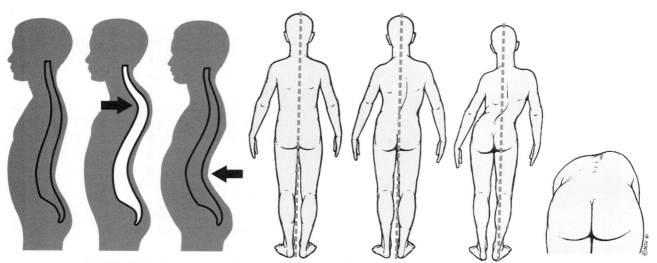

FIGURE 12-3   Scoliosis—the Bending of the Vertebral Column Sideways. In severe cases, the ribs are rotated, compressing the lungs and reducing their function; and lordosis—an increased forward curve of the lower back—occurs. The abdomen falls forward and the knees lock backward. The posture shifts weight forward; to balance weight, the child tends to carry the head and shoulders back farther than normal. This posture is common in children with hypotonia. (Redrawn from Hilt NE, Schmitt EW: *Pediatric orthopedic nursing,* St. Louis, 1975, Mosby, for Wilson D: *Wong's clinical manual of pediatric nursing,* ed 7, St. Louis, 2007, Mosby.)

will make it easier for the caregiver to dress and bathe him. The OT practitioner has taught Kevin's family members about proper body positioning to prevent contractures or scoliosis (see Figure 12-3). Finally, the OT practitioner has given Kevin a list of strengthening exercises that will help him function independently for as long as possible. (By the age of 9 years, most children with Duchenne MD need to use a wheelchair at least part of the time).

Down Syndrome

One of 2000 infants born to women who are less than 40 years of age and 1 of 40 infants born to women who are more than 40 years old have *Down syndrome.* About 95% of the individuals with Down syndrome have an extra twenty-first chromosome. The extra chromosome comes from the father 25% to 30% of the time.[10]

Early intervention, including occupational, speech, physical, and developmental therapies are an important part of helping children with Down syndrome reach their full potential. Recent research indicates that early intervention, including teaching families ways to enrich their children's environment, helps reduce developmental delays.[32]

Children with Down syndrome have characteristic facial features (slanted eyes, skin fold over nasal corners of eyes, small mouth, protruding tongue), tendency for cardiac anomalies, low muscle tone throughout, intelligence deficits, and simian creases in hands See Figure 12-4. (Box 12-8).

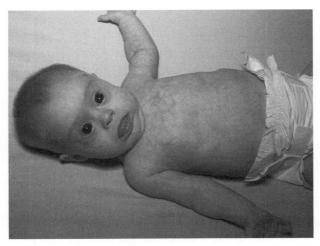

FIGURE 12-4 Child With Down Syndrome. Note the low muscle tone evidenced by the barreled chest and open mouth. Other noticeable features include large, protruding tongue and shoulder instability. (From Hockenberry MJ: *Wong's essentials of pediatric nursing,* ed 7, St. Louis, 2005, Mosby.

CLINICAL *Pearl*

Children who have Down syndrome often tongue thrust (i.e., force tongue forward) when eating. Placing food to the sides of the mouth helps them control this forward movement. Caregivers should be encouraged to place small spoonfuls of food to the side of the mouth or 2/3rd of the way into the mouth (on the tongue) with slight pressure to encourage lip closure.

CASE *Study*

Dennis, 15 years old, has Down syndrome. When he was 12 years old, the OTA gave him a prevocational assessment at the occupational therapist's request. The occupational therapist and the OTA together developed a plan of care to improve Dennis's prevocational skills through vocational readiness classes at school. Dennis now works at a local grocery store two half-days a week as part of the vocational training program. His short, stubby fingers and hands move slowly when he carefully sorts and places items in grocery sacks. His tongue sometimes protrudes, and it seems large for his mouth. His face is full and round. Behind his glasses is a fold of skin on either side of his nose. Dennis is about 5 feet 6 inches tall. His chest is round. When he pushes grocery carts to customers' cars, he walks with a wider base of support and his feet roll in. He politely chats with the customers he helps. Dennis is a confident young man and seems to enjoy his work.

OT intervention for children with Down syndrome focuses on helping children engage in ADLs, self-care, play, education, and social participation. Early intervention services are aimed at enhancing the child's developmental abilities, including improving muscle tone for movement and feeding ability (decreasing tongue thrusting and promoting lip closure). Children with Down syndrome may require adaptations to participate in regular classrooms.

Cri du Chat Syndrome

Cri du chat syndrome (*cri du chat* means "cry of the cat") is a rare genetic condition caused by the absence of part of chromosome 5. The baby or the young child with this genetic disorder has a weak, mewing cry. Classic body features documented in children with cri du chat syndrome include microencephaly; widely spaced, down-slanting eyes; cardiopulmonary abnormalities; and failure to thrive.[9] Children with cri du chat syndrome experience intellectual deficits and developmental delays .

Physical Characteristics of Down Syndrome

- Shortened limbs and fingers
- Slanted skin fold over nasal corners of eyes
- Small mouth; protruding tongue
- Straight line across palm of hand (simian line)
- Heart defects (congenital, high incidence)
- Intellectual disability (usually mild or moderate)
- Atloaxoid instability (important factor for children who engage in sports); can cause quadriplegia after minor neck injuries
- Floppy muscle tone
- Hyperextensibility of hips, limbs, and fingers
- Sensory processing problems
  - Diffuse tactile discrimination difficulties
  - Tactile sensitivity
  - Gravitational insecurity
  - Hyperactive postrotary nystagmus
  - Poor bilateral motor coordination
- Changes in developmental reflexes in infants (caused by altered sensory processing)
  - Reduced suck reflex
- Increased gag reflex (eventually resulting in food selectivity or intolerance and chewing problems)
  - Diminished palmar grasp reflex
  - Prolonged and exaggerated startle reflex
  - Prolonged flexor withdrawal and avoidance reactions in hands and feet
  - Delayed placing response in hands and feet
  - Lack of primary standing or air response*
  - Poor optical righting
- Poor body-on-body righting delayed equilibrium responses, particularly in quadruped and standing positions

*Normally, when infants' feet touch a supporting surface, they support their body weight against the surface with their feet. Infants with Down syndrome pull their feet away from the supporting surface.
Data from Crepeau EB, Neistadt ME, editors: *Willard and Spackman's occupational therapy*, ed 6, Philadelphia, 1998, JB Lippincott–Raven.

CLINICAL *Pearl*

During clinical practice, two children who had the medical diagnosis of cri du chat syndrome were encountered by one of the authors of this chapter. Both children tended to have low muscle tone, feeding issues, behavioral problems, and significant cognitive limitations.

Fragile X Syndrome

Fragile X syndrome affects boys more often than girls. Children present with limited brain development, abnormal skull, joints, and feet structures.[19] They exhibit typical structural features, including elongated faces, prominent jaws and foreheads, hypermobile or lax joints, and flat feet. Children with fragile X syndrome may be intellectually delayed.

Prader-Willi Syndrome

Prader-Willi syndrome involves chromosome 15. Children and adolescents who have Prader-Willi syndrome exhibit varying degrees of intellectual deficits, overeating habits, and self-mutilating behaviors such as picking sores until they bleed or biting their fists until large calluses develop.[20]

CLINICAL *Pearl*

To avoid excessive weight gain and obesity in children and adolescents who have Prader-Willi syndrome, a strict diet and eating schedule must be established and maintained.

General Interventions

OT practitioners working with children with genetic or chromosomal disorders address the occupational performances of these children (Table 12-5). For example, children with fragile X syndrome may have intellectual disabilities and thus will require assistance to develop ADL skills. They may require adaptations to be independent, structure to engage in leisure activities, and training to participate in work. Children and adolescents with Prader-Willi syndrome require intervention for social participation because their behaviors such as picking sores and overeating are not socially acceptable. OT practitioners may provide the families of these children with strategies to help their children function to their full potential.

The OT practitioner working with children with genetic or chromosomal disorders evaluates their abilities to perform occupations and addresses any related issues. Children with genetic disorders have physical appearances that are different from those of typically developing children, and many have associated intellectual and developmental disabilities. For example, children with Down syndrome exhibit low muscle tone interfering with movement. OT practitioners consider the specific features of the disorder when designing interventions.

OT interventions for genetic or chromosomal conditions frequently involve the following:

- Analysis of occupational performance, including the child's strengths and weaknesses and how this influences the child's performance

TABLE 12-5

Genetic and Chromosomal Disorders: General Intervention Considerations

CONSIDERATION	DEFINITION AND EXAMPLE(S)
Failure to thrive	Many genetic disorders have associated feeding difficulties. These may be due to motor, cognitive, or structural functions. The OT practitioner should evaluate and treat them through training, compensation, adaptive technology, or remediation.
Developmental delays	Many genetic disorders have associated delays in motor, social, language, and self-care skills. OT practitioners can help children learn the skills needed for their occupations through intervention.
Cognitive delays	Lower cognitive abilities are frequently a part of genetic disorders. Children may learn skills at a slower rate and may show difficulty in problem solving and with abstract thought and reasoning. Practicing occupations in a variety of contexts helps children generalize skills.
Congenital anomalies	Children with genetic disorders may exhibit certain physical features (short stature, flat hand arches) which interfere with motor skills. OT practitioners can help them compensate or adapt to perform occupations.
Psychosocial/emotional issues	Children with genetic disorders also experience a range of emotional and psychological issues. OT practitioners can help them cope with everyday situations, deal with periods of stress, adapt to life changes, and work with their strengths.
Social participation/behaviors	OT practitioners work with children, families, and communities to help the children engage in occupations. Children with all levels of ability benefit from social participation. OT practitioners can assist them in fitting into groups by helping them develop socially appropriate behaviors.

- Developmental interventions to facilitate achievement of milestones and to promote occupational performance
- Interventions to increase strength and endurance for activities
- Behavioral modification techniques to develop socially appropriate behaviors
- Task-specific activities to teach child-specific skills for daily living
- Adaptations or compensation for limited problem-solving, memory, or generalization abilities

NEUROLOGIC CONDITIONS

The neuromuscular system includes the nervous system and the muscles of the human body. The nervous system can be subdivided into the **peripheral nervous system** (PNS) and the **central nervous system** (CNS). The CNS includes the brain and spinal cord. The PNS consists of the nerves that originate from the spinal cord and innervate the muscles of the neck, trunk, arms, and legs. Children born with problems in the brain or spine (CNS) have congenital neurologic conditions. These conditions may also be acquired from trauma or infection at the time

of birth or in the early months of life. The more common neurologic conditions seen by the OT practitioner are discussed in the following sections. Table 12-6 describes other CNS conditions.

Spina Bifida

Spina bifida, a condition in which one or more of the vertebrae are not formed properly, is the most common type of congenital spinal abnormality.[6] Spina bifida is classified into three types: (1) occulta, (2) meningocele, and (3) myelomeningocele (Figure 12-5). The meninges (the covering of the spinal cord) or both the meninges and the spinal cord push out through an abnormal opening in the vertebra in the meningocele and myelomeningocele types of spina bifida, respectively. The amount of resulting disability can range from minimal, as in individuals with spina bifida occulta, to severe, as in individuals who have a myelomeningocele. The OT practitioner typically sees children with the myelomeningocele type because their limitations and disabilities are the most severe of the three.

Spina bifida occurs in about 1 of 1000 births. Its cause may be genetic, or it may result from high maternal

TABLE 12-6

Other Common Central Nervous System Conditions

CONDITION	SYMPTOMS OR SIGNS
AGENESIS OF THE CORPUS CALLOSUM	
Absence or poor development of the central part of the brain that connects the two hemispheres	Deficits ranging from mild learning problems to severe physical and mental problems
	Possible vision or hearing problems
	Possible sensory processing problems
	Possible eye–hand coordination problems
	Intellectual disability and epilepsy (common)
MICROENCEPHALY	
Literally, "small head"	Head that appears small for body
	Moderate to severe intellectual disability
	Moderate to severe motor problems
	Possible seizure disorder

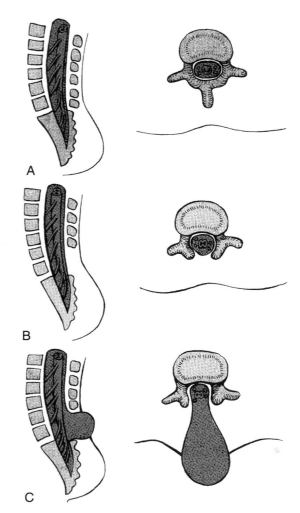

FIGURE 12-5 Normal Vertebral Column and Three Forms of Spina Bifida. **A,** *Normal*: intact vertebral column, meninges, and spinal cord. **B,** *Spina bifida occulta*: bony defect in vertebral column. This type of spina bifida can be diagnosed only by X-ray and often goes undetected. **C,** *Meningocele*: bony defect in which meninges fill with spinal fluid and protrude through an opening in the vertebral column. **D,** *Myelomeningocele*: bony defect in which meninges fill with spinal fluid, and a portion of the spinal cord with its nerves protrude through an opening in the vertebral column. This type of spina bifida is the most severe and can be detected at birth. (From Wong DL: *Whaley and Wong's nursing care of infants and children*, ed 6, 1999, St. Louis, Mosby.)

body temperatures or insufficient folic acid in the mother's diet. The amount of resulting physical disability is related to the size and location of the defect.[27] The higher the level of the spinal opening, the greater is the disability. Eighty percent of children born with spina bifida have hydrocephalus caused by excessive cerebrospinal fluid. To drain the fluid, a shunt is placed in the ventricles of the brain. The tube (which is similar to small aquarium tubing) runs down the neck to the abdomen, where the extra fluid drains. Scoliosis or **kyphosis** may be present at birth or may develop later (see Figures 12-3 and 12-6). In the early months of life, proper positioning of the paralyzed legs is important to prevent the development of contractures. Because of their immobility, these children are unable to engage in the normal sensorimotor experiences that influence development. OT practitioners help children with spina bifida engage in developmentally appropriate activities to promote body self-concept, comfort with movement, tactile discrimination, eye–hand control, and motor planning. Infants and toddlers with spina bifida benefit from a home program that encourages sensory enrichment activities.

CASE *Study*

Ten-year-old Niki was on the school playground playing catch when she began to feel ill. When she got off the bus with a fever and headache her father rushed her to the emergency room (Box 12-9). Today, she is in the hospital recovering from surgery to repair a shunt that had been previously placed to control her hydrocephalus. Niki was

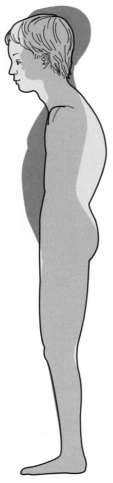

FIGURE 12-6 Congenital Kyphosis—a Backward Rounding of the Spine in the Chest Area That Can Be Caused by Malformed Vertebrae. Changes in the spine cause the head and shoulders to be carried forward. The front of the body bends forward, compressing the internal organs.

born with spina bifida and has had many surgeries, most of which were to repair her shunt. Others were to repair the hole in her back and her congenital clubbed feet. Her legs are paralyzed, and she has no bowel or bladder control. She has learned to use a catheter to empty her bladder and uses a special bowel program to eliminate. When she was younger, Niki walked with crutches and braces but was always frightened of being on her feet. As she got older, she gained weight, which made it hard for her to walk. Now Niki uses a manual wheelchair to move around.

OT practitioners address the multiple issues affecting the ability of a child with spina bifida to perform daily occupations. Physical issues such as lack of movement, lack of sensation, and positioning, as well as visual perception skills and fine motor skills, are addressed. As

---

these children get older, they are responsible for self-catheterization that requires adequate fine motor skills. OT practitioners address mobility issues in the school and community and also help the children develop body image and self-concept. OT practitioners help the children with spina bifida meet the requirements at school, play, home, and in the community. Interventions include positioning equipment, adapted technology, compensatory techniques, and developmental strategies. OT practitioners must be aware of the signs of shunt malformations and educate children, family members, and caregivers on signs and symptoms.

Traumatic Brain Injury

A *traumatic brain injury* (TBI) is a serious injury to the brain, also known as a *closed head injury* (CHI) or *head injury* (HI). Traumatic brain injury results from damage to the CNS as a result of forces coming in contact with the skull. Damage to the nerve tissue occurs both during and after the immediate trauma.[14,28]

Children and adolescents with TBIs are referred for OT because of their inability to function in the areas of occupation (ADLs, IADLs, education, work, play, and social participation) (Box 12-10). The trauma to the brain typically results in motor, cognitive, and emotional changes. Motor deficits may include abnormal muscle tone (changes in the resting state of a muscle typically resulting in increased muscle tone), hemiplegia (involvement of the arm and leg on one side of the body), and quadriplegia (involvement of both arms and legs). As the swelling of the brain begins to heal, some of the deficits may improve. The affected children and adolescents may need to relearn motor patterns. They may require orthoses of the extremities to maintain and improve the range of motion (ROM). OT practitioners work with children and adolescents who have sustained TBIs to help them relearn movements.[28] OT practitioners address cognitive changes such as loss of memory, word-finding problems, and poor abstract thinking and reasoning. These children and adolescents may

BOX 12-10

Neurologic Disorders: Signs and Symptoms of Traumatic Brain Injury

- Loss of consciousness
- Lethargy
- Vomiting
- Irritability
- Motor: loss of balance, abnormal muscle tone, weakness
- Processing, memory loss
- Communication/interaction impairments: slurred and/or slowed speech, word-finding problems
- Severe headache
- Confusion
- Personality changes
- Flat affect

Data from Rogers S. Common conditions that influence children's participation. In Case-Smith J, O'Brien J: *Occupational therapy for children*, ed 6, St Louis, 2010, Mosby.

experience perceptual deficits that include lack of awareness of their surroundings and poor sequencing and timing skills. They may experience emotional changes such as lability (moods ranging from happy to tearful or angry), inappropriateness (e.g., cursing, touching, disrobing), and personality changes. Children and adolescents who have had a TBI may demonstrate a "flat" affect, showing little or no emotion. Aggressiveness and irritability occur during recovery.[28]

OT practitioners working with children and adolescents who have had a TBI work closely with their parents and a team of professionals, comprised of speech and language pathologists, physical therapists, a rehabilitation specialist, a physiatrist, nurses, psychologists, and teachers. (Table 12-7). The OT practitioner is a key player on this team and has the responsibility of addressing the child's ability to function in everyday occupations.

CLINICAL *Pearl*

Muscle tone in a child or adolescent who has sustained a traumatic brain injury is different from that in a child who has cerebral palsy. The abnormally high tone is more resistant to handling and inhibitory techniques.

Shaken Baby Syndrome

Infants who are violently shaken by adults sustain serious brain damage, which is referred to as *shaken baby syndrome*. When an infant is shaken, it causes the brain to hit the inside of the skull so hard that it bruises the brain or causes bleeding and thus can be considered a traumatic brain injury.[1] The exact number of shaken baby cases is not known because of a lack of information in general about child abuse. Some instances may be subtle and may go undetected. Many cases show that the children have suffered previous abuse. Members of lower socioeconomic groups and younger adults are more likely to shake infants too hard, and the person shaking the infant has usually been previously abused. Most of the cases of shaken baby syndrome involve children younger than 2 years of age; about 25% of these children die.[15] Only a small percentage of infants who survive a severe shaking regain normalcy after the abuse.[1] Children with disabilities are at greater risk for being abused and

TABLE 12-7

Neurologic Disorders: General Intervention Considerations (Traumatic Brain Injury)

CONSIDERATION	DEFINITION AND EXAMPLE(S)
Preparatory activities	Prepare the child for activities by making him or her more ready to interact with the environment. "Normalize" sensory awareness/response and muscle tone. The child participates in sensory games, rubbing objects with different textures, and awareness activities.
Enabling activities	Build up skills needed for engagement in occupations (e.g., arm strength, visual attention, memory). Examples include weight-bearing and weight-shifting activities and development of arm strength through repetitive activities (e.g., weight training, lifting plates, picking up laundry).
Purposeful activities and occupations	Facilitate performing the actual occupation or activity in an environment closest to the natural one. Examples include unbuttoning the shirt in preparation for evening shower and preparing lunch at the clinic.

neglected; they are at least twice as likely to be mistreated compared with children without disabilities.[15,16]

Children with shaken baby syndrome experience neurologic damage that results in developmental delays, visual impairments, mild learning problems, or profound mental impairments (Box 12-11). The head trauma may result in loss of muscle control or cerebral palsy (see Chapter 16). The injury to the eyes may heal within weeks; however, if the visual area of the brain is damaged, the children may demonstrate permanent visual impairments or **cortical blindness**. Because the eyes are not actually damaged in children with cortical blindness, they see images as if they were looking through several layers of plastic wrap.

OT practitioners working with children with shaken baby syndrome evaluate and facilitate the child's development in all areas of occupational performance. OT practitioners examine visual perceptual skills to determine if the deficits may be interfering with the child's ability to perform daily occupations. The OT practitioner examines the child's motor abilities. The children may have cerebral palsy caused by the brain damage sustained while shaken. A child may exhibit intellectual deficits caused by the brain damage.

Erb's Palsy

During birth, stretching or tearing of the peripheral nerves that supply the arm and shoulder can cause *Erb's palsy*. Erb's palsy occurs in about 2% of births.[33] Infants who are born feet first or are too large for the birth canal are at risk for this type of injury. Erb's palsy can generally be diagnosed in the first 24 hours after birth. The paralysis usually goes away, even if untreated, in a few days or weeks (40% of infants), although the symptoms get worse in 35% of children by the time they are 18 months old. These toddlers experience delays in the

---

development of gross and fine motor skills.[19] Infants who are not treated early may develop elbow flexion contractures, and the affected arm is noticeably shorter than the other one.

OT practitioners working with infants and toddlers who have Erb's palsy begin by examining the infant's movement of the extremity and teaching parents how to support the extremity. This involves holding the arm close to the infant's body and encouraging the infant to touch the extremity and bring his or her hand to the mouth. As the infant develops motor skills, the OT practitioner promotes weight-bearing activities and exercises for ROM and strengthening of the extremity. As movement improves, the OT practitioner facilitates bilateral hand activities. Fabricating an orthosis may help the child support the extremity and regain function. Slings may be helpful as a way to protect the infant's arm. Care should be taken never to pin slings to the baby's clothes (pins may open up) or leave the sling on when the infant sleeps (may cause strangulation) (Figure 12-7).

Seizures

Approximately 2% of the general population experience *seizures* of some type.[10] One fourth of those have ongoing repeated seizures or epilepsy. Epilepsy occurs more often in children than in adults, and many children outgrow

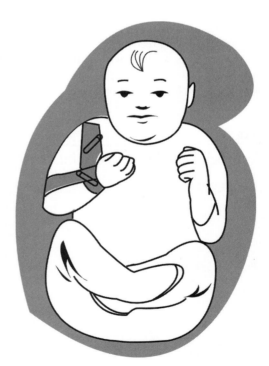

FIGURE 12-7 Sling for Infant With Erb's Palsy. The sling is made of a cotton stockinette. It is wrapped around the infant's shoulder in a position that keeps the affected hand near the infant's face.

> **BOX 12-11**
>
> *Possible Injuries From Shaken Baby Syndrome*
>
> - Injuries inside the brain
> - Brain swelling
> - Diffuse nerve cell damage
> - Shear injury
> - Bleeding
> - Injuries outside the brain
> - Retinal bleeding (75% to 90%)
> - Rib fractures
> - Bruises
> - Abdominal injuries
>
> Adapted from Alexander RC, Smith WL: Shaken baby syndrome, *Inf Young Childr* 10:3, 1998.

these seizures.[4] Most people who have seizures have only one type, which is usually grand mal (Table 12-8). About a third experience both grand mal and petit mal types.[10] Children with congenital brain damage, including those with cerebral palsy (particularly hemiplegia), spina bifida, and microcephaly, may have seizures.

Seizures may be provoked by fast spinning movements, flashing lights, and spinning visual stimuli. The OT practitioner who observes a child having a seizure documents the child's behavior during the seizure, the duration of the seizure, and the child's behavior before and after the seizure. The OT practitioner should contact the parents and the child's physician and give a description of the event. Some children have frequent unprovoked seizures, which should always be documented. While a child is having a seizure, the OT practitioner ensures that the child is safe but does not place anything in the child's mouth.

CASE *Study*

Ryan is a 6-year-old diagnosed with right hemiplegic cerebral palsy and a seizure disorder. During a busy day in the clinic, Ryan and Jill, his OTA, were working on putting a shirt on Ryan. Ryan was having difficulty putting on his shirt; then he gave a high-pitched cry, his head went back, and he fell off the stool. Jill knew Ryan had a history of uncontrolled seizures and knew right away what had happened (Box 12-12). She immediately removed the stool from the area so that his flailing arms and legs would not hit it. She turned his head to the side and tucked a cushion under it. She carefully watched his breathing and skin color, timed the seizure, and waited for it to subside. In a few minutes, Ryan began to regain consciousness but was groggy. Jill knew that the OT session for that day was over and that Ryan needed a nap. She documented the entire seizure episode and informed the parents and physician about it.

General Interventions

OT interventions for neurologic conditions frequently involve the following:

- Analysis of occupational performance, including the child's strengths and weaknesses and how they influence the child's performance
- Developmental interventions to facilitate achievement of milestones and to promote occupational performance
- Interventions to increase strength and endurance for activities
- Behavioral modification techniques to develop socially appropriate behaviors

TABLE 12-8

Seizures

TYPE OF SEIZURE	CHARACTERISTICS
Grand mal seizures	Possible crying out or mood change before the seizure
	Loss of consciousness for 2–5 min
	Falling; shaking of arms, legs, and body
	Possible loss of control of bowels and bladder
	Afterward, possible deep sleep, headache, or muscle soreness
Absence (petit mal) seizures	Mostly in children
	Most likely to occur many times a day
	Brief loss of consciousness (10–30 s)
	Possible eye or muscle fluttering
	No loss of muscle tone
	Sudden cessation of activity; restarts a few seconds later
Febrile seizures	Mostly in children 3 mo–5 yr
	Most common in children with existing neurologic problems
	In individuals with fever but no brain infection
	Varying duration; brief or up to 15 minutes
Infantile spasms ("salaam" seizures)	Seen in children under 3 yr with obvious brain damage
	A few seconds in duration but occur several times each day
	Sudden flexion of arms, extension of legs, and forward flexion of the trunk
Akinetic or drop seizures	Brief and sudden
	Complete loss of consciousness and muscle tone
	Danger of head injury because the child will suddenly fall to the ground

Data from Berkow R, editor: *The Merck manual*, ed 17, Rahway, NJ, 1999, Merck.

- Task-specific activities to teach child-specific skills for daily living
- Adaptations or compensation for deficits in motor, cognition, emotional or social functioning
- Motor relearning, including wearing orthoses and ROM, weight-bearing, and strengthening exercises
- Improving hand functioning for occupational performance

BOX 12-12

Caring for a Child Who Is Having a Seizure

- If the child is flailing, make sure nothing is close by that could cause an injury if hit with his or her body.
- Place something soft under the head.
- Do not place anything in the mouth; it may damage the teeth.
- Do not put a finger in the mouth. It will be bitten—hard.
- Roll the child on the side to avoid inhalation of vomitus.
- Call for emergency medical help if the child's skin begins to turn blue.

BOX 12-13

Developmental Disorders: Signs and Symptoms

- Delays in motor, processing, and communication/interaction skills
- Impaired body functions
- Limited repertoire of behavior
- Stereotypical behaviors
- Decreased attention to purposeful activities and occupations
- Children not reaching milestones
- Infants showing decreased exploration and interest in environment

---

DEVELOPMENTAL DISORDERS

A developmental disorder is a mental and/or physical disability that arises before adulthood and lasts throughout a person's life. Pervasive developmental disorders (PDDs) constitute a group of pediatric health conditions affecting a variety of body functions and structures with a wide range of severity. Autism is the most well known of the PDDs. Other examples include Rett syndrome, attention deficit hyperactivity disorder (ADHD), and developmental coordination disorder (DCD) (Box 12-13).

Autism

Autism is characterized by severe and complex impairments in reciprocal social interaction, communication skills, and the presence of stereotypical behavior, interests, and activities.[3] The Centers for Disease Control (CDC) estimates that four times as many boys as girls are diagnosed as having autism.[15] Children with autism come from all racial, ethnic, intellectual, and socioeconomic backgrounds.[3,4,14] Autism affects a child's ability to participate in occupations at home and in the community. The behavioral characteristics of autism that are critical to its diagnosis are presented here.[3]

- Disturbances in social interaction that affect the child's ability to meaningfully interact with people as well as inanimate objects
- Disturbances in communication that may be mild (minor disarticulation) to severe (absence of meaningful speech)
- Disturbances of behavior reflective of intolerance, evidenced by resistance to change, stereotypical behavior, and bizarre attachments to objects
- Disturbances of sensory and perceptual processing and associated impairments; problems of sensory and

perceptual processing that may be either registration (acknowledge/orient to sensation) or modulation (control over input).

Children with autism present with a variety of signs and symptoms that range in severity. While therapy for each child varies, certain considerations may be beneficial (see Box 12-14). Children with autism require a structured environment and clear expectations. Behavior management programs using positive reinforcers (such as the use of stickers) work well. OT practitioners working with children who have autism must be able to read verbal and nonverbal cues quickly. Since these children have difficulty expressing themselves verbally, they may experience frustration when OT clinicians do not "listen" to them. This may cause escalation of poor or acting-out behavior.

Children who have autism experience difficulty processing sensory information; they may benefit from a sensory integration approach (see Chapter 24). The OT practitioner carefully monitors the child's reaction to activities; it may be difficult for the child to select from several activities. Therefore, asking a child with autism to choose between only two activities facilitates decision making.

Communication with children who have autism may include the use of simple signs, verbal expressions, demonstrations, pictures, and communication systems. OT practitioners will need to consult with speech/language therapists, teachers, parents, and other professionals to determine the most effective way(s) to communicate.

OT practitioners work with children with autism to improve their ability to participate in ADLs, IADLs, education, work, play, and social participation (Box 12-15). Since these children typically experience deficits in all of these areas, OT clinicians must prioritize and identify

BOX 12-14

Signs of Autism or Pervasive Developmental Disorder

INFANTS

- Stiffen when picked up or do not physically conform to the adult's body when held
- Do not calm when held; may prefer to lie in the crib
- Startle easily when touched or when the bed is bumped
- Hate baths, dressing, or diaper changing
- Have poor sucking ability or are hard to feed
- Have poor muscle tone; bodies feel floppy
- Do not have age-appropriate head control or age-appropriate ability to sit, crawl, or walk

CHILDREN

- Seem unaware of surroundings
- Do not make eye contact
- Have general learning problems
- Do not relate to others
- Only eat certain food textures
- Refuse to touch certain textures (e.g., mud and sand)
- Have sleep problems such as difficulty getting to sleep or staying asleep
- Are hyperactive
- Are withdrawn, miserable, anxious, or afraid
- Display repetitive behavior or speech patterns
- Fixate on one object or body part
- Compulsively touch smooth objects
- Show fascination with lights
- Flap arms when excited
- Frequently jump, rock, or spin self or objects
- Walk on tiptoes
- Giggle or scream for no apparent reason
- Eat strange substances (e.g., soil, paper, toothpaste, soap, rubber)

BOX 12-15

General Intervention Techniques for Children With Autism

- Provide structure and consistency.
- Keep the same routine.
- Read the child's nonverbal as well as verbal cues.
- Communicate through signs, pictures, communication boards, and/or singing.
- Work with the child at his or her level.
- Follow the child's cues.
- Redirect when the child begins self-stimulation.
- Listen to the parent(s) to learn about the child's preferences.
- Provide a quiet setting.
- Allow the child to play with other children.
- Use positive behavioral reinforcers.
- Use sensory integration techniques.
  - Tactile
  - Vestibular
  - Proprioceptive
  - Olfactory
  - Gustatory (Children with autism may enjoy very spicy or sour tastes instead of bland tastes.)
- Provide the child with choices (may have to start with only two).
- Allow the child time to respond.
- Keep your talking to a minimum—use simple directions.
- Use behavioral management techniques.
- Realize that children have "off days" (may have to change the plan).
- Realize that practitioners have "off days"—spend some time thinking about what could have been done differently.
- Listen to the parents!
- Work on occupation-centered goals so that therapy is meaningful to the child and to the family.

meaningful goals. These goals are most effectively developed by collaborating with parents and/or teachers. For example, holding a spoon during mealtime is easily understood as addressing feeding goals. It would be harder for parents and/or teachers to understand how grasping a cube will help with feeding.

Attention Deficit Hyperactivity Disorder

Attention deficit hyperactivity disorder (ADHD) is the most common neurobehavioral disorder. It occurs in males three times more often than in females. Children who have ADHD have issues such as difficulty

with attention, hyperactivity, distractibility, and impulsivity (Box 12-16). Others include sleep disorders, emotional lability, poor self-esteem, and poor frustration tolerance.[3,9,14]

Children with ADHD benefit from organization and structure. OT clinicians and psychologists can provide parents with strategies and/or techniques to help their children with behavior problems. They can provide sensory strategies that help these children relax and concentrate. Physical activity may help them modulate their behaviors and pay attention more effectively in class. In fact, some schools have walking programs for all children before the start of classes.

BOX 12-16

Characteristics of Children With Attention Deficit Disorder or Attention Deficit Hyperactivity Disorder

- Are very active or fidgety; talk non-stop
- Are impulsive; act without thinking of consequences
- Make careless mistakes
- Lack focus; daydream
- Have difficulty following directions
- Have difficulty completing tasks
- Have racing thoughts
- May interrupt frequently
- Are inattentive during activities they consider boring or unexciting (which often include doing schoolwork)
- Are slow to wake up in the morning; are disorganized or grumpy unless anticipating an exciting activity
- Are slow to fall asleep
- Are spatially dyslexic (write mirror-image reversals of letters; have difficulty with left–right discrimination; have difficulty properly sequencing letters, words, or numbers)
- Have episodic temper tantrums that include hitting, biting, and kicking
- Are bed wetters
- Are inexplicably emotionally negative

Adapted from National Institute of Mental Health : ADHD http://www.nimh.nih.gov/health/publications/attention-deficit-hyperactivity-disorder/complete-index.shtml#pub2 Accessed June 14, 2010.

Rett Syndrome

Rett syndrome is a progressive neurologic disorder that occurs only in females. The infant or toddler seems to be developing normally until 6 to 18 months of age, at which time regression in all skills is observed. Microencephaly, seizures, abnormal muscle tone, intellectual disability, and stereotypical patterns of behavior (especially hand wriggling) emerge. Adolescents who have Rett syndrome are generally nonambulatory and do not have functional hand use.

Developmental Coordination Disorder

Developmental coordination disorder (DCD) encompasses a wide range of characteristics, but an essential feature is that the children's motor coordination is markedly below their chronologic age and intellectual ability and significantly interferes with ADLs.[3] The diagnosis of DCD cannot be the result of physical, sensory, or neurologic

impairments.[21,24] In addition, children are diagnosed with DCD only if the criteria for PDDs are not met.[3] If intellectual disability is present, the motor difficulties must be in excess of those usually associated with the level of severity of intellectual disability.

Children with DCD have difficulty forming letters quickly and precisely; this is often manifested in an inability to keep up with classmates and complete assignments efficiently.[21,29] For example, a child with DCD may be able to complete only one simple sentence in the time allotted, while other children are able to complete full paragraphs. The extra energy and time that children with DCD spend on the mechanics of writing often interfere with their ability to manage other classroom tasks. They take longer and are less efficient in carrying out everyday self-care tasks, which include such things as brushing teeth and getting dressed. Tasks that other children accomplish easily (e.g., fastening clothing, tying shoes, or organizing homework) may be problematic for a child who has DCD.[26] These children also often exhibit low self-esteem, show frustration, and begin to expect failure.[18] Feelings of low self-esteem develop as early as 6 years of age,[7,36] a time when these children experience difficulty keeping up with their peers and struggle with sports and play activities. The feelings associated with perception of low physical competence and inadequacy in performing tasks that other children take for granted can, and often do, result in emotional problems.[25,29,36,38]

Many professionals suggest that they will outgrow these coordination deficits, but evidence indicates that children who have DCD continue to have difficulty in adolescence and adulthood.[7,27,37] Losse et al monitored a group of children for 10 years and reported significant differences in verbal IQ, performance IQ, and academic performance between children with DCD and their peers.[27] Those who had DCD experienced more behavioral problems, had more difficulty with handwriting, art design, and technology, demonstrated trouble with home economics, and exhibited lower performance in practical science lessons.

The motor deficits exhibited by children with DCD are many and varied. Among other things, they exhibit poor balance, postural control, and coordination and are more variable in their motor responses.[43] Timing and sequencing deficits and slower movement times have also been reported for children who have DCD.[20,43] These children tend to rely more on visual than proprioceptive information, fail to anticipate or use perceptual information, and do not use appropriate rehearsal strategies.[43] This, in turn, impairs quality of movement, especially in situations in which the child has to react to a changing environment. According to sensory integration theory, the primary basis for the poor motor performance of children with DCD lies in the central processing of information related to the planning, selecting, and timing of movement. These children have been shown to have difficulty processing tactile, vestibular, and proprioceptive information.[6,7,13]

The treatment of children with DCD may follow a motor control (see Chapter 23) or sensory integration (see Chapter 24) approach.

CLINICAL *Pearl*

Children who have sensory processing deficits may experience the signs and symptoms of attention deficit hyperactivity disorder (ADHD). OT practitioners can provide sensory strategies and intervention that may help children modulate their attention and function within the home and the classroom. Diet may also cause ADHD behaviors (this has not been proved; but ask any parent). Overstimulating or anxious environments may cause children to exhibit the behaviors of ADHD. Those experiencing emotional trauma may exhibit the signs of ADHD.

CLINICAL *Pearl*

Developmental dyspraxia is a disorder characterized by an impairment in the ability to plan and carry out sensory and motor tasks. Children with this problem may have trouble starting or stopping a movement. They may be able to do routine activities but have trouble with new ones. Sometimes the force of their movement is too strong or too weak to be effective, or they may have trouble with balance, vision, or short-term memory.

General Interventions

OT Interventions for developmental disorders (Table 12-9) frequently involve:

- Analysis of occupational performance, including the child's strengths and weaknesses and how they influence the child's performance
- Developmental interventions to facilitate achievement of milestones and to promote occupational performance
- Motor development and refinement of abilities
- Cognitive–behavioral techniques to facilitate goal setting and occupational performance
- Interventions to increase coordination and motor planning abilities for occupations
- Sensory diet to help regulate the child's emotional and attentional states

- Successful achievement to develop self-concept and positive self-esteem
- Organizational strategies
- Behavioral modification techniques to develop socially appropriate behaviors
- Task-specific activities to teach child-specific skills for daily living
- Adaptations or compensation for limited problem-solving, memory, or generalization

CARDIOPULMONARY SYSTEM

The cardiopulmonary system consists of the cardiac (heart and vessels) and respiratory (trachea, lungs, and diaphragm) systems, which are located in the thoracic area of the human body. The following health conditions affect the cardiac and respiratory body structures and consequently one's ability to participate fully in life's roles and occupations (Box 12-17).

CASE *Study*

The OT clinic receives a referral from a physician to evaluate and treat the feeding ability of a 7-month-old child on the pediatric cardiac unit. The child has undergone surgery for the repair of a heart defect. The occupational therapist and the OTA, who will be working together, study cardiac disorders so that they can be informed before evaluating the child.

Cardiac Disorders

Cardiac disorders are conditions that involve the heart and/or vessels (Figure 12-8).

Congenital heart diseases and dysrhythmias are examples of pediatric cardiac health conditions. The referral of children who have cardiac disorders to the pediatric OT practitioner is typically based on secondary deficits associated with the child's primary diagnosis. Oral–motor and feeding issues or sensory processing problems may necessitate a referral to a pediatric occupational therapist.

Congenital Heart Disease

Most pediatric health conditions that involve the heart or major vessels are congenital. Cardiac health conditions can be serious and sometimes life threatening. The cause of congenital cardiac health conditions can be unknown. Certain cardiac health conditions are associated with specific syndromes, especially with genetic disorders. Examples of congenital heart disorders include atrial septal defects (ASDs), ventricular septal defects (VSDs), and tetralogy of Fallot (TOF).

TABLE 12-9

Developmental Disorders: General Intervention Considerations

CONSIDERATION	DEFINITION AND EXAMPLE(S)
Behavior management programs	Provide programs to promote appropriate daily actions by identifying target behaviors, establishing positive reinforcers, and implementing a behavioral plan and follow-up with data collection.
Structured environment	Set up clear routines with consistency to allow the child to understand and practice daily occupations.
Total communication approach	Use a variety of systems to relate to the child, such as a communication board, sign language, verbal language, pointing/gesturing, and facilitative communication.
Sensory integration intervention	Use suspended equipment to provide a controlled sensory input so that the child can make an adaptive response. SI theory postulates that this will help with CNS development.
Practice occupations	Repeat skills and occupations such as using backward or forward chaining. Children learn through repetition.
Teach and repeat	Simplify occupations to allow the child to participate and increase ability to reach milestones.
Education	Teach the child how to perform occupations. Educate parents, teachers, and others about the child's condition and techniques to support child's occupations.
Promote interests	Provide novelty to promote interests and exploration.
Emotional/psychosocial issues	Address the child's self-concept, self-awareness, and body awareness by providing opportunities for exploration and success.

SI, sensory integration; *CNS,* central nervous system.

BOX 12-17

Cardiopulmonary Disorders: General Signs and Symptoms

- Decreased tolerance for exercise
- Increased occurrence of respiratory infections
- Shortness of breath
- Decreased endurance
- Small physical size for age
- Cyanosis (bluish discoloration of skin and mucous membranes)
- Poor distal circulation
- Failure to thrive
- Persistent cough or wheezing
- Pain or discomfort in joints and muscles

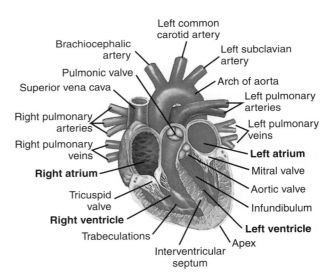

FIGURE 12-8 Frontal section of the heart. (From Canobbio MM: *Cardiovascular disorders,* St. Louis, 1990, Mosby.)

Atrial Septal Defects

Atrial septal defects (ASDs) are abnormal openings between the atria of the heart. The severity of the signs and symptoms of an ASD is dependent on the size and location of the hole (Figure 12-9, A). Typically, the right side of the heart receives deoxygenated blood from body structures and sends it to the lungs for oxygenation.

When an ASD is present, increased amounts of oxygenated blood are present on the right side of the heart. The primary symptom of an ASD is a heart murmur. Unless the ASD is severe and life threatening, the preferred medical intervention is surgical repair during middle childhood.[3]

Ventricular Septal Defects

Ventricular septal defects (VSDs) are the most common among congenital heart diseases. The defect is an opening in the septum that separates the left and right ventricles of the heart (see Figure 12-9, *B*). The opening permits oxygenated blood to flow into the right ventricle and then into the pulmonary artery and lungs. A small VSD is asymptomatic and will close spontaneously. A large VSD will require surgical repair during early childhood. Symptoms associated with a large VSD include irritability, poor weight gain, recurrent infections, and congestive heart failure.

Tetralogy of Fallot

The congenital heart disease known as *tetralogy of Fallot* (TOF) consists of four distinct defects observed in the heart and its associated blood vessels: (1) a VSD, (2) misplacement of the aorta, (3) narrowing of the pulmonary artery, and (4) abnormally large right ventricle (see Figure 12-9, *C*). Collectively, these defects lead to decreased blood flow to the lungs. Symptoms of TOF include cyanosis (body structures turn blue), failure to thrive (difficulty with feeding and weight gain), and a heart murmur. Medical intervention involves surgical repair during the first year of life.[4]

> **CLINICAL** *Pearl*
>
> Older children who know that they have an atrial septal defect (ASD) are likely to avoid exercise and activity because of fear and decreased endurance.

Dysrhythmias

A normal heart has recurrent expansion and compression of the chest that maintains proper circulation of the blood and respiration, which collectively are known as *cardiac rhythm. Dysrhythmias* are irregular cardiac rhythms. Examples of dysrhythmias include bradydysrhythmia (an abnormally slow heartbeat) and tachydysrhythmia (an abnormally fast heartbeat).

Children with cardiac disorders may experience difficulty with strength (due to the lack of practice), endurance (due to a cardiac disorder), and/or pain or discomfort in the joints and muscles (due to the lack of use or decreased oxygen). These difficulties may result in impaired functioning in the areas of occupation, including education, social participation, play, and self-care (Table 12-10).

> **CLINICAL** *Pearl*
>
> Infants with cardiac disorders may not be able to hold a regular-sized rattle. They can successfully hold small, lightweight rattles that can be found in pet shops. OT practitioners may start with these rattles until the child builds up strength and endurance.

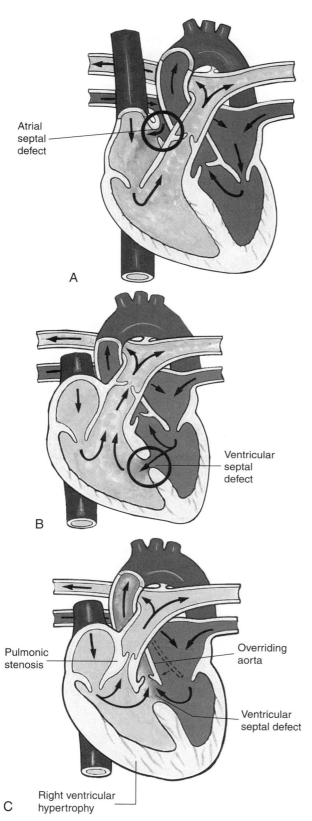

FIGURE 12-9 A, Atrial septal defect. **B,** Ventricular septal defect. **C,** Abnormally large right ventricle. (From Hockenberry MJ: *Wong's essentials of pediatric nursing,* ed 7, St. Louis, 2005, Mosby.)

TABLE 12-10

Cardiopulmonary Disorders: General Intervention Considerations

CONSIDERATION	DEFINITION AND EXAMPLE(S)
Breathing exercises	Exercises that promote optimal respiration rate by exerting the muscles involved in breathing, including the diaphragm and the oblique muscles.
Relaxation techniques	Techniques such as controlled breathing to promote decreased heart rate, lower metabolism, and decreased respiration rate. Additional relaxation methods include visualization of pleasant experiences, yoga, exercises, and biofeedback.
Energy conservation techniques	Principles and methods that promote using the least amount of energy and movement to perform activities. Sitting rather than standing while making a sandwich is one example of an energy conservation technique.
Balance/pacing of activities	Principles and methods that promote equal consideration between work and rest.
Balanced diet	Eating and drinking food with nutritional value to promote physical health and well-being.
Avoidance of internal and environmental "triggers"	Attempting to lower exposure to internal (e.g., stress, lack of rest) and external (e.g., pollen, smoke, dust) stimuli that initiate a negative cardiopulmonary response.
Strength and endurance activities	Techniques to increase participation time in activities through increased repetition and decreased breaks.
Emotional/psychosocial issues	Address the child's self-concept, perception of their abilities, interests, and so on. Help children gain an appreciation of their strengths.

CLINICAL *Pearl*

Children who fail to thrive may benefit from high-calorie foods and drinks. Consultation with a dietitian or nutritionist is helpful in determining the appropriate food for infants and children.

Pulmonary Disorders

Pulmonary disorders are conditions that involve the lungs and one's ability to breathe. Examples of pediatric pulmonary diseases include asthma and cystic fibrosis. Children with these diagnoses are referred for OT when they experience problems that interfere with ADLs, IADLs, education, play, and social participation.

Asthma

Asthma is a chronic respiratory condition that is characterized by sudden, recurring attacks of labored breathing, chest constriction, and coughing. It is a reactive disease of the small-airway structures in the lungs. Environmental and internal stimuli can trigger an attack in a child or adolescent who has asthma. Examples of environmental triggers include changes in atmospheric pressure, cold air, and cigarette smoke. Examples of internal triggers are exercise and stress. During an asthma attack, the muscular walls of the airway structures undergo spasm, and excessive mucus is secreted. These occurrences result in laborious breathing. Children with asthma have described feeling as if they were drowning in their own saliva and unable to catch their breath. Most children and adolescents anticipate oncoming attacks and are able to prevent a trip to the emergency room or doctor by following previously prescribed intervention procedures. Medical intervention often involves inhalant and/or drug therapy.[8]

Cystic Fibrosis

Cystic fibrosis (CF) occurs primarily in Caucasians and is diagnosed during infancy or early childhood. It is an inherited (genetic) disease that affects the exocrine (externally excreting) glands. The pancreas, the respiratory system, and the sweat glands are the most affected. The secretions from these glands are abnormally clammy or sticky. Symptoms of CF include frequent greasy stools, failure to thrive (problems in feeding and weight gain), frequent colds, and pneumonia with chronic coughing or wheezing. Chronic obstructive pulmonary disease (COPD) is the most serious complication of CF. Symptoms of COPD include wheezing, infections, and recurrent pneumothorax (partial collapse of a lobe of the lung).

Medical intervention for this pediatric health condition includes antibiotics for infections, inhalant therapy, and supplemental oxygen. Physical therapy may be required to assist with postural drainage, which, in turn, decreases the excessive buildup of sticky mucus in the lungs.

Hematologic Disorders

Hematologic disorders are conditions of the blood. Human blood is a fluid that consists of plasma, blood cells, and platelets. The purpose of blood is to carry nutrients and oxygen to the tissues of the body and to carry waste materials away from the tissues. *Anemia*, a pathologic deficiency in the oxygen-carrying component of the blood, deprives body tissues of necessary nutrients and oxygen. Anemia also leads to a buildup of waste products in human tissue.

Sickle cell anemia is one type of hematologic disorder that occurs in the black people of Africa or those of African descent. The red blood cells of an affected person are crescent shaped. It is characterized by exacerbation (flare-ups) and remission (lack of symptoms). During exacerbation, the person who has sickle cell anemia may experience pain in the joints, fever, leg ulcers, and jaundice (Figure 12-10). Depending on the severity of the disease, secondary complications might arise, including a hemorrhage or cerebrovascular accident (CVA). Discussions of CVA and other potential secondary complications of sickle cell anemia are beyond the scope of this text.

General Interventions

OT interventions for infants, children, and adolescents who have cardiac disorders focuses on helping them gain strength and endurance for and tolerance to activity so that they may participate in these occupations (Table 12-10). Because children with cardiac disorders may experience failure to thrive (secondary to poor endurance and/or inadequate oral–motor strength), intervention begins with providing compensatory techniques during feeding so that the child may be more successful. This may include adaptive nipples, holding the infant's cheeks to help him or her hold on to the bottle, and providing frequent breaks during feeding. OT practitioners may also focus therapy on improving the infant's ability to play for longer periods. Older children may benefit from compensatory techniques to conserve strength and endurance at home or school or during play. Those with cardiac disorders benefit from building endurance through short activity periods with frequent breaks and moving toward longer activity periods with fewer breaks. OT practitioners must be aware of signs of fatigue (e.g., bluish skin coloring, coughing, wheezing, shortness of breath).

Children and adolescents who have pulmonary disorders (such as sickle cell anemia) may be referred for OT because of an inability to function in ADLs, IADLs, education, play, and social participation due to pain in the joints. They may require assistance in organizing schoolwork because of missed school days during exacerbation of the disease. Children and adolescents may benefit from energy conservation techniques to handle the flare ups more efficiently. OT practitioners may provide adaptive positioning, night orthoses, and other assistive technology services and devices to help the child or adolescent through the flare up periods. Clients may also benefit from support groups in order to cope with the impact of the disease on daily functioning.

OT interventions for cardiopulmonary disorders conditions frequently involve the following:

- Analysis of occupational performance, including the child's strengths and weaknesses and how they influence the child's performance
- Participating in activities for longer durations (to build cardiac endurance)
- Activities designed to improve strength (e.g., more repetitions) and endurance
- Compensatory and adaptive strategies to help the children participate in daily activities
- Energy conservation and work simplification techniques
- Orthoses to support joints and to help the children rest
- Techniques and strategies to organize materials to meet occupational roles
- Cognitive–behavioral techniques to facilitate goal setting and occupational performance

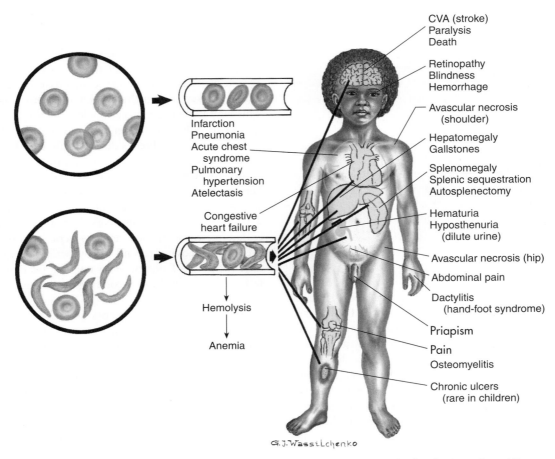

CVA (stroke)
Paralysis
Death

Retinopathy
Blindness
Hemorrhage

Avascular necrosis
(shoulder)

Hepatomegaly
Gallstones

Splenomegaly
Splenic sequestration
Autosplenectomy

Hematuria
Hyposthenuria
(dilute urine)

Avascular necrosis (hip)

Abdominal pain

Dactylitis
(hand-foot syndrome)

Priapism

Pain
Osteomyelitis

Chronic ulcers
(rare in children)

Infarction
Pneumonia
Acute chest
syndrome
Pulmonary
hypertension
Atelectasis

Congestive
heart failure

Hemolysis

Anemia

G.J.Wassilchenko

FIGURE 12-10   Sickle cell anemia. (From Hockenberry MJ: *Wong's essentials of pediatric nursing*, ed 7, St. Louis, 2005, Mosby.)

- Expose children to a variety of interesting activities to develop volition and feelings of self-efficacy
- Help the children succeed in educational and leisure activities despite missing opportunities due to illness
- Successful achievement to develop self-concept and positive self-esteem

SENSORY SYSTEM CONDITIONS

Sensory system conditions include those involving vision impairments (seeing impairments) and auditory system impairments (hearing impairments). Children may also have processing problems or deficits in other sensory systems, including the tactile (touch) system, the vestibular (balance and movement) system, and the proprioceptive (position sense) system (see Chapter 24).

Vision Impairments

About 1 in 4000 children is legally blind. One in 20 has significant but less severe vision problems. Thirty percent of children with multiple handicaps have some sort of vision problem.[12] Because a large proportion of children who have handicaps also have vision problems, the vision of all children with special needs should be monitored closely (Box 12-18). Discovering vision problems early can alert OT practitioners and family members to the need for appropriate intervention. Glasses may ease developmental and motor delays if the problem is detected early. Children who are identified early as having a vision problem may be referred to special organizations for help.

Children who are legally blind may be able to see objects if they are close enough. People who are totally blind have no perception of light. Children with **cortical blindness** have physically functional eyes, but the visual processing part of their brain has been damaged in some way, resulting in images that look as if they are being seen through several layers of plastic wrap. Less severe vision problems must also be considered during therapy. **Visual perception** is the understanding of what is being seen. It can affect eye–hand coordination. Crossed eyes cause double vision because the image seen by each eye does not fuse into one image. A lazy eye can affect depth

Signs of Undetected Visual Problems

- Parents notice that the child does not focus on his or her face or toys.
- The child holds objects close to his face.
- Gross and fine motor skills are poor.
- The child has crossed eyes or jerky eye movements.
- The child closes one eye to focus on an object.
- The child tilts his or her head while looking at specific objects.
- Older children perform poorly in school.

Data from Russel E & Nagiashi P. Services for children with visual or hearing impairments. In Case-Smith J, O'Brien J: *Occupational therapy for children*, ed 6, St. Louis, 2010, Mosby.

perception because only one eye is working at a time. Many of the more minor problems can be improved by performing eye exercises prescribed by a developmental optometrist. These minor problems are identified in 80% of children with reading problems.[31]

The intervention plan for children who have vision impairments depends on the severity of the impairment (Table 12-11). Legally blind children may be able to see quite well with corrective lenses; many of the interventions used for totally blind children also often benefit these children. Legally blind children may have problems with sensory integration, particularly with tactile defensiveness (being extremely sensitive to certain textures) and vestibular processing. Playing with various textured materials helps normalize the feeling of different textures in the hands and reduce the aversion to touch.

Opportunities to experience movement are important. To help children who are blind tolerate movement, start with gross motor activities that involve little movement and increase the amount of movement slowly. Many playground toys can be adapted for this purpose by the OT practitioner. Infants and younger children who are blind do not know to reach out for objects in the environment. By tying toys to strollers, chairs, or cribs and guiding these infants to feel for objects with their hands, these children can be taught to "look" for objects around them. Teaching the children to look for objects in increasingly larger areas can enhance this skill.

Vision is a learned skill. Any residual vision the child has should be used. The more the child uses the visual pathways, the better the vision becomes. Treating the child in a darkened room with a spotlight on the activity helps him or her see better by reducing other visual distractions. Emphasizing the visual contrasts between or among the surfaces of objects also increases the child's ability to see. For example, outlining a container's opening with a dark marker, sewing a bright ribbon around

TABLE 12-11

Suggestions for Working With Children With Visual Impairments

METHOD TO USE	PURPOSE OF THE APPROACH
Use the children's names.	Helps reduce the feeling of isolation; alerts children that they are included in what is going on around them
Explain what is going to occur.	Helps create a relationship as well as helps children understand what is going on
Describe the room.	Helps children associate sounds, smells, and shapes
Walk the children to locations when possible.	Helps children develop space perception
Reduce extra noise.	Helps children identify sound clues
Use touch to introduce new things; brush objects on the back of the hand first.	Helps identify location and function of objects; helps children develop independence; and teaches children that their actions have a cause and effect
Explain new activities and surroundings.	Helps calm children who do not understand a new activity; helps them understand what is going to happen
Talk *to* the children, not *about* them.	Prevents underestimating the children's ability to understand what is said to them
Never assume that children with vision impairments see something.	Prevents assuming that children can see you and understand you

Data from Harrell L: *Touch the baby. Blind and visually impaired children as patients: Helping them respond to care*, New York, 1984, American Foundation for the Blind.

the neck and arm openings of a shirt, and reducing clutter on a desk surface are ways to improve contrast.

Children with total blindness often fill the void left by lack of visual stimulation with other forms of sensory self-stimulation called *blindisms*. Blindisms are consistent, repetitive movements that are proportional to the degree of blindness. Blindisms can take the form of body rocking or head shaking, which stimulates the vestibular system, or eye poking, which stimulates the optic nerve. These activities can become socially unacceptable, so more accepted forms of stimulation should be taught to these children.

CLINICAL *Pearl*

It is not unusual for children with cortical blindness to need corrective lenses or glasses because they are nearsighted or farsighted. A developmental optometrist can determine whether glasses would be beneficial.

CLINICAL *Pearl*

All children should have their eyes examined by age 3. A visual evoked response test that detects brain activity during visual stimulation can be administered to infants who are suspected of having vision problems.

CLINICAL *Pearl*

A fun and useful team game for children with vision impairments is "flashlight hide-and-seek." Darken a room and "hide" toys around the room. Shine a flashlight on one of the toys, and ask one of the children to find it. The team that finds the most toys wins. This is a great competitive game and a good way to stimulate children's visual pathways.

Hearing Impairments

About 28 million Americans have hearing loss, and about 2 million are profoundly deaf.[41] Few occupational therapists work with people who are deaf unless those individuals have other disabling conditions. Hearing loss accompanies many other developmental problems and can be caused by maternal infection during pregnancy. An undetected hearing loss causes developmental delays. Because a critical period exists for the acquisition of language skills, early detection of a hearing loss is very important.

Most OT services for individuals with hearing impairments address the related developmental delays. The first 4 years of life are the most important for language development. Impaired language skills affect all other areas of development, including social and environmental interactions and identification of objects. Early detection and treatment of hearing loss are essential for normal development in these areas. A vigilant therapist is aware of and able to identify the signs of hearing loss in children (Box 12-19). Parents often begin to suspect that their infant has a hearing loss when he or she is not awakened by loud noises or does not turn toward a noisy toy. Older infants who do not hear well will not pay attention to simple commands or give feedback to questions. Any infant or child who is suspected of having hearing loss should be referred for hearing testing. Younger infants can be given an evoked response audiometry test, which is a record of brain waves that occur in response to test sounds.

Several methods can be used to communicate with those with hearing impairment. "Total communication" includes lip reading, using oral speech, signing, and using gestures (Box 12-20). **American sign language** (ASL) is a rich and unique language but is often difficult for hearing parents to learn. Spradley recommends that children who have hearing loss "catch" ASL from friends at school who also have hearing loss and "catch" English

---

BOX 12-19

Possible Indications of Hearing Loss in Infants and Children

- Newborn has no startle reflex when hearing a loud noise.
- Three-month-old does not turn the head toward toys that make noise.
- Infant stops babbling around 6 months of age.
- Infants between 8 and 12 months old do not turn toward sounds coming from behind.
- Two-year-old does not use words.
- Two-year-old does not respond to requests such as "show me the ball."
- Three-year-old's speech is mostly unintelligible.
- Three-year-old skips beginning consonants of words.
- Three-year-old does not use two- or three-word sentences.
- Three-year-old uses mostly vowels.
- Child of any age speaks too loudly or too softly; voice has poor quality.
- Child always sounds like someone with a cold.

Adapted from Russel E & Nagiashi P. Services for children with visual or hearing impairments. In Case-Smith J, O'Brien J: *Occupational therapy for children*, ed 6, St. Louis, 2010, Mosby.

Suggestions for Total Communication

- Face the child at eye level.
- Be directly in front of the child so that your face and hands can be easily seen.
- Get the child's attention.
- Use good overhead lighting.
- Speak in a normal tone of voice.
- Say a word and sign it at the same time.
- Use appropriate pauses.
- Sit close to the child.
- Keep instructions simple.
- Be consistent.
- Talk to the child. Hearing impaired children need to "hear" the same amount of language as an average child.

Adapted from Russel E & Nagaishi P. Service for children with visual or hearing impairments. In Case-Smith J, O'Brien J: *Occupational therapy for children,* ed 6, St Louis, 2010, Mosby. pp. 772–774.

from parents by signing exact English (SEE), which is completely different from ASL.[22] Learning the seemingly foreign language of ASL is a huge task for new parents of children with hearing loss. While they are learning it, the vocabulary available from SEE enables communication between parent and child. Parents who know that their infants have hearing impairments can begin using SEE in the early months of the child's life. This allows the infant to "catch" English from the parents, making the infant bilingual as ASL is learned. The OT practitioner aids this process by using the signs taught in the home and introducing new signs for identifying new objects or activities during therapy. The signs chosen should relate to items or ideas the child understands, such as objects the child can see or touch or actions such as eating and dressing. Constant communication between the OT practitioner and the parents is vital to prevent confusion and to foster language growth in the child and everyone who is working with the child.

Helping a child to accept using a new hearing aid may be difficult because of tactile defensiveness (a physical and tactile over-reaction to objects). The head is often the most sensitive part of a child's body. The younger a child is fitted with hearing aids, the easier it is for the child to accept them. The aids must be thought of as clothing—necessary items that are put on each morning. An older child may need to start using new hearing aids during quiet times in speech-related activities. Hearing aids have recently undergone significant changes. Audiologists can now make more precise fittings to accommodate certain types of hearing loss. The aids are programmable and can be adjusted for factors such as background noise or voice levels. Because hearing aids are sensitive pieces of equipment, practitioners must be able to recognize their common malfunctions. Batteries often expire in approximately a week, depending on how much they are used. Batteries can also stop working because of corrosion or incorrect installation. An audible squeal coming from the hearing aid can be caused by a loose ear mold or incorrectly set switches. Ear molds often become plugged with wax, which blocks sound transmission.

General Sensory Disorganization

In some conditions, all of the child's sensory systems transmit information poorly, causing the perception of the world to be frightening. Changes in any one of the sensory systems affect development, making it difficult for these children to make sense of gross or fine motor activities or even their surroundings. For example, one way that the infant learns about the mother is through the sense of touch; if the perception of touch is not normal, the infant may perceive touch as painful or frightening. If the vestibular system (which detects movement) is not responsive, the infant may be happy only when he or she is moving or when held by someone who is walking. If several sensory systems are not functioning properly, behavior and development can be adversely affected as well as the relationship between infants and their parents or caregivers.

Fussy Baby

Infants can be fussy for many reasons, including maternal drug or alcohol abuse during pregnancy. (See sections titled "Effects of Cocaine Use" and "Fetal Alcohol Syndrome" in this chapter.) Infants with genetic problems such as Down syndrome may have general sensory disorganization. Children with a history of autism, ADD, ADHD, or learning disabilities were often fussy infants (Box 12-21). Families who already have members with learning disabilities, ADD, or ADHD are more likely to have fussy infants.[10,17]

The formal assessment of a fussy baby who is between the ages of 4 and 18 months is the Test of Sensory Functions in Infants (TSFI). The TSFI measures infants' reactions to touch or movement and their use of vision to locate the source of touch or respond to objects in their visual field. The test also evaluates their ability to move the body while playing. The results indicate how well infants use sensation to understand their environments and bodies. The level of functioning in the tested areas can affect all areas of learning throughout life.

Infants who cry constantly, particularly past the age of 3 months, may have problems with sensory

BOX 12-21

Characteristics of a Fussy Baby

- Having sleep problems
- Taking more than 20 minutes to fall asleep and waking up several times during the night
- Being difficult to calm; mother spends many hours trying to calm the infant during the day
- Being unable to calm self by putting hand in mouth or by looking at or listening to toys such as an infant mobile or music boxes
- Having feeding problems
- Not having an eating schedule
- Vomiting, refusing food, or having other problems unrelated to allergies
- Experiencing overarousal
- New types of stimulation or situations causing the infant to become overwhelmed and appear intense, wide eyed, or jittery

Data from DeGangi GA, Greenspan SI: *Test of sensory functions in infants*, Los Angeles, 1989, Western Psychological Services.

regulation (see Chapter 24) and not colic. Some characteristics of fussy babies are listed in Box 12-21. If these characteristics are recognized early, treatment can help the infant be more satisfied and less "fussy" or irritable. CNS calming techniques include, wrapping the infant in a warm blanket, swaddling, slow rocking, dimming lights, reducing noise, and giving a warm bath

or a gentle massage. Some children may calm down with sucking or when rubbed or patted on the back. OT practitioners work with family members to identify the infant's cues that he or she is becoming overstimulated or unhappy. Responding to the infant's cues may help reduce the infant's irritability. The results from the TSFI give a good indication of the level at which treatment should begin, but observing infants who are less than 4 months old and questioning their parents is also helpful (Table 12-12).

Language Delay and Language Impairments

Children develop language problems due to many reasons. Some children eventually learn to talk, others may learn only a few sentences, and still others may never learn any words at all. Children are often nonverbal because of other developmental problems caused by genetic disorders or because of neurologic conditions such as cerebral palsy. Major language delays seem to occur more often in boys, who often have several areas of sensory processing problems. Children with language delays can develop learning problems later.

OT practitioners model patience with children who do not talk or have trouble understanding speech. Most children use "prelanguage" before they start using speech as a form of communication; they point to an object to indicate that they want it or pull the parent or caregiver, for example, to the cookie jar to indicate

TABLE 12-12

Fussy Babies: Common Problems and Intervention Strategies

REACTION (PROBLEM)	POSSIBLE CAUSE	INTERVENTION STRATEGIES
Pulls away from the nipple	Very sensitive to touch in mouth	Use infant's fingers to rub lips, working into mouth and to gums and tongue. The baby eventually begins using own finger or a cloth to do same procedure.
Flails arms and legs and screams	Frightened by movement	Swaddle infant with baby blanket.
Hates wind-up swing, stroller, or other moving things; has a strong startle reaction to movement during activities such as dressing; scares self when moving independently	Frightened by movement	Swing the infant in "blanket hammock." Start with tiny swings and build up slowly to larger ones. Sit on a therapy ball, hold infant snuggly against chest facing you, and bounce or roll the ball slowly under hips. Start with tiny movements, and increase slowly to larger ones.
Wants bottle but is not hungry	Reduced feeling of sensation in mouth	Offer pacifier or heavily textured toys for chewing. Touch gums and tongue with pressure using cloth-wrapped finger.
Seems frightened or gags when touching some things with hands or feet	Feels the sensation too strongly or not strongly enough	Play with large pans of various materials such as rice or beans. First allow the infant to watch. Slowly encourage infant to touch the items in the pan. The goal is to get the infant's entire body into the pan.

they want a cookie. Children who are physically unable to move their limbs may indicate their needs with a smile or a gaze. Language comprehension develops before the child's ability to express himself or herself in words.

Other forms of communication can be used to reduce frustration while verbal skills are developing. Those children with fair or good hand control can learn words in ASL to aid in communication. Using signs during therapy sessions and at home may be the most convenient way for the child to communicate. Choose signs that have meaning in the child's everyday life. Another alternative for communication is a simple poster board to which pictures of people and objects commonly encountered in a particular child's everyday life are taped. In the case of young children, green- and red-colored shapes could be substituted for the words "yes" and "no," which are important for indicating choices. A more portable communication system can be created by using a small photo album with a single picture on each page.

General Interventions

OT interventions for sensory disorders frequently involve the following:

- Analysis of occupational performance, including the child's strengths and weaknesses and how they influence the child's performance
- Sensory activities to address tactile, proprioceptive, vestibular, auditory, and visual functions
- Activities designed to address sensory issues, such as visual games and auditory listening activities
- Analysis of the child's sensory needs and how to regulate his or her behaviors
- Educating family members and caregivers on the child's sensory needs
- Central nervous system strategies to change the child's sensory processing (e.g., calming techniques)
- Adaptive technology or compensatory strategies to allow the child to engage in a variety of occupations
- Techniques and strategies to help the child regulate his or her sensory processing for occupational performance
- Cognitive–behavioral techniques to facilitate goal setting and occupational performance
- Helping the child maintain and organize care of adaptive devices (e.g., hearing aid, glasses)
- Expose the child to a variety of interesting activities to develop volition and feelings of self-efficacy
- Successful achievements that will help the child develop self-concept and positive self-esteem

OTHER PEDIATRIC HEALTH CONDITIONS
Burns

Burns are a major cause of a large number of children and adolescents having to undergo prolonged, painful hospitalization. Burns result from accidents involving thermal, electrical, chemical, and radioactive agents.

A thermal burn is caused by hot objects or flames, such as heat from an open fire, an iron, stove, or the tip of a cigarette. An electrical burn results from skin or other body tissue coming into contact with electricity, such as from lightning or a direct electrical current coming from an outlet or plug. A chemical burn is caused by a chemical substance such as acid or some other poison (i.e., something or some substance that is destructive or fatal). A radioactive burn is caused by rays or waves of radiation that come into contact with body tissue.

Thermal burns are the most common of the four types.[14] Specific criteria determine the severity of a burn and the prognosis for recovery. The percentage of body area burned is assessed according to the total body surface area (TBSA) by the *rule of nines* in children older than 10. According to the rule of nines, 9% is assigned to the head and both arms, 18% to each leg, 18% to both the anterior (front) and posterior (back) of the trunk, and 1% to the perineum. The formula is modified for infants and young children because of their proportionately larger head size. (See Figure 12-11 for the percentage of distribution per area of the body.)

The American Burn Association also classifies burns as *minor, moderate,* and *severe.*[2] In minor burns, less than 10% of the TBSA is covered with a **partial-thickness** burn; these burns are adequately treated on an outpatient basis. A moderate burn is considered 10% to 20% of the TBSA covered with a partial-thickness burn; it requires hospitalization. Any full-thickness burn or greater than 20% of the TBSA covered with a partial-thickness burn is considered a major burn.[2,14]

The depth of a burn is assessed according to the number of layers of tissue involved in the injury (Figure 12-12). Superficial or first-degree burns damage tissue minimally and heal without scarring. Second-degree burns are partial-thickness burns and involve the epidermis and portions of the dermis. Although second-degree burns will heal, the process can be painful and scarring may be a result. Deep-thickness burns can be third- or fourth-degree (involving muscle) burns and require emergency and ongoing medical intervention. During the **acute medical management** of a child or adolescent who has been seriously burned, the prevention of secondary infections, wound débridement (cleaning), and wound closure are critical. During the **rehabilitation** phase of intervention, team members work closely to accomplish the outcomes of healing of the body structures involved, correction of

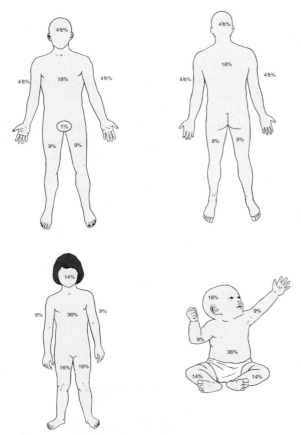

FIGURE 12-11 Percentage of distribution per area of the body. (From *Mosby's medical, nursing, and allied health dictionary*, ed 6, St. Louis, 2002, Mosby.)

cosmetic damage, reduction and management of scar tissue, restoration of function, and reintegration into the child's or adolescent's natural environment (Table 12-13).

OT clinicians working with child and adolescent burn victims begin by providing orthoses to keep the limb immobile to aid healing and later to facilitate function. They work closely with physical therapists on débridement and pain management techniques and can help with ways to compensate for physical limitations or regain physical skills. Facilitating play/leisure activities helps these children and adolescents release emotions and return to their occupations. OT practitioners may address their psychological concerns through play, self-concept activities, and discussion and help them learn, through participating in everyday occupations, how they may function despite the effects of the burns.

NEOPLASTIC DISORDERS

A *neoplasm* is an abnormal new growth of tissue (a tumor). It may be localized (in one place) or invasive (in multiple tissues and organs). It may be benign (not

immediately life threatening) or malignant (possibly cause death). Tumors are named for location, type of cellular makeup, or the person who first identified it.[4]

Leukemia

Leukemia comprises a group of pediatric health conditions involving various acute and chronic tumor disorders of the bone marrow. A child or adolescent who has leukemia may experience an abnormal increase in white blood cells; enlargement of the lymph nodes, liver, and spleen; and impaired blood clotting. These body function deficits can cause pain, fatigue, weight loss, recurrent infections, excessive bruising, and/or hemorrhaging (Box 12-22). Medical interventions may include treatment with antibiotics, chemotherapy, and blood transfusion. Referral to an occupational therapist is made because of secondary disorders and/or complications.

Tumors of the Central Nervous System

Tumors of the CNS (i.e., those located in the brain and/or spinal cord) are the most common ones of solid tissue in children and adolescents.[8,12] The causes of CNS tumors are unknown. Medical interventions vary with differential diagnoses.

Bone Cancer and Tumors

Primary (first to develop) bone tumors are rare during childhood, with the incidence peaking during adolescence. Often, *bone cancer* results from metastasis, or spreading, to bone from the primary tumor(s) located in a different body structure. Medical interventions may include surgery and radiotherapy. Children with neoplastic disorders may require OT interventions to help the child catch up with school work after missing many days due to surgery or other medical interventions (Table 12-14). These children may experience physical symptoms and require OT interventions on compensatory strategies. OT practitioners may address the emotional needs of the children and their families by instituting play therapy.

IMMUNOLOGIC CONDITIONS
Chronic Fatigue Syndrome

CASE *Study*

In the past, 14-year-old Rachel had experienced some growing pains and had felt under the weather. Lately she has been waking up tired every morning. Her symptoms started with a flu-like illness and sore throat that would not go away. Now she has tremendous difficulty just

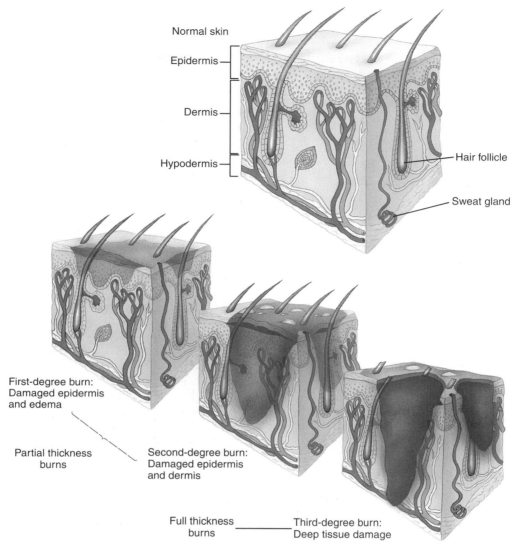

Normal skin

Epidermis

Dermis

Hypodermis

Hair follicle

Sweat gland

First-degree burn:
Damaged epidermis
and edema

Partial thickness
burns

Second-degree burn:
Damaged epidermis
and dermis

Full thickness
burns

Third-degree burn:
Deep tissue damage

FIGURE 12-12 Classification of burns. (From Thibodeau GA, Patton KT: *Anatomy and physiology*, ed 5, St. Louis, 2003, Mosby.)

getting through each day; she falls asleep every time she sits down. Despite her fatigue, she cannot sleep more than 1 or 2 hours at night before she wakes up because of muscle jerks and covered with sweat . Every morning, she gets out of bed feeling shaky. On some days, she experiences sudden weak spells and sweats. Sometimes she feels like she is going to pass out. At other times, her heart races, and she feels like she is having a panic attack. She has been having problems with an irritable bowel and experiences alternating constipation and loose stools. She has also started having trouble with bladder infections and reduced bladder control. On many days, her muscles feel stiff and sore. Nothing the family doctor tried has helped her.

One day her brother found a Web site with information describing Rachel's condition perfectly; the Web site called it *chronic fatigue syndrome* (CFS) (Box 12-23). The family doctor agreed with the diagnosis and said that Rachel was also one of the 40% of people with CFS and reactive hypoglycemia.[11] *Hypoglycemia* means a low blood glucose level, and it has been the cause of Rachel's panic attacks, sweats, shakiness, and feelings of weakness. Realizing that Rachel fatigued easily and that repetitive motions such as those used for writing could be painful, her doctor referred her for an OT consultation. The OT practitioner recommended that Rachel obtain copies of notes from her classmates, have a second set of books for home use, and an elevator pass so that she need not climb any stairs at school. The OT practitioner also prescribed a builtup pen that would help reduce Rachel's muscle fatigue while writing. The OT practitioner helped

TABLE 12-13

Burns: General Intervention Considerations

CONSIDERATION	DEFINITION AND EXAMPLE(S)
Positioning and orthotics	Orthoses in functional position to initially aid in healing and later orthoses to increase function.
ROM	Use passive and active ROM techniques to promote full AROM and PROM.
Engagement in occupations	Provide remediation, adaptation, and modification so that the child may participate in occupations.
Social participation	Help the child return to social situations.
Scar tissue management	Use orthoses, desensitization techniques, and pressure garments to decrease scarring.
Edema management	Use retrograde massage, gentle ranging, and elevation to manage edema
Self-concept	Help the child participate in occupations to develop positive self-concept.
Psychological/emotional issues	Provide a range of activities to help the child work through emotional difficulties associated with burns. Children who have burns may have issues with body image.

ROM, range of motion; *AROM*, active range of motion; *PROM*, passive range of motion.

BOX 12-22

Neoplastic Disorders: General Signs and Symptoms

- Loss of weight
- Night sweats
- Chronic fatigue
- Recurrent headaches
- Vomiting
- Changes in behavior
- Pain
- Lumps
- Misalignment of bones or joints
- Evident growths on bone

Rachel identify roles and figure out solutions so she could feel engaged in leisure and educational activities. The OT practitioner and Rachel found solutions together on how best to simplify school work so that Rachel may have some time for social activities (despite her consistent fatigue and pain).

A number of adolescents and younger children experience CFS. The symptoms develop gradually or linger after a bout of flu. At least half of the children born to parents who have CFS are suspected to also be affected.[3,9,11]

Forty percent of people with CFS also have reactive hypoglycemia.[25] Hypoglycemia can cause individuals to feel as though they are having panic attacks or are simply anxious. It can also cause racing of the heart, shakiness, and fatigue.[40] A promising medical treatment that puts this combination of conditions into remission in both children and adults is being developed (See www.FibromyalgiaTreatment.com).

Children with CFS may be also referred for OT for the treatment of attention deficit disorder (ADD) or ADHD (see Box 12-16). These conditions may be caused by symptoms of CFS, such as pain and fatigue. Children in pain may move around constantly to alleviate the pain or to wake themselves up. This distracts them from their schoolwork and activities and results in poor academic performance.[25] These children also experience difficulty with social relationships.

Children with CFS may require help with work simplification, self-care skills, or adaptive equipment because of the fatigue, cognitive problems, or pain that they experience. Once their condition has been identified, the children may benefit from the use of builtup pencils that ease finger pain and fatigue.

Taylor et al found that adolescents who developed CFS after mononucleosis infection showed equal interest in participating in a variety of activities (values) but less belief in their ability to do so (perceived competency) than did adolescents who did not develop CFS at baseline and over time.[42] Taylor et al used the Occupational Self-Assessment tool to measure values and perceived competency.[42] This study recommended that OT practitioners working with adolescents with CFS explore self-efficacy and performance in occupations.

Human Immunodeficiency Virus

Human immunodeficiency virus (HIV) causes the immune system to shut down, which results in many different problems as early as the first 1 or 2 years of life.

TABLE 12-14

Neoplastic Conditions: General Intervention Considerations

CONSIDERATION	DEFINITION AND EXAMPLE(S)
Energy conservation	Children with neoplastic conditions may benefit from learning ways to perform occupations with less physical stress. For example, sitting down while getting ready for school conserves energy.
Compensation techniques	The children may experience physical symptoms and require strategies to perform everyday tasks (e.g., using the left hand instead of the right for eating).
Psychosocial/emotional issues	The children may miss school and feel "left out." They may experience the full range of emotions and stress of a life-threatening illness. Families may be in turmoil over the illness. The children may feel alone and require intervention to help them deal with the illness so that they may engage in their occupations.
Adaptive equipment	Adaptive equipment may be recommended to assist the children in their occupations. For example, positioning young children on a bath seat may make bath time easier for the caregiver.
Engagement in occupations	Children may feel "left out" of regular activities and require participation in occupations to regain a sense of being. OT practitioners can help the children return to school, home, and play activities through education, assistive technology, and compensation techniques.

Early symptoms may be failure to thrive (FTT), fever, and diarrhea. Half of all HIV-infected infants develop full-blown *acquired immunodeficiency syndrome* (AIDS) by the age of 3 years.[10] A woman infected with HIV can pass the virus on to her infant during pregnancy, delivery, or breastfeeding. Infants born to women who are infected before or during pregnancy and who receive no medical treatment have about a 25% chance of being born with the HIV infection. Medical treatment with zidovudine (AZT) during pregnancy and labor may reduce the risk of infant infection to about 1 in 12. Mothers with HIV infection may pass the virus through breastfeeding. Treating infants with AZT for the first several weeks of life can reduce but not prevent the risk of infection.[10]

Children with AIDS may have delayed motor or cognitive development. They may not meet developmental milestones or attain certain intellectual skills and may develop microencephaly.[30] The loss of social skills and language occurs in about 20% of children with AIDS. Paralysis, tremors, spasticity, and balance problems can also develop, and major organ systems are damaged. Half of the infants born with AIDS develop pneumonia by 15 months, a common cause of death.[4] Children with AIDS-related complex (ARC) have HIV infection and some symptoms but no serious infections.[4] In the United States, 2% of all individuals with AIDS are children or adolescents. In 90% of pediatric AIDS cases, children have been infected at birth by receiving the virus from their mothers (Boxes 12-24 and 12-25).[7,12]

CLINICAL *Pearl*

Monitoring for developmental delays is one of the main goals of occupational therapy for children with acquired immune deficiency syndrome (AIDS). Because their mothers are frequently ill as well, the occupational therapist coordinates care for the mothers and their children.

Latex Allergy

Between 18% and 40% of children who have spina bifida or frequent surgeries and those who use catheters for congenital urinary tract problems are likely to develop sensitivity to latex.[34] However, anyone who has frequent exposure to latex through work or surgery can develop an allergy. A reaction can occur after breathing latex dust from an open package or contact between latex and skin, mucous membranes, open lesions, or blood. Coming into contact with a person or object that has just been in contact with latex can cause a reaction. Symptoms include watery eyes, wheezing, hives, rash, and swelling. Severe reactions can result in *anaphylaxis*, a system-wide body reaction that affects heart rate and the ability to breathe, which can be fatal.[34]

More children are developing allergies to latex since the institution of **universal precautions** that require the use of latex gloves to prevent the spread of infection; latex is also used in many health care products, such as tapes, bottle nipples, and catheters. Exposure to latex increases the chance for an allergy.

BOX 12-23

Symptoms of Chronic Fatigue, Immune Dysfunction Syndrome, and Fibromyalgia

Children may have several or all of the following symptoms or conditions:

- Growing pains
- Frequent periods of not feeling well
- Attention deficit disorder (ADD)
- Sleep disturbances or insomnia
- Irritable bowel syndrome
  - Gas or bloating
  - Periods of alternating constipation and diarrhea or loose stools
- Urinary tract problems
  - Reduced bladder control
  - Bladder infections
  - Painful urination
- Deep aches in calves and other muscles
- Frequent and severe headaches
- Lack of stamina
- Short-term memory loss
- Neurologic problems
  - Shooting leg pains
  - Restless leg syndrome (feeling a constant need to move the legs)
  - Muscle tics or twitches
  - Numbness
- Reactive hypoglycemia
  - Racing heartbeat
  - Shakiness
  - Blacking out
  - Sweats
  - Anxiety or panic attacks

From St. Amand RP: *What your doctor may not tell you about pediatric fibromyalgia*, New York, 2002, Warner Books.

BOX 12-24

Precautions for Working With Children

- Wear gloves when coming into contact with blood or secretions.
- Mix 1 oz of bleach with 10 oz of water, and use this solution to disinfect surfaces.
- Dress all cuts and sores.
- Wash your hands and/or body parts immediately after contact with blood.
- Use sharp instruments only when necessary.

Adapted from the Centers for Disease Control: http://www.cdc.gov/mmwr/preview/mmwrhtml/rr5811a1.htm Accessed June 14, 2010.

BOX 12-25

Transmission of Human Immunodeficiency Virus

Human immunodeficiency virus (HIV) does not survive well in the environment. Simply drying a surface contaminated with HIV kills 90% to 99% of the virus. HIV exists in different concentrations in the blood, semen, vaginal fluid, breast milk, saliva, and tears. Infection occurs when blood or body secretions that could contain visible blood, such as urine, vomit, or feces, come into contact with an open wound or mucous membranes, which are found inside the mouth, nose, eyes, vagina, and rectum. The concentration of the virus in saliva, sweat, and tears is low, and no case of HIV infection through these fluids has been documented.

Adapted from the Centers for Disease Control: http://www.cdc.gov/mmwr/preview/mmwrhtml/rr5811a1.htm Accessed June 14, 2010.

OT practitioners avoid using latex in the clinic by substituting Mylar balloons for latex balloons and by wearing vinyl gloves instead of latex gloves. OT practitioners and parents check the labels of tapes or any other substances that may contain rubber products. The OT practitioner cautions parents and caregivers about possible allergies and educates parents on the symptoms of allergies.

CLINICAL *Pearl*

Children who are allergic to latex may also be allergic to bananas, avocados, and kiwi fruit because they are all from the same plant family as latex. Being around latex and consuming any of these fruits may heighten the reaction.

ENVIRONMENTALLY INDUCED AND ACQUIRED CONDITIONS

Environmentally induced and acquired conditions can develop before or after birth and are directly related to factors found in the environment. Contributing factors include drugs, toxic chemicals, allergens, and viruses.

Failure to Thrive

CASE *Study*

Nathan was born 5 weeks early and weighed only 3 lb. He was resuscitated twice in the delivery room because his breathing had stopped. He left the delivery room in an incubator, and he was put on a respirator on his arrival at the neonatal intensive care unit (NICU). Because he was too weak to suckle, he was fed through the nose by a tube that went to his stomach (a nasogastric [NG] tube). Wires were taped to his chest to monitor his heart beat and to his head to measure brain activity. When Nathan was born, he was too ill to be held by anyone, including his parents. Four weeks after he was born Nathan had not grown in length and had gained only a few ounces. After all his equipment was removed, Nathan was handed to his mother for the first time. She rocked him and sang to him in the NICU. Two months later, after his parents had spent every day touching, rocking, and talking to him, Nathan weighed 4.5 lb and was able to go home with his parents.

Failure to thrive (FTT) can be a symptom of another acute or chronic condition or can be a condition in itself. When FTT is a symptom of another condition, it usually becomes obvious by the age of 6 months. Weight gain is the most accurate indicator of an infant's nutritional status. Delayed growth in height usually indicates more severe and prolonged poor nutrition. A reduced head growth rate suggests severe malnutrition because the body provides energy to the brain before it does to any other organ (Box 12-26).[10]

When infants fail to thrive but have no other physical conditions (i.e., they are physically normal at birth and have contracted no illnesses after birth), the cause usually is neglect or lack of appropriate stimulation. This type of FTT can occur at any age. Hospitalized infants or children may fail to thrive because of lack of social stimulation; an infant of a parent who is depressed or has poor parenting skills may fail to thrive. Another group of infants who may experience FTT includes those who are premature and those with feeding problems caused by neurologic or orthopedic factors (such as cleft palate) or poor sucking ability caused by cerebral palsy or sensory problems.

Children with FTT present with feeding issues such as poor suck–swallow–breathe synchrony, tactile sensitivity, delayed oral-motor skills, and decreased variability in their diets. OT personnel must provide evaluation and

---

BOX 12-26

Signs of Failure to Thrive

- Weight persistently less than 3% on growth charts
- Weight less than 80% of ideal for height and age
- Progressive loss of weight to below third percentile
- Decrease in expected growth rate compared with previous pattern

Data from Berkow R, editor: *The Merck manual*, ed 17, Rahway, NJ, 1999, Merck.

---

interventions in these areas. An important aspect of the treatment of FTT includes parental or caregiver training on feeding issues. Children who need to gain weight may require frequent high-calorie snacks throughout the day. Therefore, consultation with a nutritionist or dietitian may be warranted. Children with FTT may require interventions aimed at improving sensory modulation and development. Occupational therapists must work closely with families and caregivers to help children with FTT.

Fetal Alcohol Syndrome

The use of alcohol during pregnancy is the most common cause of birth defects. *Fetal alcohol syndrome* (FAS) occurs in 2 to 6 births out of 1000.[9,10,12] The infants of chronic drinkers are the most severely affected. Alcohol consumption during pregnancy causes intellectual disability, microencephaly, small facial features, poor development of the corpus callosum, and heart defects. Characteristic facial features include a turned-up nose and small jaws; a cleft lip or palate may be present. Children with FAS may also experience FTT and be fussy. One or more of these problems can result in developmental delays. Hyperactivity can develop and adversely affect attention span and learning. Children with FAS are frequently hypotonic, have poor coordination, and may have sensory processing difficulties.[12] Infants or children with milder cases of FAS may be referred for OT treatment for hyperactivity caused by a sensory processing disorder. Later, the children may develop learning problems as they grow older. Fine motor and visual perception skills must be assessed.

Effects of Cocaine Use

Cocaine use by the mother during pregnancy can produce malformations of the fetus's arms, legs, bowel, bladder, and genitals. It can cause poor blood flow to the placenta, causing a miscarriage or neurologic damage in developing infants. Some may experience bleeding in the brain at birth. The infants of mothers who use cocaine near the time of birth will experience withdrawal symptoms after birth. Symptoms include vomiting and diarrhea, irritability, sweating, convulsions, and hyperventilation. Tightly wrapping the infants and feeding them frequently to calm them can help alleviate the symptoms of mild withdrawal.[10]

The development of infants exposed to cocaine before birth can be unpredictable. OT practitioners carefully assess all developmental areas to determine the areas needing intervention. Because of possible neurologic involvement, sensory integration evaluation and monitoring should be included. Treatment is highly individualized so that it can meet each child's unique needs.

Lead Poisoning

It is estimated that about four million children in the United States have in them high enough lead levels that will slow their development.[23] Although many environmental toxins exist, lead is the one that most commonly affects children. Children living in older homes have a greater risk of exposure to lead in peeling paint (which children sometimes eat) and to lead used in plumbing. Lead is no longer used in these materials; however, children can eat or breathe lead from contaminated air, food, water, and soil as well. Some industries, such as battery manufacturing, produce higher air and dust levels of lead than do other industries. Parents working in these industries can carry lead home from work on their clothing. Mothers with high lead levels can pass it to their infants during gestation. Mild lead toxicity produces muscle aches and fatigue, and moderate levels cause fatigue, headaches, cramping, vomiting, and weight loss. High toxicity levels in infants causes intellectual disability, behavior problems, seizures, and sometimes death. Even low toxicity levels can affect intelligence and behavior.[3,10,12]

Allergies to Foods and Chemicals

The use of art supplies, construction materials, and various foods during pediatric OT should be carefully assessed so that children's developing bodies are not unnecessarily exposed to toxic chemicals, toxic materials, and allergy-producing foods. Always check with parents or guardians about their children's food allergies before using any food item for an art project or feeding therapy (Box 12-27). Toxic chemical fumes or materials may cause asthma, skin irritation, anaphylaxis, or other unseen damage that can accumulate over time. Always ensure that the materials used in therapy are nontoxic. Avoid using latex products when another substitute is available.

General Interventions

OT interventions for the conditions discussed above frequently involve the following:

- Analysis of occupational performance, including the child's strengths and weaknesses and how they influence the child's performance
- Activities designed to address development (e.g., gross, fine, language, cognitive, social)
- Analysis of the child's emotional needs and how to regulate his or her behaviors
- Education of family members and caregivers on how the child's condition may affect his or her occupational performance, including supports he or she may need to be successful

---

BOX 12-27

Most Common Foods Associated With Food Allergies

- Wheat
- Soy
- Corn
- Eggs
- Peanuts
- Milk
- Citrus foods
- Tree nuts
- Shellfish

Adapted from University of Maryland Medicine: http://www.umm.edu/pediatric-info/food.htm: Accessed June 14, 2010.

- Adaptive technology or compensatory strategies to allow the child to engage in a variety of occupations
- Cognitive–behavioral techniques to facilitate goal setting and occupational performance
- Helping the child maintain and organize care of adaptive devices
- Organizational strategies to help the child develop roles and occupations.
- Resources to help the family and the child achieve goals
- Awareness of allergies and environmental hindrances to development
- Exposing the child to a variety of interesting activities to help develop volition and feelings of self-efficacy
- Successful achievement to develop self-concept and positive self-esteem

ROLE OF OCCUPATIONAL THERAPY ASSISTANT AND OCCUPATIONAL THERAPIST IN ASSESSMENT AND INTERVENTION

An occupational therapist must supervise an OTA when providing OT services to infants and children. The level of supervision required depends on many variables. The occupational therapist is responsible for interpreting assessment data and developing intervention plans. The OTA may assist in collecting assessment data and help develop intervention plans with the occupational therapist. The OTA provides direct intervention and consults with the occupational therapist on the status of a plan and possible changes to it. The level of supervision depends on the OTA's level of experience and service competency as well as how well the occupational therapist and the OTA know each other's abilities. It is likely that the occupational therapist and the OTA will work more closely while developing a trusting relationship.

SUMMARY

This chapter presented an introduction to various pediatric health conditions. At the end of each section, general signs and symptoms and general intervention considerations were presented. These considerations on intervention were also presented in tables. Working with children can be a rewarding experience for OT practitioners. However, meeting the needs of children is a complex task. OT practitioners must not only meet the needs of their clients, but they must also educate their clients' families and caregivers. Knowing the common characteristics of children's conditions helps OT practitioners provide a focus for the initial assessment and intervention plan. These two components reveal that although the various conditions have some common characteristics, the needs of the children and their families are unique and must be addressed individually.

References

1. Alexander RC, Smith WL: Shaken baby syndrome. *Infants Young Child* 10:1, 1998.
2. American Burn Association: White paper: Surgical management of burn wound and use of skin substitutes, 2009. Available at: http://ameriburn.org/WhitePaperFinal.pdf. Accessed June 14, 2010.
3. American Psychiatric Association: *Diagnostic and statistical manual of mental disorders* (DSM IV), ed 4, text revision, Washington, DC, 2000, American Psychiatric Association.
4. Anderson DM et al: *Mosby's medical, nursing, and allied health dictionary,* ed 6, St. Louis, 2002, Mosby
5. Arthritis Foundation: Juvenile rheumatoid arthritis: What is it? Available at: http://www.arthritis.org/disease-center.php?disease_id=38. Accessed June 14, 2010.
6. Ayres AJ: *Sensory integration and learning disorders,* Los Angeles, 1972, Western Psychological Services.
7. Ayres AJ, Mailloux ZK, Wendler CL: Developmental dyspraxia: is it a unitary function? *Occup J Res* 7:93, 1987.
8. Barnhart SL, Czervinche MP: *Perinatal and pediatric respiratory care,* Philadelphia, 1995, Saunders.
9. Batshaw M, editor: *Children with disabilities,* ed 5, Baltimore, 2002, Paul H. Brookes Publishers.
10. Beers MH et al: *The Merck manual,* ed 18, Rahway, NJ, 2006, Merck.
11. Bell DS et al: Primary juvenile fibromyalgia syndrome and chronic fatigue syndrome in adolescents. *Clin Infect Dis* 18:21, 1994.
12. Blackman J, MacQueen JC, Biehl RI: *Mosby's resource guide to children with disabilities and chronic illness,* St Louis, 1997, Mosby.
13. Bundy A, Lanc S, Murray E: *Sensory integration: theory and practice,* ed 2, Philadelphia, 2002, FA Davis.
14. Case-Smith J, O'Brien J: *Occupational therapy for children,* ed 6, St Louis, 2010, Mosby.
15. Centers for Disease Control and Prevention: 2001. Available at: www.cdc.gov/nip/vacsafe/concerns/autism/autism-factshtm. Accessed August 28, 2010.
16. Crosse SB, Kaye E, Ratnofsky AC: *Report on the maltreatment of children with disabilities,* Washington, DC, 1993, National Center on Child Abuse and Neglect, U.S. Department of Health and Human Services.
17. DeGangi GA, Greenspan SI: *Test of sensory functions in infants,* Los Angeles, 1990, Western Psychological Services.
18. Fox AM, Lent B: Clumsy children: primer on developmental coordination disorder. *Can Fam Physician* 42:1965, 1996.
19. Fragile-X Research Foundation: About fragile X. Available at: http://www.fraxa.org/aboutFX.aspx. Accessed June 14, 2010.
20. Geuze RH, Kalverboer AF: Tapping a rhythm: a problem of timing for children who are clumsy and dyslexic. *Adapt Phys Activ Q,* 11:203, 1994.
21. Gubbay SS: Clumsiness. In Frederiks JAM, editor: *Handbook of clinical neurology: neurobehavioral disorders,* vol 2, Amsterdam, 1985, Elsevier.
22. Gustason G et al: *Signing exact English,* Los Alamitos, CA, 1994, Modern Signs Press.
23. Haan MN, Gerson M, Zishka BA: Identification of children at risk for lead poisoning: an evaluation of routine pediatric blood lead screening in an HMO-insured population. *Am Acad Pediatr* 97:84, 1996.
24. Hall D: Clumsy children. *BMJ* 296:375, 1988.
25. Henderson SE, Hall D: Concomitants of clumsiness in young school children. *Dev Med Child Neurol* 24:448, 1982.
26. Klein S, Magill-Evans J: Perceptions of competence and peer acceptance in young children with motor and learning difficulties. *Phys Occup Ther Pediatr* 18:39, 1998.
27. Losse A et al: Clumsiness in children—do they grow out of it? A 10-year follow-up study. *Dev Med Child Neurol* 33:55, 1991.
28. Michaud LF et al: Traumatic brain injury. In Batshaw M, editor: *Children with disabilities,* ed 5, Baltimore, 2002, Paul H. Brookes Publishers.
29. Missiuna C, Polatjko HJ: Developmental dyspraxia by any other name. *Am J Occup Ther* 49:619, 1995.
30. National Institute of Allergy and Infectious Diseases: Backgrounder: HIV infection in infants and children. Available at: http://www.niaid.nih.gov/news/Pages/default.aspx. Accessed June 14, 2010.
31. Optometrists Network: What is vision therapy? Available at: http://www.children-special-needs.org/vision_therapy/what_is_vision_therapy.html. Accessed June 14, 2010.
32. Prader-Willi Syndrome Association: What is Prader-Willi Syndrome? Available at: www.pwsausa.org. Accessed June 14, 2010.
33. Pronsati MP: Erb's palsy. *Adv Occup Ther* 7:19, 1991.
34. Romanczuk A: Latex use with infants and children: it can cause problems. *Matern Child Nurs* 18:208, 1993.
35. Salter RB, Dudos JP: The first fifteen years' experience with innominate osteotomy in the treatment of developmental hip dysplasia and subluxation of the hip. *Clin Orthop* 98:72, 1974.
36. Schoemaker MM, Kalverboer AF: Social and affective problems of children who are clumsy: how early do they begin? *Adapt Phys Activ Q* 11:130, 1994.

37. Sellars JS: Clumsiness: review of causes, treatment, and outlook. *Phys Occup Ther Pediatr* 15:39, 1995.

38. Shaw L, Levin MD, Belfer M: Developmental double jeopardy: a study of clumsiness and self-esteem in children with learning problems. *Dev Behav Pediatr* 3:191, 1982.

39. Shriners Hospitals for Children: Arthrogryposis. Available at: http://www.shrinershq.org/sitecore/content/Hospitals/LosAngeles/Services/Arthrogryposis.aspx?sc_database=master. Accessed June 14, 2010.

40. St. Amand RP: *What your doctor may not tell you about pediatric fibromyalgia*, New York, 2002, Warner Books.

41. Stancliff B: Silent services: treating deaf clients. *OT Practice* 3:27, 1998.

42. Taylor R et al: The occupational and quality of life consequences of chronic fatigue syndrome in adolescents. *Br J Occup Ther* (in press).

43. Williams HG, Woolacott MH, Ivry R: Timing and motor control in clumsy children. *J Mot Behav* 24:165, 1992.

REVIEW *Questions*

1. Explain the difference between a central nervous system condition and a peripheral nervous system condition.

2. What are the three types of juvenile rheumatoid arthritis? Describe them. What functional limitations are caused by each type?

3. Name the four spinal conditions discussed in this chapter. In what way does each affect the functional performance of the child?

4. Describe the reason an OTA must have a good understanding of the symptoms and signs of a child's condition before performing the initial assessment. In what way does this aid in treatment?

5. Describe two genetic syndromes. Explain the ways they affect a child's ADL skills.

6. Using information you have learned about sensory systems, explain why it is important to treat sensory system problems early.

7. What are the differences among legal blindness, total blindness, and cortical blindness? In what ways are they the same? In what ways can you make learning easier for a child who has vision impairments?

8. In what ways does an undetected hearing loss affect a child's early development?

9. Name three avoidable environmental factors that affect infants either before or after birth. Explain how these factors can cause developmental delays.

10. Describe *arthrogryposis*. In what ways can it affect a child's daily functioning?

11. What are the four types of burns? Define each, and identify which is the most common.

12. Describe intervention strategies used for children with various pediatric conditions.

SUGGESTED *Activities*

1. Visit a class of children with special needs, and observe the children at work. During your visit, observe and keep a list of the ways each child's condition affects the ability to do schoolwork. Later, make a list of suggestions you think might improve each child's ability to do schoolwork.

2. Spend some time at an outpatient clinic observing children receiving OT services. Make a list of characteristics observed in individual children. Later, try to identify each child's possible condition or which of the systems is/are involved.

3. Spend some time observing a child with a disability who is playing. Write down ways that the child's condition affects his or her ability to play.

4. Talk with a family that has a child with a disability. Before the interview, use the knowledge you have gained from this chapter to make a list of the way(s) you would expect the child's disability to affect the family. During the interview, make notes about the family's comments. Later, compare your initial list with the family's comments. How accurate were your expectations?

5. Interview a firefighter to consider the different types of fires and burns and client factors in the persons he or she has rescued.

6. Interview a family member of a child who has a diagnosis presented in this chapter. Develop a handout on the particular diagnosis for the child's siblings.

7. Using the tables as your guide, develop activities related to each type of pediatric condition described in this chapter.

Childhood and Adolescent Psychosocial and Mental Health Disorders

KERRYELLEN G. VROMAN

JANE CLIFFORD O'BRIEN

CHAPTER *Objectives*

After studying this chapter, the reader will be able to accomplish the following:

- Define psychosocial occupational therapy practice for children and adolescents.
- Recognize the signs of behavioral and mental health disorders seen in children and adolescents.
- Recognize the symptoms of behavioral and mental health disorders seen in children and adolescents.
- Assist in the occupational therapy evaluation process.
- Recognize typical assessments used by the occupational therapy practitioner to develop intervention.
- Use evaluation results to guide mental health and psychosocial practice.
- Be familiar with types of frames of reference that direct intervention in psychosocial practice.
- Select activities that support evidence-based practice.
- Be familiar with the types of group intervention for children and adolescents.

| KEY TERMS | CHAPTER OUTLINE |

Understanding Mental Health Disorders

Disruptive Behavior Disorders
ATTENTION DEFICITS HYPERACTIVITY DISORDER
PREDOMINANTLY HYPERACTIVITY: IMPULSIVE TYPE
CONDUCT DISORDER: CHILDHOOD-ONSET
OPPOSITIONAL DEFIANT DISORDER

Learning Disorders

Tic Disorders
TOURETTE'S SYNDROME

Anxiety Disorders
SEPARATION ANXIETY DISORDER
GENERALIZED ANXIETY DISORDER
PHOBIC AND SOCIAL ANXIETY DISORDERS
OBSESSIVE-COMPULSIVE DISORDER
POST-TRAUMATIC STRESS DISORDER

Mood Disorders
MAJOR DEPRESSIVE DISORDER
BIPOLAR DISORDER

Schizophrenia

Eating Disorders
ANOREXIA NERVOSA
BULIMIA NERVOSA

Substance-related Disorders
INHALANT ABUSE
IMPLICATIONS FOR OCCUPATIONAL PERFORMANCE

Data Gathering and Evaluation

Intervention
PLANNING
IMPLEMENTATION

Therapeutic Use of Self

Summary

Occupational therapy (OT) practitioners employed in all pediatric settings (early intervention programs and school systems) provide **psychosocial occupational therapy** to address children's mental health, since physical and emotional well-being through successful participation and adaptation is a fundamental goal of therapy. In addition, some children and their families are referred to OT because their mental health disorders interfere with successful occupational performance and participation. The performance problems associated with these disorders include regulating and controlling behaviors, interacting and collaborating with other children, forming and maintaining friendships, relating to and taking directions from adults, and attending to tasks.[8] Children diagnosed with mental disorders also present as having difficulties in regulating emotions, organizing thoughts, and demonstrating appropriate behaviors.

The overall focus of this chapter is mental health disorders and behavioral problems that present in childhood and adolescence. The descriptions of childhood mental health disorders in this chapter are consistent with the diagnostic criteria of the *Diagnostic and Statistical Manual of Mental Disorders (DSM-VI-TR)*.[5] These diagnostic categories assist health care professionals to describe and organize the physical, mental, and behavioral signs and symptoms to determine the most effective interventions and to measure treatment effectiveness.[5]

The chapter examines the occupational performance difficulties associated with mental health disorders and psychosocial problems and the OT evaluations and frames of references that guide individual and group therapy interventions. In addition, topics such as parents' perspective on raising a child with mental health disorders, bullying, suicide risk, and self-injury are discussed. These contextual experiences and factors can significantly affect mental health.

UNDERSTANDING MENTAL HEALTH DISORDERS

One out of five children has a mental health problem or disorder that is likely to disrupt his or her ability to perform age-related activities. These disorders include major depression, bipolar disorder, anxiety disorders, disruptive behavioral disorders, and schizophrenia (Box 13-1). In adolescence, the risk of mental health disorders increases significantly; eating disorders, aggressive and antisocial behaviors, and substance abuse are more prevalent than they are in younger children.[26] Effective treatment for mental health problems in childhood and adolescence is crucial, since mental health disorders and behavioral problems disrupt learning and social development, which, in turn, can have an effect on adult functioning. For example, disorders that develop in adolescence are associated with poorer occupational performance and adaptation in adulthood.[27]

Multidisciplinary pediatric services for children and adolescents with mental health and psychoemotional and behavioral problems are provided in a variety of settings, including psychiatric units in acute care hospitals, independent psychiatric hospitals, day treatment centers, and community mental health centers. Public schools provide psychiatric and mental health services as well. Many adolescents with mental health problems are also under the care of services such as the social welfare department or juvenile justice system and may live in a residential facility, group home, or foster care home.

In children and adolescents, mental health disorders often present as behavioral problems and/or as difficulty performing everyday activities. They are the result of the interaction of biological, behavioral, psychological, and social factors (Figure 13-1). Family history of mental illness, or sexual, physical, or emotional abuse or stresses associated with lower socioeconomic circumstances such as poverty or parental unemployment increase the risk of mental illness (Box 13-2). A biological predisposition or genetic component may make a child vulnerable to a mental health disorder, but a child will only develop a disorder when other factors are also present. Therefore, an integrative model that considers all biological, behavioral, psychological, and sociocultural dimensions is typically used to understand each child's mental health disorder.[33]

The biological dimension includes genetics, and the structures and functions of the brain such as the role of neurotransmitters, sensory processing, and the endocrine system. Some disorders have explicit genetic causes that are present at birth. These conditions are often those with multiple symptoms, including intellectual disabilities. Other disorders have genetic or biological origins that are less clearly identified. This includes disorders such as depression, anxiety disorders, and those on the autism spectrum. The psychological dimensions encompass cognitive, emotional, and personality factors, namely, characteristics of personality, learning abilities, emotional arousal, coping abilities, self-concept, and self-esteem. The social dimension includes relationships of family, friends, and other significant adults (such as teachers and extended family), while the sociocultural dimension encompasses such factors as gender orientation (see Chapter 9), ethnicity, culture, religion, and socioeconomic status.

DISRUPTIVE BEHAVIOR DISORDERS

Disruptive behavior disorders are characterized by socially disruptive behavior that is often more distressing to others than to the individual. This category includes

BOX 13-1

Quick Facts About Child and Adolescent Mental Health

- In the United States, 1 in 5 children has a diagnosable mental, emotional, or behavioral disorder (SAMHSA, 2009). However, 70% of children do not receive mental health services.
- Children and teens who have a chronic illness, endure abuse or neglect, or experience other trauma have an increased risk of depression (National Institute for Mental Health, 2000).
- Attention deficit hyperactivity disorder (ADHD) is one of the most common mental disorders in children. There are about two million children in the United States with this disorder (NIMH, 2009).
- Autism and related disorders develop in childhood and affect an estimated 3.4 per 1000 children in the United States (NIMH, 2001). It is four times more common in boys (NIMH 2008). Girls tend to present with more severe symptoms and have greater cognitive impairments (NIMH, 2008).
- It is estimated that 1 in every 33 children and 1 in 8 adolescents may have depression (Center for Mental Health Services, 1998). This is between 10% and 15% of all children and teenagers in the United States (SAMHSA, 2009).
- Depression is more common in teenage girls than in teenage boys (NIMH, 2001). Children with a parent who has depression are at an increased risk (SAMHSA, 2009).
- Approximately 750,000 children in the United States have bipolar disorder. If not treated, bipolar disorder puts children at an increased risk for drug abuse, school failure, and suicide (SAMHSA, 2010).
- Anxiety disorders are the most common mental, behavioral, and emotional conditions to affect children and adolescents This is Approximately 13 out of every 100 children aged 9 to 17 years in the United States has some form of anxiety disorder (SAMHSA, 2010).
- About 50% of children and teens with an anxiety disorder have a comorbid second anxiety or a mental or behavioral disorder, often depression (SAMHSA, 2010).
- Throughout the average lifespan, about 0.5% to 3.7% of females in the United States will develop anorexia and around 1.1% to 4.2% bulimia. Females are more at risk for developing an eating disorder than are males, but binge-eating disorders are more common in males (NIMH, 2010).
- Suicide is the third leading cause of death for 15 to 24 year olds and the sixth leading cause of death for 5 to 14 year olds in the United States (SAMHSA, 2010).
- Approximately 20% of the youths in juvenile justice facilities in the United States have a serious emotional disturbance, and most have a diagnosable mental disorder. An additional 30% of the youths in these facilities have substance abuse disorders or concurrent substance abuse disorders (OJJDP, 2000).

Data from the National Mental Health Association 2009-2010: www.nmha.org/infoctr/factsheets; National Institute for Mental Health: www.nimh.nih.gov/publicat/numvbers.cfm, or http://www.nimh.nih.gov/health/publications/the-numbers-count-mental-disorders-in-america/; United States Department of Health and Human Services: Substance Abuse and Mental Health Services Administration 2007-2009: http://mentalhealth.samhsa.gov/, Surgeon General's Report on Mental Health, 1999, Office of Juvenile Justice and Delinquency Prevention, [OJJDP] 2000.

attention deficit disorder (ADD), attention deficit hyperactivity disorder (ADHD), conduct disorder, and oppositional defiant disorder.

Attention Deficit/Hyperactivity Disorder

Attention deficit/hyperactivity disorder (ADHD) is the most common behavioral and cognitive disorder diagnosed in childhood in the United States.[7] The three types are: (1) predominantly hyperactive-impulsive type, (2) predominantly inattentive type, and (3) combined type. A diagnosis of ADHD relies on an experienced multidisciplinary health care team to make the determination that the symptoms are interfering with the child's ability to perform ADLs and that these symptoms are not the result of another medical, psychiatric, or social condition.[19] It is necessary to rule out other reasons that children have difficulty paying attention

in class, such as anxiety, sensory difficulties, feeling overwhelmed, fatigue, and boredom. Diet, routines at home, and exercise can also influence a child's ability to pay attention in class. The symptoms must be evident before age 7, last for at least 6 months, and not be associated with an anxiety disorder.[19]

CASE *Study*

Thomas is a 7-year-old boy in a regular Grade 2 classroom. He has always had trouble in school. The kindergarten teacher describes him as "fidgety, restless, and distractible." Now that he is in grade school, these symptoms are interfering with his learning. Thomas frequently stares off into space and has difficulty following multistep verbal directions. He is a shy, anxious boy. At home, his parents report that he needs frequent reminders to follow through with

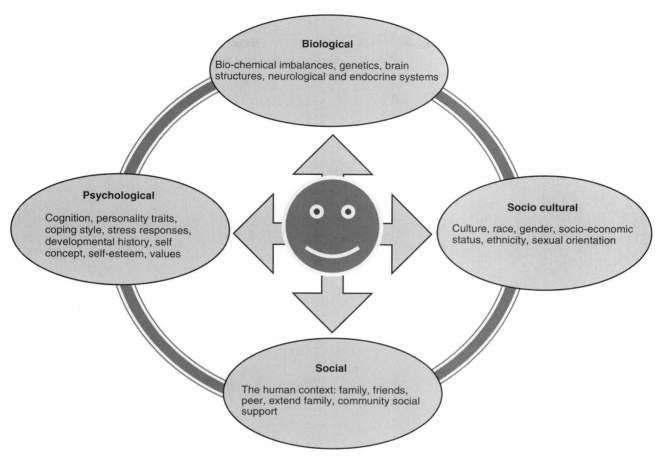

FIGURE 13-1 Multidimensional factors of mental health. (Adapted from Sue D, Sue DW, Sue S: *Understanding abnormal behavior,* ed 9, Boston, 2010, Wadsworth Cengage Learning.)

tasks. Thomas is easily frustrated and becomes bored with tasks quickly. For example, he does not brush his teeth adequately or get himself dressed in the morning. Instead, he gets distracted. His parents describe their frustrations with Thomas, his ability to lose things, forget assignments, and his untidiness.

After a comprehensive evaluation by a team of professionals (an occupational therapist, a physical therapist, a social worker, a psychologist, and a developmental pediatrician) and consultation with the teacher, the parents, and the child, Thomas received a diagnosis of *attention deficit disorder* (ADD), a form of ADHD. This type of ADHD affects both girls and boys equally. An evaluation includes a classroom visit, since one criterion for this diagnosis is difficulty in more than one situation (e.g., home and school). An OT practitioner (i.e., an occupational therapy assistant [OTA]) may observe Thomas at school or at home to establish a baseline of behaviors.

Interventions for ADD may include medication (stimulants), behavioral modification techniques, sensory

modulation, and learning strategies to help these children focus on a task. Children with ADD generally respond to lower levels of medication compared with children with ADD of the hyperactivity type.[14] Behavioral strategies can be very beneficial for these children. This may include classroom modification such as low sensory areas, which help children focus on their work and can be calming for a child when overstimulated (Table 13-1).

Predominantly Hyperactivity: Impulsive Type

Some children with ADD have excessive energy and motor activity. They are diagnosed with ADD of the predominantly hyperactivity type (referred to as ADHD), which is more common in boys and children from lower socioeconomic backgrounds.[15] Signs of ADHD include fidgeting, squirming, talking excessively, and impulsive behavior (e.g., difficulty waiting one's turn, and interrupting others who are talking). Other features associated with ADHD include sleep disorders, mood fluctuation,

BOX 13-2

Warning Signs of Sexual Abuse

These signs *do not* mean conclusively that an adolescent or child is being sexually abused. They can also be symptoms of other problems or mental health disorders. However, if these symptoms are present, sexual abuse *should* be considered a possibility and an appropriate health professional consulted to discuss the reasons for these changes in a child or adolescents. All children are at risk of sexual abuse; for example, children with disability have a high risk of sexual abuse.

Warning signs of sexual abuse in children and adults are *recent changes*, including the following:

- Sleep problems without an explanation, e.g., nightmares
- Being distracted or distant
- A change in eating habits: refusing to eat, loss of or drastically increased appetite or trouble swallowing
- A sudden change in mood or fluctuating moods: rage, fear, insecurity, or becoming withdrawn
- A new interest in discussing sexual issues or making sexual comments or exhibiting adult-like sexual behaviors, language, or knowledge
- Disturbing sexual and nonsexual content in stories, art work, or dreams
- Developing new or unusual or excessive fears of people or places
- Becoming secretive or having secrets and refusing to discuss them with an adult or older child
- Having a new friend who is older or unexplained money or other gifts
- A change in attitude to body: self as bad or body as dirty, or similar
- Complaining of pain while urinating or defecating
- Symptoms of genital infections or discomfort

Signs common in adolescents involve the development of these behaviors or symptoms:

- Self-injury (cutting, burning)
- Decline in personal appearance and hygiene
- Using drugs and alcohol to excess
- Being sexually promiscuous
- Running away from home or withdrawing from activities
- Signs of anxiety or depression, including suicide attempts
- Fear of intimacy or closeness
- Eating disorders: binge eating, anorexia, or bulimia

These symptoms should never be ignored. It may be uncomfortable to initiate a conversation about them, but the best approach is always a calm, matter-of-fact one. An abuser threatens the child or adolescent; therefore, the children need to feel safe to disclose the secret and that you will cope with what they say without judgment and will listen. Since the abuser is often someone known to the family, the child may feel safe to talk to the OT practitioner, who is a person outside the family.

This material was compiled from suggestions listed on the following sites: http://www.stopitnow.com/warning_signs_child_behavior; http://www.protectkids.com/abuse/abusesigns.htm

emotional hypersensitivity (i.e., emotional lability), poor self-esteem, and low frustration tolerance.[27] It is common for children with ADHD to experience difficulties relating to other children.

As in the case example of Thomas, a child with ADHD would receive a comprehensive evaluation before a diagnosis. The team of health care and educational personnel determines if there are any other causes for the impulsive-hyperactive behaviors. An OT practitioner observes and evaluates the child in the classroom, at home, and in the clinic and provides information on how the child's behaviors affect his or her daily functioning, especially during play and learning tasks. The OT practitioner provides strategies and modifications to help the child regulate his or her emotional arousal and manage sensory distractions. Interventions include sensory integration therapy,

accommodations and modifications in the classroom and home environment, self-regulation strategies, positive behavioral support, cognitive–behavioral therapy, and monitoring the behavioral outcomes of medication. OT practitioners work with teachers to develop therapy goals for an individualized education program (IEP). Their work with family involves developing parenting strategies to create an environment that supports a child to modify and regulate his or her behavior. The work with families and teachers is likely to involve positive behavior support strategies based on an *applied functional behavioral analysis* frame of reference (Table 13-2).[12]

The behaviors associated with ADHD, particularly the excessive motor activity and impulsivity, can frustrate parents, teachers, and other children in the family or classroom. Since these behavioral difficulties

TABLE 13-1

Classroom Modifications to Improve Attention

SPECIFIC AREA	MODIFICATIONS
General strategies	• Use a child's strengths. • Provide structure and clear expectations. • Use short sentences and simple vocabulary. • Provide supportive opportunities for success to help build self-esteem. • Be flexible in classroom procedures (e.g., allowing the use of recording device for taking notes and tests when students have trouble with written language). • Make use of self-correcting materials that provide immediate feedback without embarrassment. • Use computers for written work. • Reinforce social skills in school and at home. • Provide short breaks by allowing children to move, to stretch, or to verbalize in the classroom. • Mix up the responses required of students (e.g., Ask them to clap to the right response, sing the answer, or raise both arms). • Use positive behavior support techniques to reinforce learning.
Helping with schoolwork	• Show an interest in the child's homework. • Ask about homework; ask questions that require answers longer than one or two words. • Help the child organize homework materials. • Establish a regular time with child to do homework; develop a schedule. • Find a specific place that has plenty of light and space and is quiet where the child can do homework. • Encourage the child to ask questions and look for answers. • Make sure the child justifies answers with facts and evidence. • Practice the skills taught in school and at home. • Relate homework to the child's everyday life (e.g., teach fractions and measurements as you do other therapy activities, such as cooking). • Be a role model: Read a book or newspaper, write a letter with the child, or talk about your experiences of these activities. • Praise the child for both the small steps and big leaps in the right direction.
Language	• Have the child sit where he or she can hear you and not be distracted. • Repeat directions; remember to use gentle cuing and helpful reminders. • Provide visual cues for where to begin tasks and assignments. • NEVER embarrass students. • Phrase questions so that the student may answer "yes" or "no." • Assign shorter written language assignments. • Provide written and verbal directions for homework (so that the child does not miss assignments).
Memory	• Use mnemonic strategies: Use rhyming games; allow children to mouth or whisper reading assignments in class. • Allow the children to underline in book or circle key words. • Use a recording device for taking notes. • Older children may enjoy using their ipod to keep track of their schedule and assignments. • Have the children practice memorization before bedtime. • Elaborate on information, and relate it to prior knowledge. • Allow the children extra time on tests and assignments. • Use visual or verbal learning. • Use active learning such as role-playing and hands-on experiences. • Divide information into categories for the child.

Continued

TABLE 13-1

Classroom Modifications to Improve Attention—cont'd

SPECIFIC AREA	MODIFICATIONS
Sensory integration: coordination	• Allow the child to move around the classroom. • Ensure that the child goes to recess. • Provide the child with movement experiences. • Provide the child with quiet space when he is overly aroused. • Have the child sit in the back of the room, with few distractions. • Allow for breaks. • Provide noncompetitive games to help make all the children successful. • Work on the proximal control needed for handwriting skills. • Provide strengthening and endurance games. • Work on perceptual skills through gross motor activities (e.g., obstacle course).
Sequential processing	• Repeat instructions slowly and provide word or picture lists of steps. • Allow them to talk through or whisper the order of the steps during a task. • Anticipate difficulties. • Use a whole-word approach to reading.
Visual processing	• Provide graph paper or grid, which may help the child focus on the page. • Use tactile cues such as raised lines to help the child.
Organizational skills	• Establish routines. • Provide written as well as verbal instructions for assignments (e.g., a study guide for reading or task completion). • Outline the steps with the child so that he or she can learn the skill. • Develop strategies for taking notes (e.g., highlight key words or tasks). • Make lists, and check off the items (e.g., give the child a day planner; electronic day planners can be cool!). • Break long-term projects into small chunks.

often are the presenting problem that precedes referral to the health care team, children with ADHD sometimes are regarded as "difficult," "problematic," or "stupid." These negative labels can make these children feel inferior and create low self-esteem. They experience difficulties succeeding in school tasks and making friends, which also affect their self-esteem. As time goes on and even when others may have ceased to identify these children as problems, they may still identify themselves with the negative labels, which influences their behaviors and motivation for learning. They avoid trying because they have experienced failure. In this psychosocial dimension of therapy, the OT practitioner can help by explaining to parents and teachers how to work with the child to address his or her comprehensive needs in ways that will build confidence and self-esteem. Activities are graded (i.e., changed in some manner) so the level of difficulty is gradually increased to encourage success. Both parents and children can benefit from support groups, and the children can gain skills and confidence from participation in summer camps that focus on children with special needs.

CLINICAL *Pearl*

Teachers frequently mention to parents that their children have problems paying attention in class. This alone does not necessarily mean that the children have attention deficit disorder (ADD). The children may demonstrate attention problems for a variety of reasons. OT practitioners assist team members in determining if the attention problems are secondary to environmental, social, or sensory conditions. OT practitioners working in school systems play a role in educating teachers concerning the strategies and modifications that help these children succeed.

Conduct Disorder: Childhood Onset

CASE *Study*

Rodney is a 10-year-old boy who has difficulty getting along with other children. His parents describe him as having been an irritable baby, a difficult toddler who had tantrums, and a young child who was disruptive in the family and did not adjust easily to preschool. Now, he is inclined to bully other children, and neighbors complain about his behavior (e.g., throwing rocks at windows, fighting with other children, and stealing). Particularly distressing is his cruelty to animals and, more recently, his fascination with fire. His parents feel powerless because he does not respond to their attempts to discipline him; of late, he has started hurting his younger sister. At school, he is doing poorly in Grade 3; he was suspended recently for stealing money from his teacher's desk. The school has called a parent conference to discuss his aggressive behavior and poor school performance.

Rodney's behaviors are characteristic of a conduct disorder, characterized by long-standing behaviors that

TABLE 13-2

Psychosocial Frames of Reference

PSYCHOSOCIAL FRAMES OF REFERENCE	PRINCIPLES	STRATEGIES
COGNITIVE–BEHAVIORAL THERAPY		
This frame of reference assumes that maladaptive or faulty thinking patterns adversely influence emotions and contribute to dysfunctional behavior. Examples of this faulty thinking include overgeneralizing (i.e., if it is true in one situation, it is always true) or catastrophizing (i.e., always thinking the worst possible outcome). The greatest improvement occurs when a child or adolescent decreases his or her negative and faulty thinking. This is not achieved by changing negative thoughts to positive ones.	How one thinks and what one believes influence behavior and emotions (e.g., a child's positive or negative view of himself or herself and his or her view of the world as threatening or safe, caring, and supportive). A change in thinking can lead to improvement in function and can reduce emotional distress. The basic core and conditional beliefs are learned and become the personal rules that guide life (e.g., "if I do this (rule) the consequences are…"). It is a way of making sense of cause-and-effect relations. Focus on the present problems. Time-limited individual or group therapy focuses on a specific difficulty, condition, or skill acquisition.	Interventions include teaching a person about the relationships among their thinking, behavior, and emotions. *Interventions:* With the use of media and activities, the following techniques and skills are developed: • Identifying patterns of thinking and core beliefs and being aware of how thinking affects feelings and behavior (e.g., "I always fail") and leads to anxiety in new situations and not trying new activities because of the fear of failure. • Cognitive restructuring, also called *reframing thinking*. This involves changing beliefs and thinking patterns. • Self-monitoring and self-talk • Learning skills to reduce stress, such as relaxation • Developing problem-solving skills to address client-identified problems • Homework assignments to consolidate learning and transfer it beyond the therapy setting
SKILL ACQUISITION		
This frame of reference emphasizes that learning, practicing, and acquiring skills help children and adolescents function in social, academic, work, and family occupations.	Children develop self-efficacy, a sense of success, and skills through practice. Acquiring foundational skills can help children perform in home, school, and community settings. Skill acquisition is based on teaching-learning principles. Learning can be achieved through a therapist's instruction or in an experiential group setting through peer modeling and observation. Skill refinement occurs through specific behavioral feedback. Skills are acquired sequentially (i.e., simple to complex).	Interventions are designed to develop, modify, and refine specific skills for functional occupational performance through instructional methods such as role playing, experiential skill–based groups, practice and generalization of skill performance, modeling, and feedback on skill performance.

Continued

TABLE 13-2

Psychosocial Frames of Reference—cont'd

PSYCHOSOCIAL FRAMES OF REFERENCE	PRINCIPLES	STRATEGIES
BEHAVIOR MODIFICATION This frame of reference changes or develops behaviors required for occupational performance. The OT practitioner identifies target behaviors and shapes these behaviors using reinforcement schedules. Applied behavioral analysis is a widely used frame of reference in health and education.	Children and adolescents exhibit behaviors that can be identified and reinforced. Changing or developing behaviors will improve occupational performance. Behavior can be modified by external forces (e.g., reward or punishment schedules).	Interventions are designed to develop, modify, and refine specific behaviors. Interventions follow strict protocols that are targeted to a specific behavior to be increased or decreased (e.g., increase eye contact from a child with autism or decrease head banging in such a child). Identify behaviors to be shaped, changed, or developed. Teach, demonstrate, and practice behavioral strategies. Increase desired behaviors with rewards (e.g., praise, tokens such as stars that can later be redeemed for a toy or an activity of one's choice). Intermittent reinforcement strengthens a behavior.
PSYCHOEDUCATIONAL GROUP THERAPY The purpose of the psychoeducational group is to share information along a common focus and learn from the experiences and knowledge of group members. This process facilitates change and/or the development of skills. This approach is often used in school-based programs to develop or improve social, communication, or coping skills.	Through knowledge comes change. To develop knowledge and skills for coping with crisis events, developmental transitions, mental health disorders, or current situational challenges (e.g., parental divorce, adolescent difficulties, depression, or bullying) Draws from cognitive–behavioral principles Education is a significant component. Focuses on the here and now Intentional use of group experience for mutual and vicarious (by the examples of others and observation) learning as well as support.	Time-limited and theme-focused groups of children and adolescents with similar needs or difficulties. A well-developed curriculum with sequential instructional sessions in which a variety of teaching methods are used, such as videos, handouts, PowerPoint presentations, and blackboards. Interactive and experiential learning strategies are important components. The techniques consist of brief lectures or presentations, small-group discussions, written exercises, role playing and behavior rehearsal, peer group modeling and learning from others, and homework tasks to reinforce learning and transfer it to everyday settings.
APPLIED BEHAVIORAL ANALYSIS Positive Support Behavior: This approach consists of systemic and individualized strategies for achieving social and learning outcomes. The goal is preventing problem behavior.[12]	All behavior has a purpose for a child, and behavior is related to context. Challenging behaviors are symptoms. Interventions respect the child's preferences, dignity, and goals. Relationships are the building blocks of prosocial behaviors Learning new skills takes time.	Teach skills directly. Ask why a child is acting the way he or she is acting, as there is always a reason. Identify patterns of behavior; if problems are predicted, they can be prevented. A-B-C Model: Identify the **A**ntecedent behavior or event that precedes the child's behavior. Identify the **B**ehavior that is to be acquired or decreased, and establish **C**onsequences and teach skills.

TABLE 13-2

Psychosocial Frames of Reference—cont'd

PSYCHOSOCIAL FRAMES OF REFERENCE	PRINCIPLES	STRATEGIES
COACHING MODEL		
The premise is that children will be more successful at reaching the goals that they develop themselves. Children will learn life-long strategies through setting goals and take progressive steps toward meeting goals successfully. This child-directed model requires that the OT practitioner provide direction, support, advice, and strategies. This takes the form of coaching and mentoring.	Children and adolescents will be more successful meeting goals that they develop. Children will develop life-long strategies as they learn to analyze the steps toward goals. Providing children with support and encouraging them will facilitate progress toward goals. Children may need "coach" support or mentorship to develop abilities to meet goals. Teach children to self-evaluate and problem-solve.	Children develop goals with support from OT practitioners. Analyze the steps to meet goals. Children set realistic tasks to meet goals. Support children in addressing steps and learning skills to meet goals. Get children to practice skills. Use cueing and reminders. Act as the children's "coach" or "mentor" with weekly or daily "check-ins."

CBT, cognitive behavioral therapy; *OT,* occupational therapy.
Data compiled from Furr SR: Structuring the group experience: A format for designing psycho-educational groups, *J Specialists Group Work* 25:29, 2000; Jones KD, Robinson EH: A model for choosing topics and experiences appropriate to group stage, *J Specialists Group Work* 25:356, 2000; Kramer P, Hinojosa J: *Frames of reference for pediatric occupational therapy,* ed 2, Baltimore, MD, 1999, Lippincott, Williams & Wilkins; Sommers-Flanagan R, Barrett-Hakanson T, Clake C, et al: A psycho-educational school-based coping and social skills group for depressed students, *J Specialists Group Work* 55:170, 2000; Stein F, Culter SK: *Psychosocial occupational therapy: A holistic approach,* ed 2, New York, 2002, Delmar; Crone D, Robert Horner R: *Building positive behavior support systems in schools,* New York, 2003, The Guildford Press.

violate the rights of others and the rules of society. The following behaviors characterize conduct disorder in children and adolescents:[5,11]

- Physical aggression toward other people or animals
- Participation in mugging, purse snatching, shoplifting, or burglary
- Destruction of other people's property (e.g., setting fires)
- Breaking of rules (e.g., running away from home or skipping school)
- Impaired school performance, , especially verbal and reading skills
- Suspensions from school for behavioral problems

Boys with conduct disorder are likely to be involved in behaviors such as vandalism, stealing, and fighting, whereas girls with the disorder tend to be sexually permissive (e.g., prostitution), and engage in manipulative behaviors such as lying or running away.

Other problems associated with conduct disorder are abuse of addictive substances, reckless behavior, and temper outbursts. Children diagnosed with conduct disorders also exhibit a lack concern for others, and they show no feelings of guilt or remorse. However, despite this image of toughness, they often have poor self-esteem and experience anxiety, depression, and suicidal thoughts.

Children with conduct disorder are at high risk of poor outcomes, including dropping out of school, unemployment, and engaging in criminal behaviors and substance abuse. If left untreated, many will develop antisocial personality disorder as adults (i.e., in approximately 40% of cases, childhood-onset conduct disorder develops into antisocial personality disorder).[29] Antisocial personality disorders are associated with serious crimes, including rape, physical assault, and homicide.[5]

CLINICAL *Pearl*

It is important to praise or recognize a child when he or she is working on or exhibiting desired behaviors. This recognition should be clear, and should label the behavior of the child , for example, "Well done, you are working quietly on the task." This is better than saying, "Nice work!" This strategy helps the child feel validated and shapes his or her behavior.

Oppositional Defiant Disorder

CASE *Study*

Dwayne is a 9-year-old Grade 3 student. His mother states that he has always been a somewhat "difficult, angry" child, but his behavior has worsened over the last 19 months. He argues constantly with his parents and older sisters, loses his temper over seemingly trivial issues, and has uncontrollable rage. He blames others, refuses to obey his parents' rules, and deliberately annoys other people. He says that he hates school and his sisters and that his classmates "suck." His parents find it very difficult to set limits for him.

The primary symptoms of *oppositional defiant disorder* (ODD) are negative, hostile, and defiant behaviors that are uncharacteristic of typical children.[5] Children and early adolescents with ODD display outbursts of temper, argue, defy adults, and are especially hostile to authority figures. These children seem to be angry all the time and resent rules; they become easily annoyed and readily blame others for their mistakes. Behaviors that might be observed are frequent temper tantrums; mean, hateful talking; revenge-seeking behaviors; and deliberately annoying others. These behaviors differ in duration and intensity from the occasional "difficult" periods some children and adolescents may experience.[5] The ongoing oppositional behavior and stormy relationships with teachers and other children result in poor academic performance in school and few friendships.[10] Children with ODD may eventually grow out of it, especially if the onset occurs in preschool years. Adolescents diagnosed with ODD are more likely (75%) to have symptoms that persist into adulthood.[2]

ODD may also be an indication of underlying childhood depression or an inability to cope effectively with anger and other uncomfortable feelings. ODD differs from conduct disorder in that these children do not seriously violate the rights of others or ignore their feelings. Furthermore, they rarely engage in activities that cause physical harm to others, and as a rule, they do not engage in criminal activity. However, an initial presentation of ODD may precede a diagnosis of conduct disorder.

Interventions involve working with family and teachers to develop a comprehensive program that is consistent across settings. It will involve limit setting with explicit consequences (e.g., time out) and positive behavioral support to encourage appropriate behaviors. Because of the benefit of experiencing personal control in some aspects of their lives, therapy can provide these children with choices and participation in goal setting. Strategies that develop self-regulation of mood and anger are effective in providing a child with a sense of control and can evolve into constructive expression of emotions that, in turn, will address underlying depression and anxieties.

CLINICAL *Pearl*

The OT practitioner working with children and early adolescents with disruptive behavior disorders must possess a thorough knowledge of developmental behavior patterns.

LEARNING DISORDERS

CASE *Study*

Greg is a cooperative 8-year-old boy in Grade 3. He is reluctant to ask questions in class and avoids activities that require reading in front of other students. While the school psychologist reports Greg's IQ (intelligence quotient) score is 110, well within the normal range, his performance on writing and reading tasks falls well below this level. During a classroom exercise, the OTA observed that Greg struggled to write one sentence during "free writing" while his classmates were able to complete paragraphs. The teacher, using positive behavior support, commented to Greg, "I can see you are working hard."

Greg has a reading and writing learning disability. The school interdisciplinary team met with the teacher and Greg's parents to develop strategies to assist him in school. Greg is given additional time on writing assignments and extra help with reading, and his tests are read to him so that he can respond verbally. Other strategies include allowing him to type his assignments and no penalties for spelling or writing errors on handwritten work. It is important that his teacher provides clear and consistent expectations for class work (e.g., she will not accept one sentence if she has asked for three).

Approximately 5% of school-aged children experience a learning disability.[10] They are often aware of their difficulties, although when they are young, they may not understand or be able to describe it. The *DSM-IV-TR* criteria for a learning disorder is a severe discrepancy between ability and achievement that is not due to visual or hearing impairment, motor difficulties, intellectual disability, or environmental, cultural, or economic disadvantage.[10] The diagnosis is divided into specific disabilities: dyslexia (reading disability), dysgraphia (writing disability), and dyscalculia (math disability).

Children with learning disabilities often are referred to OT for other difficulties such as sensory processing, poor motor planning, or handwriting skills. It is the role of OT practitioners to work with the educational team to identify the learning difficulties and the underlying motor, sensory processing, or neurologic difficulties through performance assessment and develop strategies and adaptations to enhance successful learning. Frames of references and strategies used are sensory integration, coaching techniques, cognitive–behavioral therapy, or a compensatory approach that improves organization of tasks and assists memory (see Table 13-1 and Table 13-2). OT practitioners may also make environmental modifications and help improve performance with assistive devices and adaptive equipment. For example, children with dysgraphia can benefit from using a laptop computer in the classroom. As early as in Grade 1, a child can benefit from an age-related typing program.

As with any intervention, if children develop their own plans, they are more likely to use the strategies. For example, Greg was given a day-timer to keep track of his school assignments and to develop organizational skills. He frequently forgot the day-timer and was not good about writing down his work schedule. When asked about it, he said the book was too big, and while he liked the pictures and activities, he did not know where to write. Instead, he decided to use a sheet of paper attached to a clipboard. Each day he wrote the name of the class, the title of the assignment, and page number in book/workbook. He crossed the assignment off once it was completed. The system he developed worked much better for him and earned him praise from his parents. This is an example of the importance of involving children in problem solving with their own strategies.

CLINICAL *Pearl*

It is important for children to be their own advocates once they are in high school or college. Many colleges make accommodations for students with learning disabilities.

TIC DISORDERS

Tic disorders are neurologic and characterized by stereotypical, repetitive, involuntary, recurrent movements or vocalizations. They are classified as motor, phonic, vocal, or complex tics, which may involve talking to oneself, facial grimacing, or using obscene words (coprolalia). Common signs are eye blinking, neck jerking, coughing, shoulder shrugging, facial grimacing, foot stomping, touching objects, and excessive grooming. Signs of vocal tics include throat clearing, grunting, sniffing, snorting, barking, hiccupping, yelling, and the repetition of others' words (echolalia). Tics often increase in stressful situations and due to fatigue or anxiety, and they can decrease during sleep or absorbing activities such as computer games.[5] Tourette's syndrome is the most common tic disorder for which treatment is sought.[5,10]

Tourette's Syndrome

CASE *Study*

Kyle is a 7-year-old in Grade 3. Recently he has started to jerk his neck to the side and make strange faces and grunting noises. These behaviors occur intermittently throughout the day. Kyle is embarrassed that he is unable to control these movements and noises, especially since he is shouting profanities. Kyle's parents and teacher are concerned by these behaviors. His classmates are annoyed when he cannot stop and have started to avoid him and tease him. His school performance is suffering because the jerks and noises distract him.

Kyle's Tourette's syndrome is consistent with the typical onset, which is between 6 and 7 years of age and is more prevalent in boys. *Tourette's syndrome* is viewed as a genetic disorder involving repetitive involuntary motor and vocal tics. The tics may occur many times a day and must occur consistently for 1 year or more before the age of 18 for a diagnosis of the syndrome. Related comorbidity occurs with ADHD, behavioral problems, learning disabilities, or obsessive–compulsive disorder (OCD).[5] Although it is typically a chronic disorder, some children experience improvement during adolescence and early adulthood.

Tics may disrupt a child's schoolwork, participation in social activities and ADLs, and play/leisure activities. Many of these children are not significantly affected by their tics and do not require treatment. Others may require medication (antipsychotic medications, selective serotonin reuptake inhibitors [SSRIs], and benzodiazepine), but the response to medications varies. Behavioral management, anxiety management, and anger management are therapy interventions that are beneficial for some children, especially when the disorder occurs with other disorders such as OCD.

Other associated challenges are social. Kyle's experience, especially his vocal tics, is an example of how this disorder can isolate a child. The strange and obvious nature of verbal and motor tics makes children vulnerable to discrimination, and they often experience bullying or teasing.[11] It is important that the OT practitioner is aware of the bullying and includes goals for social participation in the IEP of children with this problem. See Box 13-3 for further information on bullying.

ANXIETY DISORDERS

About 13 out of 100 children and adolescents have an anxiety disorder, and this disorder is more common among girls. It is important to recognize that **anxiety** is a normal adaptive response to stress, involving feelings

BOX 13-3

Strategies for Responding to Bullying

Children with mental health disorders and disabilities, especially those that affect their social skills, are vulnerable to bullying and teasing. This bullying is often underreported, minimized, or unacknowledged in schools. In 2000, the U.S. Department of Education issued an official statement regarding harassment of those with disabilities in school. That same year, the National Center on Secondary Education and Transition provided advice and strategies on school interventions and educational programs to address and deter bullying. It specifically targeted the prevention of disability harassment (http://www.ncset.org).

OT practitioners working in the schools system can:

- Contribute to a school environment that is aware of and sensitive to disability concerns and harassment.
- Report any identified bullying to the appropriate school services.
- Be open to discussing bullying during therapy.
- Have a zero-tolerance policy toward teasing and bullying in the OT department
- Teach children and adolescents constructive strategies to stop any bullying they experience.
- Encourage parents, students, employees, and community members to discuss harassment of those with disabilities and to report it when they become aware that it is happening.
- Recommend that victims and perpetrators of harassment seek counseling.
- Participate in the school team that assesses and modifies existing harassment policies and procedures to ensure effectiveness.

From Hoover J, Stenhjem, P: *Bullying and teasing of youth with disabilities: Creating positive school environments for effective inclusion.* http://www.ncset.org/publications/issue/NCSETIssueBrief_2.3.pdf; 2003 http://www.pacer.org/publications/bullying.asp: Accessed August 20, 2008.

of apprehension and arousal of the autonomic nervous system (e.g., palpitations, perspiration, chest pain, stomach discomfort, restlessness, and/or headache).[22] It energizes and prepares a person to handle situations, especially new situations. However, anxiety is not adaptive when anxious feelings become distressing and interfere with everyday functioning. A nonadaptive stress response involves physiologic arousal (high cortisol levels, raised blood pressure and heart rate), physical sensations and symptoms (e.g., vomiting), and negative thoughts. An anxious child or adolescent may experience cognitive symptoms, such as shame, or a distorted or inaccurate view of the threat of a situation.[5] Children will describe having symptoms of anxiety such as headaches, a sick feeling, sweating hands, butterflies in their stomach, nervousness, or feary.[16] Functional problems associated with anxiety disorders are difficulties in making decisions, learning, concentrating, and accurately perceiving situations (e.g., seeing safe situations as threatening). The clinical criterion for anxiety disorders categorizes them as phobic, panic, and anxiety disorders or obsessive–compulsive disorder. Children with anxiety disorders exhibit poor school attendance, low self-esteem, and adjustment difficulties. Their social interactions are affected by poor social skills, and as they become adolescents, they are more likely to use alcohol and other drugs.

Separation Anxiety Disorder

CASE *Study*

Caitlin is a tentative, shy 5-year-old girl. Caitlin prefers to be at home, and she follows her mother around the house. She will not fall asleep at night unless her mother lies with her on the bed. She awakens during the night with "bad dreams," which have a common theme of finding herself left behind in the supermarket. Caitlin does not want to go to preschool. She cries hysterically and becomes so distressed that she vomits. At preschool, she stays close to one of the teachers and does not play with the other children.

Though separation anxiety is normal in infants and very young children, it is no longer appropriate for children of Caitlin's age. Caitlin has *separation anxiety disorder*, which is characterized by extreme anxiety when anticipating separation or separating from home or her mother. It is a disorder experienced by about 4% of children.[26] Children or adolescents with this disorder may experience extreme distress traveling away from home or may refuse to go to school or visit or sleep over at the homes of friends. In severe cases, children may refuse to attend school or participate in social and recreational activities.[5] The *DSM-VI-TR* lists as diagnostic criteria repeated nightmares involving the theme of separation, reluctance or refusal to sleep without a significant person nearby, and persistent worrying about separation or harm to major attachment figures (e.g., mother or father).[5] Separation or the anticipation of separation may trigger physical (somatic) symptoms that include headaches, dizziness, palpitation, stomachache, nausea, and vomiting.[20,22] Functional consequences are delayed social development, refusal to attend school, and experiencing anxiety while at school, all of which result in poor academic performance.[11] Separation anxiety will usually resolve or decrease in severity with time, but it may also be a precursor to other conditions such as panic disorder.

Generalized Anxiety Disorder

Generalized anxiety disorder (GAD) is diagnosed in about 3% of school children and adolescents. Symptoms include excessive anxiety and worrying (e.g., about future events, school performance, family health, world events) on most days without a specific trigger event or social situation.[20,22,26] Children with GAD cannot control their fears of numerous situations and activities, and these fears manifest as irritability, tiredness, inability to relax (i.e., feeling on edge), restlessness, apprehension, a negative self-image, difficulty concentrating, and disrupted sleep.[22] The physical symptoms described above can also occur with other anxiety or mood disorders (e.g., panic attacks, phobias or dysthymia).[22] As with all mental health disorders, the child will have difficulties in school, social situations, and all areas of occupational performance.

Phobic and Social Anxiety Disorders

When a child has specific, persistent, recurring fears, a phobic anxiety disorder or social anxiety disorder is likely to be the diagnosis. Specific phobias include intense irrational fears of things or situations, for example, dogs, injections, blood, storms, or heights. Young children will not always realize their fears are unreasonable, and they will become very distressed, have tantrums, cry, or cling to parents when near the object or in the situation that causes the fear. The response to the object or situation is one of panic. In adolescents and adults, *panic attacks* are an anxiety disorder associated with *phobias*. It is common for a parent to have a similar phobia or anxiety about the object or situation.

Older children and adolescents may develop a *social anxiety disorder*, a phobic disorder of social situations. These children are extremely self-conscious, easily embarrassed, afraid of being humiliated, and overly concerned about whether they are presenting themselves appropriately in social or public situations. Consequently, they withdraw from or avoid social contact, which further limits their social development and relationships with peers. Social anxiety disorder symptoms do not occur in situations with family members or familiar people with whom they have good relationships. Depending on the number and intensity of the phobias, this disorder disrupts routines and can restrict the children's experiences with an effect on all areas of occupational performance.

With all phobias, the avoidance of the object or the situation is the behavior that becomes disabling. Treatment involves medication (e.g., SSRIs or benzodiazepines) combined with cognitive behavioral therapy (CBT) and relaxation strategies. Using CBT principles

in play and creative activities, the OT practitioner helps these children address their fears and learn how to self-manage their anxiety.

Obsessive–Compulsive Disorder

Obsessive–compulsive disorder (OCD) is characterized by recurring, disruptive, intrusive thoughts which cause anxiety and compulsive, ritualistic, repetitive patterns of behavior that reduce the anxiety.[20,21,32] These behaviors become essential to the children, and if they try to resist them, their anxiety increases. The anxiety is a product of their persistent obsessive thoughts, which often are irrational concerns or fears, for example, disgust with dirt, germs, or bodily waste; or thoughts about terrible things happening to self or parents, friends, and siblings. There can be a preoccupation with orderliness, excessive praying, magical thinking (e.g., lucky and unlucky numbers), and forbidden yet intrusive (sexual) thoughts or images.[22] The compulsive behaviors of children and adolescents include ordering and rearranging, excessive or ritualistic hand washing or bathing routines, and checking locks or switches that may be performed with the intention to prevent harm coming to family members or self. In severe cases, this disruptive and time-consuming disorder interferes with routine daily activities. Because of the preoccupation with obsessive, intrusive thoughts, concentration and task completion are also impaired.

Post-Traumatic Stress Disorder

CASE *Study*

Chantrelle, her sister, and her parents moved to the United States from Haiti 1 month after the recent earthquake. Chantrelle, who is 6 years old, has been attending the local school. Her parents had hoped that the routine of school and living away from the chaos created by the earthquake in Haiti would help their children recover from the experience, which took the lives of their grandparents and brother. However, Chantrelle is no longer the outgoing little girl she was before the earthquake. She has not made friends, often reports feeling sick, and has little interest in food. Most nights she wakes up crying because of "bad" dreams. Her parents took her to the family doctor, who suspected PTSD and referred Chantrelle to a child psychologist who specializes in trauma disorders in children.

Acute stress disorder (ASD) and *post-traumatic stress disorder* (PTSD) are both anxiety disorders that develop in response to a traumatic event such as natural disasters (e.g., Hurricane Katrina in New Orleans or the earthquake in Port au Prince, Haiti). Other events associated with stress disorders are serious accidents, acts of terrorism, war, and physical and sexual abuse. Children who are immigrants from countries engaged in civil wars (e.g., Somalia, Sudan, or the Congo) and have lived in refugee camps frequently experience PTSD. Children separated from parents during the traumatic event(s) are most vulnerable to PTSD. ASD is an immediate stress response to exposure to trauma that lasts approximately 1 month. If the symptoms continue for longer than a month, the diagnosis is PTSD.

Symptoms of ASD and PTSD in a child differ from those of adults in that they persist longer and become more intense with time.[31] These children have recurring nightmares, repeated memories of the event, difficulty sleeping, changes in eating habits, and complaints of physical symptoms (e.g., sick feeling, headaches). They are likely to have problems focusing on activities, and their schoolwork will deteriorate. Other symptoms include being stoic about the event, withdrawal from society, isolation from other children, or engaging in more risk-taking behaviors. The most common comorbid disorders are panic attacks and substance abuse.

MOOD DISORDERS

Mood disorders are a group of disorders that involve emotional disturbances such as extreme sadness (e.g., dysphoria, depression) or euphoria (i.e., overly elevated mood with an exaggerated sense of well-being).[5]

Major Depressive Disorder

CASE *Study*

Wendy is a 12-year-old student in Grade 7. She lives with her mother and her 14-year-old brother. Typically, she is a pleasant, cooperative child, but she has been irritable and withdrawn lately. Her teacher describes her as a good student but somewhat anxious. Over the past several weeks, Wendy's schoolwork has deteriorated, and she has stopped spending time with her friends at school. Instead of playing with friends, she comes home after school, watches TV, and goes to sleep early. Her mother has noticed that she is not interested in food and that she has stopped activities she previously enjoyed (e.g., playing computer games and having friends over to play). She complains of headaches, stomachaches, and being tired. Her 18-year-old cousin recently was admitted to a hospital following a suicide attempt.

The most common of the mood disorders are major depression, minor depression, and brief recurrent depression. At any particular time, it is estimated that 15% of children and adolescents have some depressive symptoms, and between 3% and 5% meet the criteria for major depression.[9] In young children, depression reportedly is more common in boys. This changes in adolescence, and by the age of 14 years, twice as many girls as boys will have depressive disorders. Wendy's presentation is consistent with major depression, with the common symptoms of irritability and physical (somatic) complaints such as headaches and stomachaches. Other symptoms are anxiety and social withdrawal.[32] In adolescents, the symptoms of depression are more consistent with those reported by adults. Adolescents will experience thoughts of suicide (suicidal ideation), guilt, feelings of worthlessness and shame, and changes in sleep patterns and appetite.

CLINICAL *Pearl*

Never be reluctant to ask the child or adolescent in a straightforward manner, "Are you thinking about hurting yourself?" If the answer is affirmative, ask whether he or she has a plan and, if so, the details of the plan. It is important that you ask these questions even at the risk of upsetting the child. If asked directly, a child will be more likely to respond honestly, and you can take the necessary steps to make him or her safe.

Wendy's depressive symptoms are typical. She is experiencing an overall state of unhappiness, she is dissatisfied with her life, feels pessimistic, and has lost interest and pleasure in almost all her activities.[28,30] The objective signs of depression are changes in weight (either gain or loss); inability to sleep or excessive sleeping; feeling tired; slowed motor activity; and agitation. Low self-esteem, poor body image, and feelings of lack of personal control, as well as phobias, substance abuse, sexual promiscuity, and absences from school, are also associated with depression.[18,21]

CLINICAL *Pearl*

Depression can also lead to aggressive feelings toward others, including homicidal thoughts. Talking about suicide with adolescents needs to include questions about whether the teen has a desire to hurt other people, such as parents or peers at school. Depression is often an underlying problem in many children who commit violent crimes against family members, teachers, or peers.

The multidimensional model in Figure 13-1 is useful to understand depression. No single known cause for depression exists. However, biological, sociocultural, social, and psychological factors increase the likelihood of depression. Biological factors include chronic childhood illnesses (e.g., diabetes) and a family history of depression, especially in the mother. Psychosocial and cultural factors that increase the risk of depression are physical, emotional, and sexual abuse; neglect; lack of affection and support; and stress caused by factors such as poverty.[35] The presence of other mental health disorders (e.g., ADHD, learning disabilities, or eating disorders) also increases the risk of depression. Other negative events such as parents' divorce, bullying, or the death of a family member can also increase the risk.

OT practitioners need to be aware of functional difficulties associated with depression, including poor concentration, not completing tasks, learning difficulties, and aggressiveness toward others. Because children and adolescents experience apathy and fatigue, they may neglect basic ADLs such as personal hygiene and grooming. When the child or adolescent loses interest and stops participating in previously enjoyed group activities, the ensuing social isolation impairs social development and development of a positive sense of identity.[5,11]

CLINICAL *Pearl*

Depression and depressive symptoms are common and cause occupational performance deficits. Even children and adolescents with subclinical symptoms of depression (i.e., insufficient to meet the criteria for diagnosis) have significant difficulties.[32]

OT practitioners need to be able to assess suicide risk, since it is the third leading cause of death among 15- to 19-year-olds and the fourth leading cause of death among the 10- to 14-year-old age group.[1] A child or adolescent expressing suicidal thoughts or exhibiting a preoccupation with death should receive professional psychiatric help immediately and be monitored closely. Figure 13-2 is a checklist of suicidal risk signals. The OT practitioner should immediately report signs of self-mutilating behavior or suicidal ideation to the parents and/or to a supervisor or other appropriate team member (e.g., nurse, psychologist, or mental health counselor) and document this on the child's chart. Supervision and a safe environment (e.g., no access to medications and supervision of use of tools) is the best protocol when working with children who are depressed.

A child or adolescent who has recently started therapy with antidepressants can have an increased risk of suicide. The therapeutic response to a widely used antidepressant medication (e.g., an SSRI such as Prozac or Zoloft) usually takes 2 to 3 weeks before a marked improvement in mood occurs. However, ironically, the gradual improvement in energy and mood due to the medication may actually push the child or adolescent who is still depressed to act on his or her suicide thoughts. Therefore, the OT practitioner should be suspicious of sudden elation or energy in a child or adolescent diagnosed with depression. This sudden unexplained improvement is known as a "flight into health" and can signify that the decision to end one's life has been made. Other warning signs of impending suicide include getting organized, subtle good-bye gestures, and giving away personal items.

Bipolar Disorder

Bipolar disorder in children and adolescents has received more attention in the last decade and presents with symptoms similar to ADHD, anxiety disorders, childhood psychosis, and delinquency. While its prevalence in adolescents is about 1% to 1.5% of the population in the United States, its incidence in children is unknown. The characteristics of this disorder are the two extremes of mood: depression and mania. A child or adolescent with bipolar disorder will experience symptoms of major depression alternating with episodes of mania or hypomania (milder form of mania) characterized by excessive elation and energy, aggressive and disruptive behaviors, low frustration tolerance, and impulsive behavior. In both states, children may experience *delusions*, which are irrational beliefs.

While a strong genetic predisposition and usually a family history are present, the onset of bipolar disorder is multidimensional and thus requires a comprehensive treatment approach. This disorder interferes significantly with development, and while it can be managed with mood stabilizing medication, it remains a lifetime condition. The OT practitioner works with the health care team to minimize the effects of the disorder on functional abilities in all areas of occupation. The OT practitioner can also assist with diagnosis by paying attention to children who are "out of control," irritable, excitable, or have mood swings (e.g., exhibiting extreme energy and elation at one time and at other times being irritable, short tempered, sad or confused, or unable to concentrate). During manic episodes, adolescents with bipolar disorder might describe themselves being frightened because they feel "out of control," or they might not understand that a problem exists because they are feeling "high on life." They may be impulsive, take excessive risks, or have an increased interest in sex. The younger children do not always have the language to describe their emotions and instead will say that they are bored, angry, or restless; hate school; or do not like the friends they previously did. The children may be defiant; show poor judgment; be spacey at times; or talk excessively. Parents may report that their children experience sleeplessness and that they see changes in weight, appetite, and social activities. The cyclic

Suicidal Risk Signals

If you can answer "Yes" to any of the following questions about a young person, they may be thinking about suicide. Questions highlighted in bold are particularly concerning and require follow-up from a mental health professional. Be sure to document your concerns and the professionals you notified (e.g., parents, school nurse, or counselor, or teacher). Be sure that the child or adolescent is in a safe supervised situation.

Yes   No

☐   ☐   **Depression:**
—   —   Does this child/adolescent appear sad, irritable, or worthless?
—   —   Is this child/adolescent exhibiting symptoms of depression?
        (Symptoms of depression include insomnia, anorexia, withdrawn from
        others, decreased ability to concentrate, and fatigue.)
—   —   Is the child/adolescent acting out or abusing alcohol or drugs?
        (Depression can be masked by substance abuse, aggressive or risk-taking behavior.)

☐   ☐   **Preoccupation with death and dying:**
—   —   Has this child/adolescent been drawing pictures or writing poems or stories about death and suicide?

☐   ☐   **Talking about suicide:**
—   —   Has this child/adolescent been expressing a desire to die?
—   —   Has this child/adolescent been making suicidal threats?
—   —   Has this child/adolescent been listening to music with negative themes?
—   —   Has this child/adolescent been joking about suicide?
—   —   Does this child/adolescent have a plan of how he or she would carry out suicide?

☐   ☐   **Hopelessness about the future:**
—   —   Can this child/adolescent tell you about plans for the next week or next month?
—   —   Has this child/adolescent been "putting affairs in order?"
—   —   Has this child/adolescent given away special possessions or writen a will?

☐   ☐   **Changes in life situation:**
—   —   Have there been any major recent changes such as death of a parent, separation or divorce
        of parents, school problems, or boyfriend or girlfriend problems?

☐   ☐   **Previous suicide attempts:**
—   —   Has this child/adolescent previously attempted to commit suicide?
—   —   Is there evidence of self-injurious behavior (e.g., scratches, cutting)

☐   ☐   **Lack of support from family and friends:**
—   —   Has this child/adolescent expressed feeling unloved or unwanted?

☐   ☐   **Excessive use of drugs or alcohol:**
—   —   Has this child/adolescent begun or increased use of substances?

☐   ☐   **Risk-taking behavior:**
—   —   Does this person engage in dangerous behavior such as driving too fast or walking in the middle
        of the road rather than on the sidewalk?

FIGURE 13-2   Suicide risk signals. (From Hafen BQ, Frandsen KJ: *Youth suicide: depression and loneliness,* Evergreen, CO, 1984, Cordillera; Hermes P: *A time to listen: preventing youth suicide,* San Diego, 1987, Harcourt Brace Jovanovich.)

pattern, even when the positive and negative mood swings are not extreme, is an important indicator of bipolar disorder. The associated functional problems include poor school performance, few social relationships, disorganization, difficulty regulating behavior, and generally poorer long-term outcome. Therefore, early recognition and intervention are essential.

SCHIZOPHRENIA

As with bipolar disorder, *schizophrenia* is a serious chronic condition that is difficult to diagnose and has a significant genetic predisposition. It can present with symptoms of severely disturbed behavior similar to autism or a pervasive developmental disorder. It is more common in boys and can develop as early as 5 or 6 years of age.[5,17,20]

Schizophrenia of the disorganized type is seen most commonly in males in their late adolescence or early adulthood.

CLINICAL *Pearl*

Poor school performance and the developmental delays in speech and motor skills that are associated with schizophrenia are not due to intellectual disability.[22]

As mentioned, early recognition of severe mental illness and intervention are critical for long-term outcome. Before the first acute psychotic episode, an early stage of schizophrenia when the symptoms begin to develop occurs. In this *prodromal* stage, children and adolescents may begin to withdraw from activities and social contacts because of difficulty functioning in groups such as the classroom or group social settings. They may self-medicate with alcohol or illegal drugs, which can trigger the onset of their schizophrenia.

An acute psychotic state at the onset of schizophrenia is characterized by *positive symptoms*; extremely disorganized thinking, behaviors, and speech (e.g., rapid or incomprehensible speech); perceptual disturbances (e.g., hallucinations); and thought disturbances (e.g., delusions). Hallucinations involve the senses, and in children they are usually simple; nevertheless, they can be frightening. For example, auditory hallucinations involve hearing voices, which are often critical or instruct the adolescent to harm self or others, whereas visual hallucinations involve seeing changes in faces, seeing distortions of light, or seeing people who are not there. A sign of hallucinations can be the expression of emotions that do not match the situation, such as giggling without being able to explain the reason. Delusions in children can present as "magical thinking."

With the onset of schizophrenia, there is a marked deterioration in function (i.e., occupational performance). The psychotic episode and the positive symptoms typically resolve with medication, but the child or adolescent is likely to continue to have *negative* symptoms of schizophrenia, which are debilitating, as they affect the ability to communicate and to interact socially and interfere with motivation to engage in everyday activities. The negative symptoms of schizophrenia include lethargy, blunted affect (i.e., the lack of visible emotional expression in relation to a situation), poor skills in understanding social cues and body language, disorganized thinking, poor concentration, and apathy.

Negative symptoms are highly correlated with poor functioning and outcome in adulthood because they affect learning and interfere with normal development necessary to transition from adolescence to adulthood.[5,17,20]

Therefore the focus of OT is age-related skill development, especially social and life skills. This is provided within a multidisciplinary team, using groups and individual therapy based on one of the following frames of reference; psychiatric rehabilitation, cognitive disability, psychoeducation, or illness recovery and management (see Table 13-2).

EATING DISORDERS

Eating disorders occur primarily in later childhood, adolescence, and early adulthood. Dysfunctional eating behaviors characterize this group of disorders. If untreated, they result in serious physical health problems and even death.[5] For example, approximately 10% of adolescents with anorexia nervosa will die from starvation or electrolyte imbalance.[5]

The most common eating disorders are *anorexia nervosa* and *bulimia nervosa*; other eating disorders are binge eating, and body dysmorphic disorder. Even though they present more in girls, the clinical presentation for girls and boys is similar across all eating disorders. Occupational performance is generally unaffected in children and adolescents with eating disorders. They perform well in school and work settings, and ADLs are primarily intact, except for eating, food-related behaviors, and exercise routines. Social participation becomes impaired with the duration of the disorder as a preoccupation with weight and fear of rejection interferes with social relationships and participation in age-related activities. Fearing others will identify their eating disorder or finding eating with others stressful, the children and adolescents may spend their leisure time on weight-reducing activities and may avoid leisure situations that involve food.[11,25]

Adolescents with eating disorders have low self-esteem; their sense of worth has an externalized component based on their concerns of how other people judge them and their appearance and their overall self-evaluation is influenced by how they perceive their bodies and body shapes. In this section, we discuss the two most common eating disorders, anorexia nervosa and bulimia nervosa. Binge eating is discussed in Chapter 14.

Anorexia Nervosa

CASE *Study*

Jen is a 13-year-old girl in junior high school. She has very good grades, is popular, and participates in extracurricular activities such as gymnastics and cheerleading. Despite her outward appearance, she exhibits poor self-esteem and is somewhat anxious. During the past 6 months, her parents have become worried about her health. They have noticed that Jen skips meals and has become very particular about what she eats. She has lost weight and looks thin. She wears baggy clothes and loose tops with sleeves.

Despite her weight loss, Jen says she looks fat when she looks at herself in the mirror. She has always been critical of her body, but she started dieting 6 months ago to make the varsity gymnastics squad. In addition to her cheerleading and gymnastics practices, she does aerobic exercises at least 3 hours daily. Jen has not menstruated in more than 4 months and takes laxatives every day.

The two types of anorexia nervosa (AN) are restrictive and binge eating with purging. Jen has the characteristics of the restrictive type of AN. She limits her food intake, uses activity and exercise to control her weight, and shows a distorted perception of her body.

AN typically develops in early adolescence (around 13 years of age).[23] However, AN can present in younger children or older adolescents and adults. It is characterized by an intense fear of being overweight, although most often weight for age and height is well below the average. The condition is characterized by active pursuit of thinness, inability to realistically perceive the risks of weight, and self-denial of weight loss.[5,21,23] When confronted by parents or concerned friends, adolescents with AN deny or minimize the severity of the problem and resist treatment efforts. They have a distorted body image and see themselves as overweight in all or some body parts regardless of how thin or emaciated they are. Jen is critical of her body and genuinely sees herself as fat when looking in a mirror. The patterns of behavior associated with anorexia nervosa include binging on food, vigorous exercising, use of laxatives and diuretics, and purging (self-induced vomiting). The later defines *anorexia nervosa of the binge eating purging type.* Adolescents with AN are preoccupied with food, and they can enjoy preparing meals for others, even though they eat little of the food themselves.[5]

Daily food consumption may consist of fat-free yogurt and several diet drinks, and as a result AN can lead to serious medical problems associated with malnutrition. These include cessation of menstruation (amenorrhea), hypothermia (decreased body temperature), and cardiovascular impairments (e.g., bradycardia, hypotension, and arrhythmia); decreased renal function can be impaired leading to electrolyte imbalance. Vomiting of stomach acid can cause dental erosion, and osteoporosis may result from the insufficient intake of calcium and estrogen-containing foods.

Therapeutic interventions for eating disorders include medication, individual counseling, family therapy, and group programs, some of which are based on cognitive–behavioral or cognitive models. Intervention aims to address both dysfunctional eating behaviors and their associated psychological problems.[23] Hospitalization may be necessary to stabilize the medical condition when weight lost is severe. Short-term success of therapy is reported to be as high as 76%; however, long-term recovery rates are much lower.[23]

CLINICAL *Pearl*

In cooking and eating activities with clients who have eating disorders, the OT practitioner needs to be aware of problems with food that these children or adolescents may have. They may choose to hide food or purge after eating. Be aware of a teen who uses the restroom during or shortly after eating. Individuals with anorexia nervosa may enjoy cooking. It may be a way to feel in control of situations involving food; they do not perceive any pressure to eat, as it may not be a requirement for being involved in a cooking group.

Bulimia Nervosa

CASE *Study*

Kim, a high school sophomore, is slightly overweight. She seldom says anything positive about herself and lacks confidence when interacting in social groups. Her friends are concerned about her. They have noticed that she vomits in the school bathroom immediately after lunch. Kim buys cookies and other junk food and hides them. Sometimes she fasts, but when she is alone, she eats a lot of food rapidly, cramming it into her mouth in big chunks. Immediately after she has eaten excessively, she is overwhelmed with guilt and feels disgusted with herself. In an attempt to feel better, she makes herself vomit. Recently, the dental hygienist noted that she had enamel erosion on her teeth and told her that frequent vomiting will cause this to happen.

Kim has the primary characteristics of bulimia nervosa (BN). Adolescents with BN tend to have normal to above-average weight for their height and are aware that their eating patterns are abnormal.[23] For example, Kim has episodes of binge eating (e.g., eating larger than normal amounts of food, usually very rapidly) and feels she is unable to control how much she eats during these binges. Later, she becomes anxious about gaining weight and feels disgusted with herself for binging. Therefore, her binge eating is combined with drastic steps to lose weight by using laxatives, fasting, excessive exercise, and self-induced vomiting.[23] Unlike anorexia nervosa, adolescents with bulimia nervosa do not purge on a regular basis.

Bulimia shares many of the psychosocial symptoms characteristic of anorexia nervosa; feelings of inadequacy, low self-worth, poor body image, and depression. The adolescent's sense of emptiness and loneliness or the overwhelming anxiety prompts eating excessive amounts of food, usually alone. This leads to feelings of anxiety, shame, guilt, and fear. Purging temporarily eases these feelings and has a calming effect. As a result, the pattern of eating and purging becomes a way to regulate mood and cope with emotions. Adolescents with bulimia usually want to stop the pattern of binging and weight loss behaviors but feel unable to change it.

Obesity

Overeating is associated with mental health problems. Children and teens who overeat or binge eat are more likely to experience low self-worth and feelings of inadequacy. Therefore, obesity related to dysfunctional eating patterns has been proposed as a category of eating disorders in the revised *DSM-V*, which will be published in 2010 (see Chapter 14).

SUBSTANCE-RELATED DISORDERS

The *DSM-IV-TR* defines **substance-related disorders** as the misuse of drugs, toxins, and medications. The terms **substance abuse** and **substance dependence** describe the severity of substance use. Substance *abuse* classifies a pattern of use that results in adverse consequences, such as drinking alcohol and driving, or absence from school due to use of drugs or alcohol, or relationship difficulties related to drug use. **Addiction** is a term associated with substance-related disorders and refers to the intense physiologic and psychological craving for the substance being abused.[24,30,36] The terms *dependence* and *addiction* are essentially synonymous. Substance *dependence* classifies substance use that involves physical dependency on a substance (e.g., alcohol, cocaine, and other street drugs or prescription medications). In substance dependence, there is a pattern of continued use despite serious cognitive, behavioral, and physiologic symptoms and that has seven characteristics/symptoms.[5] At least three of the seven symptoms of the following must be present for a diagnosis of substance dependence.[5]

1. The development of tolerance (the need to use larger amounts of the substance to obtain the desired effect)
2. Unpleasant withdrawal symptoms when use is decreased or stopped
3. Use of the substance in increasing amounts or for increasingly longer periods of time
4. A desire to stop as well as failed attempts to stop using the substance
5. Excessive time spent in acquiring, using, and recovering from the substance
6. Neglect and a decline in occupational performance (e.g., work, leisure, ADLs)
7. Continued use despite the presence of problems caused by the substance

Among the many substances abused by children and adolescents are alcohol, amphetamines (uppers), cannabis (marijuana), hallucinogens (e.g., ecstasy and other club drugs, such as GHB and LSD), opioids (e.g., heroin, cocaine), phencyclidines (e.g., PCP, angel dust), sedatives, hypnotics, anxiolytics (e.g., Valium, Librium), steroids, and inhalants (e.g., nitrous oxide, acetone). Young people with substance dependence and abuse disorders can spend much of their time acquiring, using, and recovering from the substance.[24] As their dependence on and need for a drug grow, adolescents may become involved in illegal activities that often place them at further risk of harm (e.g., prostitution or selling drugs). Using and acquiring drugs has significant health risks, and children and adolescents entering treatment programs for substance dependence or abuse often have poor physical health and sometimes contract life-threatening conditions such as human immunodeficiency virus (HIV) infection or hepatitis from sharing needles. A strong association exists between alcohol use and suicide.

The extensive resources that are available identify specialized interventions for young people with substance abuse and dependence problems. There are residential programs that combine intensive therapy with the development of life skills and vocational skills and promote engaging in healthy activities. In this chapter, we have chosen to highlight one form of substance abuse: the use of inhalants, which is more common in children and adolescents than in adults, as these substances are easily accessible at relatively low costs.

Inhalant Abuse

CASE *Study*

Michael, a 15-year-old high school student, was found semiconscious in a local park and was hospitalized. In the preceding 6 months, Michael's parents had noticed changes in his behavior. He had appeared "spaced out and distracted and had become disinterested in his personal hygiene." They suspected that he and his friends were drinking and smoking. More recently, his mother had noticed a rash around his nose and mouth; he had become less outgoing and avoided family activities. Furthermore, Michael had failed two subjects last semester. He no longer played basketball with neighborhood boys after school and on the weekends; instead, he now spent his time "just hanging." Although he received a generous allowance, he no longer seemed to have money. Michael's admission to the hospital was the result of respiratory complications from inhalant use. His level of use may have already caused permanent brain damage.

The highest rates of inhalant use are among adolescents and children who live at or below the poverty level, and the majority of emergency consultations for inhalant-related problems are males.[5] Users refer to inhaling toxic substances as "huffing" or "sniffing." Substances commonly inhaled include gasoline, nail polish remover, solvent-based glue, paint thinner, spray paint, dry erasers and permanent markers, correction fluids, and aerosol propellants. Inhalant abuse leaves a common telltale rash around the nose and mouth and sometimes a runny nose, as noticed by Michael's mother. A cloth soaked in fluid inhalants (e.g., gasoline and paint thinner) is held over the mouth and nose and inhaled. This leaves a smell of paint or solvent on the teen's clothes, whereas aerosol substances are sprayed into a paper or plastic bag and inhaled with the bag over the mouth and nose.

The inhalant is rapidly absorbed into the bloodstream to create an almost immediate, intense "high." Psychotic experiences including auditory, visual, and tactile hallucinations (sensory perceptions incompatible with reality, such as the feeling of insects crawling beneath the skin) and delusions (beliefs incompatible with reality, such as believing parents are poisoning them). Vomiting, dizziness, generalized weakness, and abdominal pains and/or nausea are other symptoms of inhalant abuse.[5,30] The chronic use of inhalants can cause anxiety, depression, and permanent and occasionally lethal respiratory, cardiac, kidney, and liver problems.[5,30] Whatever the inhalant, its frequent use leads to significant impairment in all areas of occupational performance. Adolescent inhalant users neglect self-care, and decreased attendance and performance in school or work can occur. Changes in leisure interests such as dropping out of school activities and spending more time partying or participating in aimless activities, as with Michael's habit of "just hanging," is typical. Socially, the adolescent may stop spending time with friends who do not use substances and will develop relationships with those peers who do. In severe cases, irreversible brain damage with cognitive deficits may occur, causing long-term disability.

IMPLICATIONS FOR OCCUPATIONAL PERFORMANCE

Children and adolescents with psychosocial or behavioral disorders experience deficits in one or more areas of occupation (ADLs, instrumental ADLs [IADLs], work, education, social participation, and play/leisure).[3,13] OT practitioners examine performance patterns (i.e., habits, routines, and roles) associated with the occupational performance. For example, does the child or teen engage in self-care, attend school regularly, and participate in extracurricular activities with peers? The examination of performance patterns is combined with analysis of performance skills (i.e., motor, processing, and communication). For example, basic sharing, following rules, and peer communication skills are considered. Table 13-3 describes the effect of specific disorders on occupational performance, which is dependent on intact client factors, which are divided into mental (global and specific), neuromusculoskeletal, sensory, and systemic (i.e., cardiovascular, hematologic, immunologic, and respiratory) functions.

The OT practitioner also considers the influence of context on performance. For example, does the child or adolescent have others to play with? Do they feel safe at home and school or in other environments? Are the parents supportive physically as well as emotionally? In addition to considering the physical and social contexts, it is vital to bear in mind the child and family's cultural background. For example, there are differences in individual level of comfort with therapy and school. Differences in culture and experience may mean practitioners having to spend extra time explaining and connecting with parents so that they feel more comfortable participating with their children in the therapy settings and following recommendations. For example, parents who themselves did not have positive school experiences or did not attend school in the United States may be tentative in expressing their needs or knowing what is expected of them and their child. By demonstrating a willingness to listen and taking time for explanations, OT practitioners can help bridge cultural differences and reduce the anxiety of families. Furthermore, by creating an open and trusting relationship, practitioners may advocate for the children and their families in accessing needed resources and services. The goal is that with experience and increased knowledge, parents will become their child's advocate.

While OT practitioners examine all the client factors required to perform occupations, those working with children and teens experiencing psychosocial or mental health disorders pay close attention to global and specific mental functions. **Global mental functions** refer to consciousness, orientation, sleep, temperament and personality, and energy and drive.[3] **Specific mental functions** refer to attention, memory, perception, thought, higher-level cognition, the mental functions of language, calculation, mental functions of sequencing complex movements, psychomotor ability, emotion, and experiences of self and time.[3]

Children with impairment in global mental functions may present with low self-esteem because of frequent

TABLE 13-3

Impact of Selected Mental Disorders on Occupational Performance

PSYCHOSOCIAL DISORDER	FUNCTIONING IN ACTIVITIES OF DAILY LIVING/INSTRUMENTAL ACTIVITIES OF DAILY LIVING	SCHOOL AND WORK FUNCTIONING	PLAY AND LEISURE FUNCTIONING	SOCIAL FUNCTIONING
DISRUPTIVE BEHAVIOR DISORDERS				
Attention deficit disorder	Inattention to detail	Tardiness, absence, and neglect of school or work assignments and homework	Poor concentration, inattention, and disorganization	Inability to read social cues
ADHD	Refuses to comply with rules	Poor concentration, inattention, and disorganization	Difficulty with activity completion	Aggressive behavior toward others
Conduct disorder	Difficulty following directions	Restless and off-task behaviors	Lack of personal responsibility	Destruction of other's property, deceitfulness, and lack of remorse and guilt
Oppositional defiant disorder	Disorganization and forgetfulness	Education potentially disrupted when suspension results from defiant behavior at school or work (e.g., stealing, bullying).	Engaging in reckless activities (e.g., joining gangs) Lack of constructive leisure activities Physically aggressive or bullying Tendency to defy rules of games or sports Solitary leisure activities may not be affected.	Annoys others by being argumentative, losing temper, and blaming others for own mistakes
Learning Disorders	Seldom has problems with ADL skills, IADL skills may be disrupted by poor academic skills, disorganization, and lack of ability to maintain routines.	Specific disorder deficits (e.g., reading, writing, math) interfere with school or work performance Low frustration tolerance Poor self-efficacy in performance Additional time required for academic and work activities	Associated poor self-esteem Avoidance of sophisticated games dependent on scholastic abilities due to poor self-efficacy	Associated poor self-esteem Additional time required for academic work may interfere with social activities Feelings of low self-efficacy may result in avoidance of new social situations
TIC DISORDERS				
Tourette's syndrome	*Motor tics:* may interfere with movement during ADL/IADL *Vocal tics:* may avoid public places due to social stigma *Vocal and motor tics:* may interfere with safety because of distraction and unexpected movement	Motor and vocal tics interfere with concentration, visual scanning, writing, and communication Motor and vocal tics interfere with participation in group learning activities Difficulty finding an accepting employment/school setting	Avoidance by others Motor tics interfering with physical abilities Vocal and motor tics may interfere with safety because of distraction and expected movement Leisure activities that are engrossing and performed alone often unimpaired; in fact, the tics may decrease or disappear	Avoidance by adults and children Socially disruptive nature Embarrassment (self-imposed social withdrawal)

Continued

TABLE 13-3

Impact of Selected Mental Disorders on Occupational Performance—cont'd

PSYCHOSOCIAL DISORDER	FUNCTIONING IN ACTIVITIES OF DAILY LIVING/INSTRUMENTAL ACTIVITIES OF DAILY LIVING	SCHOOL AND WORK FUNCTIONING	PLAY AND LEISURE FUNCTIONING	SOCIAL FUNCTIONING
ANXIETY DISORDERS				
Separation anxiety disorder	Anxiety inhibiting beginning ADLs and IADLs	Anxiety inhibiting beginning tasks	Separation anxiety in attending group activities, after school activities, or play groups	Limiting relationships to significant and familiar persons
Generalized anxiety disorder	Fear of failure	Separation anxiety in attending school or work	Reluctance to take risks	Poor social self-efficacy
Phobic and social anxiety disorder	Perfectionism	Fear of failure	Anxiety inhibiting the startup of tasks	Fear of embarrassment
Obsessive-compulsive disorder	Phobias Ritualistic behaviors Inability to attain transition Intrusive thoughts	Poor self-efficacy in scholastic activities Perfectionism Phobias Ritualistic behaviors Intrusive thoughts Inability to transition Reluctance to take risks	Fear of failure Poor self-efficacy in new activities Perfectionism Phobias Ritualistic behaviors Intrusive thoughts Inability to transition or join in new groups	Reluctance to take risks Anxiety initiating social interaction Hypervigilance to social cues or oversensitivity and misinterpretation of cues Poor self-esteem Phobias Ritualistic behaviors Intrusive thoughts Lack of spontaneity
MOOD DISORDERS				
Major depressive disorder	Decreased energy and apathy Sleep and appetite disturbances Difficulty initiating and completing activities Lethargy (psychomotor retardation) Disinterest in appearance Poor self-esteem and self-loathing Somatic (physical) illness	Decreased energy and apathy Sleep and appetite disturbances Difficulty initiating and completing activities Lethargy (psychomotor retardation) Decreased concentration Difficulty with memory and following directions Difficulty with problem-solving Somatic (physical) illness	Decreased energy and apathy Sleep and appetite disturbances Difficulty initiating and completing activities Lethargy (psychomotor retardation) Decreased concentration Inability to derive pleasure Lack of spontaneity Lack of adaptive, imaginative, playfulness	Decreased energy and apathy Difficulty initiating social contact Self-imposed isolation Lethargy (psychomotor retardation) Decreased concentration Inability to derive pleasure Lack of spontaneity Poor self-esteem Slowed cognitive processing Preoccupation with ruminating thoughts

Schizophrenia	Poor concentration and inattention Disorganized thoughts Preoccupation with internal stimuli (e.g., hallucinations) Lack of awareness of reality Distractibility interferes with completing ADL/IADLs Overall lack of awareness of personal needs	Poor concentration and inattention Disorganized thoughts Preoccupation with internal stimuli (e.g., hallucinations) Lack of awareness of reality Distractibility interferes with school and work activities Tardiness, absence, and neglect of school or work assignments and homework Physical restlessness and agitation Off-task behaviors Gaps in learning Frequent hospitalization interfere with school and work performance	Poor concentration and inattention Disorganized thoughts Preoccupation with internal stimuli (e.g., hallucinations) Lack of awareness of reality Distractibility interferes with play and leisure performance	Poor concentration and inattention Disorganized thoughts making conversations difficult Preoccupation with internal stimuli (e.g., hallucinations) Lack of awareness of reality Tangential thinking Distractibility interferes with developing social relationships Sometimes inappropriate behavior Inattentive to external cues in social situations

EATING DISORDERS

Anorexia nervosa	ADL and IADL performance generally not affected with the exception of eating	Performance generally not affected unless physical health is compromised	Anorexia nervosa causing a focus on weight-controlling behaviors such as exercise	Avoids social contact for fear of having the disorder discovered
Bulimia nervosa	Inappropriate food consumption	Hospitalization leading to work and school absence	Poor body image	Poor self-esteem
Obesity	Time spent on health-related behaviors (e.g., dieting, laxative use, exercising)	Fatigue Poor concentration	Overweight teens may restrict sport and leisure activities Lack of cardiovascular fitness	Poor self-concept Avoids social events involving food (e.g., going to a restaurant with friends)

SUBSTANCE-RELATED DISORDERS

Substance-related disorders	Risky behaviors (e.g., use of illegal substances and promiscuity)	Cognitive impairment	Replacing activities with individuals who do not use substances with those associated with substance use	Limits social network to substance-using peers
Inhalant abuse	Apathy about hygiene and appearance Neglect of proper nutrition Time and money spent on substance	Tardiness, absence, and neglect of school or work assignments and homework Poor concentration Substance-induced state Consequence of poor physical health (e.g., fatigue, nausea, drug dependency symptoms) Education potentially disrupted when suspension results from criminal activity and use of illegal substances Unreliable in work setting or stealing from employer to support substance use	Dropping out of extracurricular activities to spend time "hanging out" or partying Money spent on substance Substance use dominates activities	Self-imposed social withdrawal from family

ADL, activities of daily living; IADL, instrumental activities of daily living.

failure or frustration. They may have difficulty expressing themselves through language and may show lability of emotions (frequent fluctuations in mood), which typically affects their social participation. Specific mental functions may be manifested as difficulties with memory needed for academic and ADL tasks. Similarly, specific mental functions are required for organization (e.g., dressing and other ADLs). Children with these impairments may also show poor attention to detail, resulting in errors in academic work.

The OT practitioner analyzes the child's ability to perform the occupation, paying careful attention to the global and specific mental functions that may be interfering with the child's ability to be successful. On the basis of a frame of reference, the OT practitioner designs remedial, developmental, and compensatory interventions for occupational performance problems.

DATA GATHERING AND EVALUATION

The OT practitioner has the ultimate responsibility of interpreting evaluation information.[4,19] He or she determines the specific areas of evaluation and specific assessment methods and tools. Once an OTA achieves service competency, specific aspects of the information gathering process may be given to him or her, including review of records, interviews, observations, and structured assessments. Many methods may be used to gather information about the child or adolescent's current level of functioning. OT practitioners may be assigned the task of reviewing the client's records. Inpatient and outpatient settings typically maintain medical records that provide information about the client's age, sex, academic level, family situation, cultural background, diagnosis, medical history, psychiatric history, medications, and current symptoms. In the school setting, educational records are reviewed.

CLINICAL *Pearl*

Observation skills are developed by practice. Take every opportunity to observe typical children in their areas of occupation. This provides a comparison for observing children with special needs.

Interviews with the child or adolescent and family members provide information about the individual's home environment, performance of self-care tasks, relationships with family members, and participation in leisure activities. Other members of the treatment team may provide valuable insight (verbally and as documented in the client's records) into the child's or adolescent's occupational performance. For example, in an inpatient setting, nursing staff can identify the client's specific problems with ADLs. In the school setting, teachers may be able to identify specific problems that interfere with learning and academic performance.

Observation is one of the most important evaluation tools of the OT practitioner. Much can be learned about specific client factor deficits by observing the individual's performance in ADLs, IADLs, work, education, leisure/play, and social participation. For example, by observing the child or adolescent during a classroom activity, the OT practitioner can identify specific problems in concentration, attention span, work skills (e.g., neatness and rate of completion), and behavioral deficits that interfere with learning. Observation of the child or adolescent during recess provides information about social skills, including the amount and appropriateness of interaction with peers and participation in available leisure activities. Observation is also the ongoing data-gathering process for monitoring improvement. The OTA plays a significant role in the evaluation process because he or she is the practitioner who has regular contact with the child or adolescent.

Structured evaluation tools may be used to assess the occupational performance of children and adolescents.[6,20] For example, the Piers-Harris Scale is used to determine a level of self-concept among children.[25] Many of the assessments based on the Model of Human Occupation (MOHO) provide a structured means of learning about children's and adolescents' psychosocial challenges. The Child Occupational Self-Assessment (COSA) explores an adolescent's values and how he or she perceives performance and competencies. The Volitional Questionnaire (VQ) provides practitioners with information about what the teen finds motivating and the Health Questionnaire (HQ) examines a child's perceived quality of life. These assessments may be administered by OTAs and interpreted by the occupational therapist. Many OT departments have developed facility-specific assessments by modifying and combining available tools to meet the needs of a specific setting and client population.

INTERVENTION
Planning

OT is guided by frames of reference and the best practice guidelines for the child or adolescent presenting with occupational performance difficulties (see Table 13-2). Intervention planning involves collaborating with the child or adolescent, family, and other individuals, such as the members of a health care team or an educational team. Planning considers the strengths and weaknesses of the individual in order to develop long-term and short-term goals and determine interventions (e.g., purposeful activities and strategies or techniques for implementation) as well as the frequency and duration of intervention activities. The OT practitioner capitalizes on a child's psychological, social, and behavioral strengths to determine intervention activities that will meet therapeutic goals. The goals and activities are based on the client's needs, interests, culture, and environment. The OTA contributes to this intervention planning and implementation.[4]

Long-term psychosocial goals identify the desired treatment outcome, and short-term goals identify the steps necessary to achieve the long-term goals. For example, increased social participation is a common desired outcome of therapy. Such an outcome improves the child or adolescent's ability to develop competence in age-appropriate occupational roles. Tyrone's story provides an example of one long-term goal and three short-term goals.

CASE *Study*

Tyrone is a 9-year-old boy who lives in a foster care home with his two younger brothers after the death of his mother from a drug overdose. He has been extremely withdrawn and fearful in the past 6 months. In school, he has been aggressive and socially isolated. His academic performance has dropped significantly. Tyrone has been diagnosed with depression and prescribed Paxil. He attends a before- and after-school program for children at risk.

Long-term Goal: At discharge, Tyrone will demonstrate age-appropriate social participation in peer group activities.

Short-term Goal #1: By the end of Week 1, Tyrone will verbally interact one on one with a peer during a group play activity.

Short-term Goal #2: By the end of Week 2, Tyrone will initiate conversations with peers a minimum of two times during a group activity.

Short-term Goal #3: By the end of Week 1 Tyrone will demonstrate collaborative play behaviors, as demonstrated by sharing materials and taking turns with peers in play activities.

Implementation

An effective intervention follows a set of principles and uses techniques and strategies that are based on a selected frame of reference. The purpose of following a frame of reference is to ensure that the outcomes are related directly to the method of treatment used. For example, medication combined with cognitive–behavioral therapy may be the most effective intervention for the treatment of depression.[28] This combination of interventions relieves symptoms and prevents relapse. Table 13-2 shows some of the frames of reference that direct psychosocial OT interventions.

Most OT intervention with children and adolescents occurs in groups and provides opportunities to learn and practice skills. Well-designed OT groups create an optimal environment for achieving the child or adolescent's goals, facilitating interpersonal interactions, and developing competence in a broad range of skills. Regardless of whether interventions occur individually or in groups, they typically include structure, consistency, and positive experiences. Intervention activities promote the acquisition of appropriate behavioral skills and address specific areas of occupational performance in which children perform poorly. These activities for children emphasize play and may include toys, games, and crafts that are developmentally appropriate, interesting, fun, and challenging. For adolescents, the activities have a peer group focus and may involve a variety of creative arts and role playing. The emphasis often is IADLs, self-care, and social activities that facilitate transition to adulthood.

Group interventions generally address specific problem areas tailored to a particular age group. For example, in a school setting, the OT practitioner may design a task group for children in Grades 1 through 3 who have difficulty attending to a task or demonstrate poor work skills. Children can develop or improve the skills needed to complete tasks effectively by working on individual craft projects in a structured small-group setting away from the distractions of the busy classroom. During group sessions, the OT practitioner adapts the planned activities to ensure success and to extend the skill level of the children. Additional therapeutic benefits also intentionally addressed are age-appropriate social skills (e.g., sharing equipment and materials, keeping the workspace tidy, and asking for assistance) and coping skills (e.g., dealing with frustration). Table 13-4 provides examples of psychosocial OT groups.

For many group interventions, a number of well-developed protocols and programs are available. Education, social work, OT, outdoor education, and psychology all have developed structured programs that have been shown to achieve the identified goals. This is particularly true for social skills, coping skills, assertiveness training, childhood fitness, and self-esteem and self-awareness programs. The OT practitioner needs to identify and use these resources when planning group interventions.

TABLE 13-4

Sample Occupational Therapy Groups for Children or Adolescents With Psychosocial Dysfunction

GROUP	PURPOSE	METHODS	OUTCOMES
IMAGINATIVE PLAY GROUP *Population/group membership:* Children and adolescents with difficulty enjoying or participating in play, interacting with others, problem solving, or feeling good about themselves Imaginative games may help children/adolescents decrease stress and connect with others. Playgroups can be used to work on many psychosocial issues. They help children and adolescents learn flexibility and problem solving and may teach clients how to adapt and cope with different situations.	Provide social opportunities to improve the following: • Social participation • Playfulness • Adaptability and flexibility • Problem solving • Imagination • Taking turns • Sharing	Develop a "play" in small groups that is later presented. Members discuss the play. Depending on the age of the children, pretend clothing may be used, different scenarios or role-playing. Children may be asked to act out a story or work as a team. Group storytelling Puppetry Props Music	Increased self-expression Increased playfulness (one's approach to activities) Opportunities to role-play may help with reading cues, understanding oneself and others, and dealing with issues. Improved social participation Improved stress reduction
TASK SKILLS GROUP *Population/group membership:* Children and adolescents experiencing difficulty performing occupations (e.g., ADLs, IADLs, school, work, leisure, social participation) The task skills group helps clients learn, practice, and refine the skills needed to accomplish occupations. The members receive support from the group while developing and refining the skills needed for living.	Provide opportunities to improve the following task skills. Task organization, planning, and implementation such as preparation of materials and cleanup of work area Ability to follow directions On-task behaviors Task completion Recognition of errors and problem-solving skills Ability to work with others Ability to identify steps of projects	Develop a plan as a group and carry out selected tasks. Work together toward completion of the tasks. Engage in group and individual tasks required for ADLs, IADLs, work, education, and leisure/play. Examples of types of groups include meal planning, events (e.g., dance, field trip), crafts, and planning a party.	Improve social participation, sense of belonging, efficacy, and self-confidence through completion of selected tasks as part of a team. Improve the organizational, planning, and problem-solving skills needed to complete selected tasks. Develop skills for ADLs, IADLs, education, work, leisure, and social participation.

LIFE SKILLS

Population/group membership: Typical children and adolescents with significant physical or intellectual disabilities living in a residential setting such as a group home.

Groups focusing on IADL skills are provided to older adolescents with psychiatric, intellectual, or cognitive disabilities. These adolescents may or may not be in a residential setting. Many may be undergoing transition from the home to a community residential setting such as a group home.

Teach and promote independence in basic life and self-care skills in the following areas:

- Personal care of hygiene, grooming, etc.
- Dressing
- Money management
- Functional mobility
- Community mobility
- Health maintenance
- Medication routines
- Functional communication
- Emergency response
- Sexual expression

Teach and promote independence in IADLs. These skills overlap with basic life skills but also include the ability to care for oneself and one's environment. These skills include meal preparation, home management, caregiving, care of clothes, more complex money management beyond immediate personal use, and safety procedures.

Methods include task analysis, role-playing, and behavior rehearsal.

Educational model advocates teaching, demonstrating, guiding, and practicing with supervision, followed by independent practice.

Experiential learning that involves gradual skill development is a key component in these groups. The setting can be the group home, school, or clinic.

Develop life skills

Gain age-appropriate independence.

SOCIAL SKILLS

Population/group membership: All children and adolescents

The groups work the most effectively if the children or adolescents have similar developmental and cognitive/intellectual levels as well as common problem areas.

These groups are often divided into skill areas to include specific groups in communication, relationships and supporting others, problem solving in relationships, and self-monitoring in social situations.

Develop the skills required for interacting and "getting along" with others.

Develop the skills required for effective verbal and nonverbal communication.

Learn and practice socially appropriate behaviors (e.g., manners, sharing).

Learn and practice cooperation and teamwork.

Develop positive attitudes toward others (e.g., peers, family, teachers, and authority figures such as the police).

Groups can focus on coping with specific problems such as shyness or loneliness.

Concrete activities demonstrate and practice social skills and are often based on a psychoeducational, educational, or social-cognitive model.

These structured groups use a variety of learning techniques that combine knowledge and practice of the social skills learned.

The methods include pen and paper, role-playing, practical skill demonstration sessions, films, behavior rehearsal, guided practice, homework tasks, experiential learning, and imitation.

Improvement in personal and social relationships

Increased verbal participation in classroom setting

Positive participation in group activities

Increased social interaction with peers

Increased inclusion in peer activities

Reduction in inappropriate social behavior

Continued

TABLE 13-4

Sample Occupational Therapy Groups for Children or Adolescents With Psychosocial Dysfunction—cont'd

GROUP	PURPOSE	METHODS	OUTCOMES
COPING SKILLS *Population/group membership:* Children and adolescents with no significant intellectual disabilities The groups work the most effectively if the children or adolescents have similar developmental and cognitive/intellectual levels as well as common problem areas.	Provide opportunities to improve or learn coping skills including self-regulation in the following problem areas: • Poor impulse control • Excessive motor activity • Distractibility • Low frustration tolerance • Difficulty in delaying gratification • Depression, anxiety, or hostility The groups can focus on coping with specific problems such as grief and stress.	Reflection on the techniques and/or alternatives used to perform occupations helps children and adolescents learn coping skills. Strategies for working on specific areas may benefit children and adolescents, such as stress management, homework strategies, massage, and writing assignments. The methods include pen and paper, role-playing, practical skill demonstration sessions, films, behavior rehearsal, guided practice, homework tasks, experiential learning, and imitation.	Increased self-esteem and positive self-image Increased self-efficacy in one's ability to manage emotions in a variety of situations Improvement in one's ability to interact in social settings Improvement in one's ability to share space and materials in a group setting and one on one Decrease in self-destructive behaviors and aggressive or acting-out behaviors
SELF-AWARENESS *Population/group membership:* Adolescents with no intellectual disabilities Adolescents are able to function in group settings and cope emotionally and cognitively with personal exploration.	Provide activities that increase insight and self-awareness. Facilitate self-reflection and self-evaluation in a supportive and safe context. Facilitate the resolution of inner conflicts. Develop a constructive self-concept and build self-esteem.	The methods used in self-awareness groups usually involve an activity after which the product or experience is used in a process of self-reflection. Thoughts and feelings are explored and discussed in the group setting to help the adolescents confront and gain insight into their inner feelings and conflicts. The process of self-discovery leads individuals to make connections between past experiences and current feelings, difficulties, and behaviors. Activities can be group collaborative or competitive exercises and projects as well as individual activities including art, ceramics, sculpture, dance, movement "ropes" courses and/or exercises, games, massage, writing, poetry, and drama. The discussions that are facilitated by the activity can address themes such as *who am I, caring about myself and others, understanding and confronting my problems, taking responsibility for myself, understanding the consequences of my actions, and making connections between past events and current feelings.*	Reduction in symptoms (e.g., depression) Behavioral change: Reduction in self-destructive, aggressive, or antiauthority behavior Reduction in suicidal thoughts Improvement in self-worth and ongoing development of positive self-concept Improvement in academic performance Improvement in the quality of interpersonal relationships

ADL, Activities of daily living; IADL, instrumental activities of daily living.
Data compiled from Cara E, MacRae A: *Psychosocial occupational therapy: A clinical practice,* Albany, NY, 2005, Delmar; Stein F, Cutler SK: *Psychosocial occupational therapy: A holistic approach,* ed 2, Albany, NY, 2002, Delmar.

THERAPEUTIC USE OF SELF

The benefits of an empathic (i.e., conveying to another individual that you have an appreciative sense of that individual's experience), positive relationship between a child or adolescent and adult are well recognized and are the basis of many health and educational mentoring programs (e.g., Big Brothers and Big Sisters). In the relationship between the OT practitioner and the child/ adolescent, the interaction and rapport developed is dependent on the OT practitioner's capacity to facilitate effectively a positive validating relationship and use communication and interpersonal skills in a therapeutic manner.

In a relationship with a child, the challenges include being empathetic, being consistent, and setting boundaries to create a safe and supportive environment while remaining flexible. Implicit in this relationship is respect for the child or adolescent. It is essential to give feedback that makes it clear that it is the behavior that is unacceptable or disliked not the child.

Awareness and mindfulness of how OT practitioners relate to clients is important in the OT process, and being conscious and intentional in all interactions is a necessary dimension of the therapeutic relationship. Taylor's Intentional Relationship Model (IRM) describes six modes used in therapeutic relationships: (1) advocating, (2) collaborating, (3) empathizing, (4) encouraging, (5) instructing, and (6) problem solving.[34] OT practitioners have their own favorite modes, but it is possible to use multiple modes.[34] Certain modes will be more effective for some clients than for others. Overuse of a particular mode may work against the therapeutic relationship. For example, a practitioner who solely uses the instructing mode may find that the teen stops listening. Since teens frequently rebel against authority figures, the instructing mode may feel like they are being "lectured at." OT practitioners working with teens may have more success using the collaborating or advocating modes.

OT practitioners must realize that all behavior has meaning, including that of the OT practitioner's behavior as the health care professional. Children and adolescents will ascribe meaning to the OT practitioner's actions. Individuals with poor self-esteem and low self-worth easily misinterpret interpersonal cues. For example, if the OT practitioner is consistently late for an appointment, the child may feel that he or she is not important even though thoughts and feelings are not necessarily obvious or expressed verbally. Instead, OT practitioners may observe them in the child's behaviors, affect (mood), or responses.

The therapeutic use of self requires that an OT practitioner be self-reflective, open to feedback, and aware of the influence of personal disposition, values, and culture.

Although working with children and families is rewarding, it is also emotionally demanding and at times stressful. Therefore, supervision and peer support are beneficial. Having a supportive working environment, participating in continuing education, and taking care of one's own well-being will ensure the OT practitioner's capacity to have therapeutic relationships with children or adolescents with whom they work.

SUMMARY

Children and adolescents can have psychosocial and mental disorders that affect areas of occupational performance impeding their development. Knowledge of the signs and symptoms of these disorders helps the OT practitioner design effective interventions. The goal of intervention is to provide the child or adolescent with the appropriate tools to engage effectively in occupations, be able to feel successful, and develop independence. This chapter presents the OT practitioner with practical clinical information for treating children and adolescents with psychosocial and mental health disorders.

References

1. Article Brief. Adults should heed teens' warning signs. *USA Today Magazine* 126:4, December 1997.
2. American Academy of Child and Adolescent Psychiatry. Oppositional defiant disorder. July 2009. Available at: http://www.aacap.org/cs/ODD.ResourceCenter. Accessed July 7, 2010.
3. American Occupational Therapy Association: *Occupational therapy practice framework: domain and process*, ed 2. *Am J Occup Ther* 62:625–683, 2008.
4. American Occupational Therapy Association (Screen W, compiler): Standards of practice for occupational therapy. In *American Occupational Therapy Association: reference manual of the official documents of the American Occupational Therapy Association*, ed 6, Bethesda, MD, 1996, American Occupational Therapy Association.
5. American Psychiatric Association: *Diagnostic and statistical manual of mental disorders: DSM-IV-TR*, ed 4, Washington, DC, 2000, American Psychiatric Association.
6. Asher IE: *Occupational therapy assessment tools: an annotated index*, ed 2, Bethesda, MD, 1996, American Occupational Therapy Association.
7. Banerjee TD, Middleton F, Faraone SV: Environmental risk factors for attention-deficit hyperactivity disorder. *Acta Paediatrica* 96:1269, 2007.
8. Bazyk S et al: *Occupational therapy and school mental health: American Occupational Therapy Association facts sheet*. Available at: http://www.towson.edu/etu/insider/110409/images/OT_sheet.pdf. Accessed July 7, 2010.
9. Bhatia SK, Bhatia SC: Childhood and adolescent depression. *Am Fam Physician* 75:73–79, 2007.
10. Batshaw ML: *Children with disabilities*, ed 5, Baltimore, 2002, Brooks Publishing.

11. Bonder BR: *Psychopathology and function*, ed 4, Thorofare, NJ, 2010, Slack.

12. Crone D, Horner R: *Building positive behavior support systems in schools*, New York, 2003, The Guildford Press.

13. Florey L: Psychosocial dysfunction in childhood and adolescence. In Crepeau EB, Cohn ES, Boyt Schell BA, editors: *Willard and Spackman's occupational therapy*, ed 10, Philadelphia, 2003, Lippincott Williams & Wilkins.

14. Frick P et al: Academic underachievement and the disruptive behavior disorders. *J Consulting Clin Psychol* 59:289, 1991.

15. Froehlich TE et al: Prevalence, recognition, and treatment of attention-deficit/hyperactivity disorder in a national sample of US children. *Arch Pediatr Adolesc Med* 161:857, 2007.

16. Goldman WT: *Bipolar disorder*. Available at: http://www.keepkidshealthy.com/welcome/conditions/bipolar_disorder.html. Accessed July 7, 2010.

17. Gutkind L: *Stuck in time: the tragedy of childhood mental illness*, New York, 1993, Henry Holt.

18. Hafen BQ, Frandsen KJ: *Youth suicide: depression and loneliness*, Evergreen, CO, 1984, Cordillera.

19. Hemphill BJ, editor: *The mental health assessment: an integrative approach to the evaluative process*, Thorofare, NJ, 1988, Slack.

20. Kaplan HI, Sadock BJ: *Kaplan and Sadock's synopsis of psychiatry*, ed 8, Baltimore, MD, 1998, Williams & Wilkins.

21. Lambert LW: Mental health of children. In Cara E, MacRae A, editors: *Psychosocial occupational therapy: a clinical practice*, ed 3, Clifton Park, NY, 2005, Thomson Delmar Learning.

22. Masi G et al: Generalized anxiety disorder in referred children and adolescents. *J Am Acad Child Adolesc Psychiatr* 43:752, 2004.

23. Neistein LS, Mackenzie RG: Anorexia nervosa and bulimia nervosa. In Neistein LS, editor: *Adolescent health care: a practical guide*, ed 4, Philadelphia, 2002, Lippincott Williams & Wilkins.

24. Patton GC et al: Puberty and the onset of substance use and abuse. *Pediatrics* 114:e300, 2004.

25. Piers EV: *Piers-Harris children's self-concept scale*, rev ed, Los Angeles, 1984, Western Psychological Service.

26. Robins LN, Regier DA, editors: *Psychiatric disorders in America: the epidemiologic catchments area study*, New York, 1991, The Free Press.

27. Rogers SL: Common conditions that influence children's participation. In Case-Smith J, editor: *Occupational therapy for children*, ed 5, St. Louis, 2005, Mosby.

28. Sarles RM, Neistein LS: Adolescent depression. In Neistein LS, editor: *Adolescent health care: a practical guide*, ed 4, Philadelphia, 2002, Lippincott Williams & Wilkins.

29. Searight HR, Rottnek F, Abby SL: Conduct disorder: diagnosis and treatment in primary care. *Am Fam Physician* 63:1579, 2001.

30. Sherry CJ: *Inhalants*, New York, 1994, Rosen.

31. Derrick Silove D, Bryant R: Rapid assessments of mental health needs after disasters. *JAMA* 296:576, 2006.

32. Stein F, Culter SK: *Psychosocial occupational therapy: a holistic approach*, ed 2, Albany, NY, 2002, Delmar.

33. Sue D, Sue DW, Sue S: *Understanding abnormal behavior*, ed 9, Boston, 2010, Wadsworth Cengage Learning.

34. Taylor R: *The intentional relationship: use of self and occupational therapy*, Philadelphia, 2007, FA Davis.

35. Warner V et al: Grandparents, parents, and grandchildren at high risk of depression: a three generational study. *J Am Acad Child Adolesc Psychiatr* 38:289, 1999.

36. Winter PA, editor: *Teen addiction*, San Diego, 1997, Greenhaven.

Recommended Reading

Early MB: *Mental health concepts and techniques for the occupational therapy assistant*, ed 4, Philadelphia, 2009, Lippincott Williams & Wilkins.

Early P: *A father's search through America's mental health system: crazy*, New York, 2006, The Berkley Publishing Group.

Taylor R: *The intentional relationship: use of self and occupational therapy*, Philadelphia, 2007, FA Davis.

Witkovsky MT: Child and adolescent psychiatry and occupational therapy. *Special Interest Section Quarterly Mental Health* 30, September 2007.

REVIEW *Questions*

1. What is a mental health disorder?

2. What is the *DSM-IV-TR*, and how does the OT practitioner use this classification system?

3. Describe briefly three symptoms of each of the following disorders: conduct disorder, oppositional defiant disorder, separation anxiety disorder, Tourette's syndrome, anorexia nervosa, bulimia nervosa, and major depressive disorder.

4. Describe symptoms that indicate depression in adolescents and how these symptoms would present in therapy.

5. What are five strategies you would teach a child to cope with anxiety?

6. Describe how the symptoms of each of the disorders in question 3 affect school performance.

7. What are the principles of psychoeducational groups, and when would you use them?

8. Describe important considerations when designing OT intervention for children with ADHD.

SUGGESTED *Activities*

1. Visit a few daycare centers, and observe children engaged in educational and play activities. Ask yourself questions 2 through 5 that follow.
2. Who is playing alone, what activities are the children engaged in? For example, is the play imaginative, repetitive, creative, or educational?
3. How do children transition between tasks and follow the teacher's instructions?
4. What social interactions are happening between children as they play and work?
5. Observe age-appropriate psychosocial behaviors. Do not draw conclusions about children; just observe behaviors that are functional or less functional (e.g., collaborative, aggressive, and inability to attend to play activities).
6. Visit a place where adolescents gather, such as a mall. Observe the social interaction among the adolescents, and consider their dress and choice of activities in relationship to their age.
7. Many videos that depict mental disorders in children and adolescents are available through the university or college library or health services. Watch videos on the disorders discussed in this chapter, and imagine the way you would feel if the child or adolescent were a member of your family. List the questions and concerns that come to mind. Movies and documentaries that you might watch include (a) *Precious* (2009), based on the book *Push*; (b) *Thin*, an HBO documentary (2006) about eating disorders; or (c) *Phoebe in Wonderland*, a movie about a young girl with Tourette's syndrome.
8. Contact the National Alliance for the Mentally Ill (1-800-950-6264) for information on family support.
9. Look at self-help sites for parents and teens. What are the concerns and questions that parents and teens express? Answer these questions using the chapter and other sources of information.
10. Visit the Web site of at least three mental health organizations (e.g., those of childhood depression, attention deficit-hyperactivity disorder, schizophrenia). Discuss your findings in a small group.

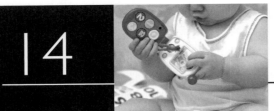

14

Childhood and Adolescent Obesity

KERRYELLEN G. VROMAN

JANE CLIFFORD O'BRIEN

CHAPTER *Objectives*

After studying this chapter, the reader will be able to accomplish the following:

- Describe the factors that cause obesity in children and adolescents.
- Recognize the behavioral and psychosocial factors associated with childhood and adolescent obesity.
- Be able to describe interventions for preventing obesity at family, school, and community levels.
- Be able to plan and implement with occupational therapy team members and other health and educational professionals a comprehensive program that promotes physical activity, healthy life style patterns, and self-efficacy for healthy behaviors.
- Be able to plan and implement with occupational therapy team members individual and group interventions for children and adolescents, with and without disabilities, who are obese or overweight.

U.S. First Lady Michelle Obama highlighted childhood **obesity** and its negative social, emotional, and health consequences in her comprehensive proposal "Let's Move Campaign." She emphasized the psychosocial consequences and, in doing so, recognized that obesity reaches beyond a child's weight. The First lady said " . . . 'overweight' and 'obese'— those words don't tell the full story because this isn't about inches and pounds, and it's not about how our kids look . . . it's about how our kids feel, and it's about how they feel about themselves. It's about the impact that this issue is having on every aspect of their life."[40] This statement affirms the perspective of obesity in occupational therapy (OT); it is not about a child's weight per se; it is about how obesity affects children's and adolescents' ability to participate successfully in age-related occupations.

Obesity affects quality of life and interferes with everyday activities, play, and social participation. Children and adolescents who are obese enjoy sport less than do peers who are not overweight. These children experience joint discomfort and problems with breathing, and they particularly dislike intense physical activity such as running.[18] They also report that they do not enjoy social activities such as shopping for clothes, eating out with friends, or dancing.[59]

This chapter outlines the biopsychosocial factors that contribute to obesity and examines specific causes and conditions associated with weight gain in children and adolescents. It includes a section on the consequences of obesity for children and adolescents and the implications of prejudicial **antifat attitudes** in OT practice. The final section presents programs and strategies an OT practitioner may use within OT to manage and prevent weight gain.

BIOLOGICAL, PHYSICAL, PSYCHOLOGICAL, AND SOCIAL FACTORS ASSOCIATED WITH OBESITY

Overweight and *obesity* are the terms used to describe weight that is well above normal for height and build. Differences in body fat between boys and girls and at various ages are taken into account.[45] For example, a child or adolescent is overweight if he or she is more than 20% over his or her ideal weight. To measure body fat, the National Institute of Health (NIH) uses the **body mass index** (BMI) as a classification system. A BMI of 30 or greater is the criteria for a diagnosis of obesity (Box 14-1). Although the BMI correlates with the amount of body fat, it is not a direct measure of body fat, and some adolescents who have a muscular body can have a BMI that identifies them as overweight.

The methods used to estimate body fat and body fat distribution include measurements of skin-fold thickness

---

BOX 14-1

Obesity and BMI

Body mass index (BMI) is a reliable tool used to measure body fat. It correlates highly with direct measures of body weight (e.g., underwater weighing-displacement). After a child's BMI is calculated, the number is plotted on the BMI for age growth chart for sex to obtain the child's percentile ranking. This ranking rates the child relative to children of the same age and sex. Some practitioners prefer to use degrees of overweight because the term *obesity* is regarded as a stigmatizing term. Others use ranges of obesity from *mild* to *severe* because this method is more informative. If the BMI index is used, the following formula is used:

$$\text{Weight (lb)}/[\text{Height(in)}]^2 \times 703$$

For a BMI calculation which will consider a child's age and sex, access the Center for Disease and Prevention (CDC) Web site calculator at http://apps.nccd.cdc.gov/dnpabmi/Calculator.aspx.

WEIGHT STATUS CATEGORY	PERCENTILE RANGE
Underweight	Less than 5th percentile
Healthy weight	5th percentile to less than 85th percentile
Overweight	85th percentile to less than 95th percentile
Obese	Equal to or greater than the 95th percentile

From www. cdc.gov, healthweight\assessing\BMI\children_BMI.

---

and waist circumference, calculation of waist-to-hip circumference ratios, and procedures such as ultrasonography and computed tomography (CT).[45]

The physiologic process that results in gaining weight is an energy imbalance, namely, energy intake (i.e., food) is greater than energy expenditure (physical activity).[61] However, this simple equation does not capture the complexity of the causal factors, since the mechanisms that underpin obesity are the interactions among biological, genetic, sociocultural, economic, and environmental factors (Box 14-2).[30] For example, interaction among genetics, diet, eating behaviors, low physical activity patterns, and sedentary lifestyle may explain the positive correlation between the weights of parents and their children.

Biological and Genetic Factors

A biological model assists in identifying children who are overweight or obese. If identified early, these children can receive personalized early interventions

Causes and Factors Associated With Childhood and Adolescent Obesity

- Childhood and adolescent individual factors (e.g., genetic disorders)
- Hormonal or endocrine (e.g., hypothyroidism)
- Diet
- Limited physical activity and preference for sedentary lifestyle
- Personal contexts: family, friends, and peer networks
  - Family stressors
  - Parent education, ethnicity, and socioeconomic status
  - Parents' limit setting concerning food choices
  - Family physical activity patterns, interests and leisure activities
  - Family preference for sedentary activity patterns
- Medications
- Chronic health conditions that restrict participation in physical activity
- Environment: schools, communities
- Availability of health care services

From Minihan PM, Fitch AN, Must A: What does the epidemic of childhood obesity mean for children with special health needs? *J Law Med Ethics* 35:61, 2007.

(pharmacologic, lifestyle, and diet measures) or preventive health care that decreases their vulnerability to chronic health disorders (e.g., diabetes, orthopedic abnormalities, and cardiovascular disease).[53]

Recent research studies, especially genome-based ones, have identified family susceptibility to obesity. Children and adolescents who are genetically predisposed to obesity will gain weight when exposed to a suboptimal diet-and-exercise pattern (e.g., poor diet and lack of exercise). Research identifying chromosomes related to weight is relatively new, and the findings are mostly provisional. Further evidence of heritable factors and the scope of knowledge of biological factors related to excessive weight gain will become more comprehensive with time.

Early-onset obesity is a symptom that occurs in some chromosomal syndromes, including the Mendelian syndromes Prader Willi syndrome, Albright hereditary osteodystrophy, and Bardet Biedel syndrome.[31] Associated characteristics with weight gain in these syndromes are small stature, low activity levels, low muscle tone (hypotonia), and intellectual disability. In other chromosomal disorders, weight

gain is a secondary problem. For example, children with Down syndrome often are overweight or obese due to low intensity of activity and other physical factors such as low muscle tone, heart defects (restricting participation in and endurance for physical activity), and hypothyroidism.[60]

Since hormonal, metabolic, and neuronal factors regulate weight, the body seeks to maintain a baseline weight, and the desire for food is adjusted accordingly through a feedback system involving the interaction of peripheral hormones, gastrointestinal peptides, and neuropeptides.[31] OT practitioners need to be aware of the biological and genetic factors that may be contributing to a child's weight. For example, hypothyroidism slows metabolic rate, and children with this disorder will need to perform high-intensity activities.

Physical Factors: Activity and Dietary Behaviors

Diet, sedentary behaviors, and lack of physical activity are modifiable causal factors of childhood and adolescent obesity. For example, insufficient physical activity is a recognized risk factor for obesity and related chronic conditions, whereas engaging in physical activity from an early age (toddlers) protects children from excessive weight gain.[28,53] These physical activity patterns established in childhood positively influence later activity patterns. Unfortunately, for many, especially girls, participation in physical activity declines across childhood and into adolescence.[48] The Centers for Disease Control (CDC) Youth Media Campaign Longitudinal Study found that 61.5% of children between the ages of 9 to 13 years did not participate in any organized physical activity in nonschool hours, and 22.3% did not participate in *any* free time activity.[13]

Low physical activity and sedentary behaviors are interrelated. However, healthy children and adolescents have a balance of low and high physical activities and derive benefits developmentally from both. For example, a child may be an avid reader, play sports, go hiking with his family, and watch TV and maintain a healthy weight. The growth in technology-based leisure pursuits such as watching TV, playing video games, and engaging in multiple forms of computer-mediated communication have contributed to sedentary behaviors and the resultant rise in obesity.[1] The problem is not that **sedentary activities** require a low expenditure of energy. Rather, sedentary activities may displace high-physical-energy activities, and children who engage in sedentary activities end up with a lower metabolic rate than their physically active peers do.

CLINICAL *Pearl*

Generally, the recommendation is that children watch no more than 2 hours of TV per day. Children and adolescents with TVs in their bedrooms watch TV more than those who do not have TVs in their rooms. Watching less TV can lead to reduction in a child's weight, but it is most effective when more physically active leisure replaces TV viewing.[41]

Numerous personal and environmental factors also lead to a predominantly sedentary activity pattern. For example, poverty contributes to higher levels of sedentary activities and poor diet. Similarly, some sedentary activities promote higher food intake and/or unhealthy eating patterns. For example, TV advertisements promote fast foods, snacks, and drinks that appeal to children, but these foods are often high in sugar and fats. Eating while watching TV encourages snacking, whereas sitting down at the table for a family meal models healthy eating patterns and helps children monitor food intake and portion size. Furthermore, family meals are associated with a higher intake of vegetables and a lower intake of such items as sodas and fried foods.[23]

Diet and eating behaviors are central to obesity; children and adolescents who are physically active are more likely to have a healthy diet.[49] Genetic, demographic, family, sociocultural, and physical factors collectively influence the foods children experience, have access to, and the patterns around food intake that they learn (Box 14-3). Eating patterns, in relation to diet and food preferences, in households where a parent is obese differ from households in which neither parent is obese.[2,48] Dysfunctional **habits** and **routines** contribute to low activity and poor diet patterns among children, adolescents, and their families.

Behavioral dietary and physical activity interventions have been shown to effectively address weight issues and the psychosocial problems associated with obesity.[54] However, interventions for children who have parents with their own challenges around diet and weight are less successful, and therefore interventions need to be family centered.[49]

Environmental Factors: Social, Economic, Cultural, and Physical

Family and peer relationships, attitudes, **education**, ethnicity, and behaviors, school/community environments and societal attitudes are the socioeconomic, cultural, and physical factors that influence activity patterns, eating behaviors, and attitudes toward food, physical activity, leisure choices, and personal weight (e.g., body image).

BOX 14-3

Diet and Physical Exercise Factors Associated With Obesity in Children

- Foods used as a reward or to soothe a child
- Inexpensive foods are cheaper, often easy to prepare, but high in calories
- Lack of healthy role modeling (eating and physical activity, and nutrition)
- Lower socioeconomic status
- Family's ethnicity, dietary choices less nutritional
- Inconsistent meals or access to healthy foods
- Limited education related to healthy nutrition and physical activity
- Occupational therapy reimbursement does not include interventions for obesity: individualized education program (IEP) goals are based on function or motor planning, and developing gross motor skills for academics
- Absence of a comprehensive approach to obesity that addresses the problems on an individual, family, school, and the community level
- Lack of effective interventions and policies

Therefore, they can contribute positively or negatively to a child and adolescent's weight.[49] For example, environmental factors may support and encourage a healthy active lifestyle, but they can equally be barriers to positive behavioral change. A 2-year study of households that restricted certain foods, especially when it involved the mother's dietary restriction, found that the weights of the children in these households increased.[17] An explanation for this finding may be that when these children managed to get access to the restricted foods, they ate more of them. In contrast, the availability of healthy foods (e.g., fruits and vegetables) in the home and the healthy eating patterns modeled by parents (and grandparents) positively influence food preferences and eating behaviors that will persist when children begin to make their own choices about the foods they will eat.[20]

Since the family environment has a significant effect on eating and exercise patterns, it is important to establish healthy eating and exercise habits early, since parental control over children's diet lessens during adolescence.[21] Adolescents are more likely to purchase foods outside the home, and these foods are often foods of convenience, which are high in sugars and fats and of questionable nutritional value. This change in diet can lead to weight gain. Peers and the media also become influential forces of behaviors and attitudes concerning weight, body image, and choices about how discretionary time is spent.

Physical environment and social trends influence activity levels and choice of activities as well. Increasingly, parents have become concerned about their children's safety, especially in urban settings. Outcomes of this trend are that children are less likely to walk or cycle to school, and less of the free time is spent playing in parks, since parents prefer to supervise their children in public spaces. Some concern has arisen that these changes are leading to less creative and less vigorous physical play.[6] At the same time, intense marketing of sedentary computer-mediated games and a decline in the availability of sports and physical education for a range of abilities continue to occur. Additionally, sport activities increasingly exclude disadvantaged children because of the cost of equipment, the lack of resources in communities, and both parents needing to work and being unable to take their children to sport activities. Fewer and fewer students at the elementary and high school levels are participating in any form of organized physical activity.[52] The national "Let's Move" initiative and many state initiatives are seeking to reverse this trend by increasing child and family activity levels and providing education to improve children's nutrition.

PSYCHOSOCIAL CONSEQUENCES OF CHILDHOOD AND ADOLESCENT OBESITY

Failure to recognize and intervene in a child's weight issues increases the risk of adult obesity and its associated morbidity and mortality.[42,51] Children or adolescents who are obese experience marginalization, which can affect their emotional well-being, although being obese does not necessarily mean that a child or adolescent will have psychological problems.[4] However, a relationship does exist between obesity and psychological difficulties such as anxiety, poor self-esteem, and depression.[59] Lower self-esteem is prevalent among children and adolescents who believe that they are themselves responsible for their overweight, and those who think that being overweight interferes with their social relationships.[43]

A significant relationship exists between dissatisfaction with physical appearance associated with obesity, namely, poor **body image**, and psychosocial problems.[26] Poor body image in girls has been shown to predict poor psychological function, depression, and binge eating.[36] Furthermore, lower levels of participation in physical activities are also associated with psychological factors. For example, children who are obese report that they enjoy sports less, especially high-energy activities such as running.

Stigma, Discrimination, and Social Exclusion

Body size is the most stigmatizing physical characteristic after race. In a study examining perceptions about disabilities, OT students ranked obesity as one of the hardest disabilities to live with.[11] Adults, adolescents, and children who are obese are viewed as unattractive in comparison with the Western ideal of physical attractiveness that is based on thinness.[10,33] Furthermore, obesity is associated with stereotypical characteristics such as laziness, self-indulgence, unreliability, untrustworthiness, and lack of self-discipline.[8,46,56] Children as young as 3 years old have been found to stereotype children who are obese as "ugly," "stupid," and "dirty."[24] These negative attitudes are also prevalent among adults working in the field of education. One fifth of high school teachers and health care workers stated that they thought obese persons were more emotional, less tidy, less likely to succeed at work, and had personalities different from those of people who are not obese.[24]

Children or adolescents who are overweight or obese are susceptible to teasing, discrimination, and social exclusion.[59] Forty-five percent of children with weight issues reported being teased, compared with 15% of children with normal weights.[24] Weight-related teasing and poor body image have been shown to be significant issues among elementary school children who are obese.[25] Besides the painful experiences of being teased or bullied, they also experience psychological, attitudinal, and behavioral negative outcomes. For example, children who experience weight-related criticism are likely to have negative attitudes toward sports and engage less in physical activities.[19] Some studies found that adolescents who reported weight-related teasing were more likely to have dysfunctional patterns of weight control such as smoking, purging, using laxatives and diuretics, and fasting than did their peers without weight-related problems. Because of the high incidence of weight-related teasing and antifat prejudicial attitudes, practitioners should assume that children who are overweight have been victimized (e.g., bullied) and are sensitive to any comments about weight.

CLINICAL *Pearl*

Make positive comments about appearance and personality traits or qualities. All children and adolescents need positive comments and praise; more often than not, those who are obese hear mostly negative comments.

Occupational Therapy Practitioners' Attitudes Toward Obesity

OT practitioners themselves are not free of the stereotypical attitudes associated with obesity.[57] Research has found that the prejudicial antifat attitudes prevalent in society are consistent with the attitudes of many health care professionals.[22,57] In a recent study, OT students were more likely to negatively evaluate and show discriminatory attitudes toward clients who were obese than toward clients who were not obese. The study showed that OT students are less likely to choose to work with clients who are obese, to view them as deserving of sympathy and understanding, and to find it easy to be empathetic toward them.[57]

Despite the ethical guidelines of the OT profession, which unequivocally states that all people are entitled to equal and compassionate care, antifat attitudes negatively influence OT practitioners' relationships with children and adolescents who are overweight. All OT practitioners need to examine their attitudes and their stereotypical beliefs concerning obesity and how these attitudes and beliefs influence their approaches to interventions for children and adolescents who are obese.

OCCUPATIONAL THERAPY AND CHILDHOOD OBESITY

Only three articles (in English) examining OT for children who are obese are found in the literature.[7,12,14] Similarly, relatively few related articles on adults who are obese are available. The American Occupational Therapy Association (AOTA) published a position paper on obesity in 2007, and *OT Practice* featured two articles on OT and disabilities associated with obesity, such as diminished ability to perform activities of daily living (ADL).[9,22,34] These articles and a chapter in *Occupational Therapy in the Promotion of Health and Wellness* (by Scaffa MS et al) explored working with clients who are obese as an emerging area of practice.[50] Weight management, lifestyle and health management, and compensatory approaches for individuals whose weight has affected their ability to engage in everyday occupations are important. However, OT practitioners rarely work with children and adolescents referred directly for their weight issues.[57] Instead, the children and adolescents tend to be referred for OT for developmental, sensory, congenital–physical disabilities, or learning problems exacerbated by excessive weight. In some cases, obesity is secondary to the disorder and is caused by reduced mobility (e.g., spina bifida, muscular dystrophy) or metabolic or behavioral conditions (e.g., Pradar Willi syndrome, Down syndrome).

Dwyer and colleagues advocated that occupational and physical therapy practitioners "embrace a broad perspective of physical activity and extend children's therapeutic and health promotion programs to include assessment of habitual level of physical activity and sedentary behaviors and promotion of recommended levels of physical activity" (p. 28).[14] Thus, pediatric OT practitioners can promote the health of children who have disabilities and clinical conditions that place them at risk for becoming overweight. In the following section, we explore a variety of individual and group programs that achieve this goal.

OCCUPATIONAL THERAPY INTERVENTIONS

The need for families to be mindful of their children's weights and levels of physical activity is not a new concern, and the primary strategies to address obesity have not changed significantly. A newspaper column written in the 1960s by Dr. R S Solomon, a family doctor in rural South Carolina, is still pertinent. In the article he stated: "One fact is established, and that is that the time to treat it [obesity] is during childhood and adolescence. The prescription is relatively simple—more exercise, the right diet, and watchful parental–doctor [health care professional] supervision . . . The human machine, like any other, functions on intake and output but must have an emotional stability in self and parent."

OT practitioners address childhood obesity as they work to help children engage in occupations. OT for children and adolescents who are obese may be categorized into three areas:

1. Obesity due to genetic or metabolic disorders
2. Obesity secondary to developmental, congenital, or chronic health disorders
3. Obesity as primary disorder

Obesity is more prevalent among children and adolescents with physical and cognitive disabilities than among peers without these disabilities.[32] In the case of children with special needs, excess weight interferes with their functioning and mobility.[32] The chronic and secondary problems associated with obesity in adolescents who are disabled can compromise their independence and limit their opportunities to participate in a variety of occupations.[47]

Since OT practitioners work with children who have disabilities, they must understand the mechanisms and consequences of obesity in these children. Effective programs and individual interventions begin with an awareness of the behavioral and environmental factors that precede weight gain.[47]

CASE *Study*

Sean is a short, clumsy, 5-year-old boy who has been diagnosed with Prader Willi syndrome. His parents are concerned about his preoccupation with food and that he is overweight. They are considering putting locks on the refrigerator and kitchen cupboards as Sean steals food. He is also having behavior problems related to food at preschool (e.g., taking food from other children and eating Play-Do and crayons).

Prader Willi syndrome (PWS) is a common genetic disorder associated with obesity. Children with this syndrome have low muscle tone and low levels of sex hormones. They constantly feel hungry, because the area of the brain that controls feelings of fullness or hunger does not work properly. As these children develop, their short stature, poor motor skills associated with low muscle tone, and patterns of overeating lead to obesity. Other problems associated with PWS are mild intellectual disability and learning difficulties.

Due to their multiple challenges, the primary focus of OT for children and adolescents who have genetic syndromes and chromosomal abnormalities is individual and family-centered therapy. The frames of reference that inform these individual interventions and group programs include *applied behavioral functional analysis* or *positive behavioral support* (see Chapter 13).

The category described above includes children whose obesity is due to sedentary or low activity level associated with their primary congenital or chronic health disorders. For example, nearly half the children with Down syndrome are obese or overweight, although obesity is not a symptom of this disorder; rather, it is associated with their activity levels and poor motor skills. Another group with a high incidence of weight problems comprises students with learning disabilities. For example, Bandini et al found that girls with learning disabilities were twice as likely to be overweight as their peers without these disabilities.[2]

CASE *Study*

Gray, an 11-year-old in Grade 6, has spina bifida (lesion in the lower lumbar area). Since starting middle school, he has preferred to use a wheelchair for functional mobility because he is too slow transitioning from class to class with his crutches. Coinciding with his wheelchair use and the new school environment, Gray has gained weight and is at the 92nd percentile on the BMI scale. The combination of increased weight and growth has made it cumbersome for him to use his crutches.

Spina bifida is a neuroskeletal structural abnormality of the spine (see Chapter 12). As children with physical disabilities such as cerebral palsy, muscular dystrophy, and spina bifida mature and the demands of their age-related activities increase, they often choose efficient means of mobility (e.g., preferring a power chair to a manual chair). The physical demands of walking or the manual operation of the chair make the activity a high-intensity activity that expends more energy. The limited strength and motor skills of children with disabilities

become more problematic with the additional demands of moving a heavier body. This pattern coincides with a typical decline in therapy exercises, physical play, and participation in organized activities (such as sports). The typical increase in sedentary academic activities and the changes in physical status combine and contribute to weight gain, increasing the likelihood of obesity.

The final category comprises children and adolescents referred to OT because of limited occupational performance due to obesity. The OT goals for this population are to improve functioning, manage weight, and develop a healthy lifestyle through behavioral changes, behavioral adaptations, and, for adolescents who are morbidly obese, compensatory approaches such as assistive devices. Since obesity limits children's movements and the opportunities to engage in occupations, OT practitioners use strategies that enable them to participate in age-appropriate occupations and to function at their optimal performance level.

Obesity may be comorbid with psychological disorders such as binge eating.

CASE *Study*

Gina is 16 years old. She has always been on some kind of diet because she her weight is slightly above average for her height, but lately she has gained weight. In the past 8 months, she has developed a pattern of compulsive overeating when she is stressed or unhappy about her parents' separation and pending divorce, her schoolwork, and not getting along well with her friends. She secretly and rapidly eats large amounts of food several times a week and then feels disgusted with herself. She feels she has no control over this behavior. Unlike individuals with bulimia nervosa, she does not purge; as a result, she is rapidly becoming obese.

The causes of obesity are numerous; not all people who are obese feel that they lack control over their eating. Binge eating only accounts for 2% to 25% of individuals who are obese. At this time, it is not a formal classification within the *DSM-IV-TR*.[62] However, although Gina's obesity is related to her psychoemotional difficulties, many children's and adolescents' weight problems do not have psychoemotional causes. The OT practitioner who works with children and adolescents seeking treatment for weight issues related to their psychoemotional difficulties will be a member of a multidisciplinary team that includes a physician, a nutritionist, a social worker, and a psychologist. The OT practitioner's role will include providing both interventions to support weight loss and strategies to reduce physical limitations and build physical skills. Psychosocial interventions will be an integral component of the OT process and will include developing skills in emotional self-regulation, stress management skills, and **self-efficacy** in social participation. Through a multifaceted approach, self-esteem can be increased, and body image and a positive self can be fostered. Psychosocial frames of reference will guide assessment and intervention.

THERAPEUTIC APPROACHES

The programs and individual interventions for children who are obese are informed by the following principles:

- Health education
- Behavioral change theory, for example, transtheoretical theory of behavioral change
- Behavioral approaches, for example, positive behavioral support
- **Cognitive–behavioral therapy**
- Social learning theory, or social cognition

As a team, the occupational therapist and certified occupational therapy assistant (COTA) will identify the approach that is effective with their population and will achieve the desired outcomes. The OT process begins with thorough evaluation and assessment of the client to identify the problem and individualize goals, interventions, and therapy priorities.

INDIVIDUAL INTERVENTION STRATEGIES
Prevention: Individual Strategies for Infants With Special Needs

Often an OT practitioner's first contact with children with specials needs is with regard to feeding, which is a crucial stage of establishing healthy eating patterns and food preferences. The first decision is whether to promote breast milk or formula. Children with feeding difficulties may need to be bottlefed rather than breast-fed, but breast milk can still be an option, since breast-feeding appears to have some protective effects against obesity. When introducing solids in a feeding program, education about healthy choices will be a component of the program. There is a tendency to give children who are difficult to feed or fussy eaters their preferred foods, which are often sweet. Some children who have special needs will not be at risk of obesity. For example, children with cerebral palsy need a high caloric intake because of the energy expenditure associated with the hypertonicity of their muscles.

In early childhood, eating routines in structured settings will begin to establish patterns and attitudes concerning food.[21] The OT practitioner works with families on setting eating patterns and how food will be viewed. For example, never using food as a reward avoids the later necessity for children having to unlearn this

behavior when they become overweight. It is better that they develop healthy snack choices that accommodate their food challenges or special needs.

Managing and Preventing Obesity

Helping children or adolescents and their families address issues of obesity requires an examination of the children's occupational profiles, including their habits and routines (Box 14-4). OT practitioners gather information on children's or adolescents' developmental, physical, psychosocial, and cognitive abilities and seek to understand cultural, familial, and physical contexts. This information is used to set goals with the children or adolescents and their families. When setting goals, OT practitioners address more than the issue of weight. Comprehensive OT interventions target the psychosocial consequences such as poor self-esteem, behavioral change to develop healthy activity and dietary habits and routines, and occupational performance through remedial strategies (such as weight management). Setting short-term goals that can easily be achieved motivates children and families.

After identifying factors that interfere with occupational performance, OT clinicians then develop strategies to improve or enhance skills. Goals are developed with the children, adolescents, and families and the practitioner works closely with them to develop family-based healthy habits and routines. The interventions may follow the principles of *behavioral* approaches by using age-appropriate **incentives** to shape and reinforce positive behaviors (see Chapter 13). Allowing the children or adolescents to participate in choosing the incentives reinforces motivation and enables them to feel a sense of control. Alternatively, a *cognitive behavioral* approach helps them identify their thinking and behaviors that may be interfering with making healthy lifestyle choices or exercising (see Chapter 13). It is necessary that the children's cognitive abilities are adequate for them to comprehend the relationships among their thoughts, feelings, and behaviors.

Social cognitive theories suggest that gaining personal motivation and self-efficacy about the ability to perform skills increases the ability to plan and carry out

BOX 14-4

Managing and Preventing Obesity

Managing and Preventing Obesity.
- Set goals that are obtainable, simple, and easy to measure
- Set one short achievable goal at a time.
- Make goals very concrete so the child sees progress. For example, provide child with a pedometer to measure distance walked. Have simple short term-goal such as walk to best friend's house or walk to the nearest store.
- Develop goals with child or adolescent. Have child set own reward system.
- Keep goals positive. For example, walk to the end of the street every other day rather than do not watch TV on Tuesdays.
- Involve friends and family in goals.
- Minimize the number of breads, sweets, soda, and replace with healthy choices such as fruit, vegetables and water at home.
- Do not completely deny child occasional sweets or soda. Otherwise, they may crave them and eat more when they are available to them.
- Address issues of health rather than weight.
- Focus on the child's volition (interests, motivation and desires) to engage in a variety of activities.
- Build on existing physical and healthy routines and habits.
- Consistently repeat new behaviors until they become part of the child's everyday behaviors.
- Encourage child to get regular sleeping hours.
- Involve child in chores that require physical effort (e.g., sweeping, taking out garbage, raking, running errands).

Sample goals:
- Mark will eat a vegetable at each meal.
- Diane will play outside with her family or friends for 1 hour each day.
- Jose and his family will drink water instead of soda during the weekend.
- Rochelle will try Frisbee and tee ball (2 new activities) at least 3 times.
- Sajay will help his parent prepare a low fat, low carbohydrate meal (once a week).

behavioral change.[5] Understanding a child's motivation is useful in designing and grading group and individual interventions. For example, developing physical skills in age-related sports will give a child confidence to participate in extracurricular physical activities. Furthermore, participation in extracurricular activities has been shown to have additional social and academic benefits for adolescents.[15]

As OT practitioners focus on bringing about behavioral changes in the children toward healthy physical activity and nutrition, an *educational* approach providing information to teachers, parents, children, and adolescents may be effective.

All approaches require that activities and programs be graded so that they are not burdensome to the family, child, or adolescent. For example, while a goal may be to provide intervention to promote high intensity physical activity, the OT practitioner may begin with a short walking program and suggest follow-up at home to increase the distance or frequency. Similarly, changing a family's dietary patterns may begin by introducing one vegetable at a time to weekend dinners.

Home follow-up programs and social support systems (i.e., family, friends, and peers) are significant to the success of individual interventions and should be components of any program (Box 14-5). Programs such as the buddy system are effective in increasing and maintaining physical activity and can increase the children's participation in after-school free play and involvement in physical activities such as baseball and soccer.

Cultural, social, and community factors exert strong influences on a child and must be integrated into OT interventions.[58] Obesity rates are higher in inner cities where no fresh produce or green space (to play) is available.[16,35,44,55] Practitioners need to be knowledgeable about community resources so that they can make appropriate and feasible recommendations (e.g., recreational departments, local YMCA, after-school programs).

Increasing Physical Activity

Children or adolescents who have disabilities are more likely to be sedentary.[47] Similarly, children or adolescents who are overweight or obese may have pre-existing motor difficulties that have discouraged them from engaging in physical activities. Instead, they are drawn to sedentary activities (e.g., watching TV, playing computer games) at which they are more likely to experience enjoyment and/or success.[47]

BOX 14-5

Recommendations for Physical Activity for All Children at Their Ability Levels

- Perform daily vigorous physical activity for at least 1 hour.
- Engage in play and activities that involve physical activity in a variety of settings: home, school, and community.
- Participate in physical activity with parents; parents can set an example and encourage physical activity as part of everyday life.
- Explore a variety of activities and choose an activity of interest.
- Participate in enjoyable, fun, and motivating activities that promote long-term activity.
- Participate in activities with peers, siblings, and parents.
- Try new activities.

CLINICAL *Pearl*

If a child has a disability, should he or she be physically active?

Physical activity is important for all children. There are appropriate types and amount of physical activities for children with disabilities. A physical activity routine should be a component of a child's individualized education program (IEP). Group physical activities in a school setting can offer important social inclusion for a child with a disability.

By understanding client factors associated with obesity, the OT practitioner can target the intervention to facilitate movement and engagement in physical activity within the children's ability levels with the "just right" challenge to promote skill development and enjoyment. By analyzing the steps to activities and making the necessary modifications, these children and adolescents may experience success in physical activities and gain confidence. This, in turn, motivates them to engage in more activities. Practitioners may design simple steps to increase a child's or adolescent's physical activity level at home by developing programs that involve walking or helping with daily household tasks and that encourage movement, such as dance.

An important component of increasing physical activity is addressing patterns and routines that discourage sedentary behaviors. Children and adolescents should be encouraged to participate in 1 hour of vigorous physical activity every day (www.letsgo.org). Planning one's use of time and providing incentives may be beneficial to maintaining behavioral changes.

CLINICAL *Pearl*

Occupational therapy practitioners can have an active role in children's and adolescents' identified opportunities for physical activity within supportive environments (e.g., teams and physical fitness programs that accommodate children with all levels of ability, including children with disabilities). Children and adolescents can also experience a variety of physical activities and gain physical skills in other settings such as summer camps and community group activities, for example, scouts. These programs have additional social and emotional benefits.

Children and adolescents are more likely to change exercise patterns if the family is proactive and involved in the process. Encouraging families to make changes, such as turning off the television and having a family evening doing alternative activities, reducing computer time, and participating in physical activity together, may all help improve the child's health. Family members can support each other and encourage success. OT practitioners working to make changes in the family system begin by suggesting simple, concrete steps toward goals that the family values. Asking children, adolescents, and families to complete just one of the steps of the program at a time will seem less overwhelming and help them experience success. For example, adolescents who drink large amounts of soda may be able to swap one soda a day for a glass of water. This goal is more achievable than not drinking any soda at all. Family members who support the adolescent by trying to increase their own water intake (over soda) can help him or her develop healthy nutritional patterns in a more effective way. See Box 14-6 for ideas to promote healthy family nutrition.

PROGRAMS: GROUP AND COMMUNITY INTERVENTIONS

Numerous programs that target childhood obesity and, to a lesser extent, adolescent obesity are available. The philosophies and emphases of these programs vary, but their core principles include the following:

- Moderate to high intensity physical activity
- Social participation
- Nutritional activity
- Health education
- Self-directedness in spontaneous play

To promote follow-through, many programs involve educating teachers and parents on topics such as exercise and nutrition. Other programmatic goals include promoting sports and extracurricular activities, encouraging hobbies, and involving families and friends in a more

BOX 14-6

BOX 14-6

Recommendations for Promoting Healthy Food Choices for Families

- Make a weekly menu.
- Use a grocery list when shopping.
- Involve children in grocery shopping and meal preparations.
- Eat meals together when possible.
- Limit the amount of soda and candy in the house.
- Establish a nutritional and/or physical goal as a family.
- Make slow transitions when changing food habits so that the changes are achievable.
- Plan and prepare meals in advance to avoid getting take-out foods when pushed for time.
- Limit availability of unhealthy choices in the home, and increase the variety of healthy snacks.
- Avoid associating unhealthy foods with fun and celebrations.
- Do not restrict sodas and candy entirely so that they become "special" foods.

active lifestyle.[37] Importantly, programs emphasize setting realistic goals as key to successful outcomes. These outcomes are not measured solely by the amount of weight loss. They can include child, adolescent, family or school satisfaction, increased knowledge of nutrition and exercise, improvement in healthy eating habits, increased levels of physical activity, and increased participation in social activities (Table 14-1).

Sample Program: The "FUN" Maine Program

OT practitioners consider the complex nature of obesity when designing a program to improve engagement in healthy occupations and routines as a way to prevent obesity. They emphasize helping children develop attitudes for overall wellness, that is, thoughts, feeling, and beliefs toward health.[27]

The Model of Human Occupation (MOHO) provides a theoretical framework for designing an effective program.[29] Kielhofner suggested that engaging children in volitionally oriented activities helps them sustain activity over time, which makes a difference in their health.[29] This model considers the multiple factors associated with childhood obesity and, thus, informs the practitioners in creating multisystem interventions.

O'Brien and colleagues designed and conducted a community after-school intervention [Fitness, yoU, and Nutrition (FUN) program] to target children's volition, habits, and performance (Figure 14-1).[38,39] See Box 14-7 for an overview of the program. The FUN program,

which aimed at developing healthy habits, encouraged the children in the study to journal their eating patterns, play activities, and exercise each week. These children received incentives (such as hula-hoops) to continue to play actively (Figure 14-2).

In the first year of this program, which was conducted after school in the community, the children were allowed easy access to healthy after-school opportunities. The program measured outcomes in terms of interest in activity (volition), habits (habituation), and performance (physical fitness, BMI). In the second year, the program expanded to include more parent input. Follow-through was enhanced by introducing workbooks with weekly goals. What distinguishes this program from other programs is its use of MOHO.

OTHER OCCUPATIONAL THERAPY–BASED PROGRAMS

The approach of using the playfulness of children has been applied innovatively to provide OT to children who are obese by introducing novel physical activity toys to Australian playgrounds.[6] The premise of the approach of Bundy and her colleagues is that play has become too "safe." The hypervigilance and protectiveness of adults is limiting children's creativity and the intensity of their activities, except in organized contexts such as a sports team. In a randomized control study, novelty play items (e.g., tires, hay) were introduced to selected schools. Although adults provided supervision, they were trained to allow children to play without interruption unless their safety was at risk.[6] The children who received this intervention in these schools (when novelty materials were on the playground) were more physically active and playful and were described as "social," "creative," and "resilient," compared with those children in the control schools where no changes were introduced to the school playground.[6] This program models an inexpensive preventive approach to changing the play environment to increase children's physical activity levels, with the additional benefits of playfulness and creativity.

Manguba et al applied an occupational therapy nutrition educational program in the school setting.[7] The authors developed both a video game and a board game based on nutritional education. Two hundred children played the video game and the board game; 27% preferred the video game, and 6% preferred the board game. The children learned facts about nutrition from both games, which suggests that play may be an effective tool in nutritional education. Since OT practitioners are skilled at examining and addressing play in children and adolescents, they are encouraged to use games and pretend play to educate children and adolescents on healthy lifestyles.

TABLE 14-1

Sample Programs for Children

NAME	DESCRIPTION OF PROGRAM	
HeartPower! http://www.americanheart.org American Heart Association	The "Heart Power!" program is a preventive health education project geared to children ages 4–7 years. It teaches children about heart disease risk factors, which may help reverse current adult trends.	HeartPower! Online is the American Heart Association's collection of free educational materials for preschool, elementary, and middle school students. Printable lesson plans, activity sheets, and teaching ideas can be used for Grades K–2, 3–5, and 6–8. These science-based online resources can introduce students to healthy habits and encourage them to live long, healthy lives by making smart choices.
Let's Go! http://www.letsgo.org/ Maine-based program	"Let's Go!" is a community-based initiative to promote healthy lifestyle choices among children, youth, and families in 12 Greater Portland communities. The goal is to increase physical activity and healthy eating in children and youth—from birth to 18 years.	*5, 2, 1, 0 slogan:* 5 fruits and vegetables 2 hours of screen time 1 hour of physical activity 0 sugar Materials and handouts are available.
Be Active Kids North Carolina http://beactivekids.org/bak/ Front/Default.aspx	"Be Active Kids" is an innovative, interactive physical activity, nutrition, and food safety curriculum for North Carolina preschoolers ages 4 and 5 years.	The program uses colorful characters, interactive hands-on lessons, and bright visuals to teach children that physical activity, healthy eating, and food safety can be fun!
Let's Move http://www.letsmove.gov/	"Let's Move!" has an ambitious but important goal: to solve the epidemic of childhood obesity within a generation.	The program will give parents the support they need, provide healthier foods in schools, help children to be more physically active, and make healthy, affordable food available in every part of the country.
ReCharge! Energizing After School http://www.actionforhealthykids. org/recharge/about/ Action for Healthy Kids and the National Football League	"ReCharge! Energizing After-School" is an after-school program designed to help students in Grades 2 to 6 learn about and practice good nutrition and physical activity habits through fun, team-based strategies. It focuses on four core concepts: 1. "Energy In" (nutrition) 2. "Energy Out" (physical activity) 3. Teamwork 4. Goal setting	The program addresses national education standards. It is designed to be practical, feasible, and adaptable to a variety of settings and program.

Besides play, education is a major occupation of children and adolescents. As such, OT practitioners who work with children and adolescents who are obese are interested in the influence of the school environment on nutritional and physical activity choices. Suarez-Balcazar and colleagues introduced system changes in Chicago schools as a way to help children and adolescents lead healthier lifestyles.[7,55] The authors described many factors involved in the school system (including students, teachers, food vendors, as well as the institution, community, and social and policy structures). They examined the barriers to system changes and implemented strategies to make these changes. In an effort to make system changes, the authors developed new school initiatives to offer healthier choices in the vending machines and introduced the Cool Food initiative (salad bar

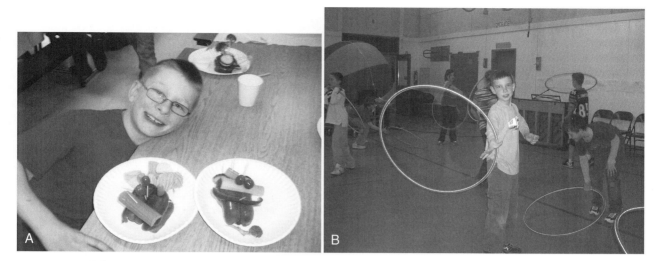

FIGURE 14-1   A, Zander is proud of his "alien" vegetables. Children in the FUN program enjoy making and eating aliens! **B,** Making decisions about how to do things, challenging oneself, and experiencing novelty all are part of volitional activities. This child uses the hula-hoop in a new way.

BOX 14-7

Fitness, yoU, and Nutrition (FUN)[38,39]

Focusing on fun after-school activities, the authors of the program encouraged children in Grades 3 and 4 to participate in physical activities and take steps toward healthy nutrition. OT students designed and implemented creative weekly sessions based on selected themes and emphasizing healthy nutrition and physical activity. Participants learned about healthy nutritional choices (e.g., the five food groups, variety in diet, importance of water, protein, grains, vegetables, and fruits). Children received incentives, such as hula-hoops, jump ropes, and frisbees. One hundred children from the Waterboro Elementary School in Waterboro, Maine, participated in the 2-year program.

The overall objectives of the FUN program include:
- *Volition*: Increase child's motivation and interest in physical activity and healthy nutrition.
- *Habituation*: Develop healthy nutritional and physical activity habits and routines.
  - Children will engage in physical activity for 1 hour daily.
  - Children will show improved nutritional habits, such as drink water instead of soda, and eat more vegetables.
- *Performance*: Achieve healthy BMI; succeed in the Presidential Physical Fitness Test.
- *Environment*: Parents will be engaged in effort to improve nutritional and physical activity habits and routines.
The FUN program will provide a free after-school program in the child's community.

SAMPLE FUN WEEKLY SESSION
Theme: Beach Day
Goal: Drink water instead of soda. Play outside with friends!
Physical Activity: Children enjoyed playing beach-type games, such as directing a "fish" into the water. This game involved holding newspapers and using arm movements to move construction-paper fish into the hula-hoops (water). Other games included hula-hoop contest to beach music and playing with the 8-foot beach ball (Figure 14-3, A).
Snacks and Drinks: Fruit kabobs (introduce children to something they might not have tried),
Incentive: Children took home with them bottled water, fresh fruit, and hula-hoops (Figure 14-3, B).

---

wagons). They provided nutrition education sessions to students as well.

These examples provide OT practitioners with strategies at the individual, group, and system levels that help children and adolescents lead healthier lives. Since the consequences of childhood obesity include type

2 diabetes, cardiac disease, asthma, apnea, and limited mobility, efforts to reduce the incidence of obesity are needed. OT practitioners are urged to use available resources such as printed handouts (see list of Internet Resources at the end of the chapter for printable worksheets). The above studies suggest that interventions

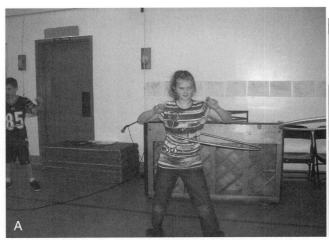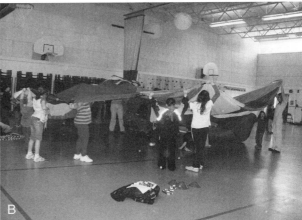

FIGURE 14-2 **A,** Hula-hooping is a great exercise. Children in the FUN program take home hula-hoops as an incentive to keep moving! **B,** Parachute games are fun for children, introduce novelty, and keep children physically active.

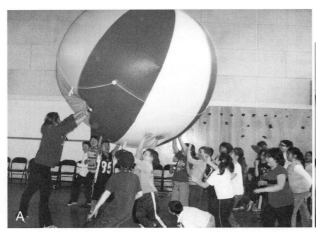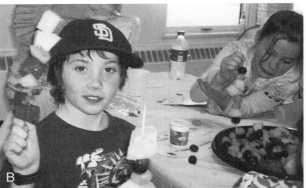

FIGURE 14-3 **A,** Children in the FUN program play different games that keep them physically active and having fun. These games are motivating and interesting to children. Beach day includes games with a giant beach ball! **B,** Making fruit kabobs is a fun and easy way to enjoy fruits. Children in the FUN program try nutritious foods while making interesting recipes. Making nutritional education fun and playful helps children learn.

such as games based on nutrition, introducing novel toys to the playground, and increasing healthy nutritional choices at school may all make a difference.

SUMMARY

Childhood obesity is on the rise. OT practitioners are in a unique position to address the multitude of factors contributing to this serious issue. Along with physical limitations such as limited movement, decreased endurance, lack of strength, and poor mobility, obesity may harm a child's or adolescent's psychosocial well-being; Children and adolescents who are obese often suffer from bullying, teasing, and low self-esteem. Environmental influences may present barriers to the ability of the child, adolescent, and family to engage in occupations. OT practitioners can help remove these barriers by introducing programs that address healthy physical and nutritional habits and routines for all children. Social after-school programs help children achieve lifestyle changes within their own communities and serve as educational and behavioral models for change. A review of the biological, physical, and psychosocial issues present in this population includes the development of self-efficacy, self-esteem, and body awareness for children and adolescents who are overweight or obese.

The authors of this chapter have presented the contributing factors to obesity, strategies for intervention planning, and sample programs to promote healthy routines and habits in children and adolescents. Case examples have been provided to illustrate key concepts.

References

1. Anderson PM, Butcher KE: Childhood obesity: trends and potential causes. *Future Child* 16:19, 2006.
2. Bandini LG et al: Prevalence of overweight in children with developmental disorders in the continuous National Health and Nutrition Examination Survey (NHANES) 1999-2002. *J Pediatr* 146:738–743, 2005.
3. Birch LL, Davidson KK: Family environmental factors influencing the developing controls of food intake and childhood overweight. *Pediatr Clin North Am* 48:893, 2001.
4. Britz B et al: Rates of psychiatric disorders in a clinical study group of adolescents with extreme obesity and in obese adolescents ascertained via a population based study. *Int J Obes Relat Metab Disord* 24:1707–1714, 2000.
5. Budd GM, Volpe SL: School-based obesity prevention: research, challenges, and recommendations. *J School Health* 76:485, 2006.
6. Bundy AC et al: Playful interaction: occupational therapy for all children on the school playground. *Am J Occup Ther* 62:522, 2008.
7. Munguba MC, Valdes MT, Silva CAD: The application of an occupational therapy nutrition education programme for children who are obese. *Occup Ther Int* 15:56, 2008.
8. Carr D, Friedman M: Is obesity stigmatizing? Body weight, perceived discrimination, and psychological well-being in the United States. *J Health Soc Behav* 46:244, 2005.
9. Clark F, Reingold FS, Salles-Jordan K: Obesity and occupational therapy. *Am J Occup Ther* 61:701, 2007.
10. Davidson M, Knafl KA: Dimensional analysis of the concept of obesity. *J Adv Nurs* 54:342, 2006.
11. Delin C: Perceptions of disability by students, the formerly obese and general community. *Psychol Rep* 76:1219, 1995.
12. Diffendal J: Growing out of control. *Adv Occup Ther Pract* 11–12, 2001. Posted May 28, 2001.
13. Duke J, Huhman M, Heitzler C: Physical activity levels among children aged 9-13 years—United States. *MMWR Morb Mortal Wkly Rep* 52:785, 2002.
14. Dwyer G et al: Promoting children's health and well-being: broadening the therapy perspective. *Phys Occup Ther Pediatr* 29:27, 2009.
15. Eccles JS et al: Extracurricular activities and adolescent development. *J Soc Issues* 59:865, 2003.
16. Evans G: The psychological environment of childhood poverty. *Am Psychol* 59:78, 2004.
17. Faith MS et al: Parental feeding attitudes and styles, and child body mass index: prospective analysis of a gene-environment interaction. *Pediatrics* 114:429, 2004.
18. Faith MS et al: Weight criticism during physical activity, coping skills, and reported physical activity in children. *Pediatrics* 110:23, 2002.
20. Field AS, Kitos NR: Social and interpersonal influences on obesity in youth: family, peers and society. In Heinberg LJ, Thompson JK, editors: *Obesity in youth: causes, consequences, and cures,* Washington, DC, 2009, American Psychological Association.
21. Fisher JO, Sinton MM, Birch LL: Early parental influences and risk for the emergence of disordered eating. In Smolak L, Thompson JK, editors: *Body image, eating disorders, and obesity in youth: assessment, prevention and treatment,* Washington, DC, 2009, American Psychological Association.
22. Foti D: Caring for the person of size. *OT Practice* 10:9, 2005.
23. Gillman MW et al: Family dinner and diet quality among older children and adolescents. *Arch Fam Med* 9:235–240, 2000.
24. Haines J, Neumark-Sztainer D: Psychosocial consequences of obesity and weight bias: implications for interventions. In Heinberg LJ, Thompson JK, editors: *Obesity in youth: causes, consequences, and cures,* Washington, DC, 2009, American Psychological Association.
25. Haines J, Neumark-Sztainer D, Thiel L: Address weight-related issues in an elementary: what do students, parents, and school staff recommend? *Eat Disord* 15:5, 2007.
26. Herbozo S, Thompson JK: Body image in pediatric obesity. In Heinberg LJ, Thompson JK, editors: *Obesity in youth: causes, consequences, and cures,* Washington, DC, 2009, American Psychological Association.
27. Heuttig C, Connor JO: Wellness programming for preschoolers with disabilities. *Teach Exceptional Child* 31:12, 1999.
28. Hill JO et al: Obesity and the environment: where do we go from here? *Science* 299:853, 2003.
29. Kielhofner G: *Models of human occupation: theory and application,* ed 4, Baltimore, 2008, Lippincott Williams & Wilkins.
30. Koplan JP, Liverman C, Kraak VI, editors: *Preventing childhood obesity,* Washington, DC, 2005, National Academies Press.
31. Markward NJ, Markward MJ, Peterson CA: Biological and genetic influences. In Heinberg LJ, Thompson JK, editors: *Obesity in youth: causes, consequences, and cures,* Washington, DC, 2009, American Psychological Association.
32. Minihan PM, Fitch AN, Must A: What does the epidemic of childhood obesity mean for children with special health needs? *J Law Med Ethics* 35:61, 2007.
33. Morrison TG, O'Connor WE: Psychometric properties of a scale measuring negative attitudes towards overweight individuals. *J Soc Psychol* 139:436, 1999.
34. Mosely L et al: Obesity and occupational therapy practice: present and potential practice trends. *OT Practice* 8, April 28, 2008.
35. Motland K et al: Neighborhood characteristics associated with the location of food stores and food service places. *Am J Prev Med* 22:23, 2002.

36. Neumark-Sztainer D, Levin MP, Paxton S: Prevention of body dissatisfaction and disordered eating: what next? *Eat Disord* 14:265, 2006.

37. Nowicki P: Physical activity—key issues in treatment of childhood obesity. *Acta Paediatr* 96:39, 2007.

38. O'Brien J et al: *FUN program (Phase II): parent involvement and behavioral changes to improve wellness in elementary school children*, Portland, 2010, University of New England.

39. O'Brien J et al: *FUN program (Phase II): development of the Fitness, yoU, and Nutrition (FUN) after school program to improve wellness in elementary school children*, Portland, 2010, University of New England.

40. Obama M: Remarks of First Lady Michelle Obama, 2010. Available at: http://www.whitehouse.gov/the-press-office/remarks-first-lady-michelle-obama. Accessed March 10, 2010.

41. American Academy of Pediatrics: Children, adolescents, and television. *Pediatrics* 107:423, 2001.

42. American Academy of Pediatrics: Prevention of pediatric overweight and obesity. *Pediatrics* 112:424, 2003.

43. Pierce JW, Wardle A: Cause and effect beliefs and self-esteem of overweight children. *J Child Psychol Psychiatr* 38:645–650, 1997.

44. Powell L, Slater SA, Chaloupka F: The relationship between physical activity settings and race, ethnicity, and socioeconomic status. *Evidence-Based Prev Med* 1:135–155, 2004.

45. Centers for Disease Control and Prevention: *Overweight and obese*, 2009. Available at: http://www.cdc.gov/obesity/defining.html. Accessed March 25, 2010.

46. Puhl RM, Brownell KD: Bias, discrimination and obesity. *Obes Res* 9:788, 2001.

47. Rimmer JH, Rowland JL, Yamaki K: Obesity and secondary conditions in adolescents with disabilities: addressing the need of an underserved population. *J Adolesc Health* 41:224, 2007.

48. Sallis JF, Prochaska JJ, Taylor WC: A review of correlates of physical activity in children and adolescents. *Med Sci Sports Exerc* 32:963, 2000.

49. Sallis JF, Rosenberg D, Kerr J: Early physical activity, sedentary behavior, and dietary patterns. In Heinberg LJ, Thompson JK, editors: *Obesity in youth*, Washington, DC, 2009, American Psychological Association.

50. Scaffa MS, Reitz SM, Pizzi MA, editors: *Occupational therapy in the promotion of health and wellness*, Philadelphia, 2010, FA Davis.

51. Serdula MK et al: Do obese children become obese adults? A review of the literature. *Prev Med* 22:167, 1993.

52. Shanklin S et al: CDC: Youth Risk Behavior Surveillance—selected steps communities, United States, 2007, MMWR, 5–7 (SS-12), 1–27, 2008.

53. Sorof J, Daniels S: Obesity, hypertension in children: a problem of epidemic proportions. *Hypertension* 40:441, 2000.

54. Steele MM, Steele RG, Hunter H: Family adherence as a predictor of child outcome in an intervention for pediatric obesity: difference outcome for self-report and objective measures. *Child Health Care* 38:64, 2009.

55. Suarez-Balcazar Y et al: Introducing systems change in the schools: the case of school luncheons and vending machines. *Am J Community Psychol* 39:335, 2007.

56. Teachman BA, Brownell KD: Implicit anti-fat bias among health professionals: is anyone immune? *Int J Obes* 25:1525, 2001.

57. Vroman K, Cote S: Prejudicial attitudes toward clients who are obese: measuring implicit anti-fat attitudes of occupational therapy students. *Occup Ther Health Care* (submitted for review).

58. Warren JM et al: Evaluation of a pilot school programme aimed at the prevention of obesity in children. *Health Promotion Int* 18:287, 2003.

59. Warschburger P: The unhappy obese child. *Int J Obes* 29:S127, 2005.

60. Whitt-Gover MC, O'Neill KL, Stettler N: Physical activity patterns in children with and without Down syndrome. *Pediatr Rehabil* 9:158, 2006.

61. Woods SC, Seeley RJ: Regulation of appetite, satiety, and energy metabolism. In Antel J et al, editors: *Obesity and metabolic disorders*, Amsterdam, 2005, IOS Press.

62. Yanovski SL: Binge eating disorder and obesity. *Int J Eat Disord* 34:S117, 2003.

Recommended Reading

Heinberg LJ, Thompson JK: *Obesity in youth: causes consequences and cures*, Washington, DC, 2009, American Psychological Association.

Smolak L, Thompson JK: *Body image, eating disorders, and obesity in youth: assessment, prevention and treatment*, Washington, DC, 2009, American Psychological Association.

Internet Resources

http://www.whitehouse.gov/blog/2010/02/09/making-moves-a-healthier-generation
Web site describing White House initiative to decrease childhood obesity across the nation.
www.mypyramid.com
Web site describing food and activity habits and routines for children. Printables and lessons for nutrition and activity for children.

STUDY *Questions*

1. What are some factors that cause obesity in children and adolescents?
2. What are the principles of interventions for preventing obesity?
3. What are the client factors that may be influenced by obesity in children who have special needs?
4. Describe antifat attitudes and stereotypes and how they might influence the OT practitioner–client relationship and treatment effectiveness.

5. How might obesity interfere with the occupational performance of children and adolescents?
6. How do interventions for preventing obesity differ at family, school, and community levels?
7. What is the OT practitioner's role in promoting physical activity, healthy lifestyle patterns, and self-efficacy for healthy behaviors?

SUGGESTED *Activities*

1. Go to www.implicit.harvard.edu/implicit/demo, the Web site for the Implicit Attitude Test (IAT), a test that measures one's attitudes toward those who are obese. Take the test to find out what your attitudes are toward people who are obese. Reflect on the findings, and discuss how you will use this information in practice.
2. Develop a physical activity and nutritional lesson plan for children or adolescents. Include handouts.
3. Keep a food and exercise diary for a week, including the weekend. What did you learn about your eating and exercise patterns? Did you meet the criteria for a healthy diet? In the following week, eat one more fruit or vegetable each day, and at the end of the

week, review your success with this behavioral change. What were the barriers, and what supported you to make this dietary change?
4. Measure the height and weight of 10 children. Determine each child's age. Calculate each child's BMI and percentile and categorize the findings. Describe your findings, and report what percentage of the children would meet the criteria for being obese or overweight.
5. Explore resources in your area for physical activities for children. Compile a list of resources, and share it with your classmates. Are any of these resources also available to children or adolescents who have disabilities?

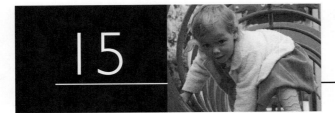

15

Intellectual
Disabilities

DANA ROTHSCHILD

DIANA BAL

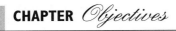

CHAPTER *Objectives*

After studying this chapter, the reader will be able to accomplish the following:

- Identify possible causes of intellectual disabilities.
- Differentiate the classifications of intellectual disabilities.
- Identify adaptive functioning for each level of intellectual disabilities.
- Identify the amount of support needed for each level of intellectual disabilities.
- Explain the roles of the occupational therapist and the occupational therapy assistant in assessments of and interventions with children who have intellectual disabilities.

KEY TERMS

CHAPTER OUTLINE

A child diagnosed with **intellectual disability** (ID) has impaired cognitive functioning that interferes with his or her ability to perform age-appropriate tasks in the areas of occupation, including social participation, education, activities of daily living (ADLs), instrumental activities of daily living (IADLs), and play/leisure. A child diagnosed with intellectual disability may or may not have an associated physical disability interfering with performance skills. Infants, toddlers, school-age children, and adolescents who have intellectual disability benefit from occupational therapy (OT) intervention to promote performance in all areas of occupation. Adults with intellectual disability also benefit from OT intervention to successfully participate in occupations over the lifespan.

DEFINITION

The former term *mental retardation* (MR) has been replaced by the current term *intellectual disability* to describe the condition in which a child has cognitive impairments that interfere with adaptive skills. The term *intellectual disability* will be primarily used in this chapter; the term *mental retardation* will be referred to when describing the classification of children with the type of disability or when referring to past sources that use this term.

An intellectual disability is a developmental disorder that occurs before the age of 18 years and is characterized by significantly below-average intellectual functioning as well as deficits in two or more adaptive skill areas (e.g., ADLs, communication, social participation, education, play/leisure, homemaking skills, and skills required to attain and maintain independence).[1] Children with intellectual disability may appear different. Some children have conditions or syndromes (e.g., Down syndrome) and present with certain physical features as well as associated intellectual disability. Other children may exhibit no atypical physical characteristics. In general, parents and professionals suspect intellectual disability when a child fails to meet developmental milestones. Some children with mild disability may not be identified until they begin school. Unlike learning disability, which affects one area of learning (e.g., math or reading), intellectual disability impacts learning in all areas of one's occupation.

The diagnosis of intellectual disability involves consideration of the child's cultural, linguistic, behavioral, sensory, motor, and communication abilities and, in particular, how those abilities may influence intelligence testing. Professionals consider the child's age, strengths, and weaknesses, along with the limitations in intelligence when examining how these factors influence adaptive functioning.[2] Health care professionals not only provide

the diagnosis, they are also interested in providing information to develop an individualized plan of needed supports that will improve the child's ability to participate in occupations.

MEASUREMENT AND CLASSIFICATION

Although *intellectual disability* is now the preferred term used to describe children with intellectual and adaptive functioning deficits, the terms *mental retardation* and *intellectual disability* are classified and defined synonymously in the *Diagnostic and Statistical Manual of Mental Disorders*, 4th edition (DSM-IV-TR).[1] Current federal and state laws contain the term *mental retardation*, and laws and public policy use this term to determine eligibility for state and federal programs.

Formal testing procedures are used to diagnose children with intellectual disability and to gather information from interviews with parents, observations of the child, and completion of norm-referenced tests. The diagnosis of intellectual disability is made when a child scores significantly below average on intelligence testing (standardized tests) and experiences deficits in two or more areas of adaptive functioning (which may be identified through tests as well). Information gathered from parent interviews and observation of the child is considered to create the child's profile and an intervention plan. The level of severity of intellectual disability is therefore determined by examining the results of intelligence testing, adaptive functioning, and mental age in conjunction with information from parents and from observation of the child.[1]

Intelligence Testing

An **intelligence quotient** (IQ) is a score derived from one of several different standardized tests designed to assess intelligence. Scores from tests of intelligence are a primary tool for identifying children who have intellectual disability. Intelligence tests are scored on a scale of 0 to 145, with the average score of 100 and a standard deviation of 15 points. Table 15-1 describes the categories of intellectual disability according to IQ scores.[4]

Scores between 85 and 115 are considered within normal limits (average intelligence quotient). Children who score between 70 and 84 fall within the borderline intellectual disability range; a score between 55 and 69 represents mild intellectual disability a score between 25 and 39 is considered to represent severe intellectual disability and children with scores lower than 25 are classified as having profound intellectual disability.[4]

IQ tests such as the revised *Wechsler Intelligence Scale* (WISC-R), *Stanford-Binet Intelligence Scale*, *McCarthy Scales of Children's Ability*, and *Bayley Scales of Infant*

TABLE 15-1

Categories of Intellectual Disability Based on Intelligence Quotient Scores

RANGE OF IQ SCORES	INTELLECTUAL DISABILITY CATEGORY
55 to 69	Mild
40 to 54	Moderate
25 to 39	Severe
Less than 25	Profound

IQ, intelligence quotient.

Development are administered by a qualified psychologist. The tests include sections on motor and verbal abilities. Administering IQ tests to children with severe disabilities can be challenging; any changes in how the test is administered tend to interfere with standardization and the results. Therefore, OT clinicians must view the results of IQ tests cautiously. Since infant and child IQ tests require motor responses, those who are physically unable to perform certain motor tasks may receive lower scores.

Along with intelligence testing, children must exhibit a deficit in two or more areas of adaptive functioning to be diagnosed with intellectual disability. Understanding the areas in which a child is able to function provides OT practitioners with information for planning interventions and providing support services.

CLINICAL *Pearl*

It is possible to estimate IQ in younger children by dividing mental age by chronological age and multiplying by 100. For example,

36 months (mental age) ÷ 72 months (chronological age) × 100 = 50.

The child in this example has an IQ of 50. (Note: This is considered an estimate.)

Adaptive Functioning

Adaptive functioning refers to the conceptual, social, and practical abilities that children rely on to adapt to changing environments and to function in their everyday lives. Conceptual skills include receptive and expressive language, reading and writing, money concepts, and self-direction. Social skills refer to self-esteem, social problem solving, and the ability to follow rules, obey laws, and avoid being victimized. Practical skills include ADLs, occupational skills, health care, travel/transportation,

schedules/routines, safety, use of money, and use of the telephone. Limitations in these areas significantly interfere with a child's ability to navigate through everyday situations.[1,2]

To measure adaptive behavior, OT professionals look at what a child can do in comparison with other children of his or her age. Adaptive skills are evaluated in many different settings, with input from the caregiver or teacher as well. A variety of scales are available to measure adaptive functioning:

- The *Vineland Adaptive Behavior Scale* uses parental input to evaluate adaptive behavior in terms of communication, daily living, socialization, and motor skills.
- The *School Functional Assessment* uses input from the teacher to assess the child's ability to perform the occupational tasks necessary in the school setting.
- The *Support Intensity Scale* (SIS) measures the pattern and level of support required for an adult with intellectual disability to lead a normal, independent life.[10] The SIS measures the support required in the medical, behavioral, and life activity areas and also addresses the frequency, time of day, and type of support required. This is beneficial when developing support plans and can assist with resource allocation and financial planning.[8]

Mental Age

Mental age refers to the age level at which the child is functioning, whereas *chronological age* refers to the child's actual age. For example, a 5-year-old child who is only able to perform tasks that a typical 3-year-old performs would be considered to have a mental age of 3. Mental age is based on and determined by performance on standardized tests. These tests allow the child's performance to be equitably compared with the chronological age standard.

ETIOLOGY AND INCIDENCE

The incidence of intellectual disability in the United States is reported to be 3 out of every 100 people.[2] Causes include genetic factors, problems during pregnancy, difficult births, and health problems. In many cases, the cause remains unknown. Children who have intellectual disability can also have physical and psychological disabilities. These deficits can include visual impairments, hearing loss, muscle tone problems, seizures, and sensory disorders (see Chapters 12, 16, and 24). Physicians often categorize the causes of intellectual disability on the basis of when they occur. Prenatal causes occur before birth, perinatal causes occur at birth, and postnatal causes occur from birth to 3 years of age.

Prenatal Causes

Prenatal (before birth) causes of intellectual disability include genetics, disturbances in embryonic development, and acquired causes (e.g., maternal toxins).

Genetic Causes

Intellectual disability may be caused by errors occurring when genes combine, by genes changing during the process (i.e., mutations), or by inheriting impaired genes from parents. Each human cell contains 23 pairs of chromosomes. Genes on these chromosomes contain deoxyribonucleic acid (DNA), the material that contains the unique physical and genetic plans for each individual. The store of DNA information on each of the genes is called the *genetic code*. The first 22 pairs are called *autosomes* and the twenty-third pair the *sex chromosomes*. During reproduction, 23 chromosomes come from the mother and 23 from the father, resulting in a cell with 46 chromosomes. When too many or too few chromosomes are present (e.g., 47 instead of 46) or an abnormal gene exists, the developing fetus is negatively affected. Genetic disorders may be inherited or caused by errors in cell division. Two common examples of genetic conditions associated with intellectual disability are Down syndrome and fragile X syndrome. Down syndrome is called *trisomy 21* because individuals with this condition have three copies of chromosome 21 instead of a pair. Individuals with fragile X syndrome have an abnormal, or "fragile," X chromosome that contains a weak area.

Acquired Causes

A **teratogen** is any physical or chemical substance that may cause physical or developmental complications in the fetus.[5] Teratogens can include prescription medications, lead, alcohol, or illegal drugs consumed by the mother; maternal infections; and other toxins. The effects of teratogens on the fetus range from congenital anomalies (defects) to intellectual disability. The type of agent, the amount of exposure, and the point at which exposure occurs during embryonic and fetal development play important roles in the outcome. Exposure to teratogens during the first 12 weeks of pregnancy can have the most dangerous consequences because it is during this time that the fetal brain, spinal cord, most internal organs, and limbs develop.

Perinatal Causes

Intellectual disability may occur during birth (perinatal) as a result of lack of oxygen (anoxia) to the neonate or due to brain trauma (e.g., bleeding) caused by undue stress on the neonate during the birthing process. Infants born prematurely or at low birth weights may experience complications that result in intellectual deficits.

Prematurity

Infants born before completion of the thirty-seventh week of gestation are considered premature.[9] Numerous factors may cause prematurity, such as poor nutrition, lack of prenatal care, toxemia, multiple fetuses, a weak cervix, numerous previous births, and adolescent mothers.[7] Although prematurity does not necessarily mean that a disability will develop, some complications caused by prematurity may result in intellectual disability. For example, prematurity can cause *respiratory distress syndrome* (RDS), a condition in which the premature infant's lungs are not yet producing surfactant, a chemical on the surface of the lungs that helps keep the lungs from collapsing. Another complication of prematurity is *apnea*, a condition in which the infant stops breathing; apnea can last from seconds to minutes. *Anoxia* refers to a total lack of oxygen, while *hypoxia* refers to a decreased amount of oxygen.[9] Intellectual disability can result when either condition affects the brain. The severity of brain dysfunction depends on (1) the location and size of the area deprived of oxygen; (2) the amount of time the area is without oxygen; and (3) the metabolic changes that take place in the body as a result of cell death in that area of the brain. Anoxia or hypoxia can occur during labor because of a small birth canal, which can result in bleeding around the baby's brain, compression of the umbilical cord, tearing of the placenta (placenta previa), or breech birth (i.e., the child is born with the buttocks presenting first instead of the head as in normal births).

Prematurity can also cause *hydrocephalus*, a condition in which the cerebrospinal fluid accumulates in the brain and can cause the head to grow disproportionately large (Figure 15-1). The extent of the infant's

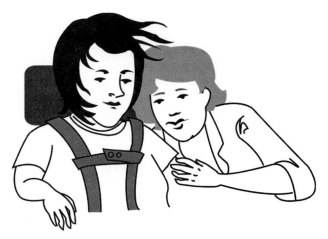

FIGURE 15-1 Adult with disproportionately sized head caused by unshunted hydrocephalus.

prematurity and associated complications affects the severity of the impairment (if any develops). Premature brain development puts infants at risk for brain hemorrhages (bleeding).

Postnatal Causes

Postnatal causes of intellectual disability include infection, trauma, tetragons, and neglect that occurs after birth.

Infections

Infections can cause brain damage and resulting intellectual disability in infants and children. *Viral meningitis* is a condition in which a virus attacks the protective covering around the brain and spinal cord, known as the *meninges*.[7] Several different viruses cause meningitis, including chickenpox virus. In small children and infants, meningitis may cause permanent brain damage that results in intellectual disability, the severity of which depends on the extent of brain damage. Inflammation of the brain, known as *encephalitis*, may be caused by complications from the mother contracting chickenpox, rabies, measles, influenza, and other diseases.[9] The severity of any resulting intellectual disability varies depending on the area and amount of the brain damaged.

Trauma

Any traumatic injury to the brain, including those sustained from an automobile accident, falls, bicycle accidents, near-drowning, and physical abuse experienced by the mother can cause brain injuries and thus intellectual impairments in the child.

Teratogens

Toxins are poisonous substances that cause particular problems when ingested.[9] Because infants and small children often place objects and substances in their mouths, certain common household substances can pose serious and life-threatening problems. For example, older homes often have lead-based paint on the walls. Inhaling, licking, or eating peeling paint can cause lead poisoning, resulting in developmental problems. Once diagnosed, lead poisoning can be treated, but residual permanent damage may exist. Other common household toxins include mercury in thermometers and cleaning agents.

Neglect

Poor nutrition and environmental deprivation (e.g., lack of physical, emotional, and cognitive support required for growth, development, and social adaptation) during infancy and early childhood may cause intellectual disability. Lack of stimulation, starvation, or poor nutrition may interfere with early brain development in children and result in intellectual deficits.

PERFORMANCE IN AREAS OF OCCUPATION

The capacity of a child with an intellectual disability to perform in areas of occupation varies depending on the severity of intellectual disability and the presence of additional deficits. Regardless of intellectual disability, "all people need to be able or enabled to engage in the occupations of their need and choice, to grow through what they do, and experience independence or interdependence, equality, participation, security, health and well being" (p. 198).[6]

CLINICAL *Pearl*

Don't judge a book by its cover! A child with even the most profound intellectual disability may be more capable than you thought (Figure 15-2). Randy is severely physically handicapped, requiring full support for his body; however, he showed great success in using an augmented communication system.

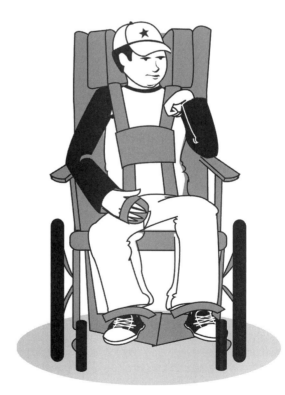

FIGURE 15-2 Adolescent with multiple disabilities and intellectual disability.

Children who have intellectual disability experience significant delays in meeting age-appropriate motor and cognitive milestones. Although learning speed may be slower for children who have intellectual deficits than it is for those who are developing typically, all children are capable of learning. OT practitioners are interested in determining how the child's limitations interfere with functional skills in occupations. Performance ability is related to the severity of the intellectual delay. The following case examples provide readers with a general description of expected capabilities based on the level of intellectual disability.

CLINICAL *Pearl*

The parents or primary caregivers of children who are developmentally delayed have valuable information concerning the children's abilities and the activities that they enjoy. This information will assist OT practitioners in developing interventions for the child and the family.

Mild Intellectual Disability

CASE *Study*

Sarah is 9 years old and is in Grade 2. When she was born, her parents found that she was "floppy" (an indicator of low muscle tone) and "weak." She had difficulty breastfeeding. Since she could not sustain a sucking pattern, a gastrostomy tube (g-tube) was placed in her stomach at 1 month. The tube was removed when Sarah was 2 years old, and she currently eats a regular diet with Ensure supplements. Sarah received early intervention services, including OT, physical therapy, and speech/language therapy until she was 3 years old. Currently, Sarah receives 2 hours of resource help daily for reading and math. Sarah has made a close friend and is able to follow daily classroom routines. Sarah reads sight words and books at Grade 1 level. Handwriting is a challenge for Sarah because she is unable to remember how to form letters, but she is able to copy print from a model. Each day Sarah's teacher has her write her name, address, and phone number three times in a designated area to promote increased speed and fluency. Sarah's individualized educational program (IEP) includes adaptations of preferential seating, a modified workload, oral testing, the use of a word processor, and extra time for completion of work as needed. For writing assignments, she uses the computer/word processor with *Co: Writer* and *Write: OutLoud* programs, which audibly read the words on the screen and provide a list of words from which she can select. Sarah is independent in school and home-related self-care tasks but requires extra time to complete them. At home, Sarah's mother encourages her to

bathe on her own and select her clothing the night before. In the future, Sarah would like to be a teacher's aide and help take care of children.

Sarah has **mild intellectual disability**.

Individuals with mild intellectual disability have IQ scores of 55 to 69 and may be further classified as "educable." Children in this category may not seem significantly different from others until they attempt to attain higher levels of cognitive skills and perform tasks that require significant abstract thinking. These children can develop social and communication skills and usually master academic skills from Grade 3 to Grade 7; however, it takes them longer than average to attain them.

They are able to achieve the following academic skills:

- Reading at the Grade 6–7 level
- Writing simple letters or lists, such as a grocery list
- Performing simple mathematical functions such as multiplication and division
- Using the computer and the Internet to perform simple research or to communicate with others

As adults, their social, vocational, and self-help skills are usually sufficient to allow them to partially or completely support themselves financially through employment. Therefore, they can live independently or in a minimally supervised setting in the community.

Moderate Intellectual Disability

CASE *Study*

Daniel is 7 years old and is enrolled in a self-contained classroom for children who have moderate intellectual disability. He is mainstreamed with typically developing peers during lunch, recess, and special areas. He is nonverbal but indicates his needs by gesturing and pointing to pictures on a simple communication board. Daniel uses a visual schedule to follow daily classroom routines. He is sensitive to certain clothing and food textures. Daniel requires minimum to moderate assistance to put on clothing, especially to get them correctly oriented. He requires moderate assistance to button and zip clothing because of inattention and the inability to follow multistep processes. He feeds himself with a fork but is a very picky eater. He is able to print his first name and sort items by size, shape, and color. An occupational therapist recommended that Daniel participate in a classroom and home sensory program to decrease his hypersensitivity. Following a consultation between the occupational therapist and the occupational therapy assistant (OTA) with regard to the intervention plan, the OTA starts to provide direct therapy and periodically consults with the school staff and the family to promote sensory modulation and oral desensitization. After 3 months, the staff and family have a better understanding of what upsets Daniel. He has begun eating a variety of foods at school and at home.

Daniel has **moderate intellectual disability**.

Individuals with moderate intellectual disability have IQ scores of 40 to 54; they may also be considered "trainable." These children need support regularly and are likely to have deficits in academic, communicative, and social skills. With special education, individuals who have moderate intellectual disability are usually able to attain the skills of a Grade 1 or Grade 2 student, including the following:

- Writing name
- Reading simple texts and emergency words
- Remembering home phone number
- Understanding written numbers and quantities (e.g., being able to select three apples from a pile of apples as directed)
- Understanding basic concepts of money

Children and adolescents with moderate intellectual disability require supervision but are able to follow a series of simple verbal directions. They may learn recurring actions such as making a sandwich for lunch. They may be able to participate in simple leisure activities. Children and adolescents with moderate intellectual disability can communicate their desires and preferences and thus should be provided with opportunities to make choices. Adolescents and adults with moderate intellectual disability may require supervision to complete ADLs and IADLs. These individuals can do some meaningful work in sheltered workshops or community-supported employment settings. Numerous adults with moderate intellectual disability live successfully in supervised living arrangements. OT practitioners can provide support and strategies to caregivers to facilitate physical routines and adapt IADLs and work activities.

CLINICAL *Pearl*

Family, caregivers, and teachers are instrumental in helping children with intellectual disability succeed. Encourage them to share their expertise with you.

Severe Intellectual Disability

CASE *Study*

Thomas is a 9-year-old boy who attends a self-contained class at his local elementary school. He is short, has low muscle tone, and appears to be unsteady when he moves about the classroom. He is able to walk, loves to eat, and has mastered feeding himself independently with a fork but is unable to open ketchup packets or milk containers. Thomas is on a toileting schedule at home and at school. He counts to two, recognizes colors, and responds to his name. In class, he scribbles on paper but tends to color the table or another student's paper if an adult is not supervising him. He is a dependent worker and requires verbal cues with supervision to stay on task. He has learned to sort silverware with a model but will stop working if not directed to continue by an adult. His favorite thing to do is bang objects on the table, rock back and forth, and take off his shirt when he has nothing to do. His language is very limited, but he is able to point to the items he wants and use some picture symbols to indicate basic needs (e.g., food, bathroom, favorite toy, and computer). He requires constant adult supervision when on the playground or walking to the lunchroom or he will roam away from the class.

Thomas has **severe intellectual disability**.

Individuals with severe intellectual disability have an IQ score between 25 and 39 and therefore require support in all areas of occupational performance on a regular basis. Functional independence depends greatly on their associated physical limitations. Habitual basic self-care skills such as feeding and hygiene tasks may be learned because of the recurring nature of these activities. Children with severe intellectual disability have difficulty generalizing skills and perform best with routine and consistency. For example, the child might be able to unzip his or her school bag but not an unfamiliar jacket.

Desires and needs can be communicated verbally or nonverbally by using communication boards or other methods. As adolescents and adults, those with severe intellectual disability may be successful in supervised prevocational training activities. They require extensive supervision and support in order to live independently. It is unlikely that these individuals will achieve any particular academic grade level in school because tasks such as reading and writing are extremely difficult for them.

With special education, the child with severe intellectual disability can do the following:

- Recognize his or her photograph
- Perform self-care skills that are routinely done (e.g., feed oneself with a spoon, pull pants up/down)
- Learn how to follow simple classroom rules that are done consistently (hang up backpack when entering classroom)

Children and adolescents with severe intellectual disability frequently also have physical disabilities, including cerebral palsy, seizure disorder, visual impairment, hearing loss, and communication disorder. OT practitioners must evaluate and address the physical demands of activities along with the global and specific mental function demands. Family members who are caring for the child may require education on handling techniques and behavior management. OT practitioners work with other family members to help them understand so that they may interact and socialize and enjoy each other.

> **CLINICAL** *Pearl*
>
> Nonverbal children with severe intellectual disability can point to pictures mounted on a place mat to indicate their wants and needs during mealtime. For example, they can point to a picture of a cup to let the caregivers know that they want more milk.

Profound Intellectual Disability

CASE *Study*

Jamie is a 5-year-old little girl who is very frail. She is unable to sit or stand because she has poor head, neck, and trunk control. She depends on others for all her care needs, including eating, toileting, and dressing. She eats pureed food and sips from a straw. Jamie drools because of her poor oral motor control. She smiles when she hears a familiar voice or music. Her eye fixation is inconsistent, and she is unable to move her body on command or respond to simple yes or no questions.

Jamie has **profound intellectual disability**.

An IQ score of less than 25 classifies individuals as having profound intellectual disability. Because of the numerous physical disabilities that may accompany profound intellectual disability, these individuals often have difficulty progressing developmentally and require constant support in all areas of occupation. Depending on the extent of their physical limitations, individuals with profound intellectual disability may learn to communicate and perform basic or routine self-care activities such as hygiene and grooming tasks. Extensive assistance is required for all other ADL skills, and continuous support is needed in living arrangements. Maintenance of the physical skills required for everyday occupations assists in preserving the overall health of the child. OT practitioners working with children who have profound intellectual disability concentrate on the basic skills required for occupations. For example, the goals of therapy may include such tasks as the following:

- Smile on approach
- Indicate food preference
- Feed oneself with a spoon
- Make visual contact

- Allow caregiver to bathe them
- Allow caregiver to touch them
- Cooperate with dressing or self-care

> **CLINICAL** *Pearl*
>
> Children who have profound intellectual disability have preferences for certain people, toys, and food and typically have a sense of humor. The OT practitioner must respect their preferences and try to discover what motivates them.

CLIENT FACTORS: FUNCTIONAL IMPLICATIONS AND OCCUPATIONAL THERAPY INTERVENTIONS

Client factors refer to the specific abilities, characteristics, or beliefs that may impact performance in the areas of occupation and include values, beliefs and spirituality, body functions, and body structures.[3] The text that follows provides examples of how client factors may be manifested in children and adolescents who have intellectual disability and provides suggestions for intervention.

Mental Function

Global mental functions are frequently delayed or absent in children and adolescents with intellectual deficits. Deficits in cognitive function and learning styles characteristic of children who have intellectual disability include poor memory, slower learning rates, attention problems, difficulty generalizing what they learn, and lack of motivation. Furthermore, these children may lack orientation to person, place, time, self, and others. Children with intellectual disability may not make eye contact or attend to activities (consciousness level). Temperaments and personalities of these clients vary, and they may experience emotional instability (e.g., quickly change from one emotion to another). OT practitioners may find that clients have difficulty choosing activities (energy and drive), have few preferences (interests), or have difficulty with impulse control.

Intervention

Intervention is not aimed at improving intelligence (it is not possible to reverse the condition); instead, it is aimed at helping the child or adolescent develop performance patterns, including habits, roles, and rituals used in the process of engaging in meaningful activities. Each client should be assessed in terms of his or her strengths and weaknesses. OT practitioners focus on the actual occupations that the child or adolescent hopes to perform as goals. (See Box 15-1 for sample goals.)

BOX 15-1

Sample Goals Showing a Variety of Functional Levels

1. Using a builtup handled spoon, Greg will feed himself independently at dinner within 2 weeks.
2. Sandy will initiate a simple conversation with another adolescent during the school picnic.
3. After demonstration and with minimal assistance, Ira will sort white and dark clothes into two separate containers within 1 month.
4. In 1 month, given minimal verbal cues, Amy will cooperate with dressing and undressing by extending her arms.
5. Given two choices, Faye will turn her head right or left to identify her food preferences for each meal, within 2 months.
6. Jerry will follow a 4-step handwashing routine, with the use of a visual schedule, by 1 month.

CASE *Study*

A typical Grade 2 health objective requires that students be able to identify the five food groups. Once students are able to identify the five food groups, teachers hope that the students will make healthy food choices. Reinhardt is an 8-year-old boy with moderate intellectual disability. The school staff would like him to eat a more balanced diet, as he only eats sweets and foods with a crunchy texture. Therefore, the OT practitioner rewrote Reinhardt's health goal to read: "The student will eat at least one bite of two food groups." In this case, rewriting the goal to include the exact occupational behavior needed is more functional and meaningful to the child and to the school staff. The intervention session would emphasize the importance of consuming at least a small portion of fruits or vegetables, bread, dairy products, or meat. The OT practitioner may decide to use a positive reinforcer (in this student's case, dessert) after she accomplishes this. (It is not wise to use food as a reinforcer in all cases. However, during mealtime, it is easy to allow dessert after the meal as a reinforcer.)

Specific mental functions that children with intellectual disability may demonstrate include the following:

- Shorter attention span
- Difficulty storing and retrieving information (memory)
- Difficulty recognizing direction and relation of objects to one another (perception)
- Slower learning ability (thought)
- Inability to recognize objects or people (thought)
- Difficulty making sense of stimuli (perception)
- Difficulty with problem solving and critical thinking (higher-level cognition)
- Difficulty generalizing information and mastering abstract thinking (thought)
- Slow, delayed, or absent language skills
- Difficulty with adding and subtracting (calculations)
- Poor motor planning (sequencing complex movements)
- Inappropriate range and regulation of emotions; self-control (emotional)
- Difficulty with body image, self-concept, and self-esteem (self and time)

Language Functions

As with physical milestones, it can take longer for children with intellectual disability to reach speech and language milestones. These children are slower to use words, put words together, and speak in complete sentences. Their social development is sometimes slow because of cognitive impairment and language deficiencies. For example, shorter memory and attention span could make recalling and retrieving words difficult, whereas difficulties with abstract thinking may make it challenging to mentally grasp certain concepts. The language and speech of children with intellectual disability may be related to associated physical problems such as inadequate oral–motor muscle tone, which results in unclear articulation, difficulty taking deep breaths, and difficulty moderating one's speech (i.e., speaking too softly or loudly). OT practitioners are responsible for referring children with intellectual disability to speech therapists as needed. Frequently, the OT practitioner and speech therapist are able to provide intervention together.

Behavioral/Emotional Functions

Children with intellectual disability are likely to exhibit behavior which may be related to specific situations that compound an impaired ability to communicate. Children with intellectual deficits may have difficulty accepting criticism, managing self-control, and displaying appropriate behaviors. They may show aggression toward others or engage in self-injurious or self-stimulating behaviors, such as hand flapping, biting, and hitting that make them stand out in typical settings. They may suck on clothing, make repetitive noises, or hop on their toes.

Children with intellectual disability may exhibit hyperactivity (impulsiveness and excessive activity that result in difficulty functioning in social situations), excessive shyness (withdrawing during familiar group activities), and distractibility (difficulty paying attention to one task). These behaviors interfere with their functioning and ability to participate in social or academic occupations. These children attain their social skills later than other children and thus may often misbehave or act in a manner much younger than that which is appropriate for their chronological age.

During adolescence, children with intellectual disability may behave inappropriately socially or sexually. Some of these children may develop psychosocial disorders such as depression, obsessive–compulsive disorder, or attention deficit disorder.

Intervention

OT practitioners use a behavioral approach to facilitate positive behaviors in children with intellectual disability. See Box 15-2 for the techniques used in this approach. The occupational therapist and the OTA can be instrumental in designing a behavioral modification plan. First, data are collected to identify the behaviors that need to be changed. The occupational therapist and the OTA use their expertise to describe these behaviors and analyze them to determine why they are occurring. They present the child's strengths and weaknesses so that the team may establish an appropriate award system. The OTA reinforces the system and checks with the school staff daily to see if they have any new concerns. OT intervention is aimed at reinforcing positive behaviors as well as working on other established goals.

BOX 15-2

Developing a Behavioral Modification Plan

1. Identify behaviors that interfere with learning, socialization, or engagement in occupations.
2. Collect data on each behavior. Consider the following when analyzing the behavior: When does the unacceptable behavior occur? How often does it occur? Under which circumstances does it occur? In what setting (quiet, noisy, dark, etc.) does the behavior occur?
3. Prioritize the behaviors that should be addressed first. Behaviors that involve safety issues are priorities.
4. With the team (e.g., parent, caregiver, teacher, staff), create a plan to reduce the behavior. The OT practitioner provides a task analysis of the behavior and identifies reinforcers or provides insight into why the behaviors occur. The plan must be simple enough to work for a variety of people with limited training. Behavioral objectives must be stated very specifically and in observable and measurable terms. Plans should be simple so that the student can incorporate them into his or her daily schedule.
5. Implement the plan. OT practitioners may be responsible for training the staff on the implementation of the plan. OT practitioners may adapt or suggest changes to the plan after a careful task analysis. Writing effective behavioral objectives require practice. Be prepared to reflect on your objectives and learn from them. You will soon find out what works and what does not work.
6. Collect data on the behavior. Evaluate the outcome, and discuss it with the team. All team members are responsible for documenting the outcome of the plan.
7. Make modifications to the behavior plan as needed to impact positive outcomes.

CLINICAL *Pearl*

Children with intellectual disabilities establish friendships and other relationships. They may experience the full range of emotions, although they may not be able to express these feelings. OT practitioners can help these children and adolescents deal with feelings of grief, sadness, (when losing someone), intimacy, and love.

CLINICAL *Pearl*

Children with intellectual disability may enjoy participating in athletic events such as the Special Olympics. These events help these children develop feelings of success by working toward an athletic goal. Children experience teamwork, achievement, and the benefits of physical activity. Events such as these promote a positive self-concept and self-esteem.

CASE *Study*

A referral was made by the school to determine why a student was throwing his tray on the floor at lunchtime. The occupational therapist met with the staff, reviewed the charts, and observed the child during lunch. The OTA then observed the child at breakfast. The OTA and the occupational therapist met and compiled their observations, discussed possibilities, and brainstormed solutions. During mealtimes, the student sat at a table with three other students with severe intellectual disability, who required one-on-one assistance to eat. This student was able to feed himself with the proper setup. He was positioned in his wheelchair at the table. He ate slowly, with a tremor. The staff was busy with other clients and did not speak to this student during the meal. The student was nonverbal but was able to point or gesture to communicate. On completion of his meal, the student threw his entire tray on the floor. The staff rushed to his side, picked up the tray, cleaned up the student, and took him back to the classroom.

The staff was frustrated with this student's lunchroom behavior but met his needs quickly when he threw his tray down. Getting quick attention thus reinforced this behavior. Both the occupational therapist and the OTA noticed that the student looked around right before he threw his tray down. They decided that the cause of the behavior was that the student was trying to communicate his need for some help and attention. Consequently, the staff changed their behavior by periodically checking to see if the student was done eating, taking the tray from him when he was ready, and bringing him back to his classroom where he enjoyed a few minutes of downtime with a few friends. The student was now getting his needs met, and the staff was reinforcing meal completion and appropriate behaviors.

Other suggestions to make mealtime more enjoyable for this student included the following:

- Limiting the number of students (with aides) at the table
- Limiting talking among aides and encouraging interaction among students
- Assigning a peer (from the regular education class) to join the student at lunch

The OTA consulted with the staff weekly. Caregivers were willing to try new strategies because the OT practitioners listened to them, addressed their concerns, and actually made their jobs easier.

Sensory Function and Pain

Children with intellectual disability may experience and process sound, taste, touch, and auditory information differently. Screenings and evaluations by health care professionals help rule out any medical problems. These children may experience adverse reactions to sensory experiences and consequently respond in an unexpected manner in certain situations. OT practitioners may be asked to evaluate these children's reactions to taste, smell, touch, movement, and body position to determine sensory preferences. OT practitioners assess sensory needs and make recommendations to help the children adapt to their environments. For example, a child may not want to eat food of a certain texture. The staff may assume that the child is not hungry when, in fact, the child does not like the texture of the food. Children with tactile sensitivity (or defensiveness) usually dislike being touched softly on areas of their bodies and/or may avoid contact with certain textures. Some children have difficulty with the modulation or self-regulation of sensory input that they receive during the day. A sensation that calms one child may excite or disturb another.

Frequently, when the children cannot handle all of the sensations bombarding them during the day, they might either act out, become hyperactive or aggressive, or even withdraw from the situation.

Intervention

OT practitioners frequently provide teams with information concerning the sensory processing abilities of children who have intellectual disability. A thorough analysis of these children's responses to a variety of sensory experiences provides insight into behaviors interfering with occupations. For example, some children with tactile defensiveness may overreact to bathing. They may dislike the feeling of water on the skin, but the staff or caregivers may interpret this reaction as uncooperative or aggressive behavior. The OT practitioner may be able to prepare the client for the bathing experience by means of a sensory program. This may be as simple as changing the time of the bath, regulating the temperature of the water, changing the soap, or establishing a brushing protocol before the bath. Other sensory modulation issues may be addressed by providing the caregiver and the child more time to accomplish the occupations; both the clients and the caregivers feel frustrated when they are rushed.

CASE *Study*

A staff member at a residential setting was responsible for waking, toileting, dressing, and feeding three adolescents with severe intellectual disability before they were transported to school. The staff member stated that giving them breakfast was an impossible task; the adolescents would not cooperate with her and frequently spat out their food. On observation, the OTA realized that the staff member was hurried, the adolescents were stressed, and they were unable to express their food preferences. One adolescent was spitting out food because of a motor deficit (tongue thrusting); the others were being served foods that they did not like. Intervention consisted of the OTA assisting the staff member in the morning until a routine was established. The OTA modeled the correct feeding techniques to help decrease tongue thrusting in the one adolescent and helped the staff identify the food preferences of the other two. The three adolescents were instructed on how to indicate their preferences instead of spitting out the food. A system change was implemented in that two staff members became responsible for the morning routines of the three individuals. This was accomplished by having one staff member come in early, which worked for her in light of her own personal/family responsibilities.

The importance of examining sensory processing can be observed as the children with intellectual disability respond to loud noises with exaggerated reactions (startle). A startle reaction may cause some children to fall or have a seizure, which is not common in typically developing children. Children with intellectual disability may have sensory problems related to body movement and muscle coordination (vestibular and proprioceptive), which lead to further motor deficits. They may not express pain proportionate to the stimuli; therefore, OT practitioners must be sensitive and perceptive to what may be perceived as pain by the child or adolescent. Children who have intellectual deficits may not understand procedures and may be fearful of new people, which makes their feelings of pain more intense. Familiar people providing medical preparation and comfort during procedures may help.

CLINICAL *Pearl*

Create opportunities for success and independence. Remember that pullover shirts, pants with elastic waistbands, and shoes with velcro make dressing easier.

CLINICAL *Pearl*

When teaching a child who has intellectual disability a new task, divide the task into small steps. Demonstrate the steps. Have the child practice the steps, one at a time. Provide assistance when necessary and immediate feedback. Practice the task in its natural context for the best carry over.

Movement-Related Functions

Children with intellectual disability often reach major physical milestones (e.g., roll, sit, stand, walk) later than usual. In fact, many infants are referred for OT because of motor delays before being diagnosed with intellectual disability. These infants and children typically exhibit low muscle tone and can exhibit a range of motor problems related to brain damage and difficulty learning complex motor tasks.

Intervention

Intervention is aimed at developing motor function and helping the children with intellectual disability adapt to or compensate for their movement problems. OT practitioners working on movement-related problems must remember that clients with intellectual deficits have difficulty finding ways to adapt to physical challenges. Since they are not able to problem solve or use cognition as readily as their peers without disability can, they will show slower progression in movement. These children

require extended practice, repetition, simple directions, and modification and/or adaptation of the requirements to succeed (see Chapter 23). Specific motor intervention is designed to address the physical problems associated with secondary diagnoses.

System Functions

OT practitioners working with children who have intellectual disability must have knowledge of how body systems affect functional ability. These children may be more susceptible to cardiac, pulmonary, blood, digestive, metabolic, urinary, reproductive, and skin disorders. For example, children who have Down syndrome experience intellectual disability and may be at risk for cardiac disorders. Food allergies and the adverse effects of medicines may affect these children. OT practitioners must be keen observers of behavior and knowledgeable about their clients' medical histories.

CLINICAL *Pearl*

Order simple and uncomplicated adaptive/positioning equipment for children and adolescents who have intellectual deficits. These children may not understand complicated equipment. The staff and family members may misplace items and become frustrated with complicated equipment demands along with those of caregiving.

ROLES OF THE OCCUPATIONAL THERAPIST AND THE OCCUPATIONAL THERAPY ASSISTANT

OT practitioners provide individualized services and supports to help children with intellectual disability develop independence by performing meaningful activities. The process includes a comprehensive evaluation that focuses on developing an occupational profile and analysis of the occupational performance (e.g., the ability to carry out ADLs, IADLs, work, play/leisure, education, and social participation).[3,7] The American Association on Intellectual Disabilities recommends that an individual's needs be assessed in nine key areas: (1) human development, (2) teaching and education, (3) home living, (4) community living, (5) employment, (6) health and safety, (7) recreation, (8) living environments, and (9) ADLs.[2] These key areas all fall within the scope of OT practice. The occupational therapist interviews the child's parents, primary caregivers, and teacher to gain information on the child's strengths and weaknesses and the contexts in which the occupations occur (e.g., physical, social, personal, cultural, temporal, spiritual, and virtual environments).

The OTA may administer standardized tests after the establishment of service competency and at the discretion of the supervising occupational therapist. The OTA and the occupational therapist work together constantly to re-evaluate and monitor the child's needs as he or she grows and learns. Infants, children, and adolescents with intellectual disability are treated in the home and at daycare centers, outpatient clinics, schools, and residential settings. Knowledge of the contexts, including community resources and environmental supports, is essential to the intervention process.

CLINICAL *Pearl*

Children with intellectual disability learn through repetition. For example, learning how to dress, bathe, or brush teeth may best be accomplished by performing the task when it naturally falls within the context of the day.

SUMMARY

Children with intellectual disabilities exhibit deficits in a range of cognitive skills that interfere with their ability to engage in occupations. OT practitioners evaluate the child's ability to perform occupations by analyzing the specific demands and client factors associated with the occupations that the child will engage in. The intervention plan is designed to maximize the child's strengths and work on the weaknesses. Children who have intellectual disability will learn, but at a much slower rate, and exhibit lifelong deficits in occupational performance. The developmental and behavioral frames of references are effective in helping these children develop abilities within their potential. The goal of OT intervention is to help the children or adolescents participate in occupations such as ADLs, IADLs, play/leisure, work, education, and social participation. OT practitioners work with team members and families and consider the overall goal of increasing the children's ability to participate in occupations. Toward this end, activities must frequently be adapted and modified to help the children succeed. OT practitioners working with these children need to be aware of community agencies for respite, social opportunities, housing, and assistance. Furthermore, children with intellectual disability may experience physical limitations that interfere with their occupations. OT practitioners educate and empower caregivers to care for their children and facilitate independence. The role of the OT practitioner in working with children and adolescents with intellectual disability is complex. They must use creativity, OT knowledge, and life skills to assist the children, adolescents, and their families in reaching the desired goals.

References

1. American Psychiatric Association: *Diagnostic and statistical manual of mental disorders (DSM-IV-TR)*, ed 4, Washington, DC, 2000, American Psychiatric Association.
2. American Association on Intellectual Disabilities: *Intellectual disabilities: definition, classification, and system of supports*, ed 10, Washington, DC, 2010, American Association on Intellectual Disabilities.
3. American Occupational Therapy Association: Occupational therapy practice framework: domain and process, ed 2. *Am J Occup Ther* 62:625–703, 2008.
4. Case-Smith J: *Pediatric occupational therapy and early intervention*, ed 2, Stoneham, MA, 1998, Butterworth-Heinemann.
5. Case-Smith J: *Occupational therapy for children*, ed 6, St. Louis, 2010, Mosby.
6. Crepeau E, Cohn E, Schell B: *Willard and Spackman's occupational therapy*, ed 11, Philadelphia, 2009, Lippincott Williams & Wilkins.
7. Mader S: *Understanding human anatomy and physiology*, ed 5, Dubuque, IA, 2004, William C. Brown.
8. Smith R: *Children with mental retardation: a parent's guide*, Bethesda, MD, 1993, Woodbine House.
9. *Taber's cyclopedic medical dictionary*, ed 21, Philadelphia, 2009, FA Davis.
10. Thompson JR et al: *Supports intensity scale*, Washington, DC, 2003, American Association on Mental Retardation.

Recommended Reading

Beirne-Smith M, Patton J, Kim S: *Mental retardation: an introduction to intellectual disability*, ed 7, Upper Saddle River, NJ, 2006, Prentice Hall.
Bernstein J: *Rachel in the world: a memoir*, Champagne, IL, 2007, University of Illinois Press.
Drew C, Hardman ML: *Intellectual disabilities across the lifespan*, ed 9, Upper Saddle River, NJ, 2006, Prentice Hall.
Osbune AG, Russo CJ: *Special education and the law: a guide for practitioners*, ed 2, Thousand Oaks, CA, 2006, Corwin Press.

Resources

The Association for Retarded Citizens of the United States (ARC)
1010 Wayne Avenue, Suite 650
Silver Spring, MD 20910
www.thearc.org.
(301) 565-3842

Centers for Disease Control and Prevention
1660 Clifton Road
Atlanta, GA
http://www.cdc.gov/.

Division on Mental Retardation and Developmental Disabilities (MRDD)
The Council for Exceptional Children
1110 North Glebe Road, Suite 300
Arlington, VA 22201-5704
(888) 232-7733
cec@cec.sped.org
www.mrddcec.org

American Association on Intellectual and Developmental Disabilities (AAIDD)
501 3rd Street, NW, Suite 200
Washington, DC, 20001
1-800-424-3688
(202) 387-1968

REVIEW *Questions*

1. How is intellectual disability diagnosed and categorized?
2. What are some causes for intellectual disability?
3. What is the role of the registered occupational therapist and the certified occupational therapy assistant in the intervention for children who have intellectual disability?
4. What are some behavioral strategies for working with children who have intellectual deficits?
5. What are the functional implications of being classified as having mild, moderate, severe, or profound intellectual disability?
6. What frames of reference work well with this population, and why?
7. How do behaviors interfere with learning in children with intellectual disability?

SUGGESTED *Activities*

1. Volunteer at a facility that specializes in working with children who have intellectual disability.
2. Attend a Down syndrome support group to learn about the challenges faced by the families and caregivers of individuals with this syndrome.
3. Volunteer your time in a school system or early intervention program. Ask to see a sample of the individual family service plan (IFSP) or individualized educational program (IEP).
4. Volunteer to babysit or provide respite care for a child who has developmental delays.
5. Volunteer in a special education classroom that has children with a variety of disabilities.
6. Volunteer in a daycare center and screen the children's developmental skills. Observe the different behaviors.
7. Analyze the tasks of a daily activity to determine the steps.

## 16

Cerebral Palsy

PATTY COKER-BOLT

TERESSA GARCIA-REIDY

ERIN NABER

CHAPTER *Objectives*

After studying this chapter, the reader will be able to accomplish the following:

- Describe the frequency, pattern, types, and classification of cerebral palsy (CP)
- Identify the impaired progression of movement associated with CP
- Describe the components of normal postural control and movement in children who have CP
- Recognize the differences among motor development, motor learning, and motor control
- Explain ways in which normal muscle tone and impaired muscle tone influence movement
- Identify the role of the certified occupational therapy assistant in the assessment and intervention of movement disorders in children who have CP
- Describe the range of interventions used with children who have CP, including medical, constraint-induced movement, complementary and alternative medicine, and splinting and casting

KEY TERMS	CHAPTER OUTLINE

Cerebral palsy (CP) is a term used to describe a range of developmental motor disorders arising from a nonprogressive lesion or disorder of the brain (Box 16-1).[3] Associated brain damage is characterized by paralysis, spasticity, or abnormal control of movement or posture. While the injury to the brain is considered static, the pattern of motor impairment may change over time, affecting development in all daily occupations of childhood. The motor disorders associated with CP are often accompanied by disturbances of sensation, cognition, communication, perception, and/or a seizure disorder.[12] The lesion or damage in the brain may cause impairment in muscle activity in all or part of the body. CP typically affects the development of sensory, perceptual, and motor areas of the central nervous system (CNS). This can cause the child to have difficulty integrating all of the information that the brain needs to correctly plan and direct the skilled, efficient movements in the trunk and extremities that are used in everyday interactions with the environment. The muscles shorten and lengthen in uncoordinated, inefficient ways and are unable to work together to create smooth, effective motion.

PROGRESSION OF ATYPICAL MOVEMENT PATTERNS

Children who have CP demonstrate difficulty in achieving and maintaining normal posture while lying down, sitting, and standing because of impaired patterns of muscle activation.[3,19] These abnormal patterns result from the decreased ability of the CNS to control coactivation and reciprocal innervation of select muscle groups. Coactivation of muscle is the result of a co-contraction of agonist and antagonist muscle groups around a joint. Simultaneous contraction of agonist and antagonist muscle groups provide stability around a joint and also affect overall body posture. Reciprocal innervations in muscle groups occur when excitatory input directs the agonist muscle to contract while inhibitory input directs the antagonist muscle to remain inactive.[12,19] These reciprocal innervations allow for movement to occur

---

BOX 16-1

Definition of Cerebral Palsy

Cerebral palsy is a movement disorder affecting smooth and coordinated movements of the body needed for participation in everyday activities such as play and self-care. Disordered movement patterns are seen in the head/neck, arms, legs, and trunk. Impairments can be seen in one or more areas of development, including fine motor, gross motor, language/communication, and overall adaptive functions.

---

around a joint and in the body. Children who have CP may develop abnormal movement compensations and body postures as they try to overcome these motor deficits to function within their environments. Over time, movement compensations and atypical motor patterns create barriers to ongoing motor skill development. Instead of freely moving and exploring the world, as children with a normally developing sensorimotor system do, children who have CP may rely on early automatic reflex movement patterns as their primary means of mobility. These early automatic reflexive movements occur without conscious control of the child and are typically elicited by a specific sensory motor action.

PRIMARY AND SECONDARY IMPAIRMENTS

Children with CP manifest *primary impairments* that are the direct result of the lesion in the CNS. Primary impairments are an immediate and direct result of the cortical lesion in the brain. The nervous system damage that causes CP can occur before or during birth or before a child's second year, the time when myelination of the child's sensory and motor tracts and CNS structures rapidly occurs. CP is described as nonprogressive, nonhereditary, and noncontagious.[12] As a nonprogressive condition, the original defect or lesion occurring in the CNS typically does not worsen or change over time. However, because the lesion occurs in immature brain structures, the progression of the child's motor development may appear to change. Normal nervous system maturation shifts control of voluntary movement to increasingly higher and more complex areas of the brain. The child who has CP exhibits some changes in movement ability that results from the expected progression of motor development skills, but these changes tend to be delayed relative to age and often show much less variety than those seen on the normally developing child.

Children with CP develop *secondary impairments* in systems or organs over time due to the effects of one or more of the primary impairments.[3,20] These secondary impairments may become just as debilitating as the primary impairments. For example, a child with CP may have a primary impairment such as hypertonia and a muscle imbalance across a joint. This abnormal muscle tone may cause poor alignment across a joint, further muscle weakness, and eventually a contracture in the joint. The resulting muscle contractures, poor body alignment, and poor ability to initiate movement would be considered secondary impairments. It is important to understand this, since the diagnosis of CP means that a child has a static nonprogressive lesion in the brain. Although the initial brain injury remains unchanged, the results or the secondary impairments are not static and change over time with body growth and attempts to move

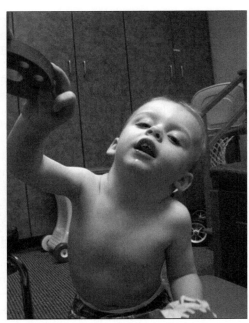

FIGURE 16-1 A child with cerebral palsy and upper extremity spasticity and tightness in his shoulder and arm as well as poor proximal stability in his trunk. During attempts to reach towards an object, the child demonstrates neck hyperextension and atypical response in his trunk. Note the open mouth posture during this reaching task.

against gravity. Children with CP may continue to rely on automatic movement patterns because they are unable to direct their muscles to move successfully in more typical motor patterns (Figure 16-1). The atypical patterns used to play or complete functional activities may become repetitive and fixed. The repetition of the atypical movement patterns prevent children with CP from gaining independent voluntary control of their own movements and can lead to diminished strength and musculoskeletal problems. The combination of impaired muscle coactivation and the use of reflexively controlled postures may lead to future contractures in muscles, tendons, and ligamentous tissues, causing the tissues to become permanently shortened. Bone deformities and alterations of typical posture or spinal and joint alignment may also occur.

FREQUENCY AND CAUSES

CP is the leading cause of childhood disability, and the reported incidence varies from 2 to 3 per 1000 live births.[12] The prevalence rate of CP has remained stable since the 1950s, in spite of dramatic improvements in prenatal and perinatal care over the last four decades.[20] According to the United Cerebral Palsy (UCP) Foundation, there are nearly 800,000 children and adults in the United States living with one or more symptoms of cerebral palsy.[21]

The accident that causes brain injury may occur during the prenatal, perinatal, or postnatal period, but evidence suggests that 70% to 80% of the causes of brain injury are prenatal in origin (Box 16-2).[3] Prenatal maternal infection and multiple pregnancies have also been associated with cerebral palsy.[12] Other prenatal factors include genetic abnormalities and maternal health factors such as stress, malnutrition, exposure to damaging drugs, and pregnancy-induced hypertension. Some gestational conditions of the mother, such as diabetes, may cause perinatal risks to the developing fetus; prematurity and low birth weight significantly increase an infant's risk of developing cerebral palsy.[19] Medical problems associated with premature birth may directly or indirectly damage the developing sensorimotor areas of the CNS. In particular, respiratory disorders can cause the premature newborn to experience anoxia, which deprives cells of oxygen that cells need to function and survive. Typical postnatal causes of CP could include conditions that result in significant damage to the developing CNS, such as malnutrition or hypoxic ischemia resulting from lack of oxygen to the brain. *Hypoxic ischemic encephalopathy* is defined as damage to cells in the CNS (brain and spinal cord) caused by inadequate oxygen. Other postnatal causes include infections and exposure to environmental toxins.

BOX 16-2

Risk Factors Associated With the Development of Cerebral Palsy

PRENATAL
- Genetic disorders
- Maternal health factors (e.g., chronic stress, malnutrition)
- Teratogenic agents (e.g., drugs, chemical exposure, radiation)

PERINATAL
- Prenatal conditions (e.g., toxemia secondary to maternal diabetes)
- Premature detachment of the placenta
- Medical problems associated with prematurity (e.g., compromised respiratory and cardiovascular systems, interventricular hemorrhage [IVH], periventricular leukomalacia [PVL])
- Multiple births

POSTNATAL
- Degenerative disorders (e.g., Tay-Sachs disease)
- Infections (e.g., meningitis, encephalitis)
- Alcohol or drug intoxication transferred during breastfeeding
- Anoxic ischemic encephalopathy (AIE)
- Trauma

POSTURE, POSTURAL CONTROL, AND MOVEMENT

To understand the functional movement problems that develop in children who have CP, the occupational therapy (OT) practitioner must be familiar with the ways that people normally control their bodies and execute skilled movements. The term *posture* describes the alignment of the body's parts in relation to each other and the environment. The ability to develop a large repertoire of postures and change them easily during an activity depends on the integration of several automatic, involuntary movement actions referred to as the **postural mechanism**, which includes several key components:

- Normal muscle tone
- Normal postural tone
- Developmental integration of early, **primitive reflex patterns**
- Emergence of **righting reactions, equilibrium reactions**, and **protective extension reactions**
- Intentional, voluntary movements against the forces of gravity
- The ability to combine movement patterns in the performance of functional activities

Disruption in the postural mechanism and the movement problems seen in children with CP are considered secondary impairments, which may be significantly reduced by OT interventions.

Righting, Equilibrium, and Protective Reactions

The functions that aid individuals in maintaining or regaining posture are *righting reactions* and *equilibrium reactions*, often referred to concomitantly as *balance reactions*. These functions can be thought of as *static* or *dynamic*. When people are sitting and not engaged in any activity, they are using static balance. When they bend to pick up an object on the floor, for example, they use dynamic balance to right themselves. Righting reactions are the foundation for all balance responses and help maintain upright postures against gravity during times when the center of gravity is moving off the body's base of support. Righting reactions help sense that the head is out of alignment with the body and produce a motor response to realign the head with the body. This requires the ability to bring the head and trunk back into "normal" skeletal alignment by using only the necessary muscle groups. When righting and equilibrium reactions are not sufficient to regain an upright posture quickly and safely, individuals use another reflexive reaction called the *protective extension reaction*. When people

fall, they frequently use this reaction, automatically reaching outward from their bodies to catch themselves or break the fall. A protective response requires the motor ability to quickly bring an extremity (i.e., arm or leg) out from the body to prevent a fall and also the strength to support the body's weight momentarily while bracing.

When movement abilities develop normally, children experience and practice many different movements and positions as they work toward mastering the upright, two-legged stance. Postural stability and the ability to demonstrate righting, equilibrium, and protective responses evolves developmentally through experimentation and play in a variety of developmental positions (e.g., prone, supine, sitting, kneeling, standing).

As children refine their control of specific postures through developmental progression, they develop the stable righting, equilibrium, and protective responses needed for a variety of skills and functional tasks. The majority of functional activities involve combinations of movement patterns of the head and neck, trunk, upper extremities, and lower extremities while moving the center of gravity off the body's base of support. Rarely do activities require isolated movements in one extremity or in a single plane of motion. Through a careful clinical analysis, the possible combinations enabling a functional activity can be described and used as a basis for making treatment decisions. For example, when a person reaches across the dinner table to pass a serving dish, that person must remain stable in the chair while going through several hand and arm motions to lift the dish, move it across the table, and then carefully release it to the person receiving the dish. Such a task requires the use of the muscles of the trunk and pelvic girdle areas as stabilizers; that is, these muscles provide postural stability as the upper extremity and shoulder girdle muscles perform the skilled movement task. In addition to the different types of muscle activity used for this task, the person must also rely on intact righting and equilibrium reactions to help keep the body upright against gravity and maintain a sitting posture in the chair while the body's weight is being shifted during the reaching task. The person passing the dish will probably lean to the left or right or forward. In this instance, just as in every executed movement, the leaning or moving from the center of gravity requires shifting of the body's weight. Each time a person shifts weight, righting and equilibrium reactions are used to counterbalance the weight shifts during the movements and help regain an upright posture with body parts correctly realigned. Vision, hearing, and other sensory inputs also provide perceptual information about whether the person is moving just the right distance when reaching and whether that person is upright in the context of the immediate surroundings.

Muscle tone

Muscle tone is the force with which a muscle resists being lengthened and can also be defined as the *muscle's resting stiffness*. It is tested by an OT practitioner passively stretching the client's muscle from the shortened state to the lengthened state and feeling the resistance offered by the muscle to the stretch. A child's ability to perform sequential movements is supported by the ability of muscles to maintain the correct amount of tension (stiffness) and elasticity during the movements. Muscle tone is highly influenced by gravity. Muscles must have enough tone to move against gravity in a smooth, coordinated motion. Emotions and mental states, including levels of alertness, fatigue, and excitement, can also influence muscle tone. Normal muscle tone develops along a continuum, with some variability among members of the typical population.

The qualities of contractility and elasticity are necessary for the muscle's accurate response to changes in stimuli experienced during movement, an event referred to as *coactivation*. Muscle tone allows muscles to adapt readily to changing sensory stimuli during functional activities. Children with CP resulting from a lesion in the CNS experience disruption in postural control; disruptions in righting, equilibrium, protective reactions; and atypical muscle tone. Decreased muscle tone, which is defined as *hypotonia*, can make a child appear relaxed and even floppy. Increased muscle tone, which is defined as *hypertonia*, can make a child appear stiff or rigid. In some cases, a child may initially appear hypotonic, but the muscle tone may change to hypertonia after several months of life and the influence of movement against gravity. An occupational therapy assistant (OTA) must possess an understanding of the ways in which postural control and muscle tone can affect normal movement patterns and everyday occupations when planning therapeutic interventions for children with CP (Box 16 -3). This knowledge is imperative for planning functional therapeutic activities that are appropriate for the child's age and physical abilities.

Primitive Reflexes

Much of the early movement patterns seen in newborns appears to be reflexive in nature and can be elicited by specific sensory motor stimulation. These early reflexes may disappear as the CNS matures and are replaced by more purposeful, voluntary, and skilled movements. The presence or absence of early reflexes is used to evaluate the health of infants. For example, when you provide gentle tactile stimulation to the cheek of a newborn, the infant will turn his or her head toward the cheek that is touched. This early reflex, referred to as the *rooting reflex*, helps newborns find the source of nutrition (i.e., breast or bottle).

Common Problems of Motor Development in Children With Cerebral Palsy

1. Abnormal muscle tone
   - Hypertonicity – increase in resting state of muscle
   - Hypotonicity – decrease in resting state of muscle
   - Fluctuating – muscle tone changes between hypertonic and hypotonic
2. Persistence of primitive reflexes
3. Atypical righting, equilibrium, and protective responses
4. Poor sensory processing
   - Decreased processing of vestibular, visual, and proprioceptive information
   - Distorted body awareness and body scheme
5. Joint hypermobility
   - Reduced limb stability and poor co-contraction across joints
6. Muscle weakness and poor muscle coactivation
7. Delays in typical progressing of motor skills and adaptive function
8. Decreased exploration of the environment

POSTURAL DEVELOPMENT AND MOTOR CONTROL

As newborns grow, they are continually developing and refining postural control. As with motor skills, the characteristics of posture vary with age. In the past 20 years, much research has been devoted to understanding motor control so that OT practitioners may provide effective neurologic rehabilitation to persons who have CP and other neurologic disorders. Motor control theory is complex, and detailed explanations of this theory are beyond the scope of this text. However, the OTA should be aware of the two main schools of thought on motor control. This knowledge can guide the OT practitioner in seeking information that can contribute to implementing effective therapeutic approaches. The theories can be grouped into two models of motor control: (1) the traditional *reflex–hierarchical models*, and (2) the more recent *systems models*.

Reflex–Hierarchical Models

Reflex–hierarchical models propose that purposeful movement is initiated only when the individual experiences a need to move.[19] When the desire to move is stimulated, the person searches his or her long-term memory for a pattern of movement that will accomplish the desired task. The movement patterns that the person has practiced the most are the most likely to be used again because they are embedded in memory. The person prepares to execute the movement, incorporating additional information from the environment to make the movements meet the demands of the task. For example, when a child is thirsty or hungry and sees food or drink, the child will become motivated to reach for or move to the desired food or drink. Long-term memory is searched for a pattern of movement that will enable the child to achieve the desired goal, that is, to reach the food or drink. Because all previous efforts to reach a bottle were stored in a generalized movement program, the child has a general history of the motor skills necessary for proper sequence, timing, and force of motor actions. Environmental factors, such as the sizes and weights of the objects, are also considerations used to determine the appropriate movement patterns. Sensory feedback determines whether the child's movement efforts have been successful (i.e., have met the task demands). The agonist muscles help lift the food or drink to the mouth, while the antagonist muscles are programmed to relax, allowing the movement of the agonist muscle to occur. Coactivation occurs when both the agonist and antagonist muscle groups work together to stabilize the container of the food or drink at the mouth in order to actually eat or drink. With continual repetition, these movement patterns can develop into motor skills. Reflex–hierarchical models support the idea that motor learning optimally occurs when a person engages in repeating the same task during frequent, regular practice; breaking down a task during frequent, regular practice into small parts is the most effective way to learn the entire task.

According to reflex models, many children with CP use tonic reflexes controlled by the lower levels of the CNS for managing most of their movements. These movement patterns are "hard wired" into the human nervous system and do not depend on the application of learned patterns for performing tasks. According to this model, children with CP lack the ability to independently learn to control movement from higher-level brain centers. Their abnormal postural mechanisms and disordered muscle tone cause them to repeatedly use and store in memory those movement patterns that are governed predominantly by the early tonic reflex patterns; these patterns inhibit the functional use of agonist and antagonist muscles during daily tasks (reciprocal innervations and coactivation). The reflex–hierarchical model has been challenged by motor theorists on several issues, including the impact of the environment on learning new motor patterns and the ability of the brain to actually store all the motor programs necessary to perform the infinite number of tasks an individual completes in his or her lifetime.

CLINICAL *Pearl*

The movement patterns of children with cerebral palsy may be influenced by primitive reflex activity, including the asymmetric tonic neck reflex, symmetric tonic neck reflex, and the tonic labyrinthine reflex affecting the acquisition of normal developmental milestones such as the ability to roll, sit unsupported, stand, and walk (Figure 16-2).

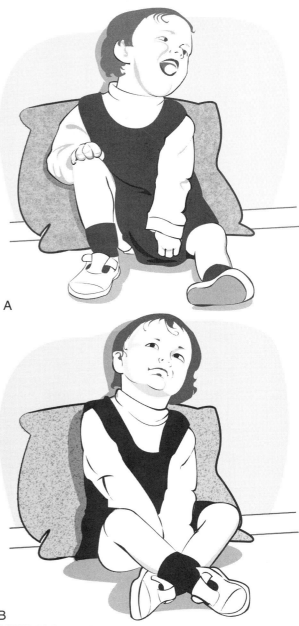

FIGURE 16-2 A, Child's head is turned to side stimulating the ATNR response (flexion on skull side and extension on the other side). **B,** Child is repositioned to help bring hands to midline and decrease the effects of the ATNR.

Dynamic System Models

The dynamic systems approach to understanding motor behavior proposes that postural control is greatly influenced by an individual's many volitional and functional daily tasks and activities.[19] Systems theorists recognize that it is impossible to understand motor control issues without understanding the external and internal forces that affect movement against the forces of gravity. Systems models purport that posture and movement must be flexible and adaptable so that a person can perform a wide range of daily activities, whereas reflex–hierarchical models state that the control of posture and movement is the outcome or product of a process. Dynamic systems models postulate that posture is anticipatory to the initiation of movement. Postural adjustments actually precede movements; they prepare the body to counterbalance the weight shifts that are caused by the movement activity. In this way, less balance disturbance occurs. Dynamic systems theorists also suggest that control of movement occurs due to the interactions of many body systems working cooperatively to achieve a desired movement goal. This concept is called the *distributed model of motor control*. Consider this example of a child trying to catch two balls, one of which is a small tennis ball and the other a large, heavy medicine ball. Before catching the balls, the child has used his or her vision to inspect them, used visual perception to make decisions about their sizes and weights, assumed an appropriate postural stance, and positioned the arms forward away from the body to be ready to catch. This anticipatory process is called *feedforward*.

According to the systems approach, feedforward actions require that posture be highly variable and subject to being affected by all the factors motivating the person to choose to catch the balls. No one right way to execute movement exists; rather, movement is strongly influenced by many variables. According to this approach, in contrast to reflex–hierarchical models, motor development follows a step-like progression, starting with primitive reflexes and progressing to voluntary movement control through the higher brain centers. The research of systems theorists has shown that motor activity is most often initiated by the interaction of sensory, perceptual, environmental, and other factors leading to task-focused, goal-directed movement.

One other concept from systems model research has important therapeutic implications for the treatment of children with CP or other neurologic disorders. Postural control and movement are at their greatest levels of efficiency, flexibility, and adaptability after randomized practice and repetition. Infants attempt to roll, crawl, stand, and walk over several hundred attempts with varied success and failure. Each attempt provides necessary feedback that will feedforward to more skilled motor responses and the eventual mastery of the motor skill.

For example, children in elementary school have many opportunities to practice learning to print their names so that the letters are neatly aligned and are of small, equal sizes. Although children practice printing during class, they are also practicing any time they spontaneously write their names during typical childhood activities and games. Over time, this repeated motor pattern develops into a skill; children can adapt the postures and movements used in the activity to fit several different tasks. They can write their names at the top of school papers while seated at their desks or at the bottom of pictures they are drawing while stretched out on the floor. By repeating this task in many different contexts, children gain the skill of motor problem solving. Systems models suggest that children with CP need to be challenged with meaningful activities that encourage repetition of motor actions that will develop motor strategies in a variety of play environments.

CLASSIFICATION AND DISTRIBUTION

CP can be defined by the location of the lesion in the CNS and by distribution of abnormal muscle tone in the trunk and extremities. Involvement of one extremity is commonly referred to as *monoplegia*, upper and lower extremities on one side of the body as **hemiplegia**, both lower extremities as **diplegia** or *paraplegia*, all limbs as **quadriplegia**, and all limbs and head/neck as *tetraplegia*. Cerebral palsy is also classified according to four main types of movement disorders: (1) spastic, (2) dyskinetic, (3) ataxic, and (4) mixed (Table 16-1).

Children with spastic CP demonstrate hypertonia and muscle spasticity. **Spasticity** is defined as a velocity-dependent resistance to stretch.[15] Resistance to range of motion will either increase with speed of force or will increase with quick movement. The effects of spasticity are often associated with *clonus*, an extensor plantar response, and persistent primitive reflexes. As a child with spastic CP attempts to move, excessive muscle tone builds up and is then rapidly released, triggering a hyperactive stretch reflex in the muscle. It may show up at the beginning, middle, or end of a movement range, but the result is poor control of voluntary movement and little ability to regulate the force of movement. Distribution of spasticity in spastic CP can be monoplegia, diplegia, hemiplegia, quadriplegia, or tetraplegia.

The second main type of CP is the **dyskinetic** type. Dyskinesias include athetoid, choreoathetoid, and dystonic CP. Distribution of tone is typically quadriplegia for all three types. **Dyskinesias** are abnormal movements—most obvious when a child initiates a movement in one extremity—that lead to atypical and unintentional movement of other muscle groups of the body. The child exhibits slow, writhing, involuntary motor movements

TABLE 16-1

Classification of Cerebral Palsy

TYPE OF MOVEMENT DISORDER	AREA OF BODY INVOLVED	PREVALENCE
Spastic	Diplegic: legs > arms	32%
	Quadriplegic: all four extremities	24%
	Hemiplegic: one-sided involvement, arm > leg	29%
	Double hemiplegic: both sides; one greater than other, arms > legs	24%
Dyskinetic	Choreoathetoid	14%
	Dystonic Athetoid	
Ataxic		<1%
Mixed		Percentages included above

in combination with abrupt, irregular, and jerky movements. Children with pure **athetosis** demonstrate a fluctuation of muscle tone from low to normal with little or no spasticity and poor coactivation of muscle flexors and extensors. Children with choreoathetosis have constant fluctuations from low to high, with jerky involuntary movement that may be seen more distally than proximally. Dystonic movements are sustained twisted postures that are absent at rest and triggered by movement (action). The movements follow a similar pattern, and these repetitive postures support the diagnosis of dystonia (unlike choreoathetosis, in which movement fluctuations are random).

The third type of cerebral palsy, **ataxia**, has less effect on muscle tone, but greatly impacts balance and coordination. Children who have ataxia may show shifts in muscle tone, but to a lesser degree than those with dyskinesias. Distribution of related muscle control issues is typically quadriplegic. Children with ataxic CP are more successful in directing voluntary movements but appear clumsy and may have tremors involuntarily and at rest. They have considerable difficulty with balance, coordination, and maintenance of stable alignment of the head, trunk, shoulders, and pelvis. These children may have poorly developed equilibrium responses and lack proximal stability in the trunk to assist with the control of hand and leg movements.

Children with CP who often show combinations of high and low muscle tone problems are considered to have the mixed type. Those who have spastic CP move their extremities with abrupt hypertonic motions but may also exhibit marked **hypotonicity** in their trunk muscles. The distribution for mixed-type CP is typically quadriplegic.

Knowledge of the degree of muscle tone abnormality and the child's cognitive, sensory, and perceptual status can help the OT practitioner establish realistic and practical therapeutic goals and interventions. The child with mild motor involvement and normal cognition has greater potential to succeed at gaining new motor skills, whereas the child with severe motor involvement and normal cognition may benefit more from assistive technologies that compensate for the absence of motor skills.

CLINICAL *Pearl*

Children with spastic type cerebral palsy may have contractures in one or more joints requiring use of orthoses to help elongate tight muscles and to correct misalignments in thumb web space, wrist, and fingers.

CLINICAL *Pearl*

Children with dyskinetic cerebral palsy often have average to above-average intelligence. Often, when these children attempt to use their arms and legs for play, self-care, or school tasks, the movements are very uncoordinated, which leads to frustration from repeated failed attempts at tasks. Occupational therapy may be successful if it focuses on a specific task (e.g., drinking from a cup) and the movements needed to complete those tasks are properly analyzed. Children should practice all the motor patterns of a task in simulated, fun activities during therapy while also practicing the actual functional activity.

CLINICAL *Pearl*

Children who have ataxic cerebral palsy demonstrate fixing of joints while attempting to reach or move due to poor balance responses. These children may also show some apprehension when trying dynamic activities in which their balance is challenged, such as reaching toward their feet to put on socks and shoes while sitting unsupported on a bench on in a low-back chair.

FUNCTIONAL IMPLICATIONS AND ASSOCIATED PROBLEMS

CASE *Study*

Tammy is a 17-year-old diagnosed with spastic quadriplegic cerebral palsy. She was recently admitted to a rehabilitation hospital to receive intensive OT and physical therapy (PT) services. She has a history of multiple orthopedic surgeries, including spinal fusion for scoliosis and bilateral tendon lengthening for wrist flexion contractures. She has a percutaneous endoscopic gastrostomy (PEG) tube in place for ingesting liquids, as otherwise she tends to aspirate thin liquids; Tammy also has significant dysarthria. She primarily uses a power wheelchair for mobility in the community. As she has gotten older, her muscle tone has affected the position of her joints and the length of her muscles. Contractures in her hips make it hard for her to stand when completing stand-pivot transfers to and from her wheelchair. Tammy also reports having trouble managing the pain in her hips. Her balance has decreased so much that she is very scared of falling and hurting herself or her grandmother, who is her primary caregiver. Her grandmother reports having difficulty with bathing Tammy because of Tammy's muscle tightness and size. Tammy's muscle tone and contractures have also caused more difficulties with toileting. Due to her hip tightness, it is hard for her to wipe herself and to pull up her pants while standing holding on to the toilet rail; she had been able to do this with just supervision when she was younger. Tammy will be working with the case manager and with her OTA to find resources in the community, such as independent living centers and home health aides, to help Tammy's grandmother with her care.

Muscle and Bone

CP can cause a host of associated changes in body structures and functions, which influence each person's functional potential. While CP is a nonprogressive condition in terms of changes in the CNS lesion, the resulting motor disorder may cause secondary impairments in the musculoskeletal system over time. Weakness and abnormal muscle tone and movement patterns can contribute to the development of muscle tissue contractures, bone deformities, and joint dislocations or misalignment. Some joint dislocations or misalignment may require surgical intervention to reposition the joint to a more functional position. As the child grows older, the potential for arthritis in misaligned joints increases, and this pain can additionally impact the person's ability to function. All of these changes further limit functional movement and can decrease the person's ability to complete activities of daily living (ADLs).

Other impairments associated with decreased functional mobility include risk of skin breakdown and decreased bone density. Individuals who are unable to assume more than a few positions or independently shift body weight risk skin breakdown. This is because body weight in these individuals is often concentrated over a few points for prolonged periods. Similarly, decreased time spent standing or ambulating can impact the strength of the individual's bones. Children diagnosed with CP are noted to have decreased bone mineral density and are vulnerable to pathologic fractures.[14]

CLINICAL *Pearl*

Positioning and orthotic programs aim to minimize the impact of muscle tone on joint position.

CLINICAL *Pearl*

The child who often keeps his or her hand in a tight fist may have hygiene issues associated with range of motion limitations.

Cognition, Hearing, and Language

Due to abnormal muscle tone and musculoskeletal changes associated with CP, children diagnosed with CP may have various problems with speech and language. These potential problems include decreased speech production, poor articulation, and decreased speech intelligibility. *Dysarthria* is the term used to describe a disorder of speech production that is secondary to decreased muscle coordination, paralysis, or weakness. In addition to speech production disorders, children who have CP may have changes in the quality of their voice due to decreased strength or control of respiratory and postural muscles. Because CP has the potential to affect areas of the brain outside of the motor system, it can cause decreased expressive and receptive language skills. This means that children with CP have difficulty processing language-based information or producing responses. Hearing loss, which can also occur in this population, is another factor that inhibits normal speech.[18]

All of these potential impairments can have a significant impact on participation in age-appropriate activities. The child's cognitive and linguistic skill level can play a significant role in his or her ability to benefit from therapeutic and educational interventions, and it can have a great effect on the types of interventions or adaptive equipment an OT practitioner chooses for the child.

Sensory Problems

Individuals who have CP experience sensory problems, including visual impairments such as blindness, uncoordinated eye movements, and eye muscle weakness in as many as 50% of children who have CP and auditory reception and processing deficits in 25%.[12] Hearing loss with both conductive hearing loss and sensorineural hearing impairments may occur if the child has been affected by a congenital CNS infection. Both vision and hearing should be tested regularly in children with CP.

Additional sensory problems include deficits in the processing of tactile and proprioceptive information. Some children have difficulty with tactile discrimination as well as fingertip force regulation during object manipulation. Children with CP may also demonstrate tactile hypersensitivities (i.e., overreacting to touch, textures, and changes in head position), causing some of them to become visibly upset when handled or moved by others. Children with multiple sensory processing problems have more difficulty understanding their environments. Some tactile sensation problems are also linked to abnormal oral movement patterns. The disorganized muscular movements that children with CP experience in their arms, legs, and trunk, may also be seen in oral–facial musculature affecting feeding experiences. Many of these children dislike certain food textures and may have problems coordinating their chewing, sucking, and swallowing movements. Those with severe problems in this area may be surgically fitted with a PEG tube for feeding. OT practitioners must consider the child's sensory limitations and strengths while setting intervention goals and determine individually which sensory experiences are likely to improve occupational performance abilities.

Hand Skills and Upper Extremity Function

Children with CP demonstrate problems with upper limb function due to abnormal muscle tone and decreased ability to maintain a stable posture when attempting functional tasks (Figure 16-3).[13] Efficient use of arms and hands depends on the proximal control and dynamic stability of the trunk and shoulder girdle. Children with CP demonstrate weakness in the shoulder girdle; may have contractures in their elbow, forearm, wrist, fingers, and thumb due to **hypertonicity**; or may move the arm and hand in synergistic patterns, as they lack the ability to isolate single joint movements. Postural instability can affect upper extremity movement also, as these children may need to use their upper extremities to support upright postures against gravity. When the upper extremities are fixed and used to help stabilize and compensate for trunk weakness, the arms and hands cannot be used for functional tasks (e.g., playing with toys at the midline of the body while challenged to sit unsupported).

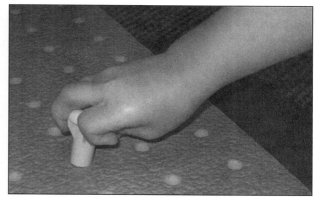

FIGURE 16-3 Note how this child with cerebral palsy uses his hand to grasp a peg. Due to thumb tightness and decreased thumb abduction and closed web space, the child is using an atypical grasp between his thumb and middle finger with wrist ulnar deviation.

Vision

A wide spectrum of visual issues affect children who have CP. Children who have more severe CP typically have greater visual impairment.[10] Regardless of the functional level of the child, issues related to vision should always be taken into consideration during performance of fine motor tasks, play, and ADLs. Vision plays an important role in the timing of grasp and release, manipulating objects, orienting materials, making eye contact, and finding needed items. Children with visual impairments may use postural adaptations, such as a head tilt or changes to the angle of gaze to compensate for visual deficits. These deficits may be oculomotor in nature, that is, the muscles of the eye do not move smoothly and synchronously or may move involuntarily. The term *strabismus* describes the misalignment of eyes due to muscle imbalance. Functionally, strabismus may cause difficulty attending to visual tasks. The child may have decreased convergence or divergence, decreased depth perception, or double vision. Other terms describing misalignment of the eyes include *exotropia* (one eye drifts temporally), *esotropia* (one eye drifts nasally), *hypertropia* (one eye drifts upward), and *hypotropia* (one eye drifts downward). The term *nystagmus* describes the constant movement of eyes in a repetitive and uncontrolled way. Functional issues associated with nystagmus include reduced acuity, difficulty fixing on a target to maintain balance, reduced target accuracy when reaching or grasping, compensatory head movements, or posturing to compensate for visual deficit. In addition to oculomotor impairments, the child may have deficits in the way the brain processes visual information. Without proper processing, the child may not understand the spatial relationships between objects, may miss part of the visual field, or not identify a partially hidden item, for example, his or her coat inside a closet.

CLINICAL *Pearl*

Children with cerebral palsy may compensate for their vision problems in a variety of ways. Turning the head to the side to use peripheral vision or fixing the body posture in a way that seems awkward to observers are examples of the adaptations used by these children to utilize the visual fields and abilities they have.

CLINICAL *Pearl*

Children with cerebral palsy may compensate for their visual impairments in a variety of ways. Placement of materials in the area of their strongest visual field can help minimize the postural compensations that they use to visually interact with their environments.

Physical and Behavioral Manifestations

Problems such as seizures and other medical conditions not directly related to the movement disorder may be experienced by children with CP. Abnormal posture and weak muscle activity may compromise cardiac and respiratory functions and prevent these systems from working efficiently. The resulting low endurance and fatigue can influence the child's capacity for activity. The OT practitioner monitors each child's physical endurance and plans therapeutic goals to increase strength and endurance.

Behavioral problems and social delays are not unusual in children with CP. They may become accustomed to receiving assistance from others, and problems such as "learned helplessness" may prevent them from attempting the developmental challenges needed for continued growth and mastery of skills. The inability to manage social and peer interactions can lead to social isolation and immaturity and a repertoire of undesirable social behaviors. The OT practitioner can often assist families and work collaboratively with the child's educational team, which may include teachers, consultants, and administrators, to suggest strategies to enhance the child's social development.

CASE *Study*

Antoine is an 8-year-old boy with a history of a seizure disorder and athetoid cerebral palsy. He uses a power wheelchair for mobility and an augmentative communication device. He attends elementary school, where he is placed in an age-appropriate classroom with accommodations and related services, including physical therapy,

occupational therapy, speech therapy, and assistive technology. Antoine's continuous body movements make it difficult for him to complete fine motor tasks, including accessing his communication device to complete class work. He tends to get frustrated when he knows the answer to a question but is not able to communicate it to his teacher and classmates. His therapy team discovers that a head stick helps Antoine improve his access to his communication device. The OTA has also worked with his art teacher to fasten a holder for tools such as a paintbrush to his head stick. Now Antoine is able to creatively express himself through a variety of mediums, including paint and pastels, which do not require a lot of pressure when drawing. Antoine also seems to have improved success in using the device when he can hold on to the armrest of his wheelchair, so his OTA experiments with a bar mounted on Antoine's tray so that he can push against it to improve his trunk stability.

ROLES OF THE OCCUPATIONAL THERAPIST AND THE OCCUPATIONAL THERAPY ASSISTANT

The occupational therapist and the OTA collaborate to provide services to children who have CP. The individual needs of the child and the family and the child's chronologic age determine each step in the assessment and intervention processes. During the child's infancy and early childhood, OT practitioners focus on family care and management issues such as feeding and bathing, mobility around the home, and family participation. During the child's early school years, the occupational therapist and the OTA assist the child with classroom participation, self-care skills, peer socialization, leisure and vocational readiness, and educational and community mobility. In the case of the adolescent with CP, OT services may focus on helping with engagement in work or other productive activities, development of independent living skills, sexual identification and sexual expression, and mobility in the community at large.

Assessment

The occupational therapist and the OTA collaboratively assess each individual child's needs. Together they evaluate areas of performance, client factors, activity demands, and contexts. The occupational therapist may use one or several standardized tests requiring specialized administration and interpretation skills and can provide the team with specific information about reflex development, sensorimotor functioning, motor skills, and developmental skill levels. The experienced, trained OTA may assist in the administration of some tests. Observation is a crucial part of the assessment process because many children who have CP cannot easily follow the directions of standardized tests because of their impaired motor skills. Both the occupational therapist and the OTA can observe the child's functional abilities at home, in school, and during leisure activities. Observation of the child's occupational performance provides the OT practitioner with data on factors influencing the child's muscle tone, reflex activity, gross and fine motor skills, sensory systems, cognition, perception, and psychosocial development. The OTA may provide information to plan the most effective OT intervention. Early identification of atypical postures can minimize the use of compensatory and dysfunctional movements that could lead to serious deformities and undesirable behaviors. More mature and typical movement patterns can be facilitated by both the OTA and the occupational therapist in order to help the child make progress in meeting typical developmental milestones.

Assessment data create a "picture" of the child's functioning and indicate his or her strengths and weaknesses. The OT practitioner uses this information (along with parental input) to formulate goals to match the child's needs and developmental abilities or potential. Examples include increasing the child's ability to participate in a classroom writing activity and teaching family members ways to reduce the hypertonicity in the child so that they can bathe and feed him or her. Goals for the adolescent might address accessing public transportation or learning ways to perform homemaking skills. Thorough OT assessment data are essential when working as part of a service delivery team. Classroom teachers may rely on the OT practitioner's expertise for help with the establishment and implementation of educational goals. Vocational skills trainers need to know the student's physical performance abilities and attitudes toward new tasks. Families may use OT input to select recreational activities for their children.

The Model of Human Occupation (MOHO) Clearinghouse provides a variety of assessments that examine the child's occupational performance. Interviews such as the Pediatric Volitional Questionnaire provide information on the child's motivation. The Child Occupational Self-Assessment (COSA) and Short-Children's Occupational Profile Evaluation (SCOPE) provide an overview of the child's volition, roles, habits, and performance within various contexts. The School Setting Interview (SSI) and the School Function Assessment (SFA) provide information on how the child is functioning at school. These assessments and others explore how the child performs his or her occupations. Motor-based assessments include the Alberta Infant Motor Scale (AIMS) and the Gross Motor Function Classification Scale (GMFCS) (Table 16-2). The AIMS is an observational assessment scale that measures the motor skills of

TABLE 16-2

Gross Motor Function Classification System (GMFCS)

LEVEL	DESCRIPTION OF FUNCTIONAL ABILITIES
I	Walks without limitations. Performs gross motor skills such as running and jumping, but speed, balance, and coordination may be impaired.
II	Walks with limitations. Includes walking on uneven surfaces, inclines, and stairs, for long distances, or in crowds or confined spaces.
III	Walks using a hand-held mobility device. Walks on even surfaces, indoors, and outdoors with an assistive device; may use manual wheelchair for long distances.
IV	Self-mobility with limitations. May use powered mobility or require assistance from a caregiver; may walk short distances with a mobility device but relies primarily on wheeled mobility.
V	Transported in a manual wheelchair. Has no means of independent mobility and relies on caregiver for all transportation needs.

infants from birth through the time when they start walking. Weight bearing, posture, and antigravity movements are evaluated. This assessment tool is often used in early intervention settings.[17]

Interventions

Individuals who have CP and receive OT services can experience a sense of empowerment and control when they successfully perform meaningful occupations, within the self-care, work, and leisure domains. OT practitioners develop and implement interventions to promote functional performance within each individual's capacity. Through training and consultation, they also assist caregivers and educators in the provision of interventions that facilitate and support the child's occupational performance. Intervention strategies include positioning and handling. (Refer to Chapter 17 for more information on positioning and handling techniques.) The OT practitioner determines the variety of postures the child can assume, maintain, and achieve independently or with physical assistance. Optimal positions are determined for ADLs. Upright sitting positions are needed for most classroom activities, while a relaxed, partially reclined position may be optimal for assisted bathing. Practitioners can also select and recommend specific types of positioning equipment, such as chairs, supine or prone standers, and sidelyers, that support the child during functional activities with the best possible postural alignment, control, and stability. Handling techniques such as slow rocking, slow stroking, imposed rotational movement patterns, and bouncing are used to enhance the child's muscle tone, activity level, and ability for independent movement (see Chapter 17). Techniques such as weight bearing and weight shifting can promote postural alignment and independent movement. A stiff, hypertonic child fixed in a strong extensor posture can be easily positioned in a wheelchair after the OT practitioner has slowly and alternately rotated the shoulders in a forward and backward motion. Handling relaxes the child's muscle tone throughout the body and is used within a neurodevelopmental treatment (NDT) approach. Each joint can move more easily, and the child can then be placed in the wheelchair with good postural alignment and comfort. Positioning and handling methods are especially important for the child with CP who is unable to move independently. These methods also help the child work toward the achievement of performance-area goals such as increased independence in dressing, feeding, playing, and doing schoolwork. An OT practitioner can learn these treatments in special training programs or under the direction of a skilled occupational therapist. The OTA can implement positioning recommendations, teach them to caregivers, and use handling methods to improve the child's functional performance by following the instructions of the occupational therapist.

Persons with CP can achieve greater independence in daily living tasks with the help of assistive and adaptive devices. The OT practitioner may recommend adapted utensils for the child with limited grasp abilities; suggest a large, weighted pen to aid a student who has tremors; or attach a large zipper pull on a coat for a self-dressing activity. The OTA consults with the occupational therapist to determine the safest and most appropriate devices to match each child's abilities. The task is particularly important in the selection of feeding equipment that can ensure safe swallowing. The OTA should become familiar with a number of assistive device vendors so that equipment recommendations can be offered for all appropriate occupational performance areas and budget considerations. With a little creative thinking, an OTA can often fabricate assistive devices from inexpensive materials. PVC plumbing pipe from a hardware store can be assembled to make an inverted U-shaped frame with suspended toys that can be placed in front of the child. This could be one way to help children with limited reaching and grasping abilities engage in a meaningful play activity.

The OTA assists clients who have CP in a variety of settings. Intervention programs can occur in the family home, a school setting, or a hospital. In each setting, the OTA is part of an interdisciplinary treatment team whose goal is to maximize the child's health, functional capacities, and quality of life. As an OT specialist, the OTA combines knowledge and skill to help each child accomplish purposeful and meaningful daily living tasks within the home, school, and community settings.

Medical-Based Interventions

A number of medical interventions exist to treat the effects of CP and are often used in conjunction with rehabilitation therapies. Common pharmacologic treatments for spasticity include oral baclofen and injectable botulinum neurotoxin (botox). Baclofen is an antispasticity medication that may be administered orally or injected into a pump that delivers the medication directly into the cerebrospinal fluid. It is a systemic medication and can reduce muscle tone throughout the person's body. Botox is a more specific approach, with injections delivered directly to a spastic muscle or muscles with the goal of reducing muscle tone. The effects of botox are short lived, lasting around 3 to 6 months. An injection is often paired with aggressive therapy to increase range of motion (ROM) and splinting to maintain gains in mobility and function. One surgical approach to spasticity management is selective dorsal rhizotomy (SDR), which involves cutting of selective sensory nerves that come from the lower limbs to the spinal cord.

Types of orthopedic surgery to address contractures and muscle imbalances include tendon transfer, muscle release, and osteotomy. Tendon transfers move the insertions of muscles to change the action that the muscle produces. For example, the child with weak or paralyzed hand musculature may have a wrist muscle moved to the hand to assist with grasp. Other types of soft tissue surgery include muscle releases or lengthenings. These procedures lengthen or release tight muscle tissue to allow increased movement of a joint. Often done in conjunction with soft tissue surgery, osteotomies are procedures in which the bone is cut to lengthen it, shorten it, or improve its alignment. All of these surgeries involve a period of immobilization initially, but early movement and physical therapy are important in maximizing functional gains from these interventions.

CLINICAL *Pearl*

To maximize the effect of medications for muscle tone management, a regime of stretching, splinting, and functional strengthening exercises may be recommended by the physiatrist.

Complementary and Alternative Medicine

The term *complementary and alternative medicine* (CAM) refers to those interventions that are not presently considered to be part of conventional medicine (Table 16-3).[16] CAM use overall in the population has grown in recent years, and it is becoming more common for parents of children with CP to seek out alternative therapies. According to the 2007 National Health Interview Survey, which gathered information on CAM use among more than 9,000 children aged 17 and under, nearly 12% of the children had used some form of CAM during the past 12 months. Children with multiple health disorders, including CP, were found to be some of the most frequent users of CAM interventions.

Constraint-Induced Movement Therapy

Constraint-induced movement therapy (CIMT) is an emerging intervention approach to address functional implications and learned nonuse or developmental disregard of the impaired upper extremity (UE) in children with hemiplegia. *Learned nonuse* and *developmental disregard* are terms used to describe how children with hemiplegic CP do not use their affected limbs because of negatively reinforced experiences despite the function that may be available.[6,22] CIMT developed out of basic experimental psychology research by Edward Taub and his colleagues, on sensory contributions to motor learning in nonhuman primates.[22] CIMT was then used in the rehabilitation of adult patients who had experienced a stroke and later was tested with children.[6]

Current implementation methods of CIMT vary but all programs have three essential features: (1) some method of constraint in the use of the unimpaired upper extremity; (2) intensive, repetitive practice of motor activities, for up to 6 hours per day, for 2 to 4 weeks; and (3) shaping of more complex, functional motor acts by breaking the desired task into its component movements and rewarding successive approximations to the target task. A variety of restraining devices such as mitts, casts, splints, and slings are used in research and clinical protocols.[4-7,11] Current literature describes home-based, clinic-based, and camp-based models of implementation.[2] Unlike occupational therapists in adult settings, pediatric occupational therapists using this approach embed repetitive task practice in play activities. Examples of play activities incorporated into a pediatric CIMT program are included in the following case study. Clearly, significant questions remain regarding optimal parameters of the protocol, including age, level of function, and cognition.

CASE *Study*

Brandon is a 4-year-old boy with hemiplegic CP. He has been receiving outpatient OT services once a week. Brandon is working on his upper extremity strength, by pulling up his pants with both hands, performing weight-bearing activities, and maintaining grasp with his affected right hand. Brandon is participating in a CIMT

TABLE 16-3

Complementary and Alternative Medicine (CAM) Programs

CAM PRACTICE	INTERVENTION DESCRIPTION
Hippotherapy	Treatment strategy that uses the help of a horse, for example, using a horse a treatment modality to help a child develop postural stability
Acupuncture/ acupressure	Stimulation of specific points on the body with pressure or needles
Massage therapy	Soft tissue mobilization
Craniosacral therapy	Mobilization of cranium/sacral bone
Myofascial release	Mobilization of interconnected fascial system
Tai Chi	Slow, graceful movement with emphasis on mind–body connection
Yoga	Body positioning, breathing, and meditation
Pilates	Breathing; core control; organization of the head, neck, and shoulders; spine articulation; alignment and posture; and movement integration
Biofeedback	Electronically utilizing information from the body to teach an individual to recognize what is going on inside of his or her own body
Dietary supplements	Substances taken by mouth to supplement the diet, including vitamins, minerals, herbs or other botanicals, amino acids, and certain other substances

program at an outpatient clinic. Brandon attends the program for 3 hours a day and wears a cast on his unaffected, stronger arm. Activities that are motivating, such as carrying a bucket loaded with toy cars and picking up the toy cars and putting them on a race track, are done at a high level of repetition. Imaginary play activities, such as pushing his affected arm through dress-up clothes, help generalize these new skills to play and ADL tasks.

Modalities

Various modalities may be used within OT sessions to improve muscle length and strength and reduce spasticity in children with CP. These treatment modalities include hot/cold therapy and electrical stimulation. Heat maybe used in conjunction with range of motion programs to improve muscle length and reduce pain, whereas cryotherapy (ice, cold packs) may be used in cases of inflammation associated with arthritis to improve patient comfort. Another modality commonly used with children with motor impairments is electrical stimulation (Figure 16-4). It may be used for a variety of reasons, including strengthening antagonist muscles, muscle re-education, pain reduction, improving coordination, increasing ROM, and reduction of spasticity.[1,15] Electrical stimulation is most effective when paired with a functional activity, such as grasping finger foods and bringing them to the mouth when stimulating the biceps or releasing toys into a container while stimulating wrist extensors.

Robotics

The area of robotics in OT takes advantage of new technology to enhance motor and cognitive performance in children with CP. Robotic therapy provides a means for repetitive practice of target movements, such as reaching in space.[8] These devices typically employ robotic arms, joysticks, or other controllers to measure the patient's performance of the targeted movement. Early studies demonstrate that patients using robotic devices in therapy sessions are motivated and make positive gains.[8,9]

Kinesio Tape

Kinesio taping (described also in Chapter 27) was developed by a Japanese chiropractor Dr. Kenzo Kase in 1973. Kinesio taping gained wide exposure when used by Japanese athletes at the Seoul Olympics in 1988. Originally used by athletes, it is now widely used in hospitals and clinics to treat adults and children with neuromuscular conditions. The kinesio tape is applied directly to the skin and works by increasing stimulation to cutaneous mechanoreceptors that facilitate muscle contraction or inhibition. This occurs due to

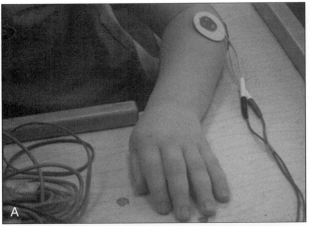

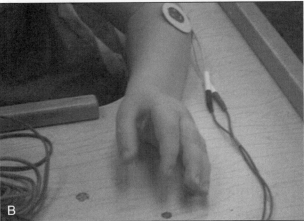

FIGURE 16-4 These pictures show electrical stimulation applied to the supinators of a child's affected upper extremity. **A,** The child's position at rest. **B,** The child's hand supinates in reaction to the electrical stimulation.

the stretch properties of the kinesio tape; this is why the amount of stretch can be important for specific muscle tapings. The degree of stimulation is determined by the degree of stretch and inward pressure. When using kinesio taping on children with CP, it is best to select a specific muscle group for rehabilitation and then apply the tape repeatedly to the same muscle group. For example, in the case of a child with CP who demonstrates tightness in wrist flexors and weakness in wrist extensors, the kinesio tape can be applied to facilitate a stronger contraction of the wrist extensors as well as to inhibit the contraction of the overactive wrist flexors. The elastic properties of the tape can also be used to reposition joints to a more appropriate alignment. Due to potential skin sensitivities in these children, it is always important to apply a small "test" strip to the child's skin to see if there is any negative reaction to the properties of the tape before fully taping an extremity.

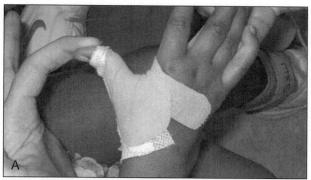

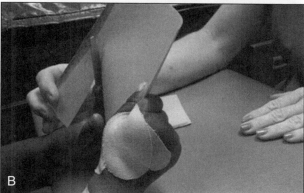

FIGURE 16-5   A, Kinesio tape applied to the child's thumb web space opens up the hand so the child can use the hand for activities. **B,** The child can now successfully hold a piece of paper while using scissors in the opposing hand.

Orthotics and Casting

Static orthoses and casts are used to help children with CP maintain a joint in one position for a variety of different goals (see Chapter 27; Figures 16-6 and 16-7). The overall objective of orthoses or casting is to improve hand function, prevent further joint contracture, improve hygiene, address pain in a specific joint, or to restrict arm and hand movement if the child is using the hands for unsafe behaviors. Serial static orthoses and casts are designed to lengthen tissues and correct deformities through application of gentle forces sustained for extended periods with the goal of reducing tightness or spasticity in a selected muscle group (e.g. elbow flexors).[13] A reduction of tightness in the muscles around a joint will allow for greater independent use of the extremity, reduce pain from contracted muscles, and improve ease of bathing and hygiene tasks provided by the caregiver. Casting and orthoses are most effective in applying low-load prolonged stretch to contracted muscle tissues. Orthoses are remolded and casts replaced at intervals, which allows the muscle tissue to respond to the lengthened position. The biomechanical effects of orthoses and casting relate to changes in the length of muscles and connective tissues, and this can reverse the effects that occur when a muscle is maintained in a shortened position. Research has shown that applying orthoses to lengthen tight contracted muscles in children with CP is most effective when applied continuously for periods greater than 6 hours.[23] Casting has additional biomechanical and neurophysiologic effects, although the exact neurophysiologic effects of casting on spasticity are not well defined at this time. It is theorized that inhibition of muscle contractions allowing lengthening of muscle tissues results from decreased cutaneous sensory input from muscle receptors during the period of immobilization. The effects of neutral warmth and circumferential contact also are believed to contribute to modification of spasticity.

Often orthoses are worn by children with CP to improve overall function. Orthoses are designed to meet specific objectives identified by the child or the parents (Box 16-4). In many instances, orthoses can compensate for functional deficits in hand grasping toys or pointing in order to get toys, holding eating utensils, holding writing implements, or accessing computing devices. Examples of this type of orthotic include using a splint to isolate a finger to point and touch a keyboard or augmentative communication device or fabrication of a joystick "goal post" on the toggle switch of a power chair to improve grasp and hand control. Lastly, orthoses are also fabricated by OT practitioners to prevent movement from the hand to the mouth in cases where the children may be engaging in self-injurious behaviors or attempting to pull out feeding tubes, intravenous lines, or tracheostomy tubing.

CASE *Study*

Missy is a 6-year-old girl. A prolonged period of anoxia during her birth resulted in spastic diplegia. Missy has moderate hypertonia throughout her lower extremities and mild muscle tone problems in her upper extremities. These problems cause difficulties with fine motor and in-hand manipulation tasks such as drawing, writing, and brushing teeth. Missy demonstrates good balance reactions from her middle trunk area upward but easily loses her balance

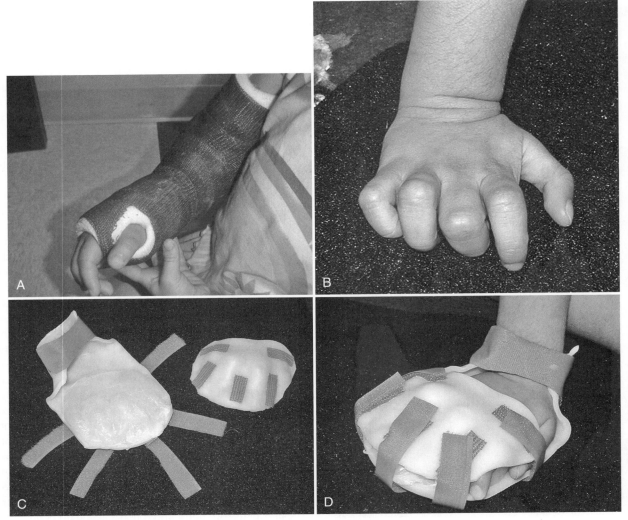

FIGURE 16-6 **A**, A full arm cast may help a child gain range of motion. **B**, A child's hand without an orthosis may not allow the child to weight bear completely. **C**, An orthosis can be applied to help the child keep the hand stable and open for activities. **D**, The orthosis stabilizes the child's joints so the child can engage in a variety of activities. (From Henderson A, Pehoski C: *Hand function in the child,* ed 2, St. Louis, 2006, Mosby.)

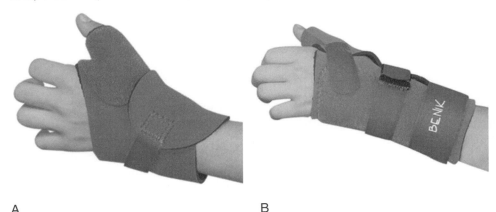

A   B

FIGURE 16-7 BENIK is a company that produces prefabricated neoprene orthoses and orthoses that are produced after proper sizing and measurement by an occupational therapist. These orthoses provide stability at the wrist as well as the thumb.

BOX 16-4

Potential Goals and Benefits of Orthoses

1. Improve overall function in play, self-care, mobility, and school related tasks
2. Improve position of a joint
   - Decrease joint stiffness and muscle contractures
   - Improve active and passive range of motion in a joint
3. Increase access to skin and allow for cleaning and hygiene
4. To protect or to help modify behavior
   - For example: Use of an elbow orthosis to keep the hands away from the face if the child is biting hands or attempting to pull on tracheostomy or feeding tubes

when seated on a chair without armrests. She frequently topples over when she tries to bend to retrieve something dropped to the floor. Missy is a bright, happy child with normal intelligence and good vision and hearing abilities. From ages 3 to 6 she attended a special preschool and kindergarten program, where she received OT and PT services. PT practitioners worked with Missy to develop functional mobility skills. She now ambulates independently with a wheeled walker, can lower and raise herself to and from the floor level using an environmental support, and can transfer on and off a preschool-size toilet. OT practitioners helped Missy increase her independence in dressing with the use of Velcro closures and zipper pulls, and they used therapeutic handling and strengthening techniques to improve her manipulation skills with drawing materials and pencils. Because Missy has been so successful in learning self-management skills, her parents and the special education team believe that she is ready to enroll in the regular Grade 1 class of her local elementary school.

OT consultation services are recommended to assist in Missy's successful school transition. Before she starts school, the OTA and the occupational therapist participate in a team meeting. Missy's parents, her new Grade 1 teacher, the school's physical education teacher, and the school principal also attend the meeting. The team members decide that the OT team will consult with the classroom teacher to address Missy's seating needs and make sure that she can participate in typical Grade 1 activities. The school district occupational therapist reviews the OT documentation from Missy's previous OT practitioners and then schedules a classroom visit for herself and the OTA, during the first week of school. During their visit, they note that the classroom desks are too high for Missy. She is not able to maintain a stable, upright posture

on a desk chair and loses her balance whenever she leans sideways. Missy also has difficulty keeping her papers firmly on the desk surface when writing and drawing. The occupational therapist and the OTA note two other problems: (1) Because of her lack of developed balance reactions in the lower body, Missy is unable to remove or put on her coat in the coatroom when she is with the other children of her class. (2) At snack time, Missy has difficulty opening her cardboard juice cartons. The teacher also tells the OTA that each student is expected to have a daily job, and she would like to get some assistance in selecting one for Missy.

The occupational therapist and the OTA review Missy's functional motor skills and muscle tone problems. They note that she sits in a regular chair with her hips rolled back, her knees and toes pointing inward, and her upper body bent forward because of the lack of postural control and stability in the pelvic area and lower extremities. The occupational therapist instructs the OTA to find a smaller chair with armrests for Missy and discusses ways to determine a good functional seating position.

The following week, the OTA and Missy's teacher locate a chair with armrests that provides Missy with good stability. Now her feet are flat on the floor, and her hips fit on the seat with a 90-degree bend. The OTA places a piece of Dycem, a nonskid rubbery material, on the seat to provide Missy with additional stability so that she can shift her weight and lean somewhat without significant loss of balance. A desk of a suitable height is found, and nonslip grips are placed under the feet of the desk so that Missy can reach a standing position easily by bracing against the desk. The OTA recommends using removable sticky putty to help Missy keep her papers in place and finds a small bench that can be positioned against the wall in the coatroom. Missy can easily manage her coat by sitting on the bench and leaning against the wall. The teacher has learned that Missy enjoys exploring the building but has fewer opportunities to do so than her classmates because she needs additional time to move around with her walker. The teacher believes that Missy would like the job of taking the daily attendance report to the school office but is not certain how she can accomplish it. The OTA suggests attaching an attractive bicycle basket of Missy's choice to her walker. The basket can also be handy for transporting other classroom materials. To solve Missy's snack time drink problem, the OTA chooses a small piece of brightly colored splinting material and fashions a ring with an inch-long pencil-like protrusion for Missy's middle finger. She can slide on the ring with the protrusion pointing down from her palm and then use the force of her open hand to punch a hole in the juice carton. The basket and ring enable Missy to be as independent as the other children at snack time.

The OTA remembers that the repeated practice of skills in a variety of situations and environments can increase a person's independent motor skills. He contacts Missy's mother, who agrees that Missy can use her ring to manage her drinks at home. After speaking with the OTA, the physical education teacher places a bench against a wall in the area where the children change into their gym shoes. Missy can now independently don and doff her gym shoes that have Velcro closures.

The OTA follows up with Missy's parents and teachers to ensure that she is meeting all the challenges. Later, he administers the Pediatric Volitional Questionnaire to ensure that the team has considered all of Missy's needs.

SUMMARY

The term *cerebral palsy* encompasses a number of postural control and movement disorders resulting from damage to the areas of the CNS that control movement and balance. Common problems associated with CP include limitations in movement options, delays in occupational skill development, muscle tone abnormalities that cause secondary problems such as contractures, and bone or joint deformities. CP can involve total or partial areas of the body, and many individuals with CP are also affected by a number of associated disorders, such as impaired vision, hearing, and communication; below-normal cognition; and seizures.

OTAs can play a vital role in helping children with CP increase their abilities to function independently and expand their repertoire of occupational performance roles. With an understanding of movement control and skill development, OTAs can apply their knowledge of positioning and handling methods to improve an individual's ability to interact with the environment. OTAs can recommend and instruct in the use of assistive devices and specialized equipment to enable children with CP to engage in purposeful activities that match their occupational roles and interests. With guidance from the occupational therapist during OT, OTAs can help the children by using techniques to develop postural control, righting and equilibrium reactions, and controlled movement against gravity. Individual therapy plans incorporate interventions that correspond to each child's unique developmental skills and occupational needs. OTAs offer service in many environmental contexts and find creative ways for each child to engage in meaningful activities at home, in the school, and in the community.

References

1. Bracciano AG: *Physical agent modalities: theory and application for the occupational therapist*, ed 2, Thorofare, NJ, Slack Incorporated, 2000.
2. Brady K, Garcia T: Constraint induced movement therapy: pediatric applications. *Develop Disabil Res Rev* 15:102–111, 2009.
3. Batshaw ML: *Children with disabilities*, ed 4, Baltimore, 1997, Paul H. Brookes Publishing.
4. Charles J, Gordon AM: A critical review of constraint-induced movement therapy and forced use in children with hemiplegia. *Neural Plasticity* 12:245–261, 2005.
5. Cope SM et al: Modified constraint-induced movement therapy for a 12-month-old child with hemiplegia: a case report. *Am J Occup Ther* 62:430–437, 2008.
6. Deluca SC et al: Intensive pediatric constraint-induced therapy for children with cerebral palsy: randomized, controlled, crossover trial. *J Child Neurol* 21:931–938, 2006.
7. Eliasson AC, Bonnier B, Krumlinde-Sundholm L: Clinical experience of constraint induced movement therapy in adolescents with hemiplegic cerebral palsy—a day camp model. *Dev Med Child Neurol* 45:357–360, 2003.
8. Fasoli SE et al: Upper limb robotic therapy for children with hemiplegia. *Am J Phys Med Rehabil* 87:929–936, 2008.
9. Frascarelli F et al: The impact of robotoic rehabilitation in children with acquired or congenital movement disorders. *Eur J Phys Rehabil Med* 45:135–141, 2009.
10. Ghasia F et al: Frequency and severity of visual sensory and motor deficits in children with cerebral palsy: Gross Motor Function Classification Scale. *Investigat Ophthamol Visual Sci* 49:572–580, 2008.
11. Glover JE et al: The effectiveness of constraint induced movement therapy in two young children with hemiplegia. *Pediatr Rehabil* 5:125–131, 2002.
12. Green L, Hurvitz E: Cerebral palsy. *Phys Med Rehabil Clin North Am* 18:859–882, 2007.
13. Henderson A, Pehoski C: *Hand function in the child*, ed 2, St. Louis, 2006, Mosby.
14. Leet AI et al: Fractures in children with cerebral palsy. *J Pediatr Orthop* 26:624–627, 2006.
15. Merrill DR: Review of electrical stimulation in cerebral palsy and recommendations for future directions. *Develop Med Child Neurol* 51(suppl 4):153–164, 2009.
16. National Institutes of Health National Center for Complementary and Alternative Medicine. (10/13/2009): *Backgrounder: CAM use and children*. Available at: http://nccam.nih.gov/health/children/#patterns. Accessed November 1, 2009.
17. Piper MC et al: Construction and validation of the Alberta Infant Motor Scale (AIMS). *Can J Public Health* 83(suppl 2):S46–S50, 1992.

18. Pirila S et al: Language and motor speech skills in children with cerebral palsy. *J Commun Disord* 40:116–128, 2007.
19. Shumway-Cook, Woollacott M: *Motor control theory and practical applications*, ed 2, Baltimore, 2001, Lippincott Williams & Wilkins.
20. Strauss D et al: Survival in cerebral palsy in the last 20 years: signs of improvement? *Develop Med Child Neurol* 49:86–92, 2007.
21. United Cerebral Palsy: *Cerebral palsy prevalence*. Available at: http://www.ucp.org/. Accessed October 23, 2009.
22. Taub E et al: Pediatric CI therapy for stroke-induced hemiparesis in young children. *Dev Neurorehabil* 10:3–18, 2007.
23. Wilton J: Casting, splinting, and physical and occupational therapy of hand deformity and dysfunction in cerebral palsy. *Hand Clin* 19:573–584, 2003.

Recommended Reading

Sutcliffe T et al: Cortical reorganization after modified constraint-induced movement therapy in pediatric hemiplegic cerebral palsy. *J Child Neurol* 22:1281–1287, 2007.

REVIEW *Questions*

1. List and describe the possible causes of CP.
2. List and describe the types of CP based on the distribution of abnormal muscle tone.
3. List and describe the types of CP based on the body structures that are affected.
4. What is muscle tone? How is tone different than muscle strength?
5. List and describe the types of abnormal muscle tone found in CP.
6. What are 3 types of traditional and nontraditional approaches to intervention while working with a child with CP?

SUGGESTED *Activities*

1. Visit a classroom in which children with CP are enrolled. Interact with the children and request permission to palpate specific muscles to feel the muscle tone and tension in the muscle.
2. Visit a summer camp for children who have special needs. Plan a simple craft activity and provide hand over hand assistance to children who need the help. Palpate the wrist and hand muscles while providing hand over hand assistance noticing the stiffness.
3. Volunteer to assist in a camp that uses constraint-induced movement therapy.
4. Palpate your biceps and triceps muscles at rest. Palpate your classmates biceps and triceps at rest and while bending and straightening the elbow. Note the tension at rest and at work.

17

Positioning and Handling: A Neurodevelopmental Approach

LISA BAILLARGEON

KATHERINE MICHAUD

KATIE FORTIER

CHOU-HSIEN LIN

CHAPTER *Objectives*

After studying this chapter, the reader will be able to accomplish the following:

- Describe the variety of positions and transitional movements children use in typical development
- Describe the characteristics of developmental positions
- Identify equipment that positions children so they may engage in their daily occupations
- Identify positioning and handling techniques occupational therapy (OT) practitioners use in intervention with children and adolescents
- Explain the key concepts and principles of neurodevelopmental treatment (NDT)
- Distinguish between positioning and handling techniques
- Understand the application of therapeutic positioning and handling principles and techniques exemplified through case examples

KEY TERMS

CHAPTER OUTLINE

Have you ever tried to eat lying down? Have you ever spent the day sitting in a chair that was too small or too big? Have you ever slept on an uncomfortable bed, or woken up feeling rather stiff from a nap?

These examples illustrate the importance of proper positioning during daily life. They also serve to highlight why OT practitioners spend a great deal of time examining children's positions and postures during different activities throughout the day.

Occupational therapy practitioners use positioning and handling techniques to help children perform in school, at home, or on the playground. **Positioning** is considered static and refers to children's ability to maintain postural control while participating in activities. For example, a practitioner may help a child sit in an adapted chair that provides additional postural stability so that he or she can write more efficiently and effectively in school. **Handling** refers to dynamic techniques used to guide children's or adolescents' movements. Handling techniques may be used to influence the state of muscle tone, promote postural stability or trigger new automatic movement responses for function. For example, an OT practitioner may gently support a child's shoulder so that the child is able to reach for objects in front of him or her. Together, positioning and handling techniques are used to help children participate in their occupations.

This chapter begins by providing readers with a description of the variety of positions prevalent in typical motor development, including the characteristics of positions and examples of equipment that help children engage in their daily occupations. After providing an overview of neurodevelopmental treatment (NDT) theory, the authors use case study examples to illustrate the principles and application of therapeutic positioning and handling techniques.

TYPICAL MOTOR DEVELOPMENT

CASE *Study*

Two-year old John loves to play with trucks in his grandmother's hallway. He lies on the floor on his belly, rolls the cars down the hall, jumps up to catch them, and runs down the hallway. Once on the other side, John kneels on one knee (half-kneels) and collects all his trucks. He then sits down, places them all in a line again, and moves on his belly, gently pushing the trucks forward one at a time.

This play scenario illustrates the many different positions that typically developing children assume during play. In this short play activity, John assumed the prone, sitting, half-kneeling, and standing positions. He also ran down the hall. A hallmark of typical development is

that children move in and out of a variety of positions with ease. Movements in and out of different positions are called **transitional movements**. For example, John moved (transitioned) from the supine position to the bipedal standing position in order to run down the hallway. He then moved from standing to sitting on the floor to prone on his stomach. Typically developing children assume a variety of positions as they engage in activities of daily living (ADLs), such as feeding, sleep, hygiene, bathing, and dressing. Children assume and move in and out of positions as they develop motor control.

Neonates are born with physiologic flexion because of their position in utero. **Physiological flexion** passively stretches all of the extensor muscles of the trunk particularly during the last trimester of pregnancy. This stretching elongates the trunk extensors and prepares the infants for active movement against gravity shortly following birth. The first voluntary movement observed in typically developing infants is neck extension while the infant is in the prone position. As the infant lifts his or her head in the prone position (extending the neck), the cervical flexors are stretched or elongated, which prepares these muscle to become active. Head control is achieved as the infant gains strength and coactivation of the cervical flexors and extensors allowing him or her to support the head at midline. The infant first rolls from the prone position to the supine position when the cervical–thoracic extension causes the infant's weight to be shifted too far to the left or right. When this occurs, the infant's whole body will accidentally roll like a log (no segmentation) from the prone position to the supine position. As the infant gains proximal stability in the arms, he or she can assume the prone-on-elbows position. As the infant places and shifts weight onto the shoulders in the prone-on-elbows position, the upper thoracic flexors are elongated. The infant gains proximal shoulder stability and upper body trunk control as the upper thoracic flexors and extensors coactivate and co-contract. This strengthening of neck, shoulder, trunk, pelvis, and leg flexors and extensors will continue as the infant continues to move and play in the environment allowing for more mature postures such as upright sitting, standing, and walking.

In the case of typically developing children, assuming and maintaining a variety of positions lead to the development of motor control. Children naturally progress as they develop postural control and muscle control for the next position. This, in turn, strengthens the muscles used for more refined movements. Children who have special needs, such as children with cerebral palsy, often require interventions to help them develop the postural and muscle control required for skilled functional movements. Positioning and handling techniques are frequently used in OT interventions to help children with abnormal muscle tone acquire the strength and typical movement patterns needed to function in everyday activities.

CLINICAL *Pearl*

Children learn as they experience different positions. They enjoy exploring in a variety of positions and gain new perspectives on things as they change positions. Parents may need to be reminded that equipment may be provided temporarily just to give their child the experience of a change in position.

GENERAL CONSIDERATIONS

The progression of motor development and motor control is necessary for skilled movements. The following section describes aspects of motor control and development that OT practitioners consider when using positioning and handling techniques to help children engage in their occupations.

Skeletal Alignment

Positioning is important toward developing postural stability, but it is also required for children to participate in daily occupations. When the skeletal system is aligned and children are positioned symmetrically, each side of the body develops adequate muscle strength needed for postural stability. **Symmetrical** alignment helps children maintain the full range of motion (ROM) for movement. Therefore, symmetrical positioning with head, neck, trunk, and pelvis aligned, allows children to move the arms and legs efficiently, bring the hands to midline to

work with objects, and maneuver the legs. Positioning children symmetrically provides physical comfort, reduces fatigue, and promotes stability so that they may engage in occupations such as feeding, dressing, and playing. Thus, one of the first principles of positioning is to make sure that children are symmetrical and well aligned. OT practitioners may use positioning devices to support children in symmetrical positions. Often providing external support helps children maintain a position to perform daily occupations (Figure 17-1).

Typical Development

When helping children maintain a position, OT practitioners consider typical development and the many different positions children assume as they interact with their environments. OT practitioners provide a variety of options for positions so that children experience a full range of experiences. For example, OT practitioners understanding typical development realize that infants (between 7 and 10 months) begin to explore their surroundings by crawling. Thus, the OT practitioner provides positioning opportunities that promote the prone-on-extended-arms position and support the infant's efforts to crawl. Similarly, infants at this age enjoy sitting, and some may require external support to maintain the upright position.

Perception and Body Awareness

Not only does assuming and maintaining various positions promote motor development, they also stimulate perceptual development and body awareness. For example, moving from the sitting position to the standing position provides children with a different viewpoint, engages the vestibular system, and enhances children's

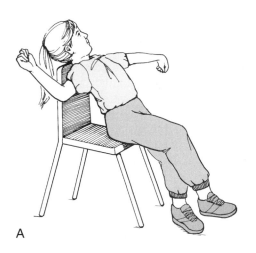

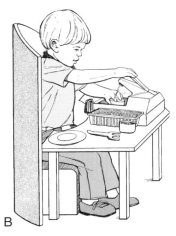

FIGURE 17-1 A, A child in asymmetrical position and showing abnormal posture has difficulty reaching for toys. **B,** Using external supports from a chair allows a child to sit in a symmetrical position to reach for toys. (From Case-Smith J, O'Brien J: *Occupational therapy for children,* ed 6, St. Louis, 2009, Mosby.)

A   B

perception of the surroundings. Each new position provides different opportunities and experiences that help children make sense of their bodies and their environments. Children develop **perception** and **body awareness** as they make sense of their position in space and view things from different angles. For example, infants' early feeding experiences occur while they are in the reclining position, whereas toddlers feed in the upright sitting position, and older children may eat while lying in front of a television.

Changing positions stimulates different sensory experiences. For example, weight bearing on hands provides infants with tactile sensations and experiences that are important for later hand development. Children develop body awareness as they experience proprioceptive feedback from their muscles and joints about where their bodies are in space. As children develop the ability to sit upright, they see things at different angles; they feel different sensations; and they develop a sense of balance, which helps promote postural stability for mobility and functional activity (Figure 17-2).

Postural Control for Balance and Functional Activity

Maintaining positions requires *postural control*, which refers to the ability to sustain the necessary trunk control to use the arms, hands, and legs and efficiently carry out skilled tasks, such as playing, coloring, or feeding. See Box 17-1 for a description of the relationship between stability and mobility. Along with adequate muscle tone

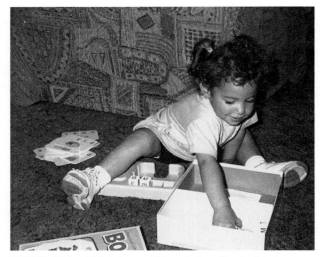

FIGURE 17-2　Child sits upright and plays. She is able to move to reach for objects. (From Parham LD: *Play in occupational therapy for children,* ed 2, St. Louis, 2007, Mosby.)

BOX 17-1

Stability and Mobility

The ability to control movements occurs within the framework of stability and mobility. *Stability* is defined as the ability to maintain or stabilize a posture. *Mobility* is defined as the ability to move into or assume a posture. Infants are born with the ability to move, and mobility will be present before stability. Infants must gain strength and co-contraction between opposing muscle groups (e.g., trunk flexors and trunk extensors) in order to stabilize postures. Once a stable posture is established, an infant can learn to control movements within that position or posture.

and skeletal alignment, children need a sense of balance to maintain postural control. **Balance**, also referred to as **postural stability**, refers to the ability to maintain the center of gravity over the base of support. The *center of gravity* is the point where the total body weight is most evenly distributed over the base of support. The center of gravity is also referred to as the *center of mass* when it relates to the child's center of distribution. Children must first sense changes in the center of mass before they are able to respond to these changes. Children respond to changes in balance through righting and equilibrium reactions. **Righting reactions** are those reactions that bring the body back to midline position and are defined as the maintenance of the proper alignment of the head and trunk in space. For example, righting reactions are present as an infant moves his head upright and vertical when tilted to the side (righting the head on the neck). Another example of righting reactions is when the head, trunk, and pelvis rotate on an axis, as seen in rolling to maintain alignment of the body segments (head, trunk, pelvis). This is observed as infants turn their bodies in alignment to roll toward a toy. An infant develops head righting reactions in the first few months of life in response to visual and vestibular sensory input. **Equilibrium reactions** help one maintain balance when the body's center of mass is shifted too far over the base of support. Equilibrium reactions may require the use of the head, trunk, arms, and legs to flex or abduct in order to adjust the body's center of mass over the base of support to prevent a fall. The maturation of equilibrium reactions occurs in an orderly sequence—prone, supine, sitting, quadruped, and standing—as the infant gains antigravity muscle strength and postural control (Figure 17-3). Equilibrium reactions may also involve subtle changes in muscle tone to maintain position. For example, equilibrium reactions can be observed as a child maintains balance when standing on one foot. This

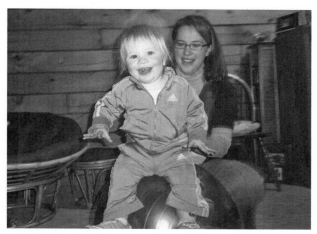

FIGURE 17-3 Playing on a ball can help to elicit equilibrium reactions in children.

involves subtle adjustments in muscle tone to maintain the upright position. **Protective extension** reactions occur when the body's center of mass is shifted too far off the base of support and righting and equilibrium reactions cannot bring the body back to midline. They involve extending an arm or a leg forward to "save face" when the change in balance is so extreme that children feel unable to correct their position to avoid falling. Protective extension can be observed as a child quickly places a hand on the floor to catch himself or herself when pushed off balance suddenly. (Refer to Table 17-1 for a description of the development of postural reactions.)

All movement requires an initial weight shift. The term **weight shift** refers to the change in the center of mass so that one can move a body part. During a lateral weight shift in the sitting or standing position, the side that accepts the weight will respond with trunk elongation, and the side that is unweighted will respond with trunk shortening. This allows a person to maintain an upright position with the head remaining in proper alignment with the body and avoid falling into gravity during shifts of the body's center of mass. Children may also initiate cephalo-caudal (head to tail) or caudal-cephalo (tail to head) weight shifts. For example, a cephalo-caudal weight shift is required when initiating movement from the supine position to the prone position. Anterior–posterior weight shifts involve tilting the pelvis. The posterior weight shift is used when moving from the quadruped position to the tall-kneel position.

OT practitioners examine the components of children's movement so they can determine pieces that may be missing or atypical. Intervention is frequently aimed at helping children perform typical movement.

TABLE 17-1

Postural Reactions

BALANCE REACTIONS	AGE (mo.)
RIGHTING REACTIONS	
Neck on Body	
Immature	Birth
Mature	4–5
Body on Body	
Immature	Birth
Mature	4–5
Body on Head	
Prone (partial)	1–2
Mature	4–5
Supine	5–6
Landau	
Immature	3
Mature	6–10
Flexion	
Partial (head in line)	3–4
Mature (head forward)	6–7
Vertical	
Partial (head in line)	2
Mature (head to vertical)	6
PROTECTIVE REACTIONS	
Forward	6–7
Lateral	6–11
Backward	9–12
EQUILIBRIUM REACTIONS	
Prone	5–6
Supine	7–8
Sitting	7–10
Quadruped	9–12
Standing	12–21

From Case-Smith J, O'Brien J: *Occupational therapy for children,* ed 6, St. Louis, 2010, Mosby.

POSITIONING AS A THERAPUETIC TOOL

OT practitioners position children so that they can actively engage in daily occupations, such as feeding, dressing, bathing, or play. Positioning children in the upright sitting position may promote socialization, independence in feeding, and successful engagement in academics and play. Some children may require external supports to assume and maintain positions. OT practitioners use the principles of positioning to evaluate postures and offer solutions to help children engage in age-appropriate occupations.

The principles of positioning children include the following:

- Providing the child with a variety of positioning options throughout the day
- Placing the child in positions that enhance function
- Avoiding positions that restrict the child's movement
- Providing positions that are comfortable for the child.
- Considering safety when prescribing positions (e.g., do not leave a child unattended in a positioning device)
- Ensuring proper skeletal alignment and symmetry during positioning of the child
- Recommending positioning equipment that provides external stability to facilitate movement

As previously stated, generally, children develop movements in the following sequence of positions: prone, supine, prone-on-elbows, prone-on-extended-elbows/arms, side-lying, sitting, quadruped, half kneel, kneel, standing.[2,7] The following paragraphs describe the development of positions and provide examples of equipment that may be used to help children assume and maintain these positions.

Prone Position

The *prone position* (on-tummy position) facilitates neck and trunk extension and thus helps children build muscle strength and stability in the neck, upper back, shoulders, arms, and hands. Once a child develops strength and stability, he or she is able to develop muscle control. Prone position leads to higher-level motor skills such as prone-on-elbows, prone-on-extended-elbows, and quadruped positions.

Placing a firm foam wedge under an infant's upper body, with the edge of the wedge just below the axillary area encourages the prone-on-elbows or prone-on-extended-elbows position, depending on the height of the wedge. OT practitioners determine the correct degree of incline according to the infant's ability to independently hold his head up during the selected activity. Neck extension below a 45-degree angle is recommended, as this prevents the head movement

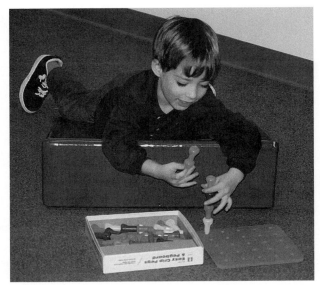

FIGURE 17-4   Child in prone position over a wedge. Note the axillary position, wedge height, and amount of neck extension.

from triggering hyperextension throughout the body. A pillow or towel may be placed between the knees to separate them if necessary (Figure 17-4).

The OT practitioner can use his own arms or legs to promote prone positions while working with infants and toddlers. Bolsters and balls can be used to promote weight bearing and weight shifting in the prone position.

CLINICAL *Pearl*

(1) The prone position is a good one to use when dressing and undressing a child or infant. Place the small child or infant prone across your lap to dress or undress him or her. (2) Make sure that the wedges and rolls are not so high that they cause excessive extensor tone or so low that those with very low muscle tone or strength cannot lift their heads.

Supine Position

Infants develop physiological flexion in utero to maintain the supine position. Within the first months of life, as cervical extension develops, physiologic flexion becomes less and less. The cervical flexors become elongated and, as such, become active. Once the cervical extensors and flexors are both active, head control is possible. The supine position (on back) helps the infant further develop neck and abdominal muscle control, and this postural support makes it possible to bring the head, hands, and feet to midline. In the supine position, the infant further develops strength in the neck flexors by engaging in play that encourages downward visual gaze and active head turning. During play activities to maintain head at midline, the infant begins to activate both neck flexors and extensors (Figure 17-5). This co-contraction of neck flexors and extensors will provide the stability needed to maintain the head at midline in the supine, prone, sitting, and standing positions.

Infants are frequently held in the supine position when swaddled in a blanket or positioned in a car seat or infant seat. Some seats cradle the infant in the supine position (e.g., in a car seat), whereas other seats (e.g., strollers) require maintaining the supine position. The infant may be positioned on a flat or inclined surface using wedges, pillows, rolls/bolsters, or towels to provide support. OT practitioners promote positioning infants in the supine position with the head at midline and flexed slightly forward for optimal visual exploration of the environment. Rolled towels under the infant's knees encourage flexion and are therefore recommended for premature infants (who have less or diminished physiological flexion).

CLINICAL *Pearl*

When working with an infant or child who is in the supine position, support the child's head in a flexed-forward position. Flexing the child's knees and hips minimizes the effects of extensor tone and encourages the use of abdominal muscles.

Prone-on-Elbows and Prone-on-Extended-Arms Position

The infant begins to stretch out the tightness in the hip flexors and develop head control in the prone position as the center of gravity shifts posteriorly to the pelvis allowing lifting of the head and weight bearing on elbows. The prone-on-elbows position allows the infant to observe the environment differently. As the infant develops improved head and trunk control from maintaining the position, he or she is able to shift weight further back (toward the feet) and assume the prone-on-extended-arms position. Once in the prone-on-extended-arms position, the infant receives proprioceptive and tactile input to the hands, important for future hand development. Playing in these positions further encourages weight shifting so that the infant can reach for objects. The prone position stretches the hip and knee flexor muscles, which is necessary for more advanced motor skills (e.g., crawling, walking) (Figure 17-6.)

As with the basic prone position, wedges, rolls, and towels propped under the children's trunk work to encourage the prone-on-elbows and prone-on-extended-arms positions.

Side-Lying

The side-lying position is a natural and comfortable position for children, especially during sleep or while lying on the couch. Children who have motor and sensory control issues may require external support to maintain alignment in the side-lying position. This position

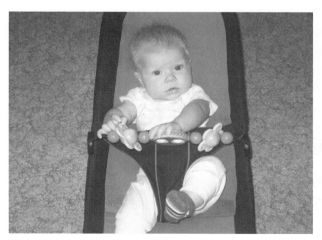

FIGURE 17-5   The supine position requires some neck and leg flexion and helps children develop the abdominal muscles.

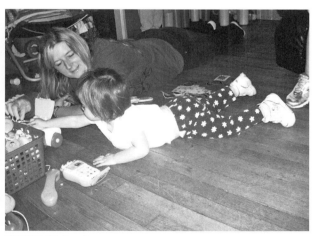

FIGURE 17-6   Children begin to bear weight on elbows before moving to the prone-to-extended-arms position. This position encourages exploration and hand development.

requires coactivation of the head and trunk flexors and extensors. The side-lying position requires children to maintain their head at midline; this promotes their hands being placed in the line of vision and toward the midline, which is important for gaining an understanding of the overall body scheme and the relationship of body parts to their functions. Body scheme awareness promotes successful engagement in functional activities, such as bringing the hands to the mouth or manipulating a toy bilaterally (Figure 17-7).

Commercially made side-lyers (e.g., Tumble forms) are available. Bolsters, wedges, pillows, rolled towels, and benches help children assume the side-lying position.

CLINICAL *Pearl*

When placing a child in the side-lying position, remember the following points:
1. Alternate the sides.
2. Use small rolls or pillows to help the child maintain the position; for example, use a towel roll in front of a child who tends to push back into extension. This cues the child to lean forward and reduces the extensor tone influence.
3. Provide adequate padded surfaces for shoulders and hips to prevent pressure sores and diminished circulation.
4. During play and social interaction, make sure that toys and people are presented well below the child's eye level to encourage flexion (and discourage extension).

Sitting Position

Children must develop sufficient head and trunk control to be able to sit upright. Typically developing children begin to assume the sitting position and stay in it without assistance around 6 to 7 months of age.[2,7] The sitting position requires children to maintain postural control of the head, trunk, and extremities against the pull of gravity and requires coactivation of the trunk flexors and extensors. Once children assume a stable sitting posture without having to brace upright using the arms, they can shift weight away from the center of gravity to reach, retrieve, and manipulate objects. This helps refine balance and establish hand dominance. The sitting position provides visual and kinesthetic experiences that advance children's perceptual and cognitive development as well. Many occupations such as feeding, toileting, schoolwork, and play are performed in the sitting position. OT practitioners frequently evaluate children's sitting posture and provide interventions to facilitate the correct postures so that children can participate in chosen occupations (Box 17-2).

Children assume a variety of sitting positions, including long-sitting (legs straight with knee extension), ring-sitting (legs formed in a circle), tailor-sitting (legs bent and crossed), and side-sitting (both legs to one side) positions (Figure 17-8). Ring-sitting and tailor-sitting positions offer more stability to children who have weaker trunk muscle tone or balance. The long-sitting position may be difficult for children who have abnormal muscle tone or tightness in the hamstring muscles in the lower extremity. Side-sitting requires greater strength and activity from the trunk muscles due to the asymmetrical positioning of the lower extremity and weight shift toward one side of the body. W-sitting or sitting with the knees bent inward such that the legs form a W is a stable position that is developmentally appropriate at 10 to 12 months of age, but it is not recommended for children older than 1 year, as it may cause hip dislocation and tightness and misalignment in the hip and leg muscles (Box 17-3).

Many adapted seats facilitate sitting positions and promote participation in activities such as feeding, dressing, playing, and academics. *Corner chairs* promote scapula protraction (shoulders forward), humeral internal

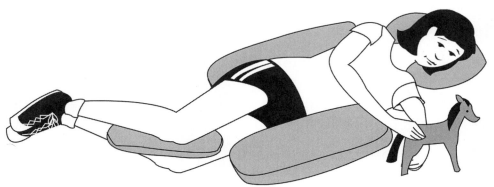

FIGURE 17-7   The side-lying position encourages the child to bring the hands together to play with a toy.

BOX 17-2

Basic Sitting Position

Occupational therapy practitioners help develop sitting options for children using the following guidelines:

- Hips and knees are flexed to 90 degrees.
- Back rests against chair back.
- The trunk is vertical.
- The body is symmetrical.
- The head is aligned with the trunk, at midline, and flexed slightly forward.
- All three back curves (cervical [neck], thoracic [middle], and lumbar [lower]) are present and in good alignment. A small, rolled-up towel or a lumbar roll can be used to help maintain the normal curves in the back.
- Both feet are positioned flat on the floor or supported on a raised surface in neutral.
- The tabletop or lapboard is positioned at elbow height. Elbows are flexed at 90 degrees position on armrests, if available.

From Crepeau E, Cohn E, Boyt-Schell B: *Willard and Spackman's occupational therapy*, ed 11, Philadelphia, 2009, Lippincott Williams & Wilkins.

rotation, and trunk stability by providing lateral supports in the seated position (Figure 17-9). Consequently, this type of chair encourages children to bring their hands to the midline within their visual field, which promotes the holding of objects (e.g., books, toys, feeding utensils). Many corner chairs have trays that further promote the use of hands in the sitting position. These trays may be positioned in such a way to help children bear weight through the elbows to facilitate hand movements if necessary. Some corner seats provide the option to sit directly on the floor so that they can participate in certain activities, for example, during story time at school; raised corner seats allow for knee flexion in addition to hip flexion in the seated position (e.g., allowing children to sit at table height with peers in the classroom).

Bolster chairs are frequently used to decrease muscle tone in the hip adductors and internal rotators. As such, these chairs promote hip abduction and external rotation as children straddle the bolster in the seated position, allowing them to maintain better stability to use their hands for play, academics, or ADLs

Wheelchairs

Wheelchairs provide the means for mobility to children with mobility issues and also access to their environment. The OT practitioner, the family, and the team

decide whether a child needs an electric wheelchair or a standard wheelchair on the basis of many factors. The team makes decisions concerning other features of the wheelchair, for example, the type of frame, push handles, rear wheels, front casters, arm rests, leg rests, and wheel locks (Figure 17-10). The appearance of the chair is important to the child, so he or she may participate in selecting the style, fabric, and color.

Wheelchairs come in ultralight, light, and heavy-duty weights. The type of seat selected is important for the fit of the chair. While some children are able to use a solid seat, others may require customized seating cushions; and some may need to use a sling seat.

The rear tires may be solid or filled with air (pneumatic). Air-filled tires are easier to push over sandy or rough terrain, but they are not as durable as solid tires. Arm rests can be fixed or removable, full length, desk length, or elevated. Removable armrests make it easier to transfer the child in and out of the wheelchair; full-length armrests provide more stable support for mounting trays or other devices.

It is important for the wheelchair to fit the child correctly. Some lending programs may allow the use of a temporary wheelchair while waiting for the permanent chair to arrive. OT practitioners may help parents and other caregivers adapt strollers to use as temporary mobility devices for very young children.

MOBILITY

OT practitioners consider the ability of the child to move around his or her environment. Children of all ages learn through exploration. For example, infants roll and crawl to investigate their environments; this provides them with new opportunities and experiences to learn and relate to others. OT practitioners may suggest strollers, scooters, adapted tricycles, or other equipment to encourage movements in children (Figure 17-11).

CLINICAL *Pearl*

When ordering a wheelchair for a young child or an adolescent, consider the required modifications for the use of the wheelchair at home or in school. For example, a large powered wheelchair cannot be carried up the stairs. While the chair may fit the child adequately, the parents may need help to bring it into their house or apartment. It may be necessary to build a ramp or to recommend a different type of chair, depending on the child's environment.

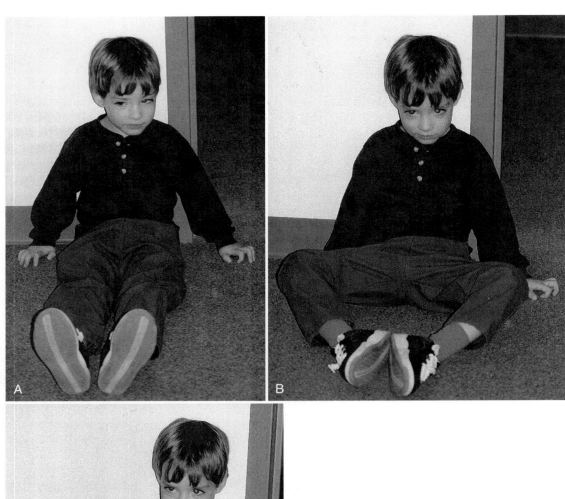

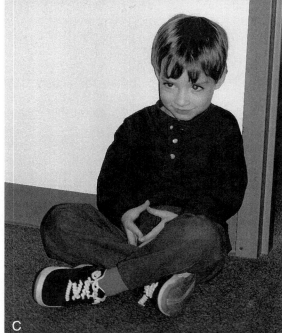

FIGURE 17-8   A, Long-sitting position. **B,** Ring-sitting position. **C,** Tailor-sitting position.

BOX 17-3

Sitting Positions

Children with poor trunk stability may favor a W-sitting position, since the lower extremities are positioned to provide a wide base of support. W-sitting does not require trunk strength or stability and thus makes it easier for children to manipulate objects and play on the floor. However, W-sitting may lead to orthopedic problems, including increased risk of hip dislocation, joint deformities, and the aggravation of muscle tightness. W-sitting does not allow for rotation, weight shifting, or the opportunity to cross midline. Therefore, OT practitioners discourage W-sitting by promoting other sitting positions that engage children's postural system and encourage the use of trunk muscles. Alternatives to W-sitting include tailor-sitting; long-sitting; side-sitting; tailor-sitting or sitting on the therapist's lap, on a bench, or on a ball.

Quadruped Position

Once children have sufficient head and trunk control as well as stability at the shoulder and pelvic girdles, they can shift weight from side to side in the prone-on-extended-arms position and will often try to assume the quadruped position and move forward. The quadruped position allows children to reach for objects and attempt to move toward motivating toys. OT practitioners frequently work with children on the stabilization and strengthening of the trunk, shoulders, and hips and on balance by encouraging them to shift weight while playing in the quadruped position. After learning to assume the position, children begin to shift weight, often by lifting a hand off the floor to reach for an object. Initially, this weight shift is brief and may result in a fall. However, after some time, children are able to reach forward and grasp an object without falling. Often this helps them discover that repeating this movement provides momentum, and they begin to rotate to the same side. Practice helps children learn that this position affords them with some locomotion. Children enjoy this new quick movement toward interesting objects and the quadruped position becomes a precursor to *creeping* (forward movement on belly) and *crawling* (forward movement on hands and knees). This forward movement involves dissociation of the hip and shoulder muscles as well as dissociation of movements on the right side of the body from those on the left side. For example, the right hip flexes while the right shoulder extends; meanwhile the left shoulder flexes while the left hip extends.

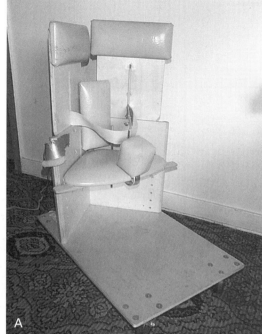

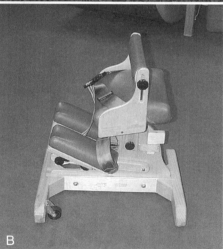

FIGURE 17-9 Two examples of adapted seating systems that help inhibit spasticity and compensate for limited postural control.

Rolls, bolsters, and scooter boards can be used to facilitate quadruped position (Figure 17-12).

Half-Kneel/Kneel Position

Children typically assume the half-kneeling or the tall-kneeling position before they attempt to stand. Tall kneeling is easier than half kneeling, since with the former children have a more secure base of support with both lower legs in contact with the support surface. The

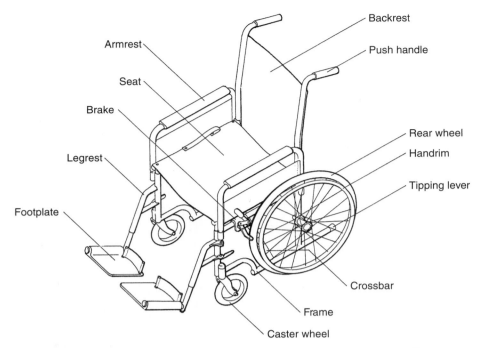

FIGURE 17-10 Conventional wheelchair: the major parts of supporting and propelling structures. From Ragnarsson RT: Prescription considerations and comparison of conventional and lightweight wheelchairs. *Rehab Res Dev 2* (suppl): 8, 1990.)

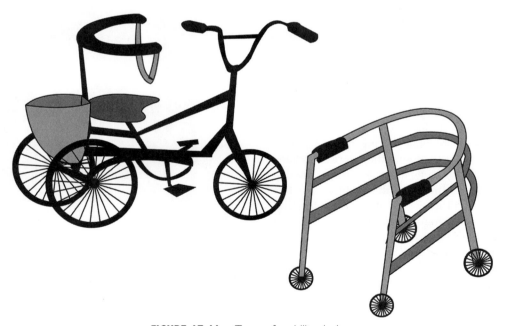

FIGURE 17-11 Types of mobility devices.

tall-kneeling position requires less work from the trunk to maintain balance during weight shifts while playing in this position. Children must develop stronger trunk stability and more mature equilibrium reactions in the sitting and tall-kneeling positions before they are able to maintain the

half-kneeling position. Gradually, as children gain more motor and balance control, they move from tall kneeling to half kneeling to standing without difficulty.

Since knees are vulnerable to injury, the tall-kneeling and half-kneeling positions are typically used

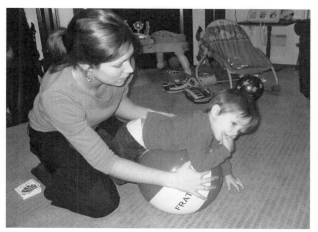

FIGURE 17-12   OT practitioners can use a ball to facilitate the quadruped position.

during transitions from sitting to standing during play activities, but prolonged kneeling is usually not encouraged. OT practitioners help children assume the half-kneeling and kneeling positions to do such things as reaching for objects low to the ground or putting on the shoes. These are temporary positions. Frequently, OT practitioners help children with finding external supports (e.g., a wall or perhaps a small table on which they can lean) that they can hold on to in order to maintain balance while bending down from the standing position to the half-kneeling position.

Standing Position

The standing position involves full weight bearing through the hips and lower extremities and promotes bone growth, muscle development, and blood circulation. Standing is typically a prerequisite skill for walking and higher level mobility. Once children gain internal stability in the standing position, they are able to use both hands for play.

Children who need positioning assistance to stand may benefit from supine and prone standers. *Standers* support the body from either the back (supine stander) or the front surface (prone stander) and can be secured in a vertically tilted position. A stander can be reclined if necessary for children who require additional trunk support (i.e., children who are unable to maintain the reclining position on their own). Children with increased trunk muscle extensor tone may benefit from having the stander tilted slightly forward to decrease the muscle tone so that they can maintain the head at midline.

Freedom standers, *standing boxes*, and *parapodiums* provide external support to children who have limited

trunk control and stability. These positioning devices allow children to stand upright and use their arms and hands to play, feed, write, or read (Figure 17-13).

THERAPEUTIC POSITIONING

The goal of therapeutic positioning is to provide the necessary support to promote children's active engagement in occupations, not as a way to improve motor control or strength. Therefore, therapeutic positioning provides external support required to promote function in play and self-care tasks. Consequently, after considering the occupations that children hope to engage in, the OT practitioner helps children maintain positions that allow them to succeed.

The goal of therapeutic positioning is to provide children with safe, efficient, and effective postures that enable them to participate in social, academic, family, and self care activities. For example, the OT practitioner provides a corner seat to help a child sit upright during story time at school. When evaluating the usefulness of the seat, the OT practitioner considers that the child will remain in the seat for 15 minutes (the period for story time). The OT practitioner provides a seat with plenty of support and one that ensures the child's success. Thus, the therapeutic value of the positioning equipment is that it allows the child to participate in story time with his peers. (Even though the seat may improve the child's trunk strength and stability over time, depending on *how* the child sits in it, that is not the goal of the device.)

CASE *Study*

Nathan is a 2-year-old boy who has been diagnosed with the quadriplegic–spastic type of cerebral palsy. Nathan keeps both his hands fisted, forearms pronated, elbows flexed, and shoulders internally rotated. His hip and knees are flexed and internally rotated, the pelvis is posteriorly

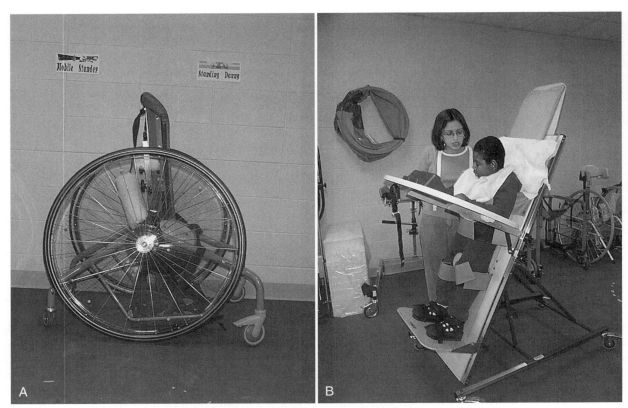

FIGURE 17-13 **A,** Mobile prone stander. **B,** Supine stander.

tilted, and the feet are plantar flexed. He has difficulty sitting unsupported. Nathan prefers to play lying prone on his belly. He reaches for objects with his right arm, but he is inaccurate. He is able to pick up objects placed close to him. The OT practitioner is working with Nathan to help him sit and play with toys, feed himself, and explore his environment through play.

Nathan has difficulty sitting upright during mealtime; he collapses forward or totally extends back into his chair. His mother reports that she has to hold him during meal time. The OT practitioner provides an adapted insert (corner seat type) for the highchair that helps to position Nathan with his hips flexed forward (anterior tilt) and provides external rotation of his knees and hips and a footrest to support his feet in flexion. The lateral supports provide adequate trunk support. The OT practitioner adds a pummel for Nathan to hold with his left hand, which provides Nathan with enough stability, so he can use his right hand to hold the spoon or pick up food. The OT practitioner provides Nathan with a small stepstool to sit on when undressing at bedtime. The stool is placed up against a corner of the room, which provides Nathan with external stability as he attempts to doff his socks and pants. The stool has arm rests, which Nathan can use to stabilize his left hand and use his

right hand more effectively. Sitting on the stool braced against the wall increases his success at dressing tasks as this supports his sitting posture; it also improves the position of his pelvis and reduces his atypical posturing. These positioning devices help Nathan engage in more independent feeding and dressing activities in his home.

OT practitioners use positioning and handling techniques to help children engage effectively in their occupations. The term *positioning* refers to static placement designed to improve function. Conversely, OT practitioners use *handling* techniques to promote improved motor control. As such, handling involves continual evaluation of children's responses to the OT practitioner's input (i.e., cues and touching) as it relates to the desired motor movement. All of this occurs within a dynamic setting and therefore requires the OT practitioner to be aware of how he or she is influencing children's motor and emotional responses. The following section describes handling techniques as described within the framework of neurodevelopmental treatment (NDT). The authors begin with a definition of NDT emphasizing the principles of the theory and conclude with a description of handling techniques, including a case application.

NEURODEVELOPMENTAL TREATMENT
What Is NDT?

NDT was developed by Karel and Berta Bobath as a technique to help children with functional limitations. "NDT is a problem-solving approach to the examination and treatment of the impairments and functional limitations of individuals with neuropathology, primarily children with cerebral palsy."[3-5,8] The goal of NDT is to help children perform skilled movements more efficiently in order to carry out life skills.[7]

Therefore, OT practitioners using NDT must have an understanding of typical movements and how they change across a person's lifespan. Once OT practitioners understand typical movements, they are able to analyze how abnormal muscle tone and abnormal postures interfere with children's movements. OT practitioners then facilitate normal postures so that children are able to "feel" typical movements. NDT theorists believe that moving in typical movement patterns improves neural pathways; this makes movements more automatic, which, in turn, helps children perform daily occupations.

NDT Principles

The principles of NDT are based on the theory of brain plasticity, meaning that through repetition of movement, children develop improved neural pathways to help them move efficiently and accurately.[6,7,8] OT practitioners using NDT help children "feel" normal movements through handling and gentle facilitation at **key points of control**. Proximal key points of control include the shoulders, hips, trunk, and pelvis, where the practitioner places his or her hands to guide the children through the movements. Distal key points of control include hands, feet, or head. Through handling and guidance, new neural pathways develop and thereby improve the quality and accuracy of movements.[3-5,7]

Frequently, OT practitioners begin NDT sessions by inhibiting the abnormal muscle tone. *Inhibitory techniques* are used to reduce hypertonicity (increased muscle tone) in children. In the presence of hypotonicity, OT practitioners use *facilitation techniques* to increase muscle tone to a more normal level (Table 17-2). Once a child's muscle tone has reached a more normal state, the OT practitioner facilitates movement, typically through handling during play. The OT practitioner follows the child's lead and uses key points of control to guide the child through the movement. The OT practitioner is careful to allow the child to actively perform as much of the movement as possible on his or her own and provides support where necessary so the child is successful.

The following list provides a summary of NDT principles that guide intervention:[4,7,10]

- Intervention should be individualized and focused on functional outcomes.

TABLE 17-2

Indicators for Use of Inhibition and Facilitation Techniques

REQUIRED TECHNIQUE	CHILD INDICATORS	STRATEGIES
INHIBITION	Hypertonicity Active primitive reflexes Excessive activity and motion Behavioral excitation Excessive sensitivity or reactivity to handling and touch	Sustained pressure to tendon Slow stroking of spine while child is in prone position Rotational movement (trunk and hip rotation) Slow rocking or rolling Heavy joint compression Sustained weight bearing Slow holding movements Wrapping, swaddling calm music, warm colors, soft noises, dim lights, warm temperatures
FACILITATION	Hypotonicity Inactive primitive reflexes, lack of balance reactions Excessive relaxation, semiconscious state Behavioral nonresponsiveness, flat affect Decreased reactivity to handling and touch	Light moving touch Tapping, sweep tapping, alternate tapping to activate contraction Fast vestibular input Heavy joint compression Active weight shifting Quick, variable movements Upbeat music, cool colors, louder noises, bright lights, cool temperatures

- Normalize muscle tone before and during movement.
- Analyze musculoskeletal limitations interfering with movement and function.
- Facilitate normal movement patterns, including both passive and active movements, that are meaningful to children.
- Emphasize quality of movement (e.g., accuracy, quickness, adaptability, and fluency).
- The goal of NDT intervention is increased active use of the trunk and involved extremities for meaningful activity.
- Experience is a driving force for children. New activities build on previous sensorimotor experiences (typical and atypical).
- Use therapeutic handling and positioning of children to facilitate movement.
- Target postural control and movement by using key points of control. Proximal points of control (e.g., hips, trunk, pelvis) provide more support to children, while distal points of control (e.g., head, hands, feet) require children to perform more of the movement.
- Engaging children in "typical" movement develops neural pathways.
- Movement occurs within children's environments.
- Consider children's motivation and active problem solving in coordinating movements for a purpose.

Therapeutic Handling

Therapeutic handling is a dynamic process used to help children participate in their daily activities. The benefits of handling include assisting children with learning movements, allowing children to feel functional movements, and facilitating or inhibiting muscle tone that may interfere with movements.[3-5,7,8] Therapeutic handling allows the OT practitioner to feel children's responses to changes in postures and movements and to modify handling as necessary to assist children in successful motor responses (Figure 17-14).

Therapeutic handling is used to facilitate normal postural control and movements so that children are able to engage in meaningful and age-appropriate activities.[6] Handling enables the OT practitioner to notice and feel changes in postures and/or movements. Consequently, handling is used both in assessment and intervention.[8] OT practitioners following an NDT approach use facilitation and inhibition to correct children's incorrect patterns of movements or positions before they lead to secondary deformities and/or dysfunction.[6]

Children with cerebral palsy or other neurologic disorders experience muscle tone abnormalities interfering

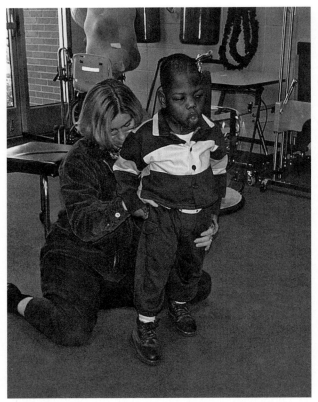

FIGURE 17-14   Handling at key points of control can facilitate movement.

with posture and movement. Abnormal muscle tone affects the children's ability to engage in play, self-care, academics, mobility, and communication. NDT theorists hypothesize that these children experience difficulty "feeling" or "sensing" typical movements and therefore are at risk for developing secondary deformities and/or dysfunctional movement.[1,9] Children who have muscle tone abnormalities are frequently unable to correct for changes in posture. They do not feel the changes in movements or may experience a delay in sensing these changes. A delay in the reaction to changes or the absence of sensations, along with abnormal muscle tone, may cause frequent falls, inaccurate movements, or slow clumsy movements.

NDT therapists use therapeutic handling at key points of control to help children feel the typical movements. Through practice and repetition of typical movements that occur in meaningful activities, children develop more accurate and efficient movements. They sense typical movements and understand intuitively how it feels to perform movements correctly. Current NDT theory also emphasizes targeting children's motivations and interests for activities during interventions.[7]

Handling Technique

The OT practitioner provides gentle cueing by placing his or her hands on the child at specific key points of control and in a certain manner. The OT practitioner uses hands to provide the child with a directional cue or assist in the weight shift (Figure 17-15). Handling may be used to stimulate a muscle group to contract or relax. The OT practitioner is careful to allow the child time to respond and to gently guide the child's weight shifts. The goal of handling is to improve the child's success and motor control through practice of the movement during the activity and within the actual context of the activity. As the child gains movement control, the practitioner lessens his or her handling or cueing. The goal of NDT is that the child actively performs the movement.

Practice Application

NDT intervention is an individual approach to examining and improving movements and begins with an assessment of the child's current level of performance. OT practitioners use knowledge of typical development to analyze the child's current movement patterns. In particular, OT practitioners analyze what might be interfering with the child's ability to participate in those activities that he or she desires. After observing the child in a variety of play scenarios, the OT practitioner examines the child's muscle tone and postural reactions and develops goals and objectives with the interdisciplinary team.

As a preparatory method, the OT practitioner may use certain techniques to either inhibit or facilitate muscle tone, depending on the need of the child. Next, the OT practitioner helps the child repeat normal patterns of movement while playing by facilitating movements at

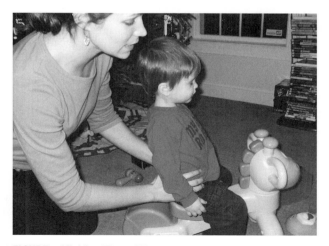

FIGURE 17-15 The OT practitioner uses gentle cueing techniques to facilitate the desired movement.

key points of control and guiding the child's movements through handling. Repeating typical movements helps the child develop neural pathways and eventually the movements become automatic. The OT practitioner uses activities that are meaningful and motivating to the child. An intervention is also most effective when performed in the typical or actual context of the activity. For example, playing with peers on the playground may be more reinforcing than playing alone in a classroom.

The OT practitioner places his or her hands on the child at either proximal or distal key points of control to help the child maintain postures for movements. The OT practitioner facilitates movements by providing the least amount of support needed for the child to be successful. The key to intervention is for the child to correctly perform as much of the movement as he or she is able to. The OT practitioner acts as a guide, working to make sure that abnormal movements are inhibited. OT practitioners are sensitive to the child's movements and are careful to limit extraneous sensory stimulation or cues.

OT practitioners examine the child's movements by carefully analyzing how the child moves in and out of positions, maintains positions, and responds to changes in his or her environment. OT practitioners examine muscle tone, joint integrity, ROM, and postural control during movements. Furthermore, they explore the child's motivations for movements and his or her ability to initiate and terminate movements. The quality of movements is also considered.

OT practitioners facilitate a weight shift by gentle cueing in the direction of the desired weight shift through handling. They do not grab the children but rather place their hands gently on the children to guide their movements. For example, when helping children move from the sitting position to the quadruped position, the OT practitioner may decide to guide the children in making a lateral weight shift by providing a directional cue to the lateral oblique muscles (flexors) of the trunk (see Figure 17-15).

When examining a child's movement, the OT practitioner considers that all movements begin with a weight shift. Thus, children must be able to initiate a lateral (to the side), cephalo-caudal, caudal-cephalo (head to toe, toe to head) or anterior–posterior weight shift. Children also use righting, equilibrium, and protective extension reactions during movements. The OT practitioner examines the child's ability to use flexion, extension, or rotational patterns during movements. The OT practitioner understands that children first develop gross movement control, or random movement, followed by stability, and then controlled and fine movement.

OT practitioners help children assume positions, maintain positions, and transition in and out of positions by facilitating the appropriate weight shift, muscle action (i.e., flexion, extension, rotation), and/or postural reactions (i.e., righting, equilibrium, protective extension). NDT intervention involves continual assessment of how children are moving. The OT practitioner adjusts his or her handling throughout the session according to the child's motor and sensory responses. As with any effective OT session, the OT practitioner facilitates movements through motivating and meaningful activities. NDT intervention involves creative intervention planning, flexibility, and the ability to read the children's cues.

The following case study applies the principles of NDT intervention to practice.

CASE *Study*

Christina is a 2-year-old girl who has cerebral palsy of the right spastic–hemiplegic type. Consequently, she has hypertonicity throughout her right upper and lower extremities. Christina avoids using her right hand during play. She holds her right arm in a flexed position; her hand is clenched, with her thumb inside her palm and her wrist flexed. She does not like to bear weight on her right and becomes irritable when touched on her right side. Christina pulls herself up to stand on her left side, leaving her right toe internally rotated and lightly touching the ground. She screams when the OT practitioner tries to facilitate a weight shift to the right.

Christina loves stuffed animals, especially dogs, and she enjoys music; she will try to dance to all types of music. The OT practitioner at the early learning center observes Christina on the playground and during indoor play activities. Christina plays alongside one other girl, but does not like to be touched (especially on her right side). Christina quickly crawls away when approached.

The OT practitioner decides to use an NDT approach to help Christina use both hands for play and move her body in and out of play positions with ease. The long-term goals of OT are as follows:

- Christina will use her right hand as an assist when playing with toys, as measured by her holding a large ball in both hands consistently.
- Christina will rotate her body to both sides in the sitting position to reach a toy.

To address these goals, the OT practitioner designs an intervention session using an NDT approach and decides to motivate Christina by having her play with stuffed animals during the session. Using facilitatory and inhibitory techniques, the OT practitioner decreases the spasticity in her right upper and lower extremities by gently and playfully stretching them. Next, the OT practitioner facilitates some weight bearing to the right, by placing her hands on Christina's hips (as a key point of control) and asking Christina to reach for the stuffed animal. Christina begins to get tearful as she senses this weight shift. The OT practitioner quickly praises her efforts and asks Christina to try to get to the stuffed animal from the other side. Meanwhile the OT practitioner helps Christina open her right hand, by pressing it into her own hand to normalize tone. Christina is able to bear weight leaning on the OT practitioner, and the OT practitioner is able to modify the stretch. As Christina shows signs of fatigue, the OT practitioner changes her position and allows Christina to move to the prone-on-elbows position. In this position, Christina must also bear weight on the right side. The OT practitioner continues to facilitate an open hand posture, by bringing in more stuffed animals. They end the session with a musical game in which Christina stands (supported at the hips) and shows off her latest dance move!

The OT practitioner encourages the mother to follow through with these play activities at home.

SUMMARY

OT practitioners work with children with cerebral palsy or other neuromuscular conditions whose poor postural control and movement patterns limit their active participation in daily occupations. OT practitioners use their knowledge of positioning and handling techniques to help these children succeed. Providing external stability through positioning equipment may allow these children to be successful in a variety of occupations, such as feeding, bathing, play, and academics. OT practitioners using NDT frequently prepare the children for movements using sensory techniques to inhibit or facilitate muscle tone to a more normal level. OT practitioners gently guide the children by placing their hands at key points of control and facilitating weight shifts and typical movement patterns. While facilitating movements, OT practitioners inhibit abnormal muscle tone and provide supports so that children are able to engage in meaningful activities. Positioning and handling techniques are used to help the children engage in social, academic, self-care, and play activities.

References

1. Barthel K: A frame of reference for neuro-developmental treatment. In Kramer P, Hinojosa J, editors: *Frames of reference for pediatric occupational therapy*, Philadelphia, 2009, Lippincott Williams & Wilkins.
2. Bly L: *Motor skills acquisition in the first year. An illustrated guide to normal development*, San Antonio, 1994, Therapy Skill Builders.
3. Bobath B: The very early treatment of cerebral palsy. *Dev Med Child Neurol* 9:373–390, 1967.

4. Bobath K: *A neurophysiological basis for the intervention of cerebral palsy*, London, 1980, Heinemann Books.
5. Bobath B, Bobath K: The neuro-developmental treatment. In Scrutton D et al, editors: *Management of the motor disorders of children with cerebral palsy. Clinics in developmental medicine*, Oxford, 1984, Spastics International Medical Publications.
6. Case-Smith J et al: Foundations for occupational therapy practice with children. In Case-Smith J, O'Brien J, editors: *Occupational therapy for children*, ed 6, St. Louis, 2010, Mosby.
7. Howle J: *Neuro-developmental treatment approach: theoretical foundations and principles of clinical practice*, ed 3, Laguna Beach, CA, 2007, NDTA.
8. Neurodevelopmental Intervention Association: *What is NDT?* 2008. Available at: http://www.ndta.org. Accessed March 23, 2009.
9. Schoen S, Anderson J: Neurodevelopment treatment frame of reference. In Kramer P, Hinojosa J, editors: *Frames of reference for pediatric occupational therapy*, Philadelphia, 2009, Lippincott Williams & Wilkins.
10. Shumway-Cook A, Woollacott M: *Motor control: translating research into clinical practice*, Philadelphia, 2007, Lippincott Williams & Wilkins.

REVIEW *Questions*

1. What is the typical development of positions?
2. What are the principles for the proper sitting position?
3. What are some examples of equipment that support positions?
4. What are the principles of neurodevelopmental treatment (NDT)?
5. What are some handling techniques?
6. How do OT practitioners use positioning and handling techniques in therapy for children with cerebral palsy?

SUGGESTED *Activities*

1. Practice different facilitation and inhibition techniques on your classmates.
2. Practice removing and replacing the detachable pieces on several different wheelchairs.
3. Research four types of positioning equipment that promote 1) side-lying 2) sitting, and 3) standing.
4. Using your hands and key points of control transition a classmate from prone to standing positions. Try to keep your hands on the same key point of control so you can better feel how to guide a person. Ask your partner to give you feedback on your technique.

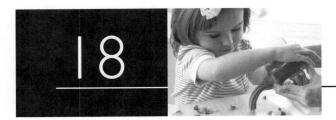

Activities of
Daily Living

MICHELLE DESJARDINS

JULIE SAVOYSKI

CHAPTER *Objectives*

After studying this chapter, the reader will be able to accomplish the following:

- Describe the progression of activities of daily living (ADLs)
- Describe a collaborative approach to help children develop the ability to engage in ADLs
- Develop intervention strategies to improve engagement in ADLs in children and youth
- Understand the concept of co-occupation as it relates to designing and implementing intervention for ADLs
- Describe remediation, compensatory, and adaptive strategies to help children perform ADLs
- Identify adaptive equipment and devices that help children perform ADLs

CASE *Study*

Ashley, a 10-year-old girl, and her family were returning home after visiting family members out of town during school vacation. Her family's car was struck by an oncoming vehicle, ejecting her through the front windshield from the passenger seat. Emergency personnel immediately transported Ashley by ambulance to a local hospital, where she was assessed and transferred via helicopter to a large pediatric acute care hospital. During her hospital stay, Ashley's medical team determined that she had sustained a traumatic brain injury (TBI) and an incomplete C6-C7 spinal cord injury (SCI). After multiple diagnostics, surgeries, and daily skilled inpatient rehabilitation, Ashley was discharged to a local pediatric unit within an acute rehabilitation facility.

After completing your new employee orientation and training period, today is your first day treating a full caseload as an occupational therapy assistant (OTA). The supervising occupational therapist gives you Ashley's chart to review and reminds you that she is first on your schedule. Her parents drove in early this morning to observe your occupational therapy (OT) session. They are concerned about Ashley's self-care abilities. What is your plan?

This chapter addresses **activities of daily living (ADLs)** in children and youth. Specifically, in accordance with the *Occupational Therapy Practice Framework: Domain and Process*, 2nd Edition, ADLs, an area of occupational performance, will be addressed in reference to the pediatric population. ADLs comprise meaningful activities that encompass self-care: bathing and showering, bowel and bladder management, dressing, eating, feeding, functional mobility, personal device care, personal hygiene and grooming, sexual activity, sleep/rest, and toilet hygiene.[2] This chapter addresses developing the OT intervention plan, implementing therapy, measuring progress, and planning for discharge. Specific intervention strategies and case examples are provided throughout to promote learning.

PEDIATRIC OCCUPATIONAL THERAPY AND ADLs: A COLLABORATIVE APPROACH

OT practitioners working in pediatrics are faced with a diverse caseload of clients with complex medical and developmental issues. Infants, children, and adolescents may present with multiple diagnoses and symptoms related to conditions that influence their overall level of functional independence in occupational performance. OT practitioners address individuals' holistically, regardless of age, disease, or disability and therefore individualize the intervention plan to meet the unique needs of each child and his or her family.

Regardless of the setting (e.g., acute care, community, school), disruption or interference with the process of development affects not only the pediatric client but also family members, caregivers, and friends within the client's physical and social environments. *Client-centered* and *family-centered* approaches are integral to the OT process, and meaningful activities should complement cultural values and beliefs.[6] Viewing the client holistically, as an *occupational being* who has individual habits, roles, and routines is considered part of the dynamic OT process.[11]

OT practitioners working with infants, children, and adolescents have the opportunity to facilitate skill acquisition so that children and adolescents can engage in a variety of ADLs. As development typically occurs in a sequential pattern, OT practitioners working with children and adolescents are challenged to think "outside the box" to determine how internal (e.g., motivation, cognition, emotions, muscle tone) and external (e.g., cultural, physical, environmental) variables interfere with development. For example, a child diagnosed with a congenital anomaly, acquired disability, or developmental disorder may present with symptoms that interfere with the maturation of functional skills. The child's condition or symptoms may interfere with his or her ability to learn both basic and higher-level skills, which may result in deficits in functional skill development and transfer of learning across multiple contexts.[20]

Pervasive developmental disorder, congenital anomalies, developmental delays, rare genetic disorders, acquired disabilities, and psychological conditions are examples of diagnoses seen by the OT practitioner who works with children and adolescents. Regardless of the symptoms related to the client's diagnosis, the OT practitioner views the individual as an occupational being who needs "to be able or enabled to engage in occupations."[23] OT practitioners working in pediatrics must possess knowledge of the theory and principles of intervention and understand the dynamics of the child and the family. Understanding their life stories and their expectations for future occupational participation is integral to the OT process.

As the OT process unfolds, analysis of occupational performance guides practice. The OT practitioner provides the groundwork for intervention by collaborating with the OTA, the child, and the family. Using a *collaborative team approach* enhances occupational performance outcomes (e.g., independence in ADLs). Under the direct supervision of the occupational therapist, the OTA may be responsible for assisting with goal development, selection of intervention approaches, determination of the means of service delivery, and selection of outcome measurements within the intervention planning process, depending on his or her level of service competence. Once the initial intervention plan begins to be implemented, OT practitioners are responsible for establishing therapeutic rapport, incorporating meaningful activities into treatment, consulting with various professionals, and providing education to the client, family, facility, and community.

A DEVELOPMENTAL PERSPECTIVE OF ADLs

Infants and toddlers rely on others to ensure that their basic needs are met. As they grow older, they begin to engage in self-care tasks such as bathing, feeding, dressing, and bowel and bladder control. They begin to move around the environment (to explore their surroundings) and sleep or rest. They learn to tolerate sensations, listen to body cues, and use their hands to manipulate objects. Infants born with congenital anomalies or inherited disorders and those born prematurely may experience difficulty tolerating, managing, and learning the skills needed to perform ADLs.

Infants, toddlers, and adolescents have many opportunities to engage in ADLs in natural settings and across multiple contexts (e.g., home, daycare, community). Peers and siblings often demonstrate how to initiate, sequence, and complete ADL tasks. Parents and teachers play essential roles in teaching children how to engage in ADLs.

Adolescents and teens experience internal variables (e.g., emotions, self-concept, motivation, initiation) and external variables (e.g., peer pressure, social expectations) that influence ADL performance. Social attention, peer pressure, *body image*, and *sexuality* influence occupational performance in activities such as hygiene, dressing, and sexual activity.

CO-OCCUPATION

The term **co-occupations** refers to occupations shared by at least two individuals.[14,24] A naturally occurring co-occupation involves a parent calming his or her child. In this case, the child is responding to the parent (social participation), and the parent is engaging in the caregiving role. Infants rely on others (such as caregivers, parents) to provide sensory stimulation, opportunities to develop relationships, and exposure to sensorimotor opportunities for skill acquisition. OT practitioners address deficits in co-occupational performance and consider the complexities of relationships when developing interventions for ADLs.[14,24]

OT practitioners work with children who come from diverse environments and cultures, including children who have been adopted from orphanages outside the United States. Exploration of the environment in early childhood is essential for optimal sensory and motor development. Many children deprived of early sensory experiences (such as those in orphanages) experience long-lasting sensory (such as vision and touch processing) and motor difficulties.[3,12] Children from orphanages who are institutionalized for prolonged periods may exhibit motor planning, sensory discrimination, and sensory modulation issues.[12] Working collaboratively to support the co-occupations of families is helpful to children and may promote the development of ADL skills.[24]

EVALUATION TO INTERVENTION

The OT practitioner completes an *occupational profile* to better understand a child's strengths and weaknesses and develop functional goals addressing occupational performance deficits. The occupational profile provides an overall picture of the child's functioning, including contraindications, signs and symptoms, and performance skills. The OT practitioner considers the child's family, culture, and environment while planning the intervention.

The following guidelines may help practitioners design various interventions to address ADLs (Box 18-1).

BOX 18-1

Guidelines to Design Interventions to Address ADL Performance

- Review the occupational profile, including goals and recommendations.
- Ensure all contraindications are taken into consideration during intervention planning and implementation.
- Be comfortable explaining the role of an OTA (in nontechnical terms) to the client and/or the family.
- Use *universal precautions* during interventions.
- Address the performance deficits and environmental modifications that enable children to be successful in participating in occupations such as ADLs.
- Encourage active client participation, and involve caregivers.
- Remember that the pediatric OT process is a dynamic one and that alterations to the intervention plan may be indicated over time.
- Consult with the supervising occupational therapist, the client, and the team (including family, caregiver, and staff members) throughout the OT process regarding goals and progress.
- Document progress clearly.
- Report any concerns about the intervention process to the supervising occupational therapist.
- Utilize available professional resources for assistance.
- Collaborate with all team members during discharge planning to ensure that the consistency of care will continue.

INTERVENTION STRATEGIES FOR THE PEDIATRIC OCCUPATIONAL THERAPY PRACTITIONER
Bathing and Showering

Bathing and showering are occupations that comprise multiple tasks and sequences, including "obtaining and using supplies; soaping, rinsing, and drying body parts; maintaining bathing position; and transferring to and from bathing positions."[2] Infants and toddlers are at the beginning stages of concept development in that they are just learning the purposes and functions of objects and activities. They have not yet ascribed meaningfulness to the act of being bathed. For infants and toddlers, bath time provides an opportunity to play and enjoy the sensations while making sense of objects. Bath time may also be a fun time for those with special needs to work on performance deficits (e.g., range of motion [ROM], stretching, positioning). Some adolescents view bathing and showering as a meaningful self-care activity that ensures health. For teens, bath time provides the OT practitioner and caregiver(s) the opportunity to work on remediating or compensating for performance skill deficits.

Children and adolescents may have difficulties with bathing and showering for many different reasons (e.g., motor, sensory, cognitive, behavioral, developmental). The OT practitioner begins with an analysis of the client's strengths and areas for growth (obtained from the occupational profile) to determine the best intervention. The following examples illustrate intervention strategies for bathing and showering.

CASE *Study*

Molly, a 3-year-old toddler, is referred to pediatric OT following a right proximal humerus fracture with no medical precautions. Areas for growth, identified from the occupational profile, include right upper extremity active ROM and strength, independence in self-care, and endurance during functional play tasks involving right upper extremity use. Molly's mother is worried about bathing her as she is hesitant to hold her and move her right arm.

What is your intervention plan? Develop a list of at least three therapeutic activities for the OT session. List four recommendations for Molly's mother addressing both therapeutic handling and safety.

With children such as Molly who are in need of remediation techniques for motor or praxis skill deficits, the focus is on meeting the client where he or she is currently functioning, facilitating the return to previous functional status, and improving overall independence. *Remediation* techniques include upper extremity therapeutic exercises (ROM and strengthening) and therapeutic activities to increase active participation and independence. *Grading* the location of bath supplies on shelves by altering the shelf height or the placement of supplies on the shelves will provide the child with reaching opportunities prior to entering the bath tub or shower area. Use of warm water creates a therapeutic environment for exercises. Some children may perceive showering or bathing as a calming, leisure-based occupation.

OT practitioners may incorporate functional activities, for example, they may have the child reach above shoulder height to retrieve their favorite toys, while physically supporting them in the bath tub as needed. Games such as various-sized water toys, weight, and resistance support the child's intrinsic motivation for play while improving bathing and showering skills. Involving the caregiver in the session helps with carryover or incorporating the OT strategies into the child's daily routines and also serves as an intervention strategy. Educating the caregiver on positioning, handling techniques, and overall safety is essential.

Children presenting with neurologic, sensory–perceptual, emotional regulation, and cognitive deficits may have difficulty with aspects of bathing and showering and require remediation. They may benefit from intervention techniques to improve motor performance to complete ADL activities guided by control or motor learning, neurodevelopmental therapy, sensory integration, or developmental frames of reference. For example, **preparatory activities** for a client with low muscle tone include stimulatory activities such as vibration, whereas calming tasks such as rocking are indicated for clients with spasticity.[17] Cold increases muscle tone, and neutral warmth relaxes muscle tone. These basic concepts are important as the activity demands of bathing and showering call for the ability to retrieve, manipulate, and use various supplies; maintain body position (i.e. standing up against gravity with water resistance or bathing in supine moving within the water); transfer between positions; and washing and drying self.[2]

Cognitive skill remediation includes analyzing tasks into small steps via forward or backward chaining (Table 18-1).[16] The OT practitioner facilitates the process by having the child or adolescent initiate the first step of a sequence or complete the last step of a sequence, depending on the chosen intervention approach. The OT practitioner continues to gradually increase the level of difficulty over time. The multicontextual frame of reference emphasizes learning skills and transferring skills to the natural context.[20]

TABLE 18-1

Forward and Backward Chaining Techniques

	DEFINITION	EXAMPLE
Forward chaining	The OT practitioner encourages the client to initiate the first step and complete the process as much as possible before the OT practitioner completes the process. The OT practitioner repeats the steps until the client completes them all.	Child takes clothes off, steps into bath, and washes self in tub; caregiver dries child off, dresses child, and empties tub water.
Backward chaining	The OT practitioner assists the client until the last step of the process and then allows the client to perform the last step; the OT practitioner repeats the process allowing the client to complete the next to last step and the last step until the client completes them all.	Caregiver takes child's clothes off, washes child in tub, dries child off. Child dresses self and empties tub water.

CASE *Study*

A 14-year-old adolescent, who has been diagnosed with schizophrenia and major depression, presents with flat affect, decreased socialization skills, and lack of motivation to complete daily grooming tasks prior to school. On the basis of the information obtained while completing the occupational profile, the OTA plans and implements a sensory inventory to gain more information about the child's sensory preferences for intervention. The adolescent reports a strong preference for warm sensations. The OTA, the adolescent, and the mother work together, coming up with a strategy to increase the adolescent's motivation and frequency for showering. The collaborative decision to have the adolescent's mother turn on the shower 2 minutes before wake-up time, paired with the verbal cue "Your warm shower is ready," helps the adolescent tolerate the shower three times during the first week. The adolescent's motivation to engage in bathing and showering is facilitated by the intrinsic motivation for experiencing sensations involving warmth and hearing her supportive mother's voice. The adolescent and the mother both report a sense of progress in accomplishing ADLs—a true example of successful co-occupational performance.

In addition to remediation, OT intervention may include *compensatory techniques*. For example, children with deficits that interfere with ADL performance (such as congenital anomalies resulting in delayed growth) may benefit from the following:

- Self-care training using assistive devices or adapted techniques, including long-handled self-care supplies (i.e., sponge), shower chairs, reachers, nonslip tub mats, safety bars, and/or removable shower heads

- Staff supervision and implementation of a *visual schedule* for an adolescent with cognitive skill deficits residing in a group home setting, which is another possibility for support during occupational participation
- Labeling items in large print and contrasting colors to support pediatric clients with low vision
- Incorporating adaptive techniques such as using a container with one U-shaped side to rest against the client's head for washing hair to eliminate the need to tilt the head backward, which may cause distress.
- Ensuring a smooth transition from a bath or shower with a snug towel wrap to help the client handle increased sensitivity to change in temperatures and to provide the sensory supports to maintain an optimal level of arousal
- Education to parents, caregivers, and staff members on the level of supervision needed throughout bathing and showering as necessary
- Rearrangement of a client's bathroom to accommodate a wheelchair and/or shower chair as necessary
- Education on *work simplification* or *energy conservation* to support co-occupation and prevent caregiver "burnout," especially when the child's needs are complex and physically taxing for the caregiver

Assistive technology may help children succeed in performing ADLs. Computer-simulated programs for self-care tasks may assist the children in learning the required sequences for bathing and showering prior to attempting the multistep task in the natural context. Using the computer for organizational purposes may be beneficial as well. Having a concrete visual schedule that includes the day and time for bathing and showering is an additional means of cognitive support.

Multiple modes of functional communication may promote self-advocacy in the child or adolescent. For example, a young child who is nonverbal may use an alternative augmentative communication (AAC) device. The OT practitioner facilitates self-advocacy by ensuring that the means of communication is readily available and accessible at all times.[18] A voice output device may allow children with neurologic conditions such as cerebral palsy to express preferences for occupations, including activities throughout the bathing and showering process, that do not compromise breathing.

Bowel and Bladder Management

Bowel and bladder management encompasses both the voluntary control of bowel and bladder movements as well as the utilization of alternative methods, including the use of equipment, to support bladder control.[2,21] In order to optimally manage bowel and bladder functions, which include processes of both volition and intention, an intact neurologic system is essential.[9]

Infants and toddlers begin developing the concept of bowel and bladder functions in addition to processing sensations before developing motor control abilities for the volitional control of their actions. As with all development, some children will mature in this domain at an earlier stage of life than will others. Young children, through either structured or nonstructured programming, have environmental affordances such as education, caregiver assistance, peer-modeling opportunities, and physical setup to support the development of functional skills. During the school-age years, children develop and participate in a consistent routine. Continued adaptations are made in accordance with daily scheduled activities throughout adolescence and the teenage years.

CASE *Study*

Destiny, an 11-year-old child, attends a private day school for children with complex needs, including behavioral and sensory issues. According to her occupational profile and individualized education program (IEP), Destiny's primary medical and educational diagnoses are visual impairment, hearing impairment, and autism. She relies primarily on her *tactile, proprioceptive,* and *vestibular* sensory systems for information regarding where she is physically in space as well as in proximity to other persons and objects within her physical environment. In addition to OT, she receives speech and language therapy and physical therapy services. Destiny also works with a certified orientation and mobility specialist,

who teaches those with visual impairment and has advanced training in teaching those with hearing impairments

Destiny's educational team members are concerned about her new behaviors this week. Today is the third consecutive day of inconsistent behaviors with regard to bowel and bladder management. The para-professional who works with Destiny and her teacher inform you that Destiny's requests to use the bathroom have been inconsistent with her previous behaviors. Previously, she required only check-ins, but now she requires one-on-one constant supervision because of her tactile-seeking behaviors, including smearing feces on the bathroom walls. The team members also report that her stools are loose and that she has been having multiple "accidents" during the day. They ask you for guidance, since Destiny's sensory-seeking behaviors interfere with her safety and hygiene. In addition, the team is wondering if Destiny's new behaviors are intentional to get attention and have something to do with arrival of a new student in her classroom this week. What are you going to suggest to the team?

You contact her caregiver and learn that over the weekend Destiny had experienced difficulty with bowel management due to constipation. Her caregiver reports that Destiny was given an over-the-counter stool softener; misreading of the dosage instructions had led to too much of the medication being given and consequently loose stools for the past 3 days. According to the caregiver, this is the first time Destiny has had bowel difficulties since she developed independence in bowel and bladder management. Her pediatrician has suggested stopping the stool softener and encouraging Destiny to drink a lot of water throughout the day. Does this additional information change your intervention plan?

CLINICAL *Pearl*

Collecting and using as much background information as possible is an essential skill throughout the pediatric OT process.

OT practitioners work with children and adolescents who have difficulties with bowel and bladder management. Common symptoms such as increased urinary frequency, lack of voluntary bowel control, and decreased sensory awareness are associated with multiple diagnoses, especially those associated with injuries to the brain, spinal cord, and/or nerves (e.g., shaken baby syndrome, spinal cord injury [SCI]).[9] Regardless of etiology, bowel and bladder management may be an integral occupation for remediation and/or compensation during the pediatric OT intervention process.

CLINICAL *Pearl*

When working with pediatric clients who have a diagnosis of spinal cord injury (SCI) at or above the T6 level, monitor for signs and/or symptoms of *autonomic dysreflexia (AD)*. AD occurs when noxious stimulation is unable to reach the brain. Instead, the information (i.e., a full bladder) reaches the spinal cord, which triggers a reflex that results in constriction of blood vessels below the injury leading to increased blood pressure. The brain attempts to send signals to dilate blood vessels, but the information cannot travel past the level of injury. Consequently, blood vessels above the injury dilate but are unable to decrease the overall increase in blood pressure. AD has the potential to result in a heart attack or death. Signs and symptoms include the following:

- Red blotches above the level of injury
- Hypertension
- Nasal congestion
- Chills
- Sweating

If a child or adolescent demonstrates signs or symptoms of AD, the OT practitioner immediately follows procedures in place at the facility regarding medical attention. When indicated, the child may benefit from being positioned into the **Semi-Fowler's position** to support abdominal relaxation and breathing.[9] The pediatric client's head should be elevated (30 to 45 degrees), and knees are to be in either flexion or extension bilaterally.[9] OT intervention addressing bowel and bladder management may help prevent future episodes of AD.[16]

CASE *Study*

Ashley, the young girl in the previous case study, who had sustained a spinal cord injury (SCI) at the C6-C7 level, lost the sensation and volitional control of both bowel and bladder functions. In addition, she has short-term memory loss due to the traumatic brain injury (TBI). She is returning to school full time in 1 month. Ashley needs strategies to recall the steps of her bowel and bladder program. Ashley is especially concerned that she will forget the steps for optimal bowel and bladder management and experience embarrassment. What strategies might the OT practitioner working in a home-based practice implement to help Ashley re-learn the multistep sequence for bowel and bladder management?

In early infancy and toddlerhood, parent education is essential for learning bowel and bladder management and handling techniques. Bowel and bladder management may be a sensitive topic to children and adolescents. For children who have experienced acute trauma, discussing self-catheterization or having a caregiver complete tasks for them may cause feelings of embarrassment and frustration. Privacy and dignity are integral aspects of intervention.

Remediation techniques for bowel and bladder management may include therapeutic handling during diaper changes to deal with fluctuating muscle tone, development of an individualized toileting program, and implementation of a behavioral reward program. Compensatory strategies include use of pull-ups or adult diapers, and adult-directed timed schedule. A pediatric client who has sustained a hip fracture may benefit from a raised toilet seat to avoid hip flexion. Children and adolescents may need to be trained in catheterization. This training is usually a collaborative effort between the OT practitioner, the nurse, the caregivers, and the child.

Dressing

Dressing is an occupation that involves multistep processes and is influenced by both internal and external variables. Selecting appropriate clothing and accessories in accordance with external variables, including weather conditions, special occasions, and/or times of day, requires intact higher level cognitive processes.[2] Perceived self-image, sense of style, and sensory preferences are some potential internal variables that may influence the dressing process. Typically, the sequence of dressing includes retrieving clothing items from a storage area and completing dressing/undressing tasks as appropriate. Developmentally, as gross motor movements precede fine motor movements, using fasteners, adjusting clothing and shoes, and the application and/or removal of devices occur after the child is able to complete dressing and undressing tasks. See Chapter 7 for the sequence of dressing skills.

Infants rely on caregivers to dress/undress them. Toddlers play dress-up and begin to develop basic skills to dress and undress. Children move from play-based dressing activities to occupations requiring specific dress codes, for example, dance and soccer, which require conformity to a costume or specific attire. The school-aged child moves from relying on caregivers to choose clothing to developing an individualized style or preference for certain clothing. Favorite colors, textures, and styles begin to drive a child's intrinsic motivation to independently go through the dressing process. Teens may change clothing preferences in response to peer pressure to look a certain way. The OT practitioner considers a child's motor and sensory skills, and motivations (e.g., preferences for style) when developing a dressing intervention program.

CASE *Study*

Megan, a 6-year-old child, with a diagnosis of "status post–left cerebrovascular accident (CVA)," with right hemiparesis and right neglect, has trouble dressing. Megan has difficulty completing the fine motor aspects of dressing. She is able to don and doff large, loose-fitting clothing items with minimal physical assistance and requires moderate verbal cues to use her right upper extremity as an assist during dressing.

Megan presents with right upper extremity spasticity, and her fist remains in full flexion. Despite the cold weather, she comes to the clinic without wearing a jacket. The OT practitioner observes her walking down the hallway. Megan appears comfortable wearing only a sweat shirt and jogging pants; yet, the right side of her waist band is twisted, and the back of her shirt is bunched up at her waist line. She continues walking to the OT room without verbalizing or demonstrating signs of discomfort.

Once in the OT room, Megan's mother reports that Megan has had difficulty getting ready for school this week. Reportedly, she is frustrated with even simple dressing tasks such as zipping her jeans and buttoning large buttons. Megan states that she "hates buttoning and zipping" and does not want to work on using her hands, as the right one is "no good anyway." Megan's mother rolls her eyes and states that Megan must learn how to dress herself.

Megan's current short-term goals include fastening four or five large buttons (one inch in diameter) with minimal physical assistance for accuracy and zipping her jacket with set-up and minimal verbal cues. What is your intervention plan? Describe your intervention plan and expected outcomes.

You decide to work on increasing Megan's motivation to dress herself by discussing her preferences for styles, colors, textures, and clothing. Once you both select an outfit more like that of her teen peers, Megan becomes interested in dressing. She seems more concerned about her appearance.

Dressing involves a complex sequence of events. Many children and adolescents with special needs experience difficulties completing the various aspects of the dressing process. OT practitioners apply their knowledge of typical development when working with children who need remediation, compensation, and education on dressing (Figures 18-1 through 18-3).

Remediation strategies include helping children who exhibit motor and *praxis* skill deficits through practice with repetition and variation, as described in the section on motor control/motor learning.[17] In addition, symptoms related to neurologic conditions, for example, *visual neglect*, changes in muscle tone, and diminished sensation, require the OT practitioner to incorporate therapeutic handling techniques, including muscle tone facilitation and/or inhibition techniques in the neurodevelopmental treatment (NDT) approach.[17] Conditions resulting in such symptoms as weakness require the pediatric OT practitioner to grade the *activity demands*. For example, a child with fair bilateral upper extremity strength may benefit from therapeutic ROM and strengthening activities, as derived from the biomechanical frames of reference.[5]

The OT practitioner working with children may have the opportunity to address dressing issues within a natural context, such as when a child changes into a bathing suit for an aquatic therapy sessions. Some children are unable to consistently demonstrate the same abilities across different contexts. Many rehabilitation centers have pools with locker rooms and bathroom/shower facilities that provide grab bars and shower chairs. Providing OT services within the child's natural environment is ideal, as the task of dressing/undressing has a sense of purpose.

A child or adolescent with sensory processing issues may present with a broad range of symptoms. As praxis is an end product of sensory integration (SI), the ability to develop even the idea of how to begin dressing can be a major area of difficulty for some children.[3] For example, some children have difficulty tolerating certain fabrics and types of clothing. Children with sensory processing difficulties may become agitated with clothing that is too snug or has tight waist bands or wrist bands. Some children need to have their new clothes washed before wearing them. Box 18-2 provides some dressing strategies for children who are sensitive to certain textures.

BOX 18-2

Strategies for Children Who Have Sensory Processing Issues

- Wash new clothes in familiar detergent before having the child wear them.
- Use detergent with mild or no fragrance.
- Allow the child to pick his or her clothing.
- Be sensitive about the waist bands, wrist bands, and neck region.
- Cut out tags completely before the child wears the clothes.
- Some children prefer "gently used" clothes; others want new clothes.
- Not all children will prefer loose clothing; some may prefer tighter-fitting clothing.
- Be aware of each child's individual clothing preferences.
- Ask children to express themselves through colors and styles of clothing.

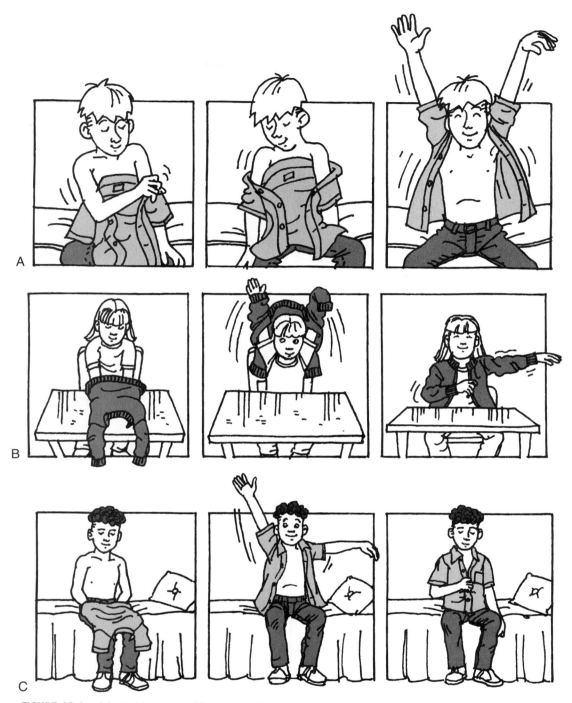

FIGURE 18-1   Adapted Methods of Putting on a Shirt. **A,** Lap and over-the-head hemiplegic method. **B,** Front lap and facing-down method. **C,** Front lap and facing-down hemiplegic method.

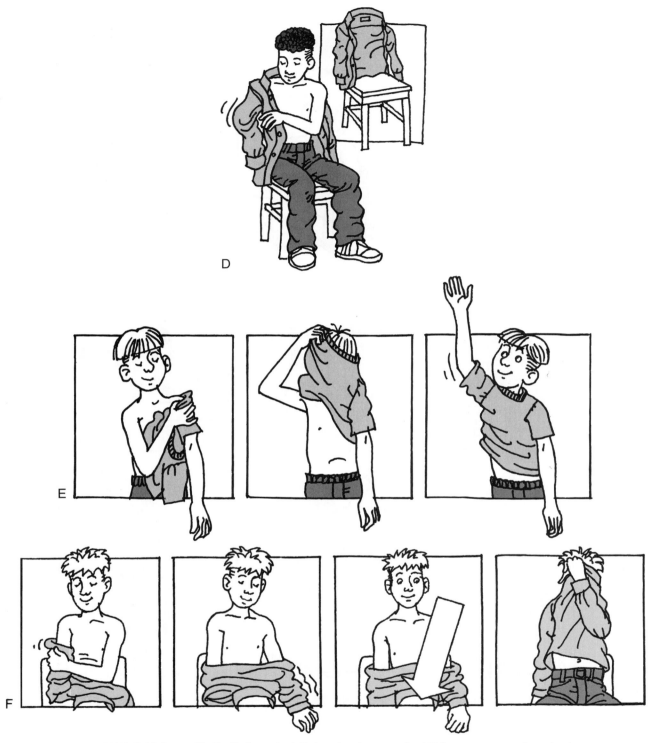

FIGURE 18-1, cont'd D, Chair method. **E,** Arm-head-arm method. **F,** Lap-arm-arm-neck method.

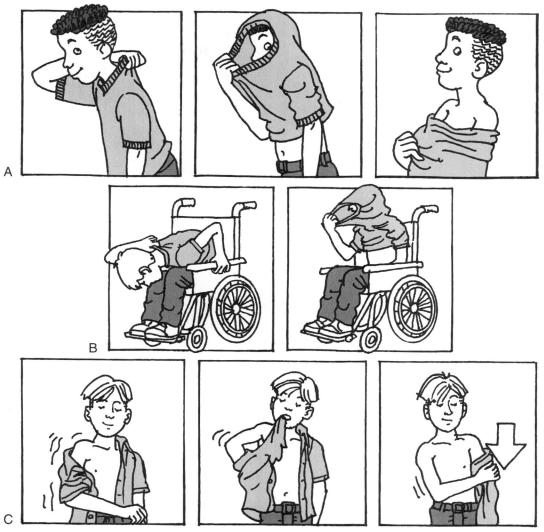

FIGURE 18-2 Adapted Methods of Taking off a Shirt. **A,** Over-the-head method. **B,** Duck-the-head-and-sit-up method. **C,** Arms-in-front method.

Compensatory strategies that may be beneficial to children include assistive devices (ADs) and adaptive equipment (AE), such as pediatric-sized reachers, button hooks, leg raisers, sock-aids, loops for clothing, shirts and pants without tags, socks without seams, and Velcro fasteners. OT practitioners must be sure that children and their caregivers demonstrate competency in using equipment and devices before recommending them. Children may benefit from utilizing ADs or AE for more immediate gratification.

Children may benefit from visual supports during the dressing process as initiation, sequencing, and activity completion.[20] OT practitioners consider motor, cognitive, and emotional factors as well as the contexts (e.g., cultural, temporal) when designing dressing intervention.

Eating/Swallowing

Eating includes the ability to maintain and control food and/or fluid in the mouth as well as **swallowing**.[2] The terms *swallowing* and *eating* are used interchangeably in some of the literature; the term *swallowing* will be used here for consistency. Swallowing is a specialized area in OT practice.[2] Some OT practitioners may work with premature babies in the neonatal intensive care unit (NICU) setting, and others may work in a community-based OT program that involves maturation of swallowing skills. Swallowing is a complex process that requires intact sensory, motor, and voluntary actions. The OT practitioner typically provides intervention as part of a feeding team. In addition to the infant, child or adolescent, team members may include the caregiver(s), physician, nurse, speech and

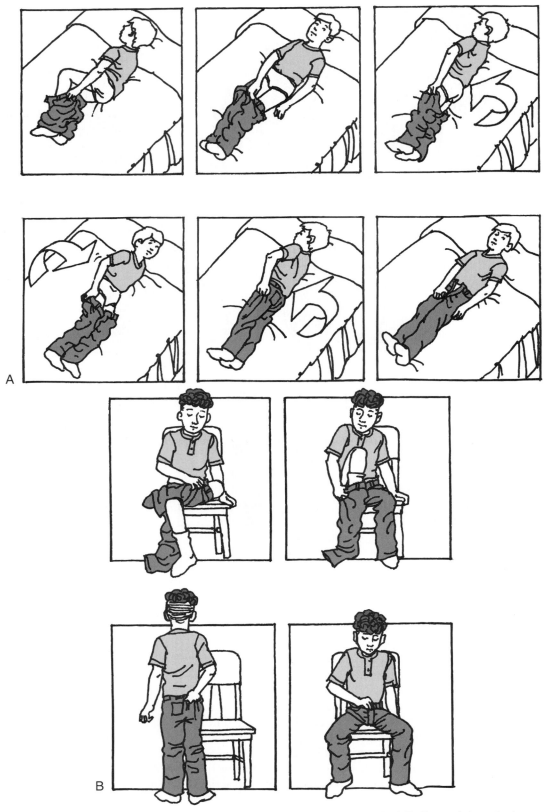

FIGURE 18-3 Adapted Methods of Putting on Pants. **A,** Supine-roll method. **B,** Sit-stand-sit method.

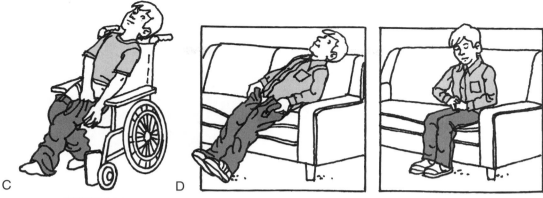

FIGURE 18-3, cont'd C, One-side bridge-sitting method. **D,** Bridge-sitting method.

language pathologist (SLP), SLP assistant, educator, and para-professionals.

From a developmental perspective, the suck–swallow–breathe synchrony typically emerges as the first self-regulatory activity during the prenatal period.[3] Caregivers provide sensory exploration opportunities to the infant when novel foods and liquids are introduced.[8] Toddlers develop feeding preferences, and fears of new foods arise.[8] With continued opportunities to explore, try, and develop early swallowing skills, the toddler matures his or her ability in attempting and/or accepting varied foods. During the school-aged years and into adolescence, food selection follows a narrower trend, as personal preferences emerge.[8] The teenager continues to change preferences based on variables such as peer group preferences. Culture influences the choice of foods as well.

Children who have difficulty swallowing foods and/or liquids are frequently referred for OT. The role of the OT practitioner may include providing intervention within a feeding group, monitoring a child for signs and symptoms of aspiration during lunch within the educational setting, and/or providing direct intervention within the acute care setting to a teen recovering from an accident that caused jaw instability .

Regardless of the context, intervention planning and implementation of OT services for children who are in need of remediation for swallowing difficulties may include oral motor/oral sensory programming, NDT muscle tone techniques, jaw rehabilitation (including jaw strengthening programming), and team/or education regarding safe swallowing.[4]

As proximal stability precedes distal mobility, swallowing is often correlated with fine motor abilities. An infant may require preparatory activities, including strategies to improve the suck–swallow–breathe synchrony.[3,4] Toddlers presenting with oral sensory defensiveness may benefit from joint compressions for increased proprioception or the Wilbarger Protocol, which includes oral proprioceptive

techniques.[22] School-aged children may benefit from biomechanical techniques to develop swallowing skills, including therapeutic exercises to increase ROM and strength.

OT practitioners may choose to use *compensatory strategies* with children and adolescents. For example, an 8 year old diagnosed with Down syndrome places food at her molars to compensate for decreased tongue coordination and low oral muscle tone. Nutrition is a major concern in the case of children with swallowing issues. Nurses and caregivers support pediatric clients with severe swallowing issues by administering G-tube and/or J-tube feedings. In addition, nurses and caregivers provide suctioning for the medically fragile pediatric client unable to manage his or her own saliva. Products to thicken liquids such as Thick-it or wheat germ, diet adaptations (i.e., puréed consistency for all foods, Pediasure for added nutritional value), change in physical context and/or type of chair for proximal support and optimal positioning may be indicated to compensate for limited and/or lack of safe swallowing. See Box 18-3 for techniques to promote swallowing.

Internal and external factors have the potential to adversely affect the pediatric client's ability to swallow safely. Internally, congenital anomalies in the oral cavity, sensory processing issues, and increased muscle tone are examples of common symptoms that interfere with optimal swallowing.

CASE *Study*

George, a 12-year-old student diagnosed with pervasive developmental delay (PDD), receives educationally based OT services on a biweekly basis. He has difficulties with saliva management and coordinating the oral phase of swallowing. His swallowing issues interfere with his personal safety and general health.

BOX 18-3

Techniques to Promote Swallowing in Children and Adolescents

- Position infants in the semi-reclined position.
- Position toddlers and teens in the upright sitting position, with the neck slightly flexed forward.
- Provide oral–motor stimulation to children who have low oral–motor musculature.
- Vibration, quick stroking (above lip, on cheeks) may improve swallowing.
- For infants with swallowing difficulties, provide jaw control to improve ability to suck on the bottle (by gently holding the fat pads on the cheeks).
- Provide jaw control to help toddlers and adolescents swallow.
- Thicker liquids are easier for most children to control and swallow.
- Do not force children to put anything in the mouth.
- Encourage children to suck on ice pop or something sour.
- Provide a calm setting for the child. Distractions may interfere with swallowing.
- Do not talk to the infant while feeding (this may distract him or her).
- Work slowly with the child. Some children may have a delayed swallow.
- Promote tongue lateralization by encouraging the child to reach both sides of the mouth for food (i.e., place cracker on one side of mouth to encourage tongue movement to side).

The OT practitioner in the junior high school observes him sitting on a bench between two of his classmates at a typical long table. For lunch, his caregiver packed yogurt, milk, a ham sandwich, and pretzels. Active ROM (AROM) of the jaw and lip closure are within functional limits during drinking through a straw or swallowing yogurt. While eating his sandwich, he takes large bites without completing a full chew–swallow cycle and pockets food in his cheeks. He sips his milk and tilts his head back, using gravity and liquid to move his food to the back of his throat. He does not observably chew his sandwich all the time. While George is finishing his meal with the small pretzel rods, the school bell rings indicating 15 minutes remaining prior to outdoor recess. George begins to rock back and forth while stuffing multiple pretzels into his mouth. He finishes early and carries his trash to the appropriate waste bucket. His cheeks are still full with some of the sandwich and pretzel rods. The final bell rings, and he places his hands over his ears and screeches. His eyes become watery, and his voice sounds wet. George has a couple of coughing episodes, and then his para-professional accompanies him out to recess.

CLINICAL *Pearl*

Children diagnosed with low vision and/or blindness may require staff and/or caregivers to provide them with information regarding foods and liquids. Ensure that these children receive accurate information and are able to express their likes and dislikes. Do not force a child to eat something that is not a preferred food.

Feeding

Feeding, which will be referred to as "self-feeding" in this chapter, involves the set-up, arrangement, and movement of food items and/or fluids from a dish/plate or cup/glass to one's mouth.[2] The process of self-feeding requires higher-level cognitive skills, including praxis (motor planning). *Ideational praxis* skills support planning for the sequential events involved in self-feeding. Task initiation, sequencing, and completion of self-feeding occur in a typical pattern. Depending on traditions followed in various cultures, the self-feeding process may include role changes, habits, and/or rituals.[11] The physical, social, and virtual contexts are important considerations in the self-feeding process. Physical accessibility, the opportunity to socialize with family and friends, as well as altering the context to include a virtual component is possible. Computer technology has provided us with the opportunity to even have dinner with a distant relative via programs such as Skype.

CLINICAL *Pearl*

Technological advancements such as computer programs (e.g., Skype) provide professionals and patients with a virtual means of video conferencing. Within the virtual context, OT practitioners can utilize computer programs to confer with colleagues and patients without being in the same physical, social, and/or temporal context.

Infants work on developing the suck–swallow–breathe synchrony, often finding pleasure in drinking from a bottle and/or breast-feeding.[3] Self-feeding provides the infant with the opportunity to bond with caregivers during occupational engagement. The toddler explores foods as well as the self-feeding process via play. A small play kitchen with a toy refrigerator and a toy oven provide the toddler and young school-aged child with the opportunity to engage in the occupation of self-feeding at both parallel and interactive levels of play. Over time, responsibility for tasks such as setting the dinner table is introduced. Habits and routines may form as the child assumes a role in the process as school-aged children may find meaning in assisting with self-feeding tasks such as set-up and clean-up. During adolescence, socialization with peers during self-feeding occurs on a more frequent basis. As the child grows, the contexts change, and transfer of learning is required as self-feeding activity occurs across multiple environments.

Many children present with immature self-feeding patterns and are in need of remediation. The young child diagnosed with developmental coordination disorder (DCD) may require practice and repetition, with variation, to succeed in carrying his milk cartons from the school kitchen to the lunch room, without dropping the tray or losing his balance. For example, a child diagnosed with Rothmund-Thompson syndrome reaches above shoulder height to retrieve plates and cups while also working on preventing joint contractures, as she may benefit from a biomechanical approach. Provided with material set-up at midline and to his left, an adolescent boy with a diagnosis of left neglect turns his head toward the left, using his functional vision, reaches for, retrieves, and places food cans on his wheel-chair tray. A teenage girl recently diagnosed with an acute brachial plexus injury engages in therapeutic upper extremity elbow flexion and extension active/assisted ROM exercises as preparation for spoon to mouth activities.

CLINICAL *Pearl*

Rothmund-Thomson syndrome (RTS) is a rare genetic disorder characterized by short stature, thumb and/or radial anomalies, juvenile cataracts, gastrointestinal issues, osteopenia, absent patella(s), alopecia, high risk of bone and skin cancers, and/or poikiloderma (skin rash); 300 cases of RTS have been identified so far in the literature.

When the OT practitioner chooses to use a compensatory approach, techniques associated with the rehabilitative frame of reference, including altering and/or adapting the task, materials, or the environment may support active engagement in self-feeding. Caregivers may engage in self-feeding as a co-occupation, setting up self-feeding items close to the child who fatigues easily during reaching tasks. ADs and/or AE including universal cuffs to hold utensils, self-feeding devices, weighted utensils, and splints (i.e., a *tenodesis* splint commonly used by a child with status–post C5-C6 SCI) support the compensatory pattern of using active wrist extension to promote a tenodesis action, in order to pick up self-feeding materials.

CLINICAL *Pearl*

Children who have sustained a neurologic injury at level C6 and/or above typically have intact active wrist extension. *Tenodesis* is a typical movement pattern that occurs as a result of the volitional ability to actively extend the wrist against gravity. During active wrist extension, the digits move into a flexion pattern. In contrast, when the child allows his or her wrist to lower (wrist flexion) with the assistance of gravity, the digits typically extend.[11a] The tenodesis action can be utilized to assist with both grasping and release of objects. A wrist–hand orthotic (WHO) such as a tenodesis orthosis helps facilitate this. OT practitioners engage children in functional activities that do not require tight digit flexion, as excessive stretching of the flexor tendons may potentially interfere with tenodesis.[11a] As a result of having the ability to utilize the tenodesis action, in addition to appropriate assistive devices and/or adaptive equipment, the child has the opportunity to increase his or her overall level of functional independence in ADLs.

Functional Mobility

Functional mobility is defined as "moving from one position or place to another during performance of everyday activities, such as in-bed mobility, wheelchair mobility, or transfers (wheelchair, bed, car, tub, toilet, tub/shower, chair, floor)."[1] Children's functional mobility can be affected in a variety of ways for any number of reasons. Some children have developmental delays that resolve with intensive early intervention services. Other children have mobility impairments and require external support in the form of orthotics or durable medical equipment (DME), such as a wheelchair, for mobility. In collaboration with the occupational therapist, the OTA determines the most appropriate intervention approach to enable a child to move from place to place to engage in meaningful activities. The child's goals (or desired outcomes), data from the evaluation, and evidence are considered when developing the intervention plan. Intervention approaches include health promotion, remediation and restoration, maintenance, modification, or prevention.[2]

Health promotion is **intervention** that seeks to create and promote activity in the context of daily life.[2] An example of health promotion related to functional mobility is the efforts of pediatricians and early intervention providers to encourage "tummy time" to promote healthy infant motor development.[10] Another example of health promotion encourages children to play outside as a reaction to rising childhood obesity statistics related to sedentary activities.[7]

For some children, the intervention approach for functional mobility may require the OT practitioner to establish, remediate, or restore specific skills.[2] As children grow, there may be a variety of factors that influence skill acquisition. A child with low muscle tone, as is commonly seen in children with Down syndrome, who shows a delay in crawling may benefit from intervention aimed at increasing trunk strength to allow him to hold his head parallel to the floor while in the quadruped position. A therapeutic session may begin with preparatory techniques designed to facilitate tone, such as playing with a vibrating toy.[13] The child might then be placed on his stomach over a therapy ball while holding his head up to enable him to play with objects of interest in his hands. Ball placement should start proximally, supporting the majority of his trunk. The OTA slowly moves the ball distally to promote increased use of trunk muscles over time. Finally, the child might be placed in a supported quadruped position on the floor to facilitate crawling to a desired object. See Chapter 17 for additional information on handling and positioning.

For some children, such as those with neurologic disorders, the use of positioning techniques and orthoses/splinting can be used to maintain skills, including those required for functional mobility. Some children may require equipment to modify, compensate for, or adapt to limited movement, such as a brace, pediatric walker, or wheelchair. The needs of the child and the family should be taken into consideration when determining the most appropriate equipment. See Chapter 27 for additional information on orthoses.

Finally, *prevention* efforts may be aimed at eliminating potential barriers to occupational performance in the area of functional mobility. A simple prevention effort for a child who is gaining functional mobility but lacks adequate safety awareness includes environmental manipulation in the form of a gate to block off access to stairs or other dangers. Another example of prevention from a therapeutic standpoint is the OTA providing education to caregivers of children with neurologic conditions such as head injury and SCI about the importance of proper bed and wheelchair positioning; ROM programs, to maintain proper joint alignment for control of abnormal tone and prevention of contractures, should also be provided.[15]

As with all areas of occupation, the needs of the child and the family will ultimately dictate the appropriate interventions for children with impairments that impact functional mobility. The pediatric OT practitioner identifies and builds on the strengths of the child and the family. When designing an intervention approach, it is important to consider the various settings and contexts where the child or adolescent is likely to engage in functional mobility.[19]

CASE *Study*

Rosalie was born prematurely at 27 weeks gestation. She qualified for early intervention (EI) services on the basis of her premature birth and other risk factors, including her mother's advanced age and use of narcotics during pregnancy, as well as the family's qualification for a number of state-sponsored welfare services. A re-evaluation has revealed that Rosalie demonstrates significant developmental delays across all domains (cognitive, self-care, personal–social, fine–gross motor, and receptive–expressive language) and confirms her need for EI services. A developmental specialist has been the service coordinator (SC) for the family. Rosalie is still not crawling at 11 months of age. The SC calls in OT services to obtain greater expertise around gross motor development. After a consultation between the SC and an occupational therapist, it is clear that Rosalie is able to sit with a wide base of support but she cannot maintain trunk control in a facilitated quadruped position. What is the best intervention approach for Rosalie?

Personal Device Care and Personal Hygiene/Grooming

Personal device care is defined as "using, cleaning, and maintaining personal care items such as hearing aids, contact lenses, glasses, orthotics, prosthetics, adaptive equipment, and contraceptive and sexual devices."[1] **Personal hygiene/grooming** is defined as "obtaining and using supplies; washing, drying, combing, styling, brushing, and trimming hair; caring for nails; caring for skin, ears, eyes, and nose; applying deodorant; cleaning mouth; brushing and flossing teeth."[2] Younger children largely depend on their parents to provide personal device care. As children get older, it may be appropriate to take a more active role in the management of their own personal device care. Additionally, managing personal hygiene and grooming becomes more important as the child grows older. This process may prove to be difficult for a child receiving services from an OTA for any number of reasons. Some children have difficulties with the process skills of temporal organization as well as organization of space and objects, which affect the ability to complete the tasks involved in grooming. A visual schedule is one treatment approach that may be helpful in remediating such issues. The role of the OTA may be to assist with creating a daily schedule to assist with personal device care and grooming tasks. The visual schedule should be individualized, and the context of the task, as it relates to the client and caregivers, should be taken into consideration. Pictures breaking down a process into steps can be posted at a logical place so that the child may utilize the visual aid. Constructing such a schedule often involves trial and error and may need to be amended many times until it works optimally for any client.

A child's or adolescent's satisfaction with his or her own hygiene may often be different from that of his or her caregiver. In such a case, it is important to educate the child on the benefits of good hygiene and work with both the child and the caregiver to come to an agreement regarding the essential tasks and the frequency of performance.

Some children require modifications due to difficulties in the performance skills of strength and effort, so adaptive equipment may be indicated to promote increased independence for completion of grooming activities. For individuals who have a limited ability to grasp small handles, a universal cuff can be used to hold a toothbrush, comb, hair brush, or razor. Some cuffs can be weighted to provide better control. For difficulties with grip strength, a built-up handle can be useful. Angled or long-handled brushes can be helpful to individuals with limited ROM. Bathroom faucet handles can be adapted to be easier to maneuver. Additional equipment that may assist an individual in completing grooming tasks include the electric toothbrush, floss holder, or water flosser.

CASE *Study*

Elliot is a 16 year old with Asperger's syndrome. His parents sought occupational therapy services because he has difficulty completing his morning and evening hygiene routines in a timely fashion. Elliot had worked with an occupational therapist who helped him develop a visual schedule—a number of pictures posted on a single large poster board—that hangs on his bedroom wall. Elliot is having difficulty accessing the visual schedule. How could the existing schedule be modified to be more accessible to Elliot?

Sexual Activity

CASE *Study*

Damyen is a 15-year-old student who lives at a residential school for students with visual impairments. In addition, Damyen has a diagnosis of autism. Since entering puberty, Damyen has started to masturbate frequently in public places. This behavior not only makes other students and the staff uncomfortable but also affects Damyen's ability to effectively perform his educational tasks. In collaboration with the school support team, an OTA, under the supervision of an occupational therapist, develops a plan to address Damyen's behavior. They begin by introducing the language of labeling "public or not private" and "private"

spaces and teaching Damyen to understand the difference. Every time he starts to touch himself in a public space, he is brought to his room or to a bathroom and he is taught that masturbation is something people do in a private place. The goal is that once Damyen understands the difference, he will ask for private time when he needs it. Once this goal is accomplished, the team slowly has him wait longer and longer. For example, when he asks for private time, the staff member says, "One more (minute, half hour, etc.)." Slowly, Damyen is able to increase the time he waits for private time so that the behavior becomes more manageable and appropriate. Damyen is better able to attend to his educational occupation.

Sexual activity is defined as "engagement in activities that result in sexual satisfaction."[2] Sexual activity becomes an area of increasing importance as children approach adolescence. Some clients the OTA encounters may engage in socially inappropriate sexual activity, for example, masturbating in public, without understanding why it makes others uncomfortable. In some cases, the role of the OTA may be to work with the child to establish and encourage the appropriate context for sexual activity. Creating a plan for appropriate times and places to experience sexual relief can be empowering to the child and help avoid awkward situations.

Sleep/Rest

CASE *Study*

Dora is 25 months old. Her parents have recently moved from one city to another for career advancement opportunities. Dora's parents are concerned about her motor development. She is evaluated by an interdisciplinary early intervention (EI) team. The evaluation results reveal that she has a gross motor delay that qualifies her for OT services through EI.

Dora's parents also express their concern that Dora has been waking up in the middle of the night and is inconsolable unless she is allowed into her parent's bed. This behavior started shortly after the move when Dora began to wake up crying in the middle of the night. Her parents felt bad about uprooting her and allowed her in their bed to comfort her; however, it has gotten out of control and has now become a nightly occurrence. This has been affecting the entire family's ability to sleep through the night. What can you suggest to the family?

Sleep/rest is defined as "a period of inactivity in which one may or may not suspend consciousness."[2] Sleep is an area of occupation in its own right, and sleep disturbances could have a serious impact on the quality of an entire family's life. Young children may experience sleep disturbances for a variety of reasons. An intervention may be suggested after the reason for the sleep disturbance is carefully evaluated. If appropriate, behavioral interventions may be proposed to help change inconvenient sleep patterns. Other interventions that can be helpful include using sensory principles, for example, calming deep pressure to help soothe the child in preparation for sleep. Sensory diets may be helpful in regulating a child's sleep–wake cycles.[22]

Toilet Hygiene

CASE *Study*

Kara is a 13 year old who was in a motor vehicle accident a month ago. She sustained a fractured right humeral head and now receives outpatient OT. Because of Kara's current limited upper extremity ROM, she requires assistance with toilet hygiene. She is mortified by her need to have anyone help her with this personal task and asks you, her OTA, if there is anything that can be done immediately to help her increase her independence to perform the task. You recall seeing a piece of equipment designed to help individuals reach behind to wipe themselves. Can you find such a device in a catalog?

Toilet hygiene is defined as "obtaining and using supplies; clothing management; maintaining toileting position; transferring to and from the toilet; cleaning the body; and caring for menstrual and incontinence needs (including catheters, colostomies, and suppository management)."[2] Toilet training can be a challenging process for any caregiver. The skilled OTA can assist children and adolescents who have difficulty with toilet hygiene by making this all important process more manageable.

A variety of adaptive equipment that may be useful for promoting increased independence for toilet hygiene is available on the market. Grab bars and toilet safety frames provide extra support for transferring onto the toilet. A raised or lowered toilet seat may also be indicated, depending on the specific needs of the child. For some individuals, a bedside commode may be beneficial. A skin inspection mirror can be helpful to individuals who have difficulty cleaning themselves. A variety of toilet tissue aids that allow individuals with limited ROM to clean themselves adequately are also available commercially. Toilet paper holders can be adapted to be maximally accessible.

SUMMARY

This chapter presented critical concepts to help children and adolescents engage successfully in activities of daily living and also discussed in depth the importance of a collaborative team approach; co-occupation from a developmental perspective; and OT evaluation and intervention to facilitate independence in age-appropriate ADLs. Case studies and guiding questions were provided to promote clinical problem solving in the classroom.

References

1. American Occupational Therapy Association: OT practice framework: domain and process, ed 2. *Am J Occup Ther* 56:609–639, 2002.
2. American Occupational Therapy Association: Occupational therapy practice framework: domain and process, ed 2. *Am J Occup Ther* 62:625–683, 2008.
3. Ayres AJ: *Sensory integration and learning disorders*, Los Angeles, 1972, Western Psychological Services.
4. Bahr DC: *Oral motor assessment and treatment ages and stages*, Needham Heights, MA, 2001, Allyn and Bacon.
5. Colangelo CA: Biomechanical frame of reference. In Kramer P, Hinojosa J, editors: *Frames of reference for pediatric occupational therapy*, ed 2, Philadelphia, 1999, Lippincott Williams & Wilkins.
6. Crepeau EB, Cohn ES, Schell BAB: *Willard and Spackman's occupational therapy*, ed 10, Philadelphia, 2003, Lippincott Williams & Wilkins.
7. Dehghan M, Akthtar-Danesh N, Merchant AT: Childhood obesity, prevalence and prevention. *Nutr J* 4:24, 2005.
8. Ernsperger L, Stegen-Hanson T: *Just take a bite: easy, effective answers to food aversions and eating challenges*, Arlington, TX, 2004, Future Horizons.
9. Francis K: Physiology and management of bladder and bowel continence following spinal cord injury. *Ostomy Wound Manage* 53:12, 2007.
10. Jennings JT, Sarbaugh BG, Payne NS: Conveying the message about optimal infant positions. *Phys Occup Ther Pediatr* 25:3–17, 2005.
11. Kielhofner G: Motives, patterns, and performance of occupation: basic concepts. In Kielhofner G, editor: *A model of human occupation: theory and application*, ed 4, Philadelphia, 2008, Lippincott Williams & Wilkins.
11a. Lashgari D, Yasuda L: Orthotics. In Pendleton H, Schultz-Krohn W, editors: *Pedretti's occupational therapy practice skills for physical dysfunction*, ed 6, St. Louis, 2006, Elsevier.
12. Lin S et al: The relation between length of institutionalization and sensory integration in children adopted from Eastern Europe. *Am J Occup Ther* 59:139–147, 2005.
13. Metcalf AB, Lawes N: A modern interpretation of the Rood approach. *Phys Ther Rev* 3:195–212, 1998.
14. Olsen JA: Mothering co-occupations in caring for infants and young children. In Esdaile SA, Olson JA, editors: *Mothering occupations*, Philadelphia, 2004, FA Davis.
15. Pearson L: *Hands on, TeamRehab Report*, 1995. Available at: www.wheelchairnet.org/WCN_Prodserv/Docs/.../9504 art2.PDF. Accessed February 6, 2010.
16. Shephard Center Learning Connections: *Education model on spinal cord injury: autonomic dysreflexia*, Atlanta, 2009,

Shephard Center Inc. Available at: https://www.myvitalconnections.org/MVCHomepage.nsf/patientpage. Accessed July 7, 2010.

17. Shoan SA, Anderson J: Neurodevelopmental treatment frame of reference. In Kramer P, Hinojosa J, editors: *Frames of reference for pediatric occupational therapy*, ed 2, Philadelphia, 1999, Lippincott Williams & Wilkins.

18. Smith Roley S, Delany J: Improving the occupational therapy framework: domain and process, ed 2. *Am J Occup Ther* 62:625–683, 2008.

19. Tieman BL et al: Gross motor capability and performance of mobility in children with cerebral palsy: a comparison across home, school, and outdoors/community setting. *Phys Ther* 84:419–429, 2004.

20. Toglia JP: A dynamic interactional approach to cognitive rehabilitation. In Katz N, editor: *Cognition and occupation across the life span: models for intervention in occupational therapy*, ed 2, Bethesda, MD, 2005, AOTA Press.

21. *Guide for the Uniform Data Set for Medical Rehabilitation (including the FIM™ instrument)*, version 5.1, Buffalo, NY, 1997, Uniform Data System for Medical Rehabilitation.

22. Wilbarger P: The sensory diet: activity programs based on sensory processing theory. *Sensory Integration Special Interest Section Newsletter* 18:1–4, 1995.

23. Wilcock AA, Townsend EA: Occupational justice. In Crepeau EB, Cohn ES, Schell BB, editors: *Willard and Spackman's occupational therapy*, ed 11, Baltimore, 2008, Lippincott Williams & Wilkins.

24. Zemke R, Clark F: *Occupational science: the evolving discipline*, Philadelphia, 1996, FA Davis.

REVIEW *Questions*

1. What is a collaborative team approach?
2. What is the most important factor that must be considered when approaching intervention from the developmental perspective? How does it differ from other approaches?
3. What is co-occupation? Provide some examples of co-occupation.
4. Identify interventions that might be used when working with a child who has difficulties with dressing.
5. What frame of reference is used when considering a compensatory technique?
6. What are the five different intervention approaches? Provide an example of each.
7. What piece of adaptive equipment may be used during hygiene tasks for a client who has difficulty with grasping small objects?

SUGGESTED *Activities*

1. Using catalogs that have assistive technology devices and adaptive equipment for pediatrics, identify a minimum of two items that may be prescribed to promote independence in the following ADLs: bathing and showering, hygiene, bowel and bladder, feeding, dressing, and functional mobility.
2. Observe a variety of children (of different ages) eating and dressing. Discuss their ease and quality of performance as well as the developmental tasks.
3. Observe a child who has special needs with regard to feeding and dressing. Discuss the motor performance and developmental tasks involved in this situation.

Identify what you can do to make the tasks easier for the child.
4. Develop a list of survey questions regarding the sexual activities of teens. Interview one adolescent who has special needs. Discuss overall findings in class.
5. Outline five strategies to improve ADLs. Describe the ADL clearly and examine the steps and motor, cognitive and sensory requirements. Consider how you would make the tasks easier or more challenging for the child. Describe other factors an OT practitioner would consider before implementing the strategies.

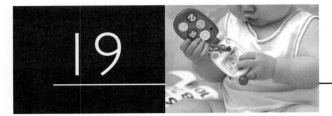

Instrumental Activities of Daily Living

CARYN BIRSTLER HUSMAN

BARBARA STEVA

CHAPTER *Objectives*

After studying this chapter, the reader will be able to accomplish the following:

- Identify the instrumental activities of daily living (IADLs) and describe how they relate to occupational performance in children and adolescents
- Describe therapeutic activities that an occupational therapy (OT) practitioner might use to address difficulties in occupational performance in the IADLs
- Describe adaptations that may be used to improve an individual's performance in the IADLs
- Describe intervention strategies that may be used to improve an individual's performance in the IADLs

The profession of occupational therapy (OT) is defined by its unique focus on "everyday life activities," known clinically as *occupation*.[2] OT practitioners work to assist adults and children in a wide variety of occupations, thus facilitating opportunities for satisfaction, competence in roles, health, wellness, and quality of life.[2]

Instrumental activities of daily living (IADLs) are defined by the American Occupational Therapy Association (AOTA) as "activities to support daily life within the home and community that often require more complex interactions than self-care used in ADL" (p. 631).[3] IADLs comprise an area of occupation that includes activities that are focused on interaction with the environment.[2]

More specifically, IADLs involve care of others, care of pets, child rearing, communication management, community mobility, financial management, health management and maintenance, home establishment, meal preparation and clean-up, religious observance, safety and emergency maintenance, and shopping. Explanations of these categories, as described by the AOTA *Practice Framework* are found in Table 19-1.

IADLs are typically multifaceted patterns of occupation. Each occupation can be divided into several tasks, each requiring specific skills. To develop individualized intervention strategies, goals, objectives, and outcomes, the OT practitioner considers the performance skills, performance patterns, and body functions; specific task

TABLE 19-1

Definitions of Instrumental Activities of Daily Living Areas

CATEGORY	DEFINITION
Care of others (including selecting and supervising caregivers)	Arranging, supervising, or providing the care for others
Care of pets	Arranging, supervising, or providing the care for pets and service animals
Child rearing	Providing the care and supervision to support the developmental needs of a child
Communication management	Sending, receiving, and interpreting information using a variety of systems and equipment, including writing tools, telephones, typewriters, audiovisual recorders, computers, communication boards, call lights, emergency systems, Braille writers, telecommunication devices for the hearing impaired, augmentative communication systems, and personal digital assistants (PDAs)
Community mobility	Moving around in the community and using public or private transportation, such as driving, walking, bicycling, or accessing and riding in buses, taxi cabs, or other transportation systems
Financial management	Using fiscal resources, including alternative methods of financial transaction and planning and using finances with long-term and short-term goals
Health management and maintenance	Developing, managing, and maintaining routines for health and wellness promotion, such as physical fitness, nutrition, decreasing health-risk behaviors, and medication routines
Home establishment and management	Obtaining and maintaining personal and household possessions and environment (e.g., home, yard, garden, appliances, vehicles), including maintaining and repairing personal possessions (clothing and household items) and knowing how to seek help or whom to contact
Meal preparation and clean-up	Planning, preparing, and serving well-balanced, nutritional meals and cleaning up food and utensils after meals
Religious observance	Participating in *religion*, "an organized system of beliefs, practices, rituals, and symbols designed to facilitate closeness to the sacred or transcendent" (p. 844)[26]
Safety and emergency maintenance	Knowing and performing preventive procedures to maintain a safe environment as well as recognizing sudden, unexpected hazardous situations and initiating emergency action to reduce the threat to health and safety
Shopping	Preparing shopping lists (grocery and other); selecting, purchasing, and transporting items; selecting method of payment; and completing money transactions

From American Occupational Therapy Association: Occupational therapy practice framework: Domain and process, 2nd edition, *Am J Occup Ther* 62:625–683, 2008.

analyses; individual values, roles, and interests; and current barriers to independence for each client. By their very nature, IADLs are optional and may be completed by a person other than oneself.[2] In particular, IADLs may be optional for children, depending on age, the family culture, and the culture of the community in which they live. However, performance in IADLs is pivotal for independent living as an adult. Therefore, the promotion of skills and independence in this area cannot be understated, especially in the case of children with disabilities as they grow.

The reader will explore the factors and considerations with regard to interventions for children and adolescents with cognitive, physical, visual, and communication challenges in the area of IADLs.

COGNITIVE AND EXECUTIVE FUNCTIONING

Due to the complex nature of IADLs, **cognitive functioning**, particularly executive functioning, must be thoroughly evaluated to develop appropriate goals, objectives, and intervention plans. Individuals with cognitive impairments often express a decreased awareness of cognitive limitations that could impact realistic goal setting and adjustment to a disability.[38] **Executive functioning** is a term used to describe a set of cognitive abilities located in the frontal cortex of the brain. More specifically, the frontal lobe provides organization and control for all cognitive skills. Cooper-Kahn and Dietzel described executive functioning as a set of processes that include the following:[13]

- *Inhibition* – the ability to stop one's actions and thoughts at an appropriate time
- *Shift* – the ability to think freely and move from one situation to another in order to respond appropriately
- *Emotional control* – the ability to regulate emotional responses by thinking and responding rationally
- *Initiation* – the ability to begin a task, generate ideas, responses, and problem-solving strategies
- *Working memory* – the ability to hold information in the mind to use for completing a task
- *Planning/orientation* – the ability to manage present and future oriented tasks
- *Organization of materials* – the ability to impose order on work, play, and storage spaces
- *Self-monitoring* – the ability to monitor self-performance and measure it against a standard of what is needed and/or expected

Individuals with challenges in one or more of these areas may struggle to plan a project, tell a story with details or in sequential order, memorize or recall information, initiate and complete tasks, and retain information while doing another task (recall a phone number while dialing). Although executive functioning is used continually in daily occupations, it is difficult to evaluate all the aspects that this term encompasses. In addition to formalized test batteries, observation and "hands-on" assessment of task completion are invaluable to the practitioner. Brown, Moore, Hemman, and Yunek found that client reports of independence and actual performance were not always consistent.[6] Real-life experiences were found to be more complex than those portrayed in simulations or in the interview process. The OT practitioner may need to adapt an activity or teach the individual to use a compensatory strategy for absent or impaired skills.

Intervention Strategies

Intervention strategies aimed at improving independence for the client with impaired cognitive skills can include deficit-specific training of cognitive skills, meta-cognitive training, compensation, social skills training, and task-specific training. *Deficit-specific training* involves restoring or improving specific cognitive tasks such as attention, initiation, and problem-solving through remedial exercises, grading of tasks, and gradually increasing demands on cognitive performance components.[39] *Meta-cognitive training* works to improve the fundamentals needed to set realistic goals by enhancing self-awareness and skills such as time management, self-control, anticipation, and self-monitoring. *Compensation* teaches the client to use alternative methods or strategies to complete a given task. Individuals can use lists, memory notebooks, electronic cuing devices, diaries, wall charts, and picture schedules. *Social skill training* involves improving interpersonal skills such as nonverbal cues, verbal and nonverbal communication skills, and conflict negotiation skills. *Task-specific training*, also referred to as *functional skill training*, involves systematic training of specific tasks required to complete an activity. A combination of these techniques may be needed to achieve the most efficient and functional outcome for the client.

When working with cognitive functioning, the OT practitioner also conducts activity analysis to break each task down into parts and determine specific skill areas the client might be lacking. The OT practitioner may use forward or backward chaining to teach a task. *Chaining* involves breaking the task down into individual steps, teaching each step, and finally putting the steps together. *Forward chaining* involves teaching the task from beginning to end, while *backward chaining* involves teaching the task from the last step to the first step. For example, tying shoe laces may be taught using forward chaining, where the client is taught first to tie the initial knot, then to make a loop, wrap the other lace around the loop, push the lace through the hole to make another loop, and finally pull both loops. When using backward chaining, clients complete only the last step of pulling the loops to finish the task. Next, they would combine the last two steps of pushing the lace through the hole and pulling the loops to complete the task. They would continue adding the previous step of the task until the task can be performed completely by the client. Another way of adapting an activity is to provide *faded assistance* or *grading*. This involves providing assistance for all, or a portion, of the activity. As the client improves, assistance is "faded" to encourage the client to perform more of the activity independently. Faded assistance could occur in the form of physical assist or grading of the activity in the form of adaptations or accommodations to the size of objects, speed, frequency or duration of the activity, height and angle at which the activity is performed, number of steps, complexity, and sensory components of the activity.

CASE *Study*

Julie is an 18-year-old girl attending high school. When she was 16, she was hit by a car while riding her bicycle without a helmet and suffered a traumatic brain injury. Although her residual physical impairments were mild, she continued to be challenged by decreased organization and memory. She has received OT services at school since returning after her injury. Julie and her educational/OT therapy team have identified goals, which include improved independence in self-organization. Julie has significant difficulty organizing herself at school with respect to homework assignments and class schedules. A memory book/daily planner was implemented to assist Julie in organizing activities, although she continued to be forgetful and leave the book in her locker or at home. She had similar issues with the "To Do" lists that were implemented. Julie enjoyed using her cell phone to text and talk with her friends and was seldom seen without the device. The OT practitioner and Julie worked together to program the phone as a memory aid. Julie learned to access and use the daily planner on the phone, "To Do" lists were set up, and an alarm was programmed to remind Julie of important events. The OT practitioner provided faded assistance in the form of verbal cues, which were then faded to written directions, to help Julie program important events and assignments into the phone. The educational team provided verbal cues to prompt Julie to use the aid during the school day, and the cues were faded as she became more independent. The team also worked with Julie's parents to develop and implement a reward program for successful use of the cell phone as a memory/organization aid. Each day, whenever Julie used her memory aid independently, she was rewarded with additional computer or video game time at home, a preferred activity that was typically time limited. Julie's independent organization improved at school and in the community. In time, Julie became more proficient at programming and accessing the aid independently.

COMMUNICATION

Communication is an integral part of participation in all daily tasks. Many clients receiving OT experience difficulty communicating due to their disabilities or injuries.[35] Communication devices compensate for that difficulty and allow for participation in work, leisure, and social occupations. Communication devices also support independence, facilitate greater engagement in learning and progress toward goals, and contribute significantly to occupational performance and quality of life.[46]

Communication devices provide **augmentative and alternative communication (AAC)** to children who are unable to communicate effectively.[34] Children who have autism, apraxia, or physical disabilities such as cerebral palsy that prevent the oral structures from being coordinated fluidly for speaking are candidates for a communication device. Persons with hearing impairments might wish to use a communication device to communicate with those outside their community without the help of an interpreter. A wide range of communication devices, from low-tech to complex high-tech options, is available. Low-tech communication devices include systems that do not require a form of power for operation. High-tech devices are able to store information and produce auditory communications.[16] These devices are also known as *speech-generating devices* or **voice output communication aids (VOCAs)**.

Although communication is classically the realm of the speech and language pathologist, occupational therapists can make a unique contribution to this area. The OT practitioner is an important team member in the selection and use of a communication device and assists with the selection of equipment that best fits the child's movement abilities by assessing range of motion (ROM), motor control, positioning, endurance, and visual–perceptual skills. The most common communication devices require the use of the upper extremity for operation. If upper extremity movement does not enable the use of a device, other available movements such as neck and eye movement should be documented. The OT practitioner determines that the child is able to discriminate between symbols to be able to use a device successfully. The OT practitioner also works with the child to determine if he or she shows a preference for a specific type of communication device.[35] Once the device has been selected, the OT practitioner sets up the child's environment to facilitate ease of use and ergonomic function and works as part of the team to train the child to use the equipment effectively.

Telephones

The telephone and the cell phone are the most commonly used communication devices. Children who have disabilities can use these devices to ensure safety and security. Cell phone features can be set up to benefit people with motor challenges. One key dialing, speaker phone, and more rugged phones may be helpful. A common cell phone adaption that is widely available is the large number pad.

Children who have disabilities may need training in the effective use of a cell phone. The child practices with the phone repeatedly to ensure that he or she will be able to access the phone when needed. Picture cards that demonstrate the steps of making a call may be helpful and can be attached to the phone by a key ring. Important phone numbers such as home and emergency numbers should be programmed for one key dialing. Other phone numbers or the key to the phone's speed dial may also be included on the card attached to the phone. If the child is unable to use the phone to call multiple numbers, the phone can be programmed to call one number only. Families can consult with their cell phone providers for further information.

Currently, individuals who cannot speak but can use technology with dexterous fingers are also able to use cell phones. Text-to-speech applications are available for the iPhone® and other devices.

Low-Tech Communication Boards

Low-tech communication boards are simple and inexpensive pieces of equipment to augment communication. They are often the first support used to increase a child's ability to communicate. Communication boards may contain pictures of items or activities a child may want or need. In the early stages, the child may use the board to make choices. This is especially effective for children with physical disabilities who are unable to access their environments independently due to motor limitations. Using a communication board, the child is able to indicate what toys or areas of the room s/he wishes to interact with.

More complex communication boards may be suitable for children who lack the motor control to speak and type quickly for communication but have the cognitive ability to communicate and spell. These boards may contain frequently used phrases and the letters of the alphabet. The children point to the letters or words with their hands or a mouth stick to indicate what they would like to communicate. Although these systems can be effective, they require an active and participating listener and can be laborious to use. However, they may also be an important first step in facilitating communication and can demonstrate the chidren's ability to use their cognitive and motor skills to communicate.

Communication boards may contain words or pictures that are hand drawn, computer illustrated, or photographic. Several programs that provide a wide range of high quality illustrations and commonly used pictures are available. Communication boards often come with Velcro so that pictures can be held in place or moved as needed. Picture books organize pictures for communication. Books allow access to a greater number of pictures than do communication boards and may be organized by topic for quick and easy location of pictures. Velcro is often placed on the outer cover of the book so that the pictures currently in use can be displayed on the front of the book. *Note:* The use of pictures for a communication board should not be confused with the Picture Exchange Communication System, which will be explained in greater detail later in this section (Tables 19-2 and 19-3).

Using Pictures to Communicate to the Client

Pictures can also be used as visual supports to assist an OT practitioner in communicating to the child.[7] These pictures will be called *visual supports* in this text to avoid confusing them with communication boards that children use to communicate their thoughts. When

TABLE 19-2

Common Methods for Using Pictures for Communication During Daily Tasks and Occupational Therapy Sessions

METHOD	DESCRIPTION
Indicating wants and needs	Pictures of daily tasks and items in the environment can allow a child to communicate when he or she is tired or hungry, needs to use the bathroom, or wants to play.
Building words or sentences	Symbols, letters, and common words are visible to build sentences by pointing to them.

Adapted from *PECS USA*, 2009 : *What is PECS?* http://www.pecs-usa.com/WhatsPECS.htm: Accessed October 13, 2009.

TABLE 19-3

Visual Supports for Participation, Regulation, and Emotional/Behavioral Development

VISUAL SUPPORT	DESCRIPTION
Activity schedule	Pictures may be placed on a strip or page to show the number and order of activities expected. When each activity is completed, the pictures are removed or shifted to another area that indicates the activity is "all done."
First/Then	Two pictures indicate activities that come first and second. This can be an effective motivator if a nonfavored activity is followed by a favorite task. For example, use the bathroom and then play a game.
Choice making	Pictures are presented so that a child can choose an activity, toy, or snack. A small or large amount of pictures can be presented, and choices can be made based on therapeutic effect and therapist intentions.
Break-down of tasks into steps for teaching and independence	Pictures represent the steps of a task. This can increase independence and attention for multistep actions and activities. Examples include grooming sequences, setting the table, or steps for production line work.
Communication of feelings	Pictures of facial expressions can assist children with understanding and identifying their emotions.
Visuals to accompany songs	Pictures that represent verses of songs allow children of all abilities to participate in songs and help explain what the words mean in a concrete manner.
Visuals for support during emotional dysregulation	When children are emotionally dysregulated, they may have difficulty taking in auditory information from others. Pictures may allow people working with them to communicate safe and regulating alternatives to unsafe behavior.
Social stories	Social stories are written about future events that may be difficult for a child to tolerate such as going to a busy store or going trick-or-treating. Pictures are frequently used to make the story easier to understand. These are especially effective for children who have autism spectrum disorders.
Support for visual impairment	Large pictures provide directions for individuals who have difficulty reading small print.

Adapted from Bryan LC, Gast DL: Teaching on-task and on-schedule behaviors to high-functioning children with autism via picture activity schedules, *J Autism Development Dis* 30(6):553–567, 2000.

pictures assist a child to function, it is important that the OT practitioner consult with teachers and parents so that the system can be used across various settings.

Visual supports are commonly used to communicate expectations, show how many activities are expected, and demonstrate the order of activities.[7] Visual supports can increase on-task behaviors; be used to teach complex topics such as arousal or excitement level by presenting symbols that young people can understand and relate to; increase self-awareness of emotions and arousal/excitement level, and also be used to augment social stories to ensure children know how to respond and act safely in challenging situations.[7]

How to Obtain Pictures for Use in Therapy Sessions

It is highly recommended that the OT practitioner consult with a speech and language pathologist on the use of pictures for individual clients (Table 19-4).

CLINICAL *Pearl*

Picture schedules can help structure the therapy session if a child is impulsive or distractible. They can also be useful when a child is avoidant of therapy tasks or has difficulty tolerating nonfavored activities.

Picture Exchange Communication System

The Picture Exchange Communication System (PECS) was created to increase communication for individuals with autism spectrum disorders.[31] PECS has also been found effective for other populations with cognitive, communication, and physical disabilities. The system is put in place by a speech and language pathologist and should only be used under the supervision and guidance of that specialist. Nevertheless, it is important for OTAs to have a cursory knowledge of the program, which is widely used.

TABLE 19-4

Using Pictures or Illustrations During Intervention

TYPES OF PICTURES	PROS	CONS
Photographs	Photographs are necessary for children who do not understand the symbolism of other pictures. They provide an exact communication of objects, people, and places.	Use of photographic pictures requires time and resources, including a compatible digital camera and computer, or actual photographs.
Programs such as Boardmaker®	These programs provide clearly drawn, universally understood symbols for communication. They may be transferred to a variety of settings and are commonly used in school settings.	The program must be purchased and may be expensive. An OT practitioner must learn the computer program for ease of use.
Pictures from the Internet or magazines	Pictures are readily available on the Internet and in magazines.	The quality of the image may vary. Copyright laws must be adhered to.
Hand-drawn pictures	Hand-drawn pictures are readily available and may convey messages for which a specific illustration does not exist.	Quality will vary with drawing skill. Some children may not understand the symbolism of hand-drawn pictures.

PECS is a systematic method for teaching initiation of communication through the exchange of pictures.[31] Through PECS, a child is taught to use communication to get his or her needs met. The goal is to teach the child to use communication independently. The system is not necessarily a replacement for speech; frequently young children who begin using the program also begin to use vocal language.[31] An OTA can continue to use language with a client who uses PECS. However, basic use of the protocol will reinforce the work done in speech therapy and may improve OT sessions and outcomes (Table 19-5).

TABLE 19-5

Phases of the Picture Exchange Communication System

PHASE	DESCRIPTION
Phase 1	The child is taught to initiate communication by presenting a picture to obtain a desired object such as a toy or a snack. The desired object is provided immediately to reinforce the communication exchange. During this phase only one picture is used, and the child is not asked to determine which picture matches what he or she wants.
Phase 2	The child is taught to initiate communication when others are not readily available and waiting for the picture exchange. To do so, the child is taught to obtain the picture and go to another person to request the object in exchange for the picture. The occupational therapist begins by standing close by and then moves farther away to make the child persist in the effort to communicate.
Phase 3	The child is taught to distinguish between pictures to get the desired item. Initially, the child distinguishes between two very different pictures such as a snack and a sock. As the child is successful, more similar and numerous pictures are presented.
Phase 4	The child is taught to use a sentence strip. A picture denoting "I want" is placed on the strip and the child must add the item or activity that he or she wants and exchange the entire strip with the other person.
Phase 5	The child is taught to respond to the question "What do you want?"
Phase 6	The child is taught to make comments about the environment such as "I see."
Continued expansion of vocabulary	The child is taught to use adjectives to describe the things he or she wants or notices.

Adapted from *PECS USA*, 2009: *What is PECS?* http://www.pecs-usa.com/WhatsPECS.htm: Accessed October 13, 2009.

High-Tech Voice Output Communication Aids

A wide range of high-tech devices and software is available to augment communication for people who have disabilities. These devices include small, handheld devices that contain a few messages; larger devices that are portable, are mountable on wheelchairs, and store large amounts of vocabulary; and complex systems that can be used with computers to export any message the individual can type.[1] The handheld and larger portable devices are usually the first high-tech devices used with children, who must learn to use the devices as they are learning to communicate and use vocabulary. It is important that their continued development is taken into account when selecting a VOCA.

VOCAs are the specific hardware that the child accesses for communication. These high-tech communication boards work in the same way as low-tech boards: the child accesses a picture or symbol to communicate with others. However, when a picture or symbol is accessed by the child on a VOCA, an audible message is given out by the device so that others can hear it when the child wishes to communicate.

Small devices present a limited number of pictures, sometimes as few as three or five.[1] When activated, the device plays a frequently used sentence or message such as "I want to play" or "I need to go to the bathroom." Some of these devices are able to record specific messages and can therefore be useful for including children who have difficulties with typical occupations of childhood such as giving an oral report or acting in a school play.[1] More complex systems comprise several menus that present words or messages within a theme. The child is able to access many words or messages for each theme. The child first selects a topic from a main menu page and then is able to access a number of words or messages about that theme. For example, the child might access a food theme, in which several choices of favorite foods and snacks are presented. Common themes for young children include foods, bathroom, greetings, weather, songs, and toys. As communication and the use of the device develop, an ever-expanding array of themes may be programmed on complex VOCAs.[1]

VOCAs can be accessed by a variety of means so that an individual can communicate using whichever part of the body he or she is best able to move. If the child has controlled movement of the upper extremity, he or she can access the symbols with fingers on a touch screen. If less volitional movement is available, the child may use a switch to select the appropriate symbol.[23] Switches can be accessed through paddles that are pushed by any part of the body where controlled movement exists. This might be the hand, elbow, or side of the head. Puff and sip configurations can be set up for the individual who is unable to move any of the limbs in a controlled manner.[23]

OT practitioners play a vital role in teaching children to use switches.[23] First, the OT practitioner provides experiences to help the child learn that the switch causes something to happen. This is most easily achieved with a cause-and-effect toy that moves, lights up, and/or makes sound when the switch it activated. Once the child understands the concept thoroughly, the switch can be used to operate a highly motivating phrase. In the case of some children, this might be "I want a snack," "Tickle me!" or simply "Hello." Next, the child works with more than one switch to produce more than one communication. In later stages, the OT practitioner works with the child to use the switch to select a picture from the screen of a high-tech VOCA. A common set-up includes a cursor on a screen that moves among various pictures. The child works to press the switch as it lands on a specific picture. In this way, the OT practitioner prepares the child to use technology to select whole words and phrases in a complex communication system.[23]

Other alternative methods for accessing VOCAs include pointers and eye-tracking devices. Pointers may utilize light beam or infrared technology to select symbols.[11] Eye-tracking devices follow the movement and gazing of the eyes to select symbols and messages.[5] These adaptations require a significant level of head and eye control as well as high-level cognitive skills.[11]

CASE *Study*

Carl began attending a special purpose preschool program soon after turning 3 years old, when he was diagnosed with autism. Carl did not use words to communicate at home or in school. When he was strongly motivated to get something, he would take an adult's hand to lead him or her to the desired object. In school, Carl rarely displayed interest in free play activities; he needed direct facilitation from a teacher or an OT clinician to engage in play activities for short periods. Carl also cried frequently and threw tantrums; at times, he was extremely difficult to console. The speech and language practitioner (SLP) introduced the PECS system to the school program. The OT practitioner first worked with the SLP to help Carl learn to use the system. The team used motivating activities and snacks to encourage Carl to use the pictures for communication. The OT practitioner incorporated short activities, cause-and-effect toys, and sensory activities to encourage Carl to participate and communicate during this phase of learning the system. After Carl learned the system, the OT practitioner carried over the use of PECS into other activities such as free play, playground time, and snack. The SLP and the OT practitioner also consulted with Carl's teacher and parents to further generalize the use of PECS. Several months later, Carl was independently accessing his PECS picture book to request food, toys, and games. He became more engaged and compliant with classroom and therapy activities. He also showed a marked decrease in crying and tantrum episodes across settings. Carl's vocal language, however, did not develop further. Therefore, he participated in an evaluation for a VOCA and was going to begin training to use the system soon.

Computer Systems for Communication

Computers allow individuals to communicate via email, blogs, and programs that convert text to audible speech.[5] Many modifications are available so that individuals can access keyboards and mouse pointers.[5]

Alternative keyboards have been created to increase the ease with which a person who has a disability can type.[5] Keyboards may be enlarged or constricted to allow for more success with the keys. The order of the letters may also be customized, so that the most frequently used keys are situated in the home row, or the most important keys clustered in the center for one finger typing. Keyboards can be designed for use with one or two hands. Further, keyboards may be programmed to produce words or phrases when a combination of keys is pressed. Other adaptations include moisture guards, overlays to increase visual contrast or tactile feedback, and rigid overlays to prevent pressing the wrong buttons.[5]

Computers may be accessed through non-traditional mouse arrangements if the user is unable to effectively use a mouse.[5] A track ball may be helpful for people who have limited movement of the upper extremity, but accurate movement at the fingers. The track ball may also be appropriate for the individual who has full range of motion, but lacks the motor control or stability to move the whole hand or arm to move a standard mouse. Alternatively, a computer screen can be accessed through the use of a switch. Again, a cursor moves between different areas of the screen and the child presses the switch when the cursor pauses on the appropriate area. An individual may also use a stick or pointer as a mouse; software is available to interpret head movement as movement of the pointer across the screen.[5] In addition, eye gaze and infrared programs are available for the individual with the ability to gaze into a camera in a controlled manner.[5,11] See Chapter 26. Assistive Technology for additional information.

COMMUNITY MOBILITY

An individual's role in regard to **community mobility** changes through the lifespan and is dependent upon the life role and interests of the individual. Progression may involve a car seat/stroller > walking > tricycle/bicycle > school bus > public transportation > driving > dependency on others for transportation and mobility.[37] The clinician assesses client factors to best prepare and modify the human and non-human aspects of the environment for access. Human factors may include disability, values or interests while non-human factors involve physical barriers and accessibility.

Developmental Stages of Mobility

The OT practitioner takes into consideration the **developmental stages of mobility** while planning intervention. The infant and toddler typically take on the role of a passenger. The young child begins to explore mobility by creeping and walking. Transportation to and from school on a school bus or on public transportation becomes a focus for the school-aged child. At this time, the child is often exploring his or her community when riding a bicycle or scooter as well. As the child grows, increased importance is placed on safety and judgment as the child begins to explore the environment more independently. Crossing the street, reading and understanding street signs and signals, and negotiating curbs and obstacles within the environment become important to independence and safe community mobility. The adolescent and young adult incorporate all of the above developed skills as they find independence and autonomy preparing to drive or navigate public transportation.[3] Ultimately, mobility is a necessary life component that leads to better quality of life, fulfillment of roles, access to leisure activities, and engagement in meaningful activities. In order to provide effective intervention, it is necessary to assess on an ongoing basis the child's strengths and needs in performance areas specific to the mode of mobility that the child is seeking. Visual perception, motor coordination, muscle strength, sensory regulation, and executive functioning can impact the successful and independent participation of an individual's mobility within the community. Adaptations in the form of mobility devices, supplemental aids, or modifications to the environment may be necessary to attain optimal independence. The child or the caregiver and the OT practitioner work together to develop individualized treatment goals, objectives, and a specific treatment plan to address the child's mobility needs.

Transportation for the Infant, Toddler, and Young Child

The National Highway Traffic Safety Administration (NHTSA; http://www.nhtsa.dot.gov/) provides clear guidelines for the safe transport of infants, toddlers, and young children. Car seat manufacturers provide detailed weight and age limits specific to each particular seat. Installation methods for car seats vary, and manufacturer instructions should be followed, without exception, when installing the seat in a vehicle. The role of the OT practitioner is to assess the child's physical needs and make recommendations as to the type of seat required. Although no adaptations or modifications should be made that will change the structural integrity of the seat, low-tech modifications, for example, towel rolls for head and trunk support, can be made to provide comfort and safety to the child.

Considerations

- *Minimum weight:* When assisting a caregiver in selecting a seat for an infant with medical needs, the minimum weight limit needs to be considered, as most commercially available car seats have a minimum weight of 5 lb. Many premature infants or infants with special needs weigh less than 5 lb, so customized seats may be required for them.
- *Car bed:* A car bed may be needed if the infant is unable to tolerate the semi-reclined position.
- *Convertible car seat:* A convertible car seat provides a rear-facing position for the infant and converts to a forward-facing seat, when appropriate, as the child grows. The infant should remain in the rear-facing position as long as possible to prevent injury in the event of a crash, since in this position the seat helps to absorb the force of the crash, whereas a forward-facing seat could cause abdominal or spinal injuries to the small child. A rear-facing seat that accommodates greater weight can be beneficial to children with issues such as small stature, developmental delay, brittle bones, Down syndrome, hydrocephalus, low muscle tone, and poor upper body control.
- *Forward-facing seat:* A forward-facing seat designed to only face forward is generally used for children at least 1 year of age *and* weighing at least 20 to 30 lb. These seats typically use a five-point harness, and, as the child grows, many can be converted into a booster seat when used in conjunction with the vehicle lap-and-shoulder belt. The booster seat systems are designed for children weighing greater than 40 lb, which generally occurs at approximately 4 years of age. These seats elevate the child to a level in which the lap-and-shoulder belts can be properly positioned. The vehicle safety belt should only be used when the child is tall enough for it to cross over the shoulder in the middle of the clavicle and pass over the sternum. The lap belt should sit low and snug across the pelvis with the lower edge sitting on the upper thigh. The child should never place the shoulder belt under the arm or behind the back. This leaves the upper body unprotected and can lead to abdominal or spinal injuries in the event of a crash.[8] As the child grows and becomes more physically adept, adaptations may be required to prevent the child from releasing the seatbelt or harness. The NHTSA offers a list of the Web sites of organizations that provide safety seat inspections to ensure proper installation and use of individual car seats (www.seatcheck.org).
- *Special car seats and harnesses:* Specialized car seats or harnesses can be purchased through certain manufacturers to accommodate more severe physical limitations (Table 19-6).

CASE *Study*

Joel is a 5-month-old (2 months adjusted age) boy born prematurely at 27 weeks gestation weighing 7 lb. He has been hospitalized since his birth due to low birth weight and multiple congenital anomalies. During his hospitaliza-

TABLE 19-6

Automobile Safety Seats for Children and Adolescents with Special Needs

DESCRIPTION	WEIGHT OF CHILD	SIZE OF CHILD	POSITION	CONSIDERATIONS

Car Bed
Dream Ride SE
(Dorel Juvenile
    Group Inc.)
	5–20 pounds	19–26 inches	Center of vehicle, with
			    head facing center of
			    vehicle
			Back or side-lying
				Inability to maintain an
				    upright position
				    due to breathing
				    difficulty

Angel Ride Car Bed
(Mercury
    Distributing)
	Less than
	    9 pounds
		Less than 20 inches	Infant should not be placed
			    on the stomach (due to
			    increased risk of sudden
			    infant death syndrome
			    (SIDS) unless instructed
			    by medical staff	

TABLE 19-6

Automobile Safety Seats for Children and Adolescents with Special Needs—cont'd

DESCRIPTION	WEIGHT OF CHILD	SIZE OF CHILD	POSITION	CONSIDERATIONS
Hippo Convertible Car Seat (Snug Seat, Inc.)			Rear- or forward-facing	Designed for children in hip casts
Rear-facing	5–33 pounds and one year of age	49 inches	Shallow seating surface and low sides and wedge positioning system	A tether is required for children weighing more than 40 pounds
Forward-facing	20–65 pounds		Forward facing seat can be used semi-reclined or upright	
Modified E-Z-On Vest (E-Z-On Products, Inc.)	2–12 years	20–100 pounds Child must fit lengthwise on vehicle bench seat	Lying down	Transport of a child needing to lie down due to hip casts Two lap belts may be required to secure the child Padding is needed to fill floor space beside the child
Forward-facing medical seats			Forward-facing	Tether required
Britax Traveler Plus (Snug seat, Inc.)	22–105 pounds	Up to 56 inches		Additional support for the larger child requiring physical support
Orthopedic Positioning Seat (Columbia Medical)	Child: 20–102 pounds Small Adult: 40–130 pounds	36–60 inches 54–66 inches		Additional restraint for children with behavioral challenges that may impact safety
The Roosevelt (Merritt Manufacturing)	35–115 pounds	33.5–62 inches		Most seats available with optional positioning features such as postural pads, wedges, seat depth extenders and stroller bases
Special Tomato (Bergeron Health Care)	Small: 20–80 pounds Large: 80–150 pounds	32.5–50 inches 50–63 inches		
Carrie Seat (Sammons Preston/ Tumble Forms)	Four sizes: 20–130 pounds	30–68 inches		
Peppino Car Seat (Reha Partner, Inc.)	20–55 pounds	33.5–47 inches		
Recaro Car Seat Reha Partner, Inc.	30–80 pounds	37–59 inches		
Upright Vests E-Z-On Vest (E-Z-On Products, Inc.)	2 years and older and 20–68 pounds		Upright in vehicle seat	Tether required Additional restraint for children with behavioral challenges that may impact safety Front or back closures available

From Indiana University, School of Medicine, 2009: *Special needs transportation: Restraints.* http://www.preventinjury.org/SNTrestraints.asp: Accessed September 14, 2009.

tion, it was found that Joel was able to tolerate the upright and semi-reclined positions for very brief periods before his oxygen saturation decreased to an unhealthy level. A referral was made to the OT practitioner for assistance with positioning to prevent deformity, parent teaching, and discharge planning. The OT clinician worked with Joel and the family to develop an intervention program consisting of position changes and activities to build Joel's tolerance to the upright position. Upon discharge from the hospital, Joel was able to tolerate the semi-reclined position for 3 to 5 minutes at a time. The OT practitioner consulted with the family and the medical team to develop a method for Joel's transportation within the community. A car bed was ordered for Joel to provide safe positioning in the back seat of the car. Joel's parents were instructed in positioning through discussion and demonstration, during which the OT practitioner positioned Joel in the car bed and placed towel rolls at his head, feet, and sides to prevent rolling with the starting and stopping motions of the car. The parents were then observed to assess their ability to position Joel. The OT practitioner re-demonstrated proper installation of the car bed in the automobile, and this was followed by parental demonstration. Joel left the hospital with his parents and continues to receive early intervention services within the home environment to address positioning and developmental skills, as appropriate.

Transportation for the School-Aged Child

School buses are designed to use compartmentalization among other features such as size, height, and weight of the vehicle to ensure the safety of its occupants and are not equipped with safety belts. Compartmentalization maintains students in a small padded space between seats with high backs. This prevents the passenger from being thrown forward, over the seat, in the event of a crash.[36] Children with medical or behavioral challenges may require special considerations when using school transportation. Safety seats, seat belts, harnesses, and wheelchair tie-downs may be required to ensure safe transportation. The OT practitioner works with the educational team, including the transporter, to develop a safe plan for transportation and an evacuation plan in the event of an emergency. Since 2002, the American National Standards Institute/Rehabilitation Engineering and Assistive Technology Society of North America (ANSI/RESNA) *Wheelchair Standards, Volume 1: Wheelchairs for Use as Seats in Motor Vehicles* (WC-19) requires wheelchairs to be dynamically crash tested and mandates specific requirements for wheelchair frames used as seating within a motor vehicle. ANSI WC-20 outlines safety requirements for the seating systems (seat pan, seat back, and attachment hardware) placed into the wheelchair frame after purchase (visit RERCWTS.org). When securing a wheelchair

within any motor vehicle, the chair should be forward facing to prevent injury to the occupant through lateral body shift and/or shearing forces applied to the wheelchair. When assessing options for school and personal transportation for an individual in a wheelchair, all other viable seating options should be exhausted before considering the wheelchair as the seating device for transportation. Individuals using a wheelchair due to poor endurance or small children using a child safety seat should be transferred out of the wheelchair into a vehicle seat or safety seat for transportation. The OT practitioner should provide training to all individuals expected to assist with these transfers to ensure proper body mechanics and safe transfers. When not being used as a transportation device, the wheelchair should be properly secured within the vehicle to prevent it from becoming a projectile in the event of a sudden stop or crash. If the individual cannot be transferred into a vehicle seat due to his or her physical limitations, the wheelchair must be secured using the four-point tie-down system and the three-point occupant restraint system. Shutrump, Manary, and Buning described in detail the requirements of school bus transportation of the student in a wheelchair.[34] Modifications to the school bus are required for proper placement of tie-down systems. The four-point tie-down system consists of four individual anchors (two front and two back) secured to the vehicle floor and then attached to the frame of the wheelchair. Tie-downs are secured to the chair frame as close as possible to the seating surface while remaining below it. Detachable parts of the chair should never be considered for placement of the tie-downs, and straps should form a direct line between the floor and the attachment point, with no wrapping or angling around other chair parts. A shoulder-and-lap belt must be used in addition to any safety belts used for positioning within the chair. The lap belt must fit low and snug across the pelvis, with the lower edge of the safety belt touching the upper thighs. This is typically achieved by threading the lap belt between the armrest and back of the chair. The shoulder portion of the belt must also be snug and positioned over the middle of the clavicle, across the sternum and connect to the lap belt near the hip. Any accessory equipment such as lap trays, backpacks, and communication devices should be removed from the wheelchair and secured separately. A power wheelchair must be restrained in this same manner, although it may require an additional set of anchors due to its weight.[34]

Transportation for the Adolescent

When the adolescent begins to attempt driving, the OT clinician evaluates cognitive, visual, physical, and sensory processing abilities that impact this life role. Obtaining a driver's license can impact an adolescent's access to employment, housing, social, educational, and recreational opportunities.[37] The evaluation and care plan for the individual considering independent mobility within the community takes into account physical ability, executive functions, visual perception, and visual motor skills, including coordination and quick use of extremities, ability to cross streets safely, managing social interactions, managing time, handling emergency situations, and caring for self independently. Other skills to consider include map reading, money management, management of emotions/feelings, and regulation of sensory input, as it pertains to tolerating sensory input on a crowded bus, in a traffic jam, and so on.

"All occupational therapists and occupational therapy assistants have the education and training necessary to address driving and community mobility as an IADL."[38] The use of clinical reasoning skills to evaluate and treat the strengths and weaknesses in the areas of performance skills, performance patterns, contexts, and client factors is viewed by AOTA as a basic role of the OT practitioner. AOTA recommends specialized training for the clinical assessment of vision, cognition, motor performance, reaction time, knowledge of traffic rules, and behind-the-wheel driving skills. The supplementary training and expertise allow the OT practitioner to provide recommendations and assistance in vehicle modifications and driver training. AOTA also requires additional, specialized training for OT professionals who want to work in the area of driver rehabilitation providing direct services to clients with health or age-related issues.[38]

CLINICAL *Pearl*

Many states require licensure as a professional driving instructor before intervention or instruction can be provided to a novice driver or to a driver whose license has expired.

Public Transportation

The adolescent begins to develop independence through the use of public transportation to access peer activities, school, and work. Physical and cognitive limitations can impair successful completion of these activities. The Americans with Disabilities Act of 1990 clearly outlines physical and structural access requirements for all public transit systems.[40] Environmental awareness, directionality, and ability to follow multistep sequences play an important role in achieving independence in this area. The individual is required to combine several skills to complete this task successfully. He or she must purchase tickets using some form of money exchange, choose the appropriate transit system to go to the correct location, and navigate the system safely, including loading and unloading if using a mobility device. Problem solving and multistep sequencing are required to determine what needs to be done during delays or rerouting. Some individuals may require preteaching on the correct way to purchase tickets and deposit coins/tokens. Anticipation and attention deficits could impact the ability to prepare for the stop and to signal the driver to stop. Treatment within the clinic setting should incorporate education on the use of the subway, the bus, and road maps. This can be done by setting up a treasure hunt or by simply asking the client to plan a route from one destination to another using a map. It is in the client's best interests to incorporate problem-solving dilemmas into the session. This encourages the client to practice cognitive flexibility and come up with problem-solving strategies. These skills should be assessed and applied to actual community mobility as much as possible, since simulated environments often do not provide for handling variables such as increased noise, crowds, delayed schedules, and alternative routing.

Wheelchair Mobility

Mobility for the individual with physical challenges must be considered when developing a care plan. Brinker and Lewis found typically developing children learn naturally occurring effects and consequences as they interact with their environments through self-initiated mobility such as creeping, walking, and biking.[4] Children limited in self-initiated mobility opportunities because of their physical challenges can demonstrate limited motivation, diminished overall independence, learned helplessness, and diminished cognitive, social, and emotional development. When providing OT intervention to a child with newly acquired limitations, progressive limitations, or limitations that are becoming more difficult as he or she grows, the clinician may work with the child and/or his or her caregivers to obtain assistive mobility in the form of a wheelchair. Butler found that independent mobility impacted an individual's spatial understanding of the environment.[9] A study conducted by Deitz, Swinth, and White found enhanced self-initiated movements and increased attempts for peer interaction after the introduction of a power mobility device.[14] Physical and cognitive impairments that can impact independent mobility, whether power or manual, can include impaired head and eye control, body control, upper body strength, spatial awareness, and motor planning. The individual should be assessed and receive instruction, as necessary, in locking and unlocking the brakes; maneuvering the chair through environments with and without obstacles; turning, starting and stopping; and the ability to open or close doors independently. Strength should be assessed for the ability to propel the manual chair over rough, smooth, and angled surfaces as well as up and down hills or ramps. Strength limitations can be addressed in direct therapy sessions through play activities such as throwing weighted beanbags at a target and through weight-bearing activities. The ability to safely maneuver the wheelchair can be addressed in simulated environments using obstacle courses. Prior to discharging a client from direct therapy services, these skills should be assessed in the natural environment to ensure that generalization of skills from the simulated tasks to the real life situation has occurred.

When selecting a wheelchair, the OT practitioner must ensure proper fit, allowing for growth adjustments, as most funding sources expect seating systems to accommodate the individual for at least 5 years. Powered mobility versus manual mobility should be evaluated with care. The powered wheelchair is less portable and requires specialized transportation due to its greater weight, is more costly, and requires adequate safety awareness, judgment, and visual perception. Control systems need to be assessed to ensure adequate control and safety. The manual wheelchair is lighter and more portable, is less costly, and can be easily propelled by the user or caregiver. Both chairs can typically accommodate specialized seating systems based on the individual's needs. Whichever type of mobility the individual uses, powered or manual , he or she should have symmetrical hip alignment with hips, knees, and ankles supported at approximately 90 degrees. The seat depth should accommodate the length of the thigh, while allowing two to three inches of space from the front edge of the seat to the popliteal fossa. The seat width should be approximately two inches wider than the widest part of the hip and thighs. The height of the seat back is dependent upon the stability and balance of the individual, with a higher back required for more stability and support. A low back, preferably below the scapula, is useful for the individual with good balance who propels the chair manually. This allows for extension at the shoulders when pushing. Leg rests that are removable are helpful for the individual who performs standing transfers. Removable armrests are typically necessary for the individual performing sliding transfers and helpful when sitting at a low table. The seat belt and lap tray are also accessories to be considered when selecting a wheelchair.

CLINICAL *Pearl*

When having difficulty seating an individual with excessive extensor muscle tone, seating that provides flexion of the hips at an angle slightly more than 90 degrees can inhibit the muscle tone. Placement of the seatbelt on the chair at a 90-degree angle to the thighs can help maintain the position.

CLINICAL *Pearl*

Ensure that children's skin is protected under lap trays, as severe sunburn can occur when using a clear lap tray in direct sunlight.

Walkers, Canes, Crutches, and Miscellaneous Mobility Devices

Physical therapists are responsible for the evaluation, selection, and training in the use of walkers, canes, and other mobility devices, and occupational therapists are involved in facilitating safety in the community and at home while using of the device during daily occupations. The anterior or posterior walker provides support to the individual and the ability to move the lower extremities, but it requires support. The upper extremities should be carefully monitored for hyperextension of the thumb and fingers and excessive weight placed on the wrists due to poor lower extremity strength and upright posture. In these cases, a walker with forearm troughs may provide better positioning and support for the individual. Canes come as straight canes or quad canes. The straight cane has a single end point to provide stability for the individual. The quad cane has a single staff with four end points to provide increased stability. Devices such as mobile standers, adapted cycles, and so on provide mobility to individuals with special needs and allow for social interaction within the community setting. Adaptations may be required to provide comfort and optimal positioning and function.

CLINICAL *Pearl*

The single walking device such as a single crutch or cane is placed in the "strong" hand or on the opposite side of the weakened lower extremity to promote reciprocal stride gait when walking.

Bicycles, Scooters, Roller Blades

As the child grows, independent mobility becomes more important to his or her autonomy. Bicycling, scootering, skateboarding, and skating require advanced development of balance and equilibrium reactions, postural control, and upper and lower extremity coordination. These skills can be assessed and any deficits treated within the clinic or community environments. Executive function skills such as attention, initiation, safety awareness, and judgment are more difficult to assess in a simulated environment. The use of safety equipment such as helmet, elbow pads, and knee pads should be taught before placing a child on a moving object and should be strictly enforced each time the child rides. Judgment and safety awareness are required when crossing a street, riding among pedestrians, and following general riding rules. Recognition of, and generalization of skills with regard to, the meanings of traffic signals and street signs can impact an individual's ability to ride safely in the community by himself or herself.

Street Safety

Children with disabilities will likely need assistance to learn to navigate their community safely. Repeated exposure and learning opportunities will likely be needed to facilitate learning and eventual independence with regard to street safety. The OT practitioner may address street safety during natural learning opportunities and through consultation with parents and teachers.

Street Safety With Young Children

Young children learn about general safety around cars, safety in parking lots, and how to cross the street. OT practitioners encounter natural opportunities to teach children about street safety during school outings, when getting on and off school buses, and when going to and from playgrounds. Although young children are not expected to navigate streets independently, they can learn to play only in safe areas such as driveways and playgrounds, walk on sidewalks and crosswalks, stop when they reach a street, avoid going into the street without an adult, and recognize when it is safe to cross a street. Young children can also be taught to pay attention to crossing guards for assistance.

Street Safety With Older Children

Older children may begin to assume independence in maintaining their personal safety when moving through their communities. These individuals learn how to understand traffic signals and road signs and how to navigate city streets. The OT practitioner ensures that they can recognize and understand street signs and traffic signals. Practice on observing street safety rules can be integrated well with community mobility interventions. Additionally, the OT practitioner ensures that children who have intellectual disabilities or communication limitations carry personal identifications, which would be vital in case they get lost; this may be attached to a belt or backpack and should include emergency contact information. Further, children who use wheelchairs are encouraged to attach reflective strips to the wheelchair and use a strobe light when traveling on the street during dusk or in the dark.

FINANCIAL MANAGEMENT, SHOPPING, AND CARE OF PETS

Challenges in the areas of financial management, shopping, pet care, and care of others often result from impaired use of one or more executive function skills. Generalization of skills across environments and tasks is necessary for the successful completion of these tasks. Treatment in this area often involves the use of external aids to assist the individual in accessing and participating in activities independently. Careful assessment of the individual's knowledge and skills in each area is necessary to determine where to begin the intervention process.

Financial Management

Financial awareness begins in early childhood with imaginary play involving shopping, money exchange, and the awareness that money is required to obtain desired items. Children in elementary school begin to learn to identify names and values of coins and paper currency. Children with learning disabilities or visual–perceptual impairment may have more difficulty distinguishing between items of similar size, for example, a dime and a penny, or a nickel and a quarter. Some children can be taught to distinguish between these items using the texture on the edges of the coins. Pennies and nickels have smooth edges, whereas dimes and quarters have rough or ridged edges. Paper currency can be folded differently to distinguish between denominations. This can, however, continue to present difficulties for the individual with impaired memory. These individuals may require a picture book or card with a picture of the bill or coin paired with the value. Coin carriers can also be useful for the individual having difficulty distinguishing between coins. Children can practice these skills in a simulated environment or in a school store, where small school items or snacks are sold. In this situation, the children are asked to interact with peers to discuss the prices of items, collect the correct amount of money, sort the bills, and provide change to the customer as necessary.

As the adolescent begins to seek employment and earn money, skills for budgeting and for using a savings or checking account become more important. The individual may require assistance in making lists and planning or sequencing the steps needed to develop a budget that fits his or her needs. The adolescent may lack awareness of the cost of items or what is required for budgeting. Money management involves check writing, depositing and withdrawing money, and use of an automatic teller machine (ATM). Check writing can be learned through practice using commercially available practice checks. For individuals with perceptual or motor difficulty that impacts their ability to maintain writing within a small space, a cardboard template can be made with cutouts in the areas requiring completion. An individual may recall the value and demonstrate appropriate exchange of the currency during the therapy session but may be unable to perform the task in an unfamiliar environment due to impaired shift or generalization across environments. The newly learned skills should therefore be assessed within the natural environment prior to discharge from therapy to ensure adequate proficiency.

Shopping

Performance skills required for successful shopping include the ability to make a list; identify where to purchase the item(s), that is, department store or grocery store; find and obtain a needed item in the store; calculate the purchase price; maneuver the shopping cart through the store; and complete the currency exchange to purchase the item(s). The client using a mobility device may need to call the store to find out about the accessibility and location of elevators. Grocery stores may provide a list of aisle numbers paired with items in the aisle or a map of the store to assist shoppers with disabilities. The client may need to practice asking for assistance from others as needed. Copies of lists with staple items or frequently used items can be prepared, with the client highlighting or circling the currently needed items before each trip. Items should be grouped (dairy, bread, soups, frozen items) as much as possible to conserve energy and increase efficiency. Picture cards can be made to assist the individual with difficulty identifying specific brands of item. Laminated picture cards can be attached to a ring before shopping and each card removed from the ring as the item is purchased. A calculator can be used to keep track of the cost of items. Individuals with visual or motor impairments may require a large-keypad calculator for successful use. Simulated environments can be set up in the clinic setting for the individual to practice maneuvering a shopping cart through obstacles and finding needed items.

Care of Pets

Many individuals experience great reward and gratification from caring for family pets. The child or adolescent is often expected to assist in the daily care of the family pet. Responsibilities could include feeding, grooming, keeping the environment clean, providing shelter and exercise as needed, and ensuring proper health care for the pet. Depending on the age of the individual, one or more of these activities may be expected. Lists and schedules can assist the individual with impaired memory skills carry out these responsibilities. Picture lists or schedules can assist the child or adolescent who is unable to read. Adaptations may be required for the individual with motor impairment. Larger tools for scooping food and cleaning up after the pet may be needed.

HEALTH MANAGEMENT AND MAINTANENCE

Managing one's health is an important IADL. To be healthy, a person must exercise, eat nutritious foods, protect the body, and manage medication regimens. Many children and adolescents do not manage and maintain their health status independently; however, this is an area in which children take an increasingly larger role as they get older. Therefore, it is important to address this area continually throughout childhood at the appropriate level for the individual.

CLINICAL *Pearl*

Adapted physical education should be recommended when the general gym class does not facilitate a child's participation because it does not meet his or her ability level or provide a safe environment. No student should be deprived of physical education and exposure to physical leisure opportunities.

Exercise

Exercise is a crucial element of health and wellness. Currently, the United States is facing the alarming challenge of increasing numbers of overweight and obese children.[10,12,15] Long-term consequences of obesity include increased risk for diabetes, cardiovascular disease, respiratory disorders, metabolic syndromes, cancers, gall bladder disease, and sleep apnea, as well as lowered self-esteem.[3,12] Further, children who have physical disabilities are at an increased risk for obesity.[10,12,15] OT practitioners can take on an important role in the prevention and remediation of obesity in children. For additional information, see Chapter 14, "Childhood and Adolescent Obesity."

New models of practice are emerging in which OT practitioners provide structures for **fitness** programs and work to change the environmental context and perceptions regarding physical activity.[3,12] The programs are especially relevant in school settings. OT practitioners can work creatively to improve access to physical occupations.[12] Occupational therapists have impacted fitness at the community level, for example, by increasing children's participation in active occupations or advocating for an open gym time at the local school.[10]

The OT practitioner can bring a unique and informed perspective to a fitness program.[10,12] The OT philosophy regarding health and wellness can be applied to create programs based on fitness and life-long participation in healthy physical activities rather than on weight loss. The OT practitioner plays an important role in determining the frequency and duration of physical activity for any individual.[12,15] When focusing on individuals with disabilities, the OT practitioner can promote activities with just the right challenge, or engage these individuals in activities that will enhance motor skills and ability to participate in social and community occupations.[15] The OT practitioner may provide consultation to a teacher or to a family regarding ways to include fitness activities in the daily routine of the client. In addition, an OT practitioner might advocate for a child with a disability to participate in sports or games to his or her ability or determine resources for adaptive sports.

CLINICAL *Pearl*

Within a school setting, advocacy for healthy choices in the cafeteria and vending machines, and the inclusion of recess and motor breaks positively impacts the health and well-being of all students and staff.

Fitness Programs

When developing a fitness program, the OT practitioner first determines the child's current level of physical activity and activity tolerance.[15] Gross motor skills are observed to determine the activities in which the child can participate with little or no assistance. The OT practitioner observes running, jumping, and climbing abilities. If these movements are not available or skilled, the OT practitioner determines what parts of the body have the most movements and designs activities and games that capitalize on those movements.[15]

Children who have significant motor impairments and lack volitional movement also need special programs for fitness such as passive range of motion (ROM) programs. An OT practitioner carries out ROM programs and teaches the program to the school staff or family members to ensure that the client receives the program each day. When teaching such a program, it is important to provide the information in more than one way and give informational materials to the learners so that they may review the lessons as needed. For example, ROM is demonstrated, explained verbally, and also explained with words and pictures on an information sheet. The OT practitioner teaches which joints should be moved

and how far and in what direction they should move. It is important to show the learner where to place the hands, how to watch for signs that the child may be in pain, and when to back off and consult with the occupational therapist. The OT practitioner ensures that the teachers and family members are able to safely provide the ROM exercises by asking them to demonstrate their ability before the learning session ends.

CLINICAL *Pearl*

If a child's range of motion decreases, consult your supervisor and/or report this change to the child's doctor. The child may need a splint to provide passive stretch during the day. In extreme cases, casting or surgeries may be necessary.

Adaptive Sports and Activities

People who have disabilities may wish to participate in competitive or club sports. The OT practitioner may play a role in identifying potential sports, providing resources and information regarding choices, and assisting with skill development or enhancement for successful participation in such an occupation. The Special Olympics provides competitive options for people with a wide range of abilities. Wheelchair sports as well as sports for those with visual impairments are available in many areas. Other options for children of varied abilities include swimming programs, karate, adapted gymnastics, and horseback riding. Physical fitness activities may be accessible via therapeutic recreational programs in the community. (See the resource list for adaptive sports at the end of the chapter.)

CLINICAL *Pearl*

Individuals with motor impairments may be better able to learn and participate in ball sports if larger equipment, such as a large ball or bat, is provided.

Nutrition

Nutrition is another area of health maintenance that OT practitioners can address during intervention, when appropriate, for the individual client.[10,27] Nutrition information can supplement other OT activities and add additional meaning. Nutrition themes can be woven in when working on handwriting, cutting, finger isolation for calculator use, or a variety of other goals. Nutrition information integrates well with OT activities for financial planning and cooking. Further, the OT practitioner can use games (e.g., board games) to teach the principles of eating well, avoiding too much snack foods and drinks, and minding caloric intake. When using the game, the OT practitioner may not only work on primary goals such as visual perception but also impact knowledge about nutrition through the theme of the game. For example, when working with matching, sorting, or identifying items from partial pictures, the OT practitioner may choose to use a healthy food as pictorial theme.

Occupational therapists have also impacted nutritious eating through novel and creative programs in school systems.[27] In one urban school, occupational therapists advocated for healthier choices at lunch and promoted healthier eating through educational programs regarding food and nutrition.[10] Within school and community settings, the OT practitioner can advocate for healthy choices in vending machines and snacks.

An OT practitioner may also be called upon to help picky eaters try new foods. When working with picky eaters, it is important to first consult with an occupational therapist trained in feeding interventions to ensure that no impairments in feeding exist.[19] Once cleared to try a variety of foods, the OT practitioner encourages pleasurable exposures to new foods. Strong pushing to try new foods should be avoided, as this can cause a power struggle and decrease the likelihood of the child increasing the food repertoire. Further, some children may withdraw from foods secondary to sensory processing disorders.[19] If a child is noted to gag at the sight or smell of food or withdraw from touching food or certain textures, sensory processing may need to be addressed before success with eating can be achieved. If this is the case, tolerance of smell and tactile experiences may be an appropriate starting point.

When working with picky eaters, it is important to expose them to new foods gradually.[19] Allow the child to enjoy mealtimes and experience pleasure through a slow introduction to new foods. New foods can also be introduced through a process known as *chaining*. First, determine what specific foods the child eats, as well as the textures, flavors, shapes, and colors of food the child currently enjoys. Next, provide exposure to new foods that share some of the characteristics of the familiar foods. For example, if the child enjoys the taste of spaghetti, he or she may be encouraged to try other dishes that have long noodles, are red and white in color, or have a tomato sauce flavor. The child might also try other shapes of pasta, other brands of tomato sauce, or other sauces. The child may also try new tastes by dipping a favorite food in new sauces.[19] Before using food chaining to increase a child's food repertoire, it would be highly beneficial to read the study report of Fraker, Fishbein, Cox, and Wilbert (Box 19-1).[19]

BOX 19-1

Sample Progression to Begin Trying New Foods and Improve Nutritious Eating

- Tolerate new foods in one's space—on the table, on another person's plate, and eventually on the child's plate.
- Touch new foods—this may occur through play, for example, feeding a toy.
- Smell new foods.
- Touch new foods to the cheek or lips.
- Lick new foods.
- Put new foods in the mouth and possibly chew the food with the option of discreetly spitting it out into a napkin.
- Chew and swallow new foods, beginning with one bite or a small bite.

Adapted from Fraker C, Fishbein M, Cox S, Walbert L: *Food chaining: The proven 6-step plan to stop picky eating, solve feeding problems, and expand your child's diet,* Cambridge, MA, 2007, Da Capo Press.

Note that the physician should be contacted immediately if the child experiences vomiting, retching, choking, spitting up, gagging, ongoing diarrhea, painful swallowing, wheezing, constipation, or lack of appetite during the intervention.[19]

CLINICAL *Pearl*

When working with picky eaters, new foods are best introduced during a planned snack time, rather than during regular meals.

Sexuality

Sexuality is a key element of life and plays a vital role in physical and emotional expression. Sexuality becomes an area of concern as children get older. It is especially important to discuss sexuality with adolescents who have cognitive disabilities or difficulty understanding the emotions or intentions of others.[33] Teenage girls and boys with cognitive disabilities may be particularly in need of consultations and coaching with regard to protecting their bodies and developing healthy sexuality.

Some OT practitioners may not feel comfortable discussing sexuality with their clients or other members of the team. However, the importance of this topic as it relates to health and safety cannot be underestimated. This issue can be addressed in several ways.[33] An OT practitioner can advocate for students with disabilities to participate in sexual education in public school at the appropriate learning level. It may be necessary for the OT practitioner to explain the importance of sex education to teachers, school administrators, or parents and guardians. Another option for dealing with this issue is direct consultation with the family. This can be achieved through written or oral communication, which might include information materials sent home with the child. Information materials on abstinence, sex education, and safe sex are readily available on the Internet.[33] It is imperative that the OT practitioner obtains consent from an individual's parent or guardian before discussing the topic of sexuality with a client who is a minor.

Medication Management

Children and adolescents require supervision to manage medication regimens. As adolescents mature, they may be able to take more and more responsibility for **medication management**.[30] The OT practitioner never works alone in teaching medication management. Rather, increasing the child's independence in medication management is a team decision. The parent or caregiver is always involved in the decision and the teaching/learning process. Some parents may desire their children's early independence in medication management. The number of children in the family and the educational level of parents may impact the decision. The severity of the disease or disorder and the developmental level of the child should always be taken into consideration.[30] Independence in managing medications cannot be taken lightly, as serious consequences may result from missing, duplicating, or misdosing medication.[17] Incorrect medication management can result in functional impairments, hospitalization, or even death.[17] When deciding if a client is ready for increased independence in medication management, the following questions must be asked:

- What would be the consequence if the medication were missed? In other words, how important is each medication dose to the person's health and well-being?[30]
- Does the client willingly take the medication? Does the client take all of the medication when it is presented?
- Can the client tell time? Can the client count correctly?
- Does the client know the names of his or her medications?
- Can the client distinguish between different medications based on size, shape, and other identifiable characteristics?[25]
- Can the client read the label on the medication container to distinguish between different medications?[25]

- Can the client independently open medication containers and manipulate individual pills effectively?
- Does the individual have problem-solving skills to be able to avoid taking too much or too little medication? Will the individual contact a caregiver or professional for help if confusion or problems arise?[21,30]

Once the team has decided to move forward with increasing the client's independence in medication management, the OT practitioner identifies the areas the client needs to work on through the questions listed above. The client may need to work on matching and sorting pills; this can be practiced with small items such as buttons or candy before moving on to pills. Fine motor skills may need to be targeted to promote efficient manipulation of the pills. In this case, grasp and in-hand manipulation are observed and addressed during the intervention.

Success with medication management is increased through assistance with effective organization of medications.[17] Therefore, intervention techniques include setting up a weekly pillbox and organizing visual reminders such as written cue cards or pictures that display the pill organization accurately that the client can work from.[25] Once the pillbox is set up, the client will need fine motor skills and motor planning to open each segment and pour the pills into the hand.

Once the client can successfully organize the medications, he or she may be ready to begin taking them with more independence. Initially, the child takes the medication independently, but under the supervision of a caregiver. Next, an effective system to remind the client to take the medication is set up.[17] Visual notes and reminders may be helpful. Computer reminders through e-mail and calendar programs may assist computer-savvy individuals.[17] Ongoing success is often dependent on the generation of routines and habits with regard to taking medications.[21]

Once the client has demonstrated success to this point, the decision to move forward with greater independence may be taken. At first, a telephone call to ensure each dose has been taken is recommended. The amount and type of support a client needs is then individualized. The OT practitioner may consult with caregivers or nurses to assist with determining the level of support that the individual requires. Some clients may need assistance to set up the weekly pillbox but may be independent in taking the medication each day. Others may be more independent with medication organization but may need assistance each month to determine which medications need refills. Regardless of the level of independence, it is important that an accurate list of all medications be maintained. It is further recommended that a pill count be regularly done to ensure that medications are being taken correctly.[21] Also, additional support is given whenever a medication regimen changes.[21]

HOME ESTABLISHMENT AND MAINTENANCE

Home management tasks frequently include activities such as cleaning, laundry, and trash disposal, as well as maintenance tasks such as repairs and yard care.[32] For children and adolescents, home management includes occupations that are typically known as *chores*. The expectations for chore completion vary depending on the family culture and the individual's capacity for engagement. Many families of children with disabilities may not require their children to do chores. However, when children participate in doing chores, even simple or adapted ones, they are learning how to complete tasks, role competence, and responsibility. Further, they will likely gain self-efficacy and confidence. Common chores include putting toys and games away, cleaning the bedroom, making the bed, doing laundry, washing kitchen or bathroom surfaces, vacuuming, dusting, and taking out the garbage. Adults with disabilities who experience difficulty with home management tasks have to rely on assistance from others in the community, or they may be unable to live alone.[32] Therefore, it is important for children to learn and practice home management tasks as they grow older to prepare them for greater independence as adults.

The OT practitioner consults with parents to suggest home management tasks that are appropriate for the individual client's abilities, assists with modifications and adaptations to improve success and independence, and provides direct intervention so that the child can learn to do the task as appropriate. OT practitioners may also address home management tasks in the school system as part of a life skills program or to prepare for transition out of the school system. Young children participate in home management through tidying up toys; they are frequently helped in doing this by a "clean-up song" or routine. Clearly marked boxes and shelves also improve performance. Older children begin doing chores at home. It is recommended that a child is allowed to master one or two specific chores that they are able to accomplish with the most independence possible before more complex chores are expected to be done in the natural environment. Such tasks may include taking out the garbage, getting the mail, or washing the kitchen table. As the child shows greater success, independence, and initiative with these tasks, the more difficult tasks are introduced. Positive reinforcements, whether verbal or monetary, increase motivation. Also note that behavioral strategies such as

---

BOX 19-2

Methods for Working With Cognitive Limitations

- Provide lists, charts, or check off sheets to indicate what tasks need to be done.
- Break tasks down into smaller components.
- Provide visuals to communicate each step.
- Provide pre-teaching for each step; it may be helpful to teach the motor plan, or physical process of getting the job done; for example, spray, wipe up and down, step to the right and do it again.
- Provide gradated assistance to get the job done, but fade assistance to increase independence. Begin with hand-over-hand if needed, then gradate physical assistance; next, fade to verbal cues, then provide visuals or check lists.
- Provide positive reinforcements, as appropriate.

---

sticker charts or tangible reward systems may be necessary.

Common barriers to independence in home management include cognitive and physical limitations. Methods for assisting individuals with general difficulties in these areas are described in Boxes 19-2 and 19-3.

MEAL PREPARATION AND CLEAN-UP

Meal preparation is an important occupation for independence. When learning to prepare meals, children often begin by simply helping adults with cooking or setting the table. As they get older, children may begin to follow a simple recipe or prepare a simple snack by themselves. Later, adolescents may learn to use the microwave, toaster, toaster oven, range, or oven. At each stage, the OT practitioner instructs clients in safety in the kitchen, techniques for handling food properly, and safety with utensils.[20] Depending on needs of the individual client, the OT practitioner may also address using specific cooking appliances, measuring ingredients, using a recipe, cleaning the workspace, and properly storing food.[20] The OT practitioner modifies and adapts tasks, tools, and workspaces to provide interventions that facilitate greater independence with meal preparation. The OT practitioner may also provide educational materials to assist with generalization of skills.[20]

Meal Preparation With Young Children

Young children benefit from assisting with preparation of snacks that do not require cooking and from assisting with obtaining and mixing ingredients for a dish which the adult will cook or bake. These tasks can be

BOX 19-3

Methods for Working With Physical Limitations

- Provide direct intervention with regard to mobility through the home or other natural environment where the tasks will take place.
- Provide adaptive equipment such as reachers, long-handled tools, tools with built-up handles, tools that have straps to affix to the hand during chores and work, or tool belts for carrying cleaning products.
- Adapt the environment to remove physical obstacles: Remove throw rugs, move unnecessary furniture that may block a pathway, store cleaning products and tools in an accessible area, and remove doors from the door frame to improve accessibility.
- Organize the environment so that the products and tools used for particular jobs are located close to the area where the job is performed.
- Recommend products for ease of use, such as self-propelling vacuums, easy spray or aerosol cleaning products, dusting rags that require no dusting spray, front-loading washing machines and dryers, accessible shelves in lieu of cabinets or deep closets for storage of linens and clothing.
- Recommend home modifications, when possible, to include accessible sink spaces, accessible home appliances, widened doorways, and lowered cabinets, counters, and shelf spaces.

integrated into an OT session, school curriculum, or parent activity. Young children might slice bananas with a dull, plastic knife, assemble a fruit salad, sequence the addition of ingredients for trail mix, slice tubes of cookie dough, roll up pieces of deli meat, or stir the ingredients for a cake or mashed potato. These activities can be used as creative ways to address many goals such as fine motor, sequencing, and pre-reading goals. They provide a natural venue for discussing healthy eating as well as cultural traditions. They also make excellent group activities. The OT practitioner can get recipe ideas for OT activities from cookbooks for young children.

Meal Preparation With Older Children

Older children may begin participating in snack and meal preparation more independently. The OT practitioner begins with a simple snack preparation and observes the child's motor and cognitive skills to determine what level of cooking suits the therapy sessions best. Older children are likely ready to prepare snacks or lunch foods that require more than one step. Examples include sandwiches, tuna and egg salads, cake mixes,

vegetable and fruit salads, and frozen foods that are cooked in the microwave. Older children may begin working on simple cutting and peeling if their fine motor skills are adequate for safe participation. Modifications and adaptations may be required for safety, independence, and success.

Meal Preparation With Adolescents

Adolescents who have achieved the skills to complete the tasks previously noted may begin participating in more complex food preparation. They may work from a recipe and prepare snacks and other foods with multiple steps. Some clients may work with printed recipes, while others may benefit from recipes that also show the steps in a picture format. They may begin learning to use appliances. The OT practitioner observes motor and cognitive skills to select the most appropriate appliances. A microwave allows individuals with physical or visual impairments to cook with greater ease and safety.[24] The toaster oven and the crockpot are convenient for individuals whose physical disabilities may prevent them from using the oven easily.[22] Additionally, these smaller and portable devices will likely be used more often than an oven when the client lives independently.[24] Therefore, the OT practitioner may choose to work with these appliances first.

Modifications and Adaptations to Assist With Meal Preparation

CLINICAL *Pearl*

When working with meal preparation, begin with simple snacks that require no heating. Increase the number of steps or ingredients that are needed to increase complexity. Move on to microwave preparation before asking the child to use the stovetop or oven.

As individuals who use wheelchairs get older, kitchen accessibility may become a priority (Table 19-7). The OT practitioner can provide consultation on kitchen modifications to make cooking easier and safer for them. Using a microwave, crockpot, toaster oven, or cook-top range (burners only) helps avoid more extensive modifications.[22] Wheelchairs need an adequate turning radius in the kitchen, ideally 5 × 5 ft. People using wheelchairs need to get close to the counters, sink, and oven. Counters can be lowered; and adaptive refrigerators, sinks, and stovetops that provide space for the cook's knees can be installed. Cabinets and cabinet doors can be removed so the cook can access the workspace while in the wheelchair.[22]

TABLE 19-7

Cooking Adaptations

ADAPTATION	DESCRIPTION
ADAPTATIONS FOR WORKING WITH ONE HAND	
Utensils with large and ergonomic handles	Provide a larger surface to grasp, hold, and carry the tools
Jar openers	Mount to wall or provide power to open jars and bottles
Electric can openers or those with shelves	Provide power or stability to open cans
Bottle and carton holders	Increase ease of pour for large liquid containers
Stationary bowls	Prevent bowl from slipping while working through suction cups or metal frames
Pot holding frames	Hold a pot onto a burner to prevent it from moving
Stationary cutting boards	Suction to the work space and hold food stationary with prongs to allow for one-handed cutting
Stationary peelers	Suction to the work space to allow for one-handed peeling
Roller or rocker knives	Allow for one handed cutting
Stationary scrubbers	Suction to side of sink basin to allow for one-handed dish washing
ADAPTATIONS FOR WORKING WITH LOW VISION	
Contrast-color cutting boards	Improve visibility of food and working materials
Liquid indicators	Indicate when liquid is reaching a certain level
Adjusting level guides for measuring	Provide a tactile method for measuring rather than relying on small printing on liquid measuring cups

Adapted from Infinitec, 2009: *Infinite potential through assistive technology.* http://www.infinitec.org/live/kitchens: Accessed January 3, 2009.

The OT practitioner also trains individuals in mobility in the kitchen. Without modifications to the environment, the client will have to approach the counter or sink sideways in the wheelchair which is not ideal. To remove items from the refrigerator, the client will have to maneuver the wheelchair sideways to the refrigerator door, open the door, and then move into the space such that the wheelchair keeps the door open and the client can reach the items in the refrigerator. The refrigerator contents must be organized in such a way that the client can reach all of the items without stretching unsafely. If the kitchen lacks the space the cook needs, chopping and cold preparation can be done in another location close to the kitchen.[22] The client can use a rolling cart to transport items, or trays can be placed strategically throughout the workspace to ensure safe mobility; cooks who use wheelchairs should never carry hot items on their laps.[22]

CASE *Study*

Robert receives OT through his school. As part of his transition planning, some goals were set—that he prepare snacks and simple meals independently. This would allow him to eat nutritious foods when home alone and participate in an independent living program after high school. When a certified OTA began working with him, Robert's personal goal was to make macaroni and cheese. The OT practitioner recommended that they start with some other foods so she could observe his skills and ensure that he would be safe using the stovetop. As they worked, the OT practitioner noted that Robert could not maintain his postural control when using both hands despite a chest strap on his chair. Robert needed to support his upper body with one arm when pouring, cutting, stirring, or transporting bowls or pots. Robert and the OT practitioner worked on his positioning to make food preparation most effective and help him expend his energy more efficiently. He worked at low tables where he could use one arm to support his body while also holding a bowl, rather than working at the higher countertop. They worked on transporting items across the counters with a sliding motion and discussed environmental modifications that would help Robert avoid having to transport bowls, especially hot bowls, over long distances. They also worked on maneuvering Robert's wheelchair to bring him close to the refrigerator and microwave so that he could reach items without compromising his posture. The OT practitioner realized that Robert would not be able to stir or flip an item on the stovetop because he would be unable to support his upper body and stabilize the pot or pan at the same time. Therefore, they decided to make microwave macaroni and cheese, and Robert could thus achieve his goal while ensuring safe cooking practices. The certified OTA also consulted with the physical therapist to determine whether a more supportive system was indicated for increased postural stability.

SAFETY PROCEDURES AND EMERGENCY RESPONSES

Individuals who have disabilities have the same needs and rights with regard to safety and emergency response as do others. In some cases, children with disabilities will require a higher level of planning, practice, adaptations, or environmental modifications to ensure their safety. The OT practitioner may consult with parents and the staff at schools or daycare centers to ensure the safety of children. Factors to consider include the use of child safety devices, fire safety, safety with strangers, and street safety. Emergency planning must also be given specific attention. Families and schools must plan for expected emergencies, for example, a storm that has been forecast, as well as sudden emergencies. Advance planning is the key to ensuring safety. Refer to the list of resources for specific publications and information on emergency planning.

Child Safety Devices

Some children with disabilities may be more prone to exploring unsafe household substances or lack the judgment to identify unsafe substances. Children with physical disabilities may also require enhanced safety while sleeping in a bed (Table 19-8).

CLINICAL *Pearl*

When recommending bed safety rails, for optimal safety, consider rails that attach at the bottom of the bed rather than at the sides. Older and large-sized children sleeping in full-sized beds may require hospital bed rails.[28]

Fire Safety

Special measures must be taken to ensure the safety of children with disabilities in the event of a fire.[41-45] These children may need to be alerted about the fire and be helped to exit safely. All families should have basic fire escape plans. Government guidelines for a safe fire escape are as follows:[18]

- Install fire alarms on each floor of the home or building.
- Create a fire escape plan with two ways to exit each room.

TABLE 19-8

Common Safety Devices

COMMON SAFETY DEVICES	USES
Safety locks and safety latches	Use to close doors, cabinets, and drawers that contain sharp objects, cleaning products, or toxic chemicals
Safety gates	Prevent children from falling down stairs, or entering rooms containing dangerous materials or tools
Door locks and door knob covers	Prevent children from entering some areas at all, such as the area with an unsupervised swimming pool
Electrical outlet covers	Prevent children from touching electrical outlets
Child bed safety rails	Prevent children from falling off the bed

Adapted from *My Child Safety*, 2010: *Child safety devices:* http://www.mychildsafety.net/child-safety-devices.html: Accessed January 3, 2009.

- Leave immediately if a fire occurs.
- Feel a door before opening; if it is hot do not open it.
- Plan a meeting place outside the house; use a specific location rather than a general "across the street."
- Never go back into the building; wait for the assistance of fire fighters.
- Know the principle of "stop, drop, and roll"; if an individual is unable to do so due to physical disability, he or she should have a small fire extinguisher readily available and be trained in its use.

Recognition of a fire is the first step to a safe escape. People who have visual or hearing impairment will need adapted fire alarms. Devices that vibrate, flash, or flash a strobe light outside the home to alert others ensure that an individual with a disability becomes aware of a fire as soon as possible.[41-45]

Escaping a burning building will be especially difficult for a child with a physical disability.[41-45] A plan of escape must be put in place and practiced repeatedly to ensure that all possible obstacles are considered and the extent of assistance that the child will need is fully understood. A family or institution may enlist the assistance of the fire department in developing a safe exit strategy. Additionally, the local fire department can be contacted in advance to provide information about the specific needs of a child with a disability when there is a fire. When formulating an exit plan, ensure that the child's mobility system, such as the wheelchair or walker, can fit through all doors of the escape route. Wheelchair ramps should be installed at emergency exits to ensure easy access for these children. Whenever possible, children with physical disabilities should be housed on the first floor of a building because they will not be able to use an elevator in the event of a fire. New buildings that have only one accessible exit are required to set up a fireproof area equipped with an emergency call system. If such an area exists, the child must be trained in how to get to the area and call for assistance. Schools must have fire escape chairs available when children in powered chairs use the upper floors of school buildings. Families and institutions may also consider making a back-up plan for the eventuality of the child being unable to escape the burning building. In this case, fire protection devices should be installed. This might include sprinkler systems and fireproof partition walls. Fireproof blankets and fire extinguishers will also be helpful in this situation.[41-45]

Safety With Strangers

All children must be taught about who they can trust and who they cannot and that they should never go anywhere with a stranger.[29] Children who have disabilities may need more intensive and repeated learning opportunities to ensure that they can maintain their safety.

Safety With Strangers for Young Children

Young children learn about dealing with strangers from their parents, preschool, early elementary school, and storybooks. Stranger safety information is easily integrated into the school curriculum and in OT interventions for fine motor or perceptual goals. This issue is commonly addressed through information about the people in the community that children are safe to trust—community helpers such as policemen, firemen, security guards, teachers, and medical workers. OT practitioners may assist children with learning about community helpers through discussions and activities that include coloring, cutting, gluing, or matching pictures of community helpers. OT practitioners may also recommend songs or storybooks to teachers and parents. It is usually the responsibility of parents and teachers to teach children not to go anywhere with strangers; however, at times, the OT practitioner may see the need to provide guidance to parents about effective methods for communicating this to their children and to teachers about methods for integrating activities to teach this safety lesson into the school curriculum.

Safety With Strangers for Older Children

Older children who have disabilities may require repeated learning opportunities and practice with strategies to ensure they understand the rules and methods for keeping themselves safe. Common methods for introducing stranger safety concepts include pictures, movies, and social stories. The OT practitioner can ensure that children know what to do if they are confronted by strangers and provide opportunities for practice through role-play activities. Children can be taught that when a community helper is not present, they can make a loud noise, scream, and yell for assistance. Some children may also carry a whistle or other emergency noisemaker if they are unable make enough noise to get assistance in an emergency.[29]

SUMMARY

The authors provide a description of instrumental activities of daily living (IADLs) which include communication, community mobility, financial management, shopping, care of pets, health management and maintenance, home establishment and maintenance, meal preparation and clean-up, safety procedures and emergency procedures. Specifically, the authors provide thorough descriptions of the IADLs and discuss how OT practitioners help children and adolescents with cognitive, physical, visual, and communication challenges engage in these activities. The authors provide intervention strategies and discuss the considerations, (e.g., family culture, community culture, age, physical setting) that practitioners examine when making clinical decisions. Specific intervention techniques such as forward and backward chaining, compensation, and assistive technology are introduced along with numerous case examples to illustrate sample intervention sessions. OT practitioners play a key role in helping children and adolescents engage in a variety of IADLs which are important in developing autonomy and life satisfaction.

References

1. Adaptive Technology Resource Centre. Inclusive Design Resource Centre. Available at: http://atrc.utoronto.ca/. Accessed July 8, 2010.
2. American Occupational Therapy Association: Occupational therapy practice framework: domain and process. *Am J Occup Ther* 56:609–639, 2002.
3. American Occupational Therapy Association: Occupational therapy practice framework: domain and process, ed 2. *Am J Occup Ther* 62:625–683, 2008.
4. Blanchard SA: AOTA's statement on obesity. *Am J Occup Ther* 60:680, 2006.
5. Brinker RP, Lewis M: Discovering the competent handicapped infant: a process approach to assessment and

intervention. *Top Early Childhood Special Educ* 2:1–16, 1982.

6. Brodwin MG, Cardoso E, Tristen S: Computer assistive technology for people who have disabilities: computer adaptations and modifications. *J Rehabil* 70:28–33, 2004.

7. Brown C et al: Influence of instrumental activities of daily living assessment method on judgments of independence. *Am J Occup Ther* 50:202–206, 1996.

8. Bryan LC, Gast DL: Teaching on-task and on-schedule behaviors to high-functioning children with autism via picture activity schedules. *J Autism Dev Disord* 30:553–567, 2000.

9. Bull MJ, Engle WA: Safe transportation of preterm and low birth weight infants at hospital discharge. *Pediatrics* 123:1424–1429, 2009.

10. Butler C: Effects of powered mobility on self-initiated behaviors of very young children with locomotor disability. *Dev Med Child Neurol* 28:325–332, 1997.

11. Cahill SM, Suarez-Balcazar Y: Promoting children's nutrition and fitness in the urban context. *Am J Occup Ther* 63:113–116, 2009.

12. Chen SC et al: Infrared-based communication augmentation system for people with multiple disabilities. *Disabil Rehabil* 26:1105–1109, 2004.

13. Clark F, Reingold FS, Salles-Jordan K: Obesity and occupational therapy. *Am J Occup Ther* 61:701–703, 2007.

14. Cooper-Kahn J, Dietzel L: *What is executive functioning?* Available at: http://www.ldonline.org/article/What-Is-Executive-Functioning%3F. Accessed January 9, 2010.

15. Deitz J, Swinth Y, White, O: Powered mobility and preschoolers with complex developmental delays. *Am J Occup Ther* 56:86–96, 2002.

16. Dwyer G et al: Promoting children's health and well-being: broadening the therapy perspective. *Phys Occup Ther Pediatr* 29:27–43, 2009.

17. DynaVox Mayer Johnson, 2009. Available at: http://www.dynavoxtech.com/products/devices.aspx. Accessed October 13, 2009.

18. Feldman PH et al: Medication management: evidence brief. *Home Healthc Nurse* 27:379–386, 2009.

19. Fire Safety: *An information resource for eliminating residential fire deaths,* 2010. Available at: http://www.firesafety.gov. Accessed Janueary 3, 2010.

20. Fraker C et al: *Food chaining: the proven 6-step plan to stop picky eating, solve feeding problems, and expand your child's diet,* Cambridge, MA, 2007, Da Capo Press.

21. Grimm EZ et al: Meal preparation: comparing treatment approaches to increase acquisition or skills for adults with schizophrenic disorders. *Occup Ther J Res* 29:148–153, 2009.

22. Haslbeck JW, Schaeffer D: Routines in medication management: the perspective of people with chronic conditions. *Chronic Illn* 5:184, 2009.

23. Infinitec: *Infinite potential through assistive technology,* 2009. Available at: http://www.infinitec.org/live/kitchens. Accessed January 3, 2009.

24. Jones J, Stewart H: A description of how three occupational therapists train children in using the scanning access technique. *Austr Occup Ther J* 51:155–165, 2004.

25. Kondo T et al: The use of microwave ovens by elderly persons with disabilities. *Am J Occup Ther* 51:739–747, 1997.

26. Kripalani S et al: Development of an illustrated medication schedule as a low-literacy patient education tool. *Patient Educ Couns* 66:368–377, 2007.

27. Moreira-Almeida A, Koenig HG: Retaining the meaning of the words religiousness and spirituality: a commentary on the WHOQOL SRPB group's "A cross cultural study of spirituality, religion and personal beliefs as components of quality of life" (62:6, 2005). *Soc Sci Med* 63:843–845, 2006.

28. Munguba MC, Valdes MTM, Da Silva CAB: The application of an occupational therapy nutrition education programme for children who are obese. *Occup Ther Int* 15:56–70, 2008.

29. My Child Safety: *Child safety devices,* 2010. Available at: http://www.mychildsafety.net/child-safety-devices.html. Accessed January 3, 2009.

30. My Child Safety: *Stranger danger,* 2010. Available at: http://www.mychildsafety.net/stranger-danger.htm. Accessed January 3, 2009.

31. Orrell-Valente JK et al: At what age do children start taking daily asthma medicines on their own? *Pediatrics* 128:e1186–e1192, 2008.

32. PECS USA: *What is PECS?* 2009. Available at: http://www.pecs-usa.com/WhatsPECS.htm. Accessed October 13, 2009.

33. Powell JM et al: Gaining insight into patients' perspectives on participation in home management activities after traumatic brain injury. *Am J Occup Ther* 61:269–279, 2007.

34. Savarimuthu D, Bunnell T: Sexuality and learning disabilities. *Nurs Stand* 17:33–35, 2003.

35. Shutrump SE, Manary M, Buning ME: Transportation for students who use wheelchairs on the school bus. *OT Practice* 13:8–12, 2008.

36. Sigafoos J et al: Supporting self-determination in AAC interventions by assessing preference for communication devices. *Technol Disabil* 17:143–153, 2005.

37. Stav W: Seatbelts on school buses, not a good idea. *OT Practice* 14:18–20, 2009.

38. Stav WB, Monahan M: *The occupational therapy role in driving and community mobility across the lifespan* (fact sheet). Available at: http://www.aota.org/Older-Driver/Professionals/Toolkit/Professional/Brochures-and-Fact-Sheets/41773.aspx. Accessed September 14, 2009.

39. Stav WB et al: Driving and community mobility. *Am J Occup Ther* 59:666–670, 2005.

40. Toglia J: Management of occupational therapy services for persons with cognitive impairments (statement). *Am J Occup Ther* 53:605–607, 1999.

41. United States Access Board: *ADA accessibility guidelines for transportation vehicles,* September 1998. Available at: http://www.access-board.gov/transit/html/vguide.htm. Accessed September 15, 2009.

42. U.S. Fire Administration: *Fire risks for the blind or visually impaired,* 1999. Available at: http://www.usfa.dhs.gov/downloads/pdf/publications/fa-205.pdf. Accessed January 3, 2010.

43. U.S. Fire Administration: *Fire risks for the deaf or hard of hearing*, 1999. Available at: http://www.usfa.dhs.gov/downloads/pdf/publications/fa-202-508.pdf. Accessed January 3, 2010.
44. U.S. Fire Administration: *Fire risks for the mobility impaired*, 1999. Available at: http://www.usfa.dhs.gov/downloads/pdf/publications/fa-204-508.pdf. Accessed January 3, 2009.
45. U.S. Fire Administration: *Fire safety for people with disabilities*, 2009. Available at: http://www.usfa.dhs.gov/citizens/disability/. Accessed January 3, 2010.
46. U.S. Fire Administration: *People with disabilities and their caregivers*, 2009. Available at: http://www.usfa.dhs.gov/citizens/disability/fswy22.shtm. Accessed January 3, 2010.
47. Watson AH et al: Effect of technology in a public school setting. *Am J Occup Ther* 64:18–29, 2010.

Resource List

ADAPTIVE SPORTS ORGANIZATIONS

Disabled Sports USA: www.dsusa.org
Dwarf Athletic Association of America: www.daaa.org
Great Lakes Adaptive Sports Association: www.glasa.org
Adaptive Sports Center of Crested Butte Colorado: www.adaptivesports.org
International Paralympic Committee: www.paralympic.org
BlazeSports America: www.blazesports.org
National Sports Center for the Disabled: www.nscd.org
National Wheelchair Basketball Association: www.nwba.org
Special Olympics: www.specialolympics.org
United States Association of Blind Athletes: www.usaba.org
USA Deaf Sports Federation: www.usadeafsports.org

DAILY LIVING AIDS COMPANIES

Daily Living Aids for People who are Blind or Visually Impaired: www.annmorris.com
Dynamic Living: www.dynamic-living.com
Independent Living Aids, Inc.: www.independentliving.com
Sammons Preston Roylan: www.sammonspreston.com

REVIEW *Questions*

1. List 5 IADLs and describe how they relate to occupational performance in children and adolescents.
2. What therapeutic activities might an OT practitioner use to address difficulties in community mobility for a child or adolescent?
3. What are the safety procedures and emergency procedures an OT practitioner may need to address with children and youth?
4. Describe some communication strategies. How would an OT practitioner consult with a speech therapy practitioner? Describe the differences in the two roles.
5. What are some intervention strategies to help a child or adolescent engage in health management and maintenance activities?
6. How might an OT practitioner help a child who has physical or cognitive difficulties with home establishment and maintenance?

SUGGESTED *Activities*

1. Choose one IADL in which you currently engage. Describe in detail the tasks involved in this IADL. Describe how you have changed in your ability since when you were a child. Discuss those things that have helped you succeed or interfered with your ability to perform. How would you help a child perform this IADL?

2. Describe some compensatory strategies to help a child or youth who is visually impaired perform IADLs. What equipment is available? Describe resources in your area.

3. Interview adolescents to better understand their health management and maintenance routines. What issues are they facing regarding sexuality, fitness, and nutrition?

4. Design a meal preparation activity for toddlers, middle-school children, and adolescents. Participate in the acitivity with a child and describe how you had to change your activity to be successful. Examine what you would do differently next time.

How did you choose this activity and whom would it benefit?

5. Review the section on community mobility and then explore the options in your neighborhood. Describe the transportation options and consider how a child or adolescent who uses a wheelchair would access such options. Explore how a child would access the typical activities (e.g., school, playground, sports, local places). Present your findings to classmates.

6. Prepare a meal using a variety of cooking adaptations (from class or from local store). Describe how the adaptations changed the task.

7. Visit a speech therapy practitioner and discuss the variety of communication devices. How does the practitioner view the role of the OT practitioner? Communicate with a child who uses a communication device. Discuss this with the speech therapy practitioner and specifically ask about techniques that would help the communication. Provide a summary of your findings to classmates.

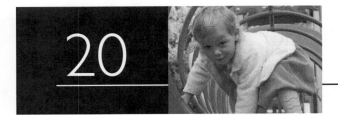

20

Play and Playfulness

JANE CLIFFORD O'BRIEN

GWENDOLYN J. DUREN

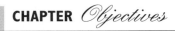

CHAPTER *Objectives*

After studying this chapter, the reader will be able to accomplish the following:

- Describe the characteristics of play and playfulness and differentiate between the two
- Identify potential barriers to play that children with disabilities may encounter
- Describe ways to facilitate play and playfulness in children who have special needs
- Describe the way that play is used as a tool in occupational therapy sessions to increase skills
- Describe how play is used as a goal of occupational therapy
- Identify occupational therapy assessments used to evaluate play and playfulness
- Describe techniques that promote play and playfulness

CASE *Study*

Think about a time in your childhood when you were playing.

- What were you doing?
- Who was with you?
- Where were you?
- How did you feel?
- What was the expression on your face?
- What did you learn?
- Was playing an important aspect of your day?

Perhaps you are thinking about a time you and your friends sat on your grandmother's porch and played house. Maybe you were playing school. Recalling these moments brings many happy memories to mind. People remember laughing, making friends, learning and testing skills (such as who could jump the highest), problem solving, and negotiating. These skills are critical to a child's development and provide a foundation for the future.

Children learn motor, social–emotional, language, and cognitive skills through play.[23,30,33,46,50] To illustrate this fact, consider a 1-year-old girl playing in the water sprinkler. The child bends down to feel the cool water in her hands. She is practicing motor planning, squatting, and balancing while receiving the tactile sensation of the water on her hands. As she cups her hands on the sprinkler, she must coordinate her tiny fingers to grasp the nozzle. Cognitively, she pays attention to the water and tries to figure out what happens when she changes her hand position. She is learning the ways in which liquid differs from the solid ground on which she stands. She problem-solves to keep the water in her hands and tries to understand the reason it leaks through. Orally, she feels the water on her tongue and swallows the droplets. She sticks her tongue out and gathers the liquid in her throat to swallow it. Her 4-year-old brother joins the play activity, and now she must share the sprinkler. He laughs and jumps. She watches and smiles and tries to imitate his skills. She is developing social skills. The children repeat the play activities. Watching them, it becomes clear that play requires many skills.

Children learn and refine skills during play.[1,5,6,17,20,27] This is demonstrated as children show off feats of strength and agility, problem-solve to play a game or perform a motor skill, and work out problems that arise. They communicate to satisfy their needs and decide on rules for the activities by negotiating with group members. Often children spend the entire play time deciding on the rules of the game or the way the story will unfold. They use their language skills and must become keen observers of nonverbal communication.[6,10]

Maximizing a child's ability to play interests occupational therapy (OT) practitioners because it is the primary occupation of childhood and critical to the development of skills.[10,28,36] To appreciate the importance of play, imagine life without it. Life would certainly be lacking without play. Parham and Primeau underscored the importance of play by stating that it may reveal what makes life worth living.[42]

With this appreciation of the importance of play, imagine making a difference in a child's ability to play. Developing a child's play skills comprehensively affects both the child and his or her family. The child is better able to interact with friends, family members, and the environment.

OT practitioners work with children to enhance their ability to play and thus can make a difference in their lives.

PLAY

Most adults smile when asked to remember a time they were playing. They reminisce about childhood memories of favorite toys and activities. They laugh and relate humorous stories such as having mud fights and conducting elaborate neighborhood play events. Adults recall historic events from childhood play such as pretending to be astronauts landing on the moon. They are able to describe the activities, feelings, and skills they gained during play. Most agree that play was, and still is, fun!

Play is generally defined as a pleasurable, self-initiated activity that the child can control. **Intrinsic motivation** is the self-initiation or drive to action for which the reward is the activity itself rather than some external reward.[10] Intrinsic motivation is demonstrated when children repeat activities over and over.[10] **Internal control** is the extent to which the child is in control of the actions and to some degree the outcome of an activity.[10] Internal control is observed when children spontaneously change the play (e.g., when a 6-year-old boy declares in the middle of a pretend game, "Now I am going to be the good guy."). Intrinsic motivation and internal control are important for the development of problem solving, learning, and socialization skills.

Another element of play is the **freedom to suspend reality**, which is sometimes seen as the ability to participate in make-believe activities, or pretend play (Figure 20-1).[10,49] **Pretend play** develops as children are able to engage in higher cognitive functioning.[46] They begin by role playing simple everyday actions such as feeding a doll. They are able to engage in elaborate make-believe scenarios as their language and cognitive skills develop.

Freedom to suspend reality also includes teasing, joking, mischief, and bending the rules.[10] Children turn old games into new ones by changing the rules, creating new situations, and using objects imaginatively during play.

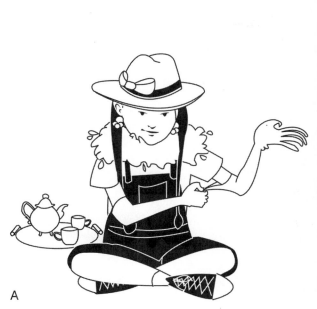
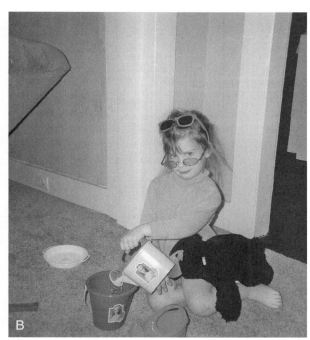

FIGURE 20-1   A, Pretend play allows children to break free from rules. **B,** A girl plants a garden with her bear.

Play is the primary occupation of children and a medium for intervention.[11,23,27,35,40,41]

Play affords skillful OT practitioners unlimited opportunities to teach, refine, and enable more successful functioning and play.

PLAYFULNESS

Playfulness is defined as one's disposition to play.[5,11] It is a style individuals use to flexibly approach problems and can be regarded as an aspect of a child's personality.[11] Playfulness, like play, encompasses intrinsic motivation, internal control, and freedom to suspend reality, all of which occur on a continuum.[10,23,33,36]

Children who are engaged in the play process are intrinsically motivated. They show signs of enjoyment and seem to be having fun.[10,14] Internal control is evidenced in sharing, playing with others, entering new play situations, initiating play, deciding, modifying activities, and challenging themselves.[10,14] Children who use objects creatively or in unconventional ways, tease, and pretend show the element of freedom to suspend reality (Figure 20-2).[10,14]

CASE *Study*

Children lacking playfulness exhibit problems fulfilling their roles as players. For example, Sam is a 6-year-old boy with sensory integrative dysfunction. He has difficulty with motor tasks and does not play well with friends. Sam is not spontaneous in activities. He requires time to plan the way he will accomplish motor tasks. Sam becomes very upset when he does not get his way. He does not like the rules to be changed and has trouble changing pace once he is involved in an activity. Moreover, he does not read the other children's cues and frequently plays roughly. He shows poor body awareness by getting too close to the other children. Sam does not initiate play with his peers. His slow and awkward movements cause him to lag behind. During the OT evaluation, Sam states that he has no friends and no one likes him. His parents are worried that Sam does not have any friends. The goal of his OT sessions is to improve his playfulness so that he can interact with friends in the home, school, and community settings.

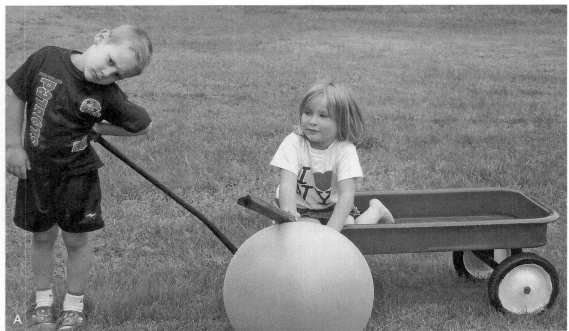

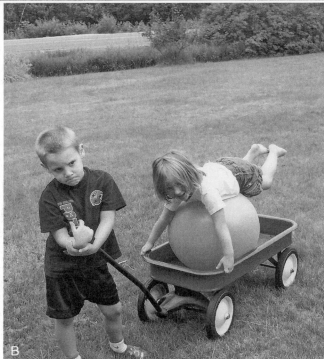

FIGURE 20-2 Children Must Negotiate and Problem-Solve During Play. **A,** A girl and a boy spend time figuring out what to do with the large ball, stick, and wagon. They must negotiate who will pull the wagon. **B,** The boy pulls the wagon while the girl is holding on tight. They challenge their motor skills (e.g., balancing on the large ball). Using objects in unconventional ways (e.g., lying on the ball in the wagon) is part of playfulness.

The OT practitioner works to develop rapport with Sam and plans fun and playful activities. Sam does not initiate play activities but is cooperative and attempts all of them. The OT practitioner strives to enable him to have fun and be spontaneous during the therapy sessions, hoping that this behavior extends to the home and school settings as well.

During one session, the OT practitioner and Sam engage in a game of Star Wars. Sam, playing Darth Vader, runs after the OT practitioner, saying, "I will get you, Luke." The OT practitioner is thrilled that Sam is initiating play. However, shortly thereafter Sam stops playing, looks at the OT practitioner, and says, "Is it time to go yet?"

Sam exhibits a low level of playfulness. He is not engaged in sustained, intense enjoyment. He focuses on the end product (completing therapy) rather than being intrinsically motivated to play. Poor internal control is characterized by an inability to enter new play situations, initiate play with peers, share, decide what to do, and challenge himself. Sam is able to engage in pretend play when acting out Star Wars with the OT practitioner but has difficulty reading others' cues, which is evident when he plays too roughly and gets too close to his peers during interactions.

Considering Sam's limitations and the long-term goal of enabling him to play with peers, his OT objectives include the following:

1. Spontaneously initiating a change in activity, at least three times, during a 45-minute supervised play situation
2. Responding positively (smiling, cooperating with the OT practitioner) when he does not get his way, at least three times during a supervised play situation
3. Entering a group of peers already playing on the playground and participating in the activity without interrupting the play, at least three times a week.
4. Engaging in a motor challenge during play, at least three times, during a supervised play situation.

Framing situations as play allows children to know what play is so that they may interact accordingly. They are free to pretend, challenge each other, and tease without malice. All of these actions require that children read nonverbal as well as verbal cues. Reading nonverbal cues allows children to realize when they have pushed a boundary too far during play.

CASE *Study*

Scott and Alison are playing in a sandbox, pouring sand on each other. They laugh and watch for cues from each other that say, "This is okay. We are still playing." The game continues, and Alison begins to pour sand on Scott's head. She receives a serious look from Scott. The nonverbal cue says, "Hey, that is a little too close to my eyes. I do not like that."

Alison responds with a smile that says, "Oops! I'm sorry," and pours sand on Scott's arm instead. Her nonverbal response says, "Okay, I'll be more careful." This exchange of cues allows the play to continue while they learn to be attentive to each other. They are learning the rules and boundaries of play.

Assessment of a child's playfulness provides information about the way the child processes, problemsolves, and manages emotional stress. These skills are important to the child's development and social well-being.

NATURE OF PLAY AND PLAYFULNESS

OT practitioners must understand the nature of play and playfulness in order to use it effectively as an intervention technique. When children play and are playful, depending on the activity, they may laugh, smile, and be active; they may also be serious, quiet, and totally absorbed in play (Figure 20-3). Play can be frustrating, and it can involve failures. The flexible and spontaneous nature of play and playfulness is demonstrated when children change themes or use toys in unexpected ways.

The process (doing) rather than the product (outcome) provides the primary source of reward in play activities.[10] Children engage in play for its own sake.[11,14] Playful children discover, create, and explore. Therefore, no way of playing is right or wrong. Play is a safe outlet for children to challenge themselves and helps them develop skills.

OT practitioners must remember to maintain the nature of play and playfulness during therapy. Children who have special needs may require additional assistance to play.[32,44] OT practitioners are knowledgeable about the abilities of children who have special needs and are therefore in an ideal position to promote play and playfulness.

PLAY DEVELOPMENT OF CHILDREN WITH DISABILITIES

The normal sequence for the development of play is often delayed in children who have special needs.[25,27,30,32,34,37] (See Chapter 7 for a discussion of this sequence.) This may be the result of limited physical, cognitive, or social–emotional skills.[27,30,34] For example, a child who is unable to bring the hands to the mouth has trouble exploring the environment. Children who are unable to experience sensations in a typical manner often require intervention to engage in play opportunities, which stimulate their growth and development. If children are not afforded these opportunities, they may exhibit poor play skills.[34,38,44] Changing or modifying the environment (such as modifying the playground for

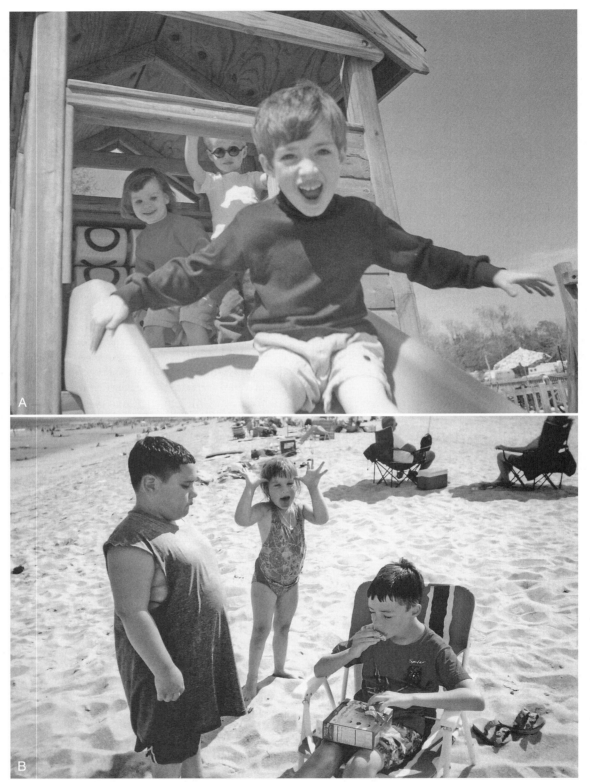

FIGURE 20-3   Playful Children May Be Silly or Serious During Play. **A,** A boy shows playfulness by his smile. **B,** His younger sister teases him.

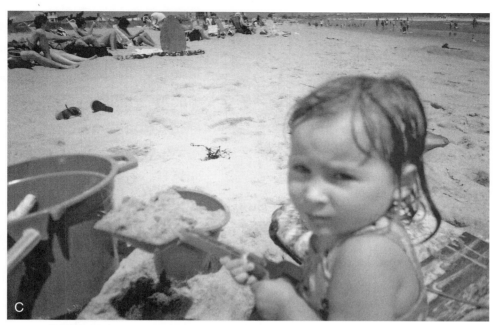

FIGURE 20-3, cont'd   C, The girl is quite serious while building a sandcastle.

wheelchair access) helps children who have special needs experience play.[34,37,38]

Children who have special needs may take longer to respond, make less obvious responses, initiate activities less frequently, and be less interactive than other children.[32,37] They are often passive in their play.[30,32,34] Children with intellectual deficits exhibit a restricted repertoire of play and language, decreased attention span, and less social interaction during play.[30,32,34] Children with visual impairments are less interested in reaching out to explore and engage in social exchanges during play.[30] Children with hearing impairments show less symbolic and less organized play.[30]

Children who have developmental and physical disabilities commonly experience difficulty playing. They do not have the same play skills as their typically developing peers, and therefore are not exposed to the same play opportunities. These barriers are believed to correlate with deficits in other areas of the child's development such as social and emotional, speech, gross motor, creativity, and problem-solving abilities. Children with disabilities often receive interventions for their diagnosed disabilities and their presenting symptoms; unfortunately, most interventions rarely focus on play.[29]

Children with attention-deficit hyperactivity disorder (ADHD) commonly experience difficulty engaging in cooperative play.[21] They tend to play for shorter periods of time, frequently change their play activity, and have difficulty returning to an activity after an interruption.[15] In structured play settings, children with ADHD often experience trouble transitioning from one activity to another and display more negative play behaviors (such as disrupting and violating established play rules).[21]

Cordier et al studied children with ADHD to determine how to effectively design a play-based intervention model.[21] They focused on the typical behaviors of children with ADHD, their play environments, and motivating these children. The impulsive and hyperactive behavior in conjunction with poor self-regulation and control may also create deficits in a child's intrinsic control and motivation, a foundational component of play. They suggested that OT practitioners use a client-centered approach to design interventions for children with ADHD focusing on improving their socials skills and reducing tendencies of disruption and domination.[21]

Children with autistic disorders display deficits in communication abilities, social interactions, and range of interests and activities. They show limited socialization and imagination, which interferes with play. They tend to prefer playing alone, and when in groups, they commonly have difficulty detecting and understanding the meaning of verbal and nonverbal social cues displayed by the other children.[48] To successfully promote play, OT practitioners strive to create interventions that are both appealing and motivating to the child.

Children with sensory processing disorder (SPD) and those with developmental coordination disorder (DCD; see Chapters 12 and 24 for explanations of these conditions) may have difficulties with play and playfulness.[15,19] These children may benefit from play environment adaptations and focus on their ability to play. SPD often interferes with a child's ability to interact with people and objects in his or her environment. Children with DCD experience gross motor delays. Furthermore, once they have mastered tasks, they repeatedly perform the tasks with little variation and show limited flexibility in their movement patterns.[15] Children with SPD also often exhibit limited variability in movements.

With respect to play, this lack of variability or flexibility causes less interest in play and participation in play groups. Bundy et al found that for children with SPD, changing the play setting seems to have more effect on play capabilities than does focusing on remediating praxis (e.g., motor planning).[15] For example, modifying a child's environment to better stimulate interest and inspire confidence may promote expansion of social play skills. Improving social skills and confidence through play may lead to parallel developments in other areas of a child's life and learning experiences.[48]

Children with cerebral palsy (CP) display impaired postural control and functional ambulation, which can be accompanied by emotional and behavioral dysfunction.[47] (See Chapter 16.) This condition affects both physical and cognitive development, including communication skills, and is present over an individual's lifespan. These functional impairments may create significant barriers to a child's development of playfulness. Modifying the play environment by reducing physical barriers helps increase playfulness in children who have CP.[13] Improving communication with parents can also positively influence playfulness.[13]

Children who have special needs require assistance in order to meet developmental challenges and learn ways to play.[26,30,32,34,37] OT practitioners must understand typical play patterns and support these children when teaching skills and facilitating play. For example, OT practitioners can increase spontaneity in children by allowing them to discover play materials that have been hidden or placed within reach.[18,34,37,44] OT practitioners must identify these children's strengths and weaknesses, as well as those of the family, to design effective interventions. Capitalizing on strengths can increase the success of therapy and facilitate development of advanced play skills.

CLINICAL *Pearl*

Children play in various physical positions. OT practitioners make sure that children with special needs spend time in many positions, such as supine, quadruped, sitting, and standing positions. Play time is not the time to work on positioning. Children should be free to use their arms and hands and feel safe.

INFLUENCE OF ENVIRONMENT ON PLAY

The environment in which play occurs influences children's play. Each child has his or her own unique style of play, which is shaped by age, gender, experiences, family, and environment.[4] Engaging in play depends on a child's feeling of safety, confidence, and interests. Therefore, a child's environment may promote or restrict playfulness.[7,16,48] For example, structuring of school days and the availability of staff members have influenced play environments and opportunities for children. Currently, many schools have restricted the allotted time for outdoor recesses and have removed equipment from playgrounds. In the past, children commonly played outdoors in wooded areas or cleared fields and mostly did not play with manufactured toys, which promoted social interactions, imaginative play, creativity, and physical activity.[13] Bundy suggested that parental responses to safety concerns have reduced the opportunities for children's play in imaginative and creative ways.[13] For example, parents and teachers promote the "correct way" to go down a slide. Children commonly play on playgrounds—play environments with static play equipment (slides, swings, climbers, etc.) that do not lend themselves to nearly as much imaginative play and creative manipulation.[12,13] For children with physical disabilities, playgrounds can create a barrier to cooperative play with their typically developing peers.

It is important for an OT practitioner to consider a child's environment when assessing play and playfulness. Models such as the Model of Human Occupation and Person–Environment–Occupation (PEO) examine how the physical or social environment supports or inhibits a child's play.[16,28] Interventions focusing on changing or modifying environmental factors can promote play skills.

RELEVANCE OF PLAY

CASE *Study*

Twelve-month-old Frankie cannot sit up because of hydrocephalus and poor trunk tone. He is nonverbal. He can move his arms but is unable to reach and grasp objects. He occasionally smiles and laughs. His vision is poor. After positioning him properly, the OT practitioner places a mercury switch attached to a flashlight on his arm. When Frankie raises his arm, the flashlight lights up his face. Frankie raises his arm soon after the switch is placed on his arm and smiles when the flashlight lights up his face. He puts his arm down and the light turns off. Frankie laughs and laughs. He repeats this activity numerous times. It is evident that he realizes he is in control of the light. His mother has tears in her eyes. She turns to the OT practitioner and says, "Frankie is playing."

OT changed this family's perception of Frankie by showing them his ability to play, which is both a powerful tool and an important outcome in OT.

CLINICAL *Pearl*

Observe the child's movements when deciding where to position a switch. Place the switch where the child can activate it by using movement patterns he or she uses automatically. This promotes play and provides the child with control and immediate success.

OT practitioners work with families, educators, and other professionals to improve the quality of life for children and their families. Play is vital to a child's development and an important outcome of intervention. OT practitioners who use play may be faced with parents and professionals who do not take them seriously.[9,11,24] Engaging parents in discussions from the beginning educates them about the importance of play during therapy sessions. OT practitioners should discuss with parents how the session went and the progress made toward the goals. OT practitioners who recognize that parents do not value play as a goal may decide to emphasize the use of play as a tool to increase the child's skills in other areas. Other professionals may take OT practitioners more seriously once they see the progress a child makes in OT. OT practitioners may frequently need to educate parents and other professionals on the purpose of the use of play.

Activities recommended for the home should be limited to those that are fun and nonthreatening for the child in order to promote play and playfulness. The child can engage in activities in which he or she can show off certain abilities to the parents. This is motivating for both the child and the parents. OT practitioners investigate the role of play in children's lives and focus on providing them with a means to play.

Play as a Tool

Play is often used as a tool to increase skill development. OT is designed around play activities that will increase skills such as strength, motor planning, problem solving, grasping, and handwriting, which are necessary for the child to function. Using play as a tool to improve a child's ability to function has many advantages. Children typically cooperate and readily engage in play. Most goals can be addressed during a play session because play encompasses a variety of activities.

The characteristics of play (i.e., intrinsic motivation, internal control, and suspension of reality) need to be present when play is used as a tool to improve a child's skills. These characteristics occur within the framework of a play setting. The OT practitioner arranges the environment so that children can choose activities that help meet their goals while having fun. The OT practitioner allows the child to tease, engage in mischief, and face challenges.

CLINICAL *Pearl*

Many household items make novel toys for the clinic and can also be used as such at home. Pots and pans can be containers, musical instruments, or even hats. They promote pretend play. Use cardboard boxes, grocery bags, and laundry baskets for a variety of play activities. Bring them into the clinic to allow children to explore and be creative with them (Figure 20-4).

Making therapy sessions fun through play is not always easy. OT practitioners must set up an environment to encourage the child to choose activities that foster therapy goals. This is considered the art of therapy.[2,11] The OT practitioner sets up just the right challenge, which is one that is neither too hard nor too easy.[2,11] The OT practitioner must know the child's strengths and weaknesses to do this effectively. Some children are competitive and enjoy such games. Others fear failure and may be easily intimidated by competitive games. Some children enjoy roughhousing, and others do not. Making a therapy session fun means observing a child's subtle cues and spontaneously adapting the session to maintain a level of excitement and motivation.

A physically and emotionally safe environment allows the child to feel in control. The OT practitioner designs activities to target specific skills. The child is only aware that the activity is fun. Often the practitioner may need to discreetly change the way the task is performed to get the maximum benefit from the activity. This must be done playfully to keep the flow of the play session going.[23] Sometimes the practice of a skill takes priority over playing.

A critical element of play is for activities to be free from rules. This does not mean that rules are not present in play activities but that they are negotiable. Children may make up new rules and change them during play. OT practitioners should provide enough rules for children to feel secure and safe without imposing so many that they do not feel free to play. Both the child and practitioner must have the freedom to change the activity. Therefore, if a child is performing an activity that does not promote therapy goals, the OT practitioner can modify the challenge. This is illustrated in a therapy session challenging the child's balance.

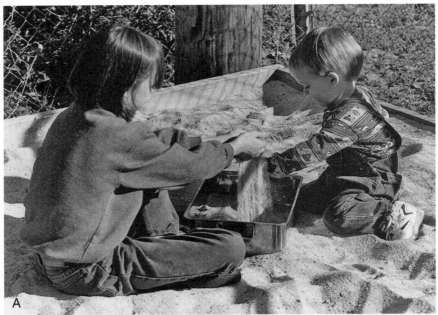

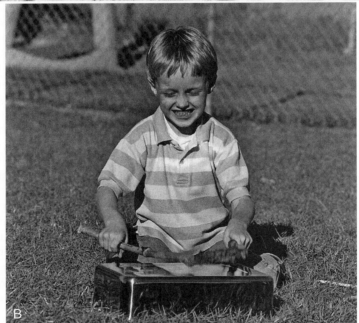

FIGURE 20-4 Everyday Household Objects Allow for Pretend Play and Creativity. **A,** A brother and sister are using a stainless steel cake pan to build sandcastles. **B,** The same cake pan is turned upside down and, with some sticks from the yard, is being used as a drum.

CASE *Study*

David is kneeling on a platform swing and propelling it forward and backward. The practitioner increases the skill level required by saying, "Oh, here come the asteroids," and throwing large balls under the swing. David looks at the OT practitioner, smiles, and says, "Hey, no fair. I didn't know that was coming." The OT practitioner responds, "The asteroids came out of nowhere! Luckily, you are Superman and were able to stay on the spaceship!" The changes are skillfully made so that the session remains playful.

Children can imagine a therapy session to be a spaceship ride, an Olympic quest, a deep sea diving expedition, a skiing event, or a leisurely stroll down the alley. Through pretend play the child gains skills in imagination, verbalization, and communication. Pretend play allows the OT practitioner to use the same equipment in countless ways that tap into the child's imagination. Teasing, joking, and mischief are parts of play. The child may teasingly throw a soft ball to hit the OT practitioner's head. Children may joke that the OT practitioner cannot perform a skill. Children develop their sense of humor during play.

Play provides an excellent tool for intervention when used correctly because children are highly motivated to participate.[11,17,18,24,30,35,37]

CASE *Study*

Angie is a 2-year-old girl with hemiplegia on the right side of her body. She lives with her two brothers aged 8 and 9 and her parents. Angie attends daycare daily. She receives OT services for 1 hour weekly. Her parents report that she does not play well with other children. She grabs their toys, pushes them, and screams in order to have her needs met. She does not like to be touched on her right side and does little weight bearing on that side. Angie has a difficult time engaging in play activities. She screams and cries when the OT practitioner touches her on the right arm. She does not initiate play. Angie exhibits decreased active range of motion (AROM) in her right arm.

The OT practitioner designs an intervention that involves play to increase Angie's use of her right side. (See Chapter 7 for a description of the sequence and development of typical play and useful information for designing this type of intervention.) The OT practitioner considers Angie's age when choosing the play activities. Based on her knowledge of 2-year-old children, the OT practitioner chooses busy and messy play activities. According to Parten, 2-year-olds usually participate in solitary play but do make an effort to interact with other children.[43,45] The OT practitioner notes that 2-year-old children enjoy sensory activities such as playing in sandboxes, water play, and working with Play-Doh. They also enjoy manipulatable toys such as Legos, pop-up toys, and blocks and gross motor toys such as balls, riding toys,

and swings. Table 20-1 includes a list of suitable toys and activities for various ages.

The child's age and gender, the setting, and the concerns of parents must be considered when writing the goals and objectives of OT. The OT practitioner considers the child's physical capabilities and the factors interfering with her ability to play. Angie has right-sided hypersensitivity. She does not bear weight on the right side. Considering Angie's limitations and the long-term goal that she will use her right hand spontaneously for bimanual activities, Angie's therapy objectives include the following:

1. She will spontaneously reach for objects placed above her head with her right hand, at least five times during a 45-minute therapy session.
2. Using two hands, she will catch a 20-inch ball tossed underhand from two feet away, at least three times in a 45-minute session.
3. She will walk at least 10 feet while holding on with both hands to a push toy such as a shopping cart.
4. She will use both hands to take apart small objects such as pop beads.

Box 20-1 contains sample objectives involving play as a tool for OT intervention.

The OT practitioner designs play activities that incorporate the use of Angie's right side. She plays games rolling a large ball, wheelbarrow racing, and climbing a ladder. She pulls pop beads apart, dresses baby dolls, pours sand and water into containers, and makes confetti out of newspaper. All these activities require Angie to use both arms. The OT practitioner stages the activities in such a way that Angie is successful. The OT practitioner frequently provides Angie with hand-over-hand assistance. She watches for cues from Angie when placing a hand on her arms. The practitioner uses humor and laughter to keep the session playful. Intervention focuses on keeping the atmosphere fun and playful while increasing the functional use of Angie's right arm. The emphasis of the intervention session is to promote bilateral hand skill development. The OT practitioner assists Angie in using her right hand during play.

Table 20-1 lists toys associated with the development of specific client factors. Angie's case demonstrates the use of play as a tool to improve a child's physical skills.

TABLE 20-1

Toys and Play Activities Designed to Target Selected Client Factors

CLIENT FACTOR	TOYS AND ACTIVITIES
SENSORY FUNCTION	
Sensory awareness and sensory processing	
Tactile	Water play, massage, Play-Doh, koosh balls, glue, beans, sand play, tactile boards, brushing, lotion games, stickers
Proprioceptive	Trampolines, jumping, pulling on ropes, climbing ladders, tug-of-war, pulling a wagon, wheelbarrow walking, pushing
Vestibular	Riding a bike, skateboarding, see-saw, sliding, swinging, Sit and Spin, rocking horse
Visual	Mobiles, toys that move, bright-colored rattles and toys, mirrors
Auditory	Musical toys, bells, rattles, CD players, songs
Gustatory	Food, gum, candy
Olfactory	Smelly markers, Play-Doh, smelly stickers, food
NEUROMUSCULOSKELETAL AND MOVEMENT-RELATED FUNCTIONS	
Strength	Ball games, bike riding, manipulative games, jump rope, Red Rover, London Bridge, swimming, sports
Endurance	Repetitive games, walking, sports, hiking, swimming, bike riding, climbing
Postural control	Trampolines, bike riding, sports, swimming, climbing, walking on uneven terrrain
Gross coordination	Outdoor playground equipment, bikes, sports, water, outdoor play
Fine motor	Manipulatives, arts and crafts, small toys, figurines, dolls, dress-up, sewing, coloring, cutting
Oral motor	Musical instruments, whistles, bubble blowers, pinwheels
MENTAL FUNCTIONS (AFFECTIVE, SELF-MANAGEMENT, COGNITIVE, PERCEPTUAL)	
Affective	
Psychological	Self-esteem board games, art projects, motor challenges
Interpersonal	Pictionary, team games, Twister, new games
Self-expression	Arts and crafts, pottery, clay, dance
Self-management	
Coping skills	Monopoly, life skills game, role playing
Cognitive	
Memory, sequencing	Board games (e.g., Memory, Clue, Monopoly, Candy Land)
Categorization	Card games (e.g., Hearts, Go Fish), sorting, matching games
Spatial operations	Puzzles, models, arts and crafts, Legos, Lincoln Logs
Problem solving	Board games, card games, arts and crafts, puzzles
Perceptual	
Perceptual processing	Puzzles, building blocks, doll houses, farms, building logs, model cars and airplanes, paper dolls, coloring books, mazes, computer games, dress-up, obstacle courses, Simon Says, Follow-the-Leader

Adapted from the American Occupational Therapy Association: Uniform terminology for occupational therapy, *Am J Occup Ther* 48:1047, 1994; American Occupational Therapy Association: Occupational therapy practice framework: Domain and process, 2nd edition, *Am J Occup Ther* 62(6):625–703, 2008.

BOX 20-1

Sample Objectives When Play Is the Tool for Occupational Therapy Intervention

- Child will catch a large object such as a beach ball with both hands, at least five times, when it is thrown directly to him or her from three feet away.
- Child will utilize a neat pincer grip to pick up 10 small objects for use in daily activities.
- Child will ride a bike at least 20 yards in a straight line without falling.
- Child will make at least 3 out of 10 baskets from the free-throw line.
- Child will put on and button a shirt independently.

The OT practitioner uses play activities to increase the ability of the child to use her right side.

Play as a Goal

OT practitioners must be careful to avoid "teaching" play. They model play, cultivate the skills needed for play, and set up the environment to facilitate play. OT practitioners must ensure that play is enjoyable. Increasing the skills required for play is important and beneficial to the child.

OT practitioners must maintain the quality of play.[11,28,45] A child who has the skills needed for play but does not engage in spontaneous and intrinsically motivated activity is at risk. That child may show deficits in play that will carry over to the school, home, and community. Play deficits in childhood may inhibit a child's ability to gain the needed skills for adulthood.[17,19,20,22,27,31,45] Therefore, it is important for OT practitioners to target play as a goal of therapy.

The OT practitioner emphasizes the child's approach to activities and the manner in which the child plays when play itself is the goal of therapy. When play is viewed as a goal of therapy rather than merely a tool of intervention, the OT practitioner notes the way Angie engages in play, not just her using her right hand to manipulate a toy. A short-term objective to increase Angie's play might be for her to spontaneously initiate play with a peer at least three times during an adult-supervised play session. Box 20-2 contains sample objectives when play is the goal of OT intervention.

CASE *Study*

Angie's OT sessions include playmates because she needs assistance playing with others. The OT practitioner designs the environment to encourage Angie to respond to

BOX 20-2

Sample Objectives When Play or Playfulness Is the Intended Outcome of Occupational Therapy Intervention

- Child will initiate one new activity during an adult-supervised play session.
- Child will enter into a play activity (already in progress) without disrupting the group during an adult-supervised play session.
- Child will stay with the same basic play theme for at least 15 minutes during an adult-supervised play session.
- Child will use an object in an unconventional manner spontaneously at least once during an adult-supervised play session.
- Child will share toys with another child (trading toys at least three times) during a 15-minute play session.

changes and be spontaneous. Angie participates in bilateral activities such as playing with balls, wheelbarrow racing, and ladder climbing. The OT practitioner facilitates a playful attitude in Angie while allowing her to pick the activities and choose the way she will perform them. The OT practitioner facilitates sharing, negotiating, and taking turns, and encourages the child's parents and teachers to facilitate the skills of sharing, negotiating, and taking turns at home and in the school, thus creating many opportunities for Angie to improve her play skills.

CLINICAL *Pearl*

Invite another child or OT practitioner to keep the play sessions exciting. This is a great way to learn new activities and methods of playing.

CASE *Study*

Angie's second session differs from the first, which targeted the use of her right hand, in that the emphasis is now on both interaction and motor skills as opposed to motor skills alone. The OT practitioner pays close attention to Angie's ability to engage in spontaneous activity, choose a variety of tasks, initiate changes, and read the cues of her peers. The Test of Playfulness (ToP) is used as a framework for the observation, evaluation, and documentation of playfulness.[8] O'Brien and colleagues were able to design play goals after a parental interview and a 30-minute observation of free play using the ToP as a guide.[39]

It is possible to use play as both a tool for therapy and a goal of therapy sessions. In Angie's case, it would be appropriate to work on increasing the use of her right side as well as improving play. This takes skill on the part of the OT practitioner, who must have the trust of the child and read his or her cues very carefully to maintain the child's engagement in play.

ROLE OF THE OCCUPATIONAL THERAPIST AND THE OCCUPATIONAL THERAPY ASSISTANT DURING PLAY ASSESSMENT

The observation of children during play provides OT practitioners with important information. Play assessment, in combination with parent, child, and teacher interviews, provides the OT practitioner with necessary information. Bryze supports the contributions of narratives in collecting information on play.[8] These narratives focus on the interviews of parents, caregivers, and children.

OT practitioners use a variety of **play assessments** when working with children with special needs. (See Appendix A of this chapter for descriptions of several play assessments.) The occupational therapist is responsible for the evaluation and analysis of information when evaluating play but can delegate portions of the assessment to the occupational therapy assistant (OTA), who can assist in interviewing the teachers and caregivers and observing the children during play. The OT practitioner uses the results of the play assessments to design therapy goals and provide effective intervention. Play assessments provide a foundation for organizing information.

It is not always possible to evaluate children with moderate to severe physical and cognitive disabilities through standardized testing. However, play evaluations may be administered to all children. These evaluations provide the flexibility needed to assess children and give measurable information concerning a child's strengths and weaknesses. For example, the ToP has been found to be reliable in measuring playfulness in children with intellectual disability; the Knox Preschool Play Scale (PPS) is reliable in measuring play skills in children with multiple disabilities. The Transdisciplinary Play-Based Assessment (TPBA) is designed to be used with all children and includes an accompanying intervention manual (Transdisciplinary Play-Based Intervention [TPBI]) to assist OT practitioners in intervention planning. The findings obtained from play evaluations are easily translated into measurable goals for therapy sessions that allow clinicians to organize intervention more deliberately, thereby benefiting the children they treat.

TECHNIQUES TO PROMOTE PLAY AND PLAYFULNESS

Fully utilizing play in OT practice is an art and a science. Just as with any intervention, OT practitioners must practice the techniques. The science of using play involves understanding the characteristics, components, and settings that facilitate it. OT practitioners must identify the desired outcome of therapy and evaluate the motor, psychological, and/or social factors interfering with the child's ability to play.

Creating a therapeutic environment involves analyzing a child's skills and determining the way(s) to adapt activities. Knowledge of the development of the motor, cognitive, language, social–emotional, and play skills of children is essential to designing effective interventions. Examination of the environment and knowledge of the child's culture help OT practitioners determine appropriate play activities.

OT using play requires the OT practitioner to find the child within himself or herself. Playful practitioners practice play and are able to support the child's playful nature. Clinical expertise in the therapeutic use of self is important for understanding the way(s) to evoke play in children and is considered part of the art of therapy. OT practitioners engage in the art of OT when they connect with the child. Skillful practitioners play effortlessly with children while challenging them to acquire and master new skills. The art of OT involves weaving clinical judgment, skill, and individual style into successful therapy sessions.

Examples of How to Improve Playfulness

- Set up the environment to facilitate playfulness in children and adolescents. The environment can be easily modified to promote playfulness.
- Set up a "tea party" theme by adding a small table, tea set, and pink table cloth.
- Use curtains or dividers to separate children's and adults' spaces if space is shared in the clinic.
- Change the themes of spaces through paintings or party items (e.g., birds, piñatas, or other decorations).
- Keep the space child-friendly.
- Music adds a playful nature to the space.
- Add the children's favorite toys to the environment. You may ask them to bring one or two to the session.
- Include an element of "pretend" in the session.
- Change the demands of the task to provide the just right challenge.
- Magnetic blocks are easier for children with coordination difficulties.

- Adaptive toys allow children to hit a switch or pull a lever to activate a toy.
- Puppets come in all sizes, so use of them can be easily gradated.
- Having a limited number of directions for the games makes it easier for children to play them.
- Change the rules to make children more successful, or bring the target closer.
- Using the finger for painting is easier than using a brush.
- Sitting in adapted chairs allows children to use their hands better.
- Allow for a variety of positions during play.
- Remember that eye contact may be overwhelming to some children. In addition, it is not imperative for children to smile to show that they are having fun.
- Allow the children to make changes to the activity.

CLINICAL *Pearl*

Get in touch with your playful side. Spend a day with a child to remember the way it feels to play. Let the child lead you and show you how to play.

Characteristics of Playful Occupational Therapy Practitioners

OT practitioners can cultivate specific characteristics in themselves that promote play (Box 20-3). They must be playful themselves if they wish to treat children effectively and facilitate play and playfulness. Children view a happy, smiling OT practitioner—one who is able to interact joyfully with them—as playful.

It is important for the OT practitioner to establish goals and to structure the intervention setting. However, the OT practitioner must be flexible enough to change the activity based on the child's responses. The OT practitioner needs to be skillful in planning and setting up a playful environment so that the child will choose activities that further the therapeutic goals. This ensures that therapy will be fun for the child. Facilitating play requires that the OT practitioner keep the goals clearly in mind while structuring the environment and adjusting the mode of interaction.[24,30]

OT practitioners acting as play facilitators pay careful attention to a child's interests, elaborate on his or her verbalizations, and model play behaviors.[30] If an activity is not challenging to a child but he or she is enjoying it, the OT practitioner may decide to continue the activity before increasing the level of the skill required. The child may need to practice the task to gain mastery.[45] Children need to be challenged in all areas of development. OT

BOX 20-3

Characteristics of Occupational Therapy Practitioners That Promote Play and Playfulness in Children

- *Playfulness:* Having warm, inviting, and sincere personalities
- *Flexibility, creativity, and spontaneity:* Ability to change activities and pace based on the needs of the child and to stop activities and create new ones if needed
- *Child friendliness:* Interacting at the child's level; being familiar with child's terms and current trends, such as Dalmatians, Power Rangers, Barney, and Teletubbies
- *Sense of humor:* Trying out silly things; laughing at self
- *Intuition:* Being able to read child's cues (nonverbal and verbal); being aware of signs of boredom, fatigue, or frustration
- *Positive reinforcement:* Offering sincere praise when child has performed well, has tried very hard, or is in need of support
- *Patience:* Allowing child to experience some frustration; helping child to work on frustration tolerance through play
- *Observational skills:* Being able to watch and not intervene at every turn; allowing child to be in control
- *Openness:* Learning new games and play activities from children; watching children in many settings to keep activities novel
- *Fun:* Smiling; laughing; playing with children

---

practitioners need to provide social, cognitive, and motor challenges.

OT practitioners need to be creative to spark children's imaginations during play sessions. (See Appendix B of this chapter for a resource list of play ideas.) A sense of humor is vital; OT practitioners may have to act silly, make mistakes, and even act as a peer to encourage a child to play. From the child's point of view, the OT practitioner may seem to demand that he or she perform tasks that are much harder to them than to the adult. For example, in one intervention session a child asked to play the role of the OT practitioner and then said, "Okay, now stand on your head and clap your hands together behind your back three times. I will time you." This suggests that the degree of challenge the child has experienced during treatment sessions was too much.

Reading a child's verbal and nonverbal cues provides OT practitioners with information that may help change the play activities. This is important in gaining the trust of the child. Children need to feel that someone is listening to them. Skillful OT practitioners use the child's cues as indicators of stress and emotion. They can assist children in learning to listen to and give cues by nodding and listening to their nonverbal and verbal feedback.

CLINICAL *Pearl*

Provide children with themes for play activities. Ask them to bring in objects from their homes and use them during therapy.

Praising children is highly effective if done properly. They appreciate honest and specific praise. They realize that play can be frustrating and not always successful. OT practitioners need to allow children with special needs to feel frustration and experience failure sometimes.

Playful OT practitioners allow children to make mistakes occasionally. Some of the most playful sessions are those in which the children make mistakes along the way. It is the process that is important.

CASE *Study*

An obstacle course in the clinic is difficult for Jon to climb without falling. He tries numerous times and each time falls into the pillows laughing. He is determined to succeed. He works on this activity until he succeeds in doing it properly. Once he masters the task, he moves on to something new. For Jon, falling into the pillows is almost as fun as staying on the course.

OT practitioners must have a sense of humor. They must take into consideration the setting and the play frame. Therefore, if the child says, "I have a laser gun," during a pretend game, the OT practitioner does not become alarmed. However, a child may be crying out for help during play. OT practitioners should take these opportunities to reach out to the child. Perhaps the most important characteristic of playful practitioners is that they have fun. Children learn the way to play from practitioners who get involved in it. They smile, laugh, and enjoy playing.

Characteristics of the Optimal Play Environment

The optimal **play environment** has specific characteristics (Box 20-4); first and foremost, it is a safe environment.[3,46]

Children must be safe and feel physically and emotionally safe. The environment should have a variety of

---

BOX 20-4

Characteristics of an Optimal Play Environment

- *Playful:* Provides cheerful, warm, and safe feeling
- *Fun and inviting:* Is child-friendly; is decorated in such a way that children enjoy being there
- *Safe:* Keeps children physically and emotionally safe so that they can feel free to explore and play; has mats available
- *Novel:* Provides various new toys and challenges
- *Flexible and creative:* Allows children to play in different ways with toys; is arranged to promote a variety of play activities
- *Encouraging:* Includes adults who facilitate play, are not directive, ensure that the children are safe, assist when needed, and disappear when appropriate
- *Creative:* Has materials and supplies that promote creativity and not necessarily have an end product,; for example, sand, water, clay, and Play-Doh
- *Quiet:* Allows children some space to be alone if they desire

---

age-appropriate toys that the child can choose from.[3,18,24,30,37] These toys need not be expensive; children enjoy playing with even ordinary household items such as pots and pans.

The OT practitioner should design an environment that promotes novelty, the opportunity for exploration, repetition, and the imitation of competent role models.[23] Novelty makes the session fun and enjoyable, fosters creativity, and creates arousal. An environment that allows for exploration requires arranging toys in such a way that children can look for them, reach them, and investigate the surroundings. They learn from repetition and should be allowed to do this during play. Repetition is encouraged by the initiation of the same activity with a different theme, goal, or object. For example, the OT practitioner may ask a child to throw a ball at a new target to continue the activity. Being a competent role model requires the OT practitioner to demonstrate playful behavior. Parents and professionals need to give children space to work out play scenarios, and this space must be safe (Box 20-5).

The play space should be arranged to promote a variety of types of play (see Chapter 7).[1,3] The ways to promote different types of play include the following:

1. *Pretend play:* This type of play promotes make-believe and may involve using the kitchen table, play food, puppets, and dress-up clothes during play.
2. *Constructive play:* This type of play is designed to allow children to build and create things and involves

BOX 20-5

Safety in the Play Environment

- **The best safety precaution is to watch all children carefully at all times.**
- Plug all electrical outlets with safety caps.
- Ensure that bookshelves are sturdy and will not topple. Anchor shelves to the wall at the top.
- Do not place toys in such a way that they will fall on toddlers' heads when they pull them down.
- Remove all cords to ensure that children do not get caught in them.
- Place mats under all the equipment.
- Pad corners of walls and furniture.
- Know how to perform infant cardiopulmonary resuscitation (CPR).
- Be sure that cleaning supplies and medications are out of reach of children.
- Be sure that water tables are closed when not in use.
- Watch for and mop up slippery surfaces.
- Have a first-aid kit available, and frequently review emergency procedures.
- Check out all equipment periodically to ensure that everything is in good working order.
- Clean and disinfect toys and surfaces after each use.
- Follow universal precautions while cleaning up spills.

the use of blocks, Legos, Lincoln Logs, and various other building toys; arts and crafts, paper; crayons, clay, markers, paint, chalk, and scissors; and wind-up toys, beads, and small manipulative toys.

3. *Reflective or reading area:* This is a quiet area, where children can read and/or write. Items placed in this area may include books, audiotapes, videotapes, paper, and pencils.
4. *Sensorimotor area:* This area is for major motor movements. Toys and equipment present in this area include mats, balls, bikes, swings, balance beams, and trampolines.
5. *Exploratory play:* This type of play includes water, sand, and other tactile play activities.
6. *Computer play:* This play area includes a computer with a variety of games.
7. *Musical play:* This type of play promotes music and involves the use of whistles, rattles, drums, pianos, rhythm games, singing, and tapes.

The OT practitioner should allow children to express their creativity and spontaneity. Toys have many uses in addition to those suggested by the manufacturer. Unless the children are being harmful to others or themselves, allow them to use toys in different ways. Some children

may not be aware of the way a toy is typically used. After they have taken some time to explore it, the OT practitioner may demonstrate the expected way without imposing only one method of playing with the toy.

Many children enjoy roughhousing. Children with special needs may also enjoy this. Gentle roughhousing can provide sensory input to them and is often therapeutic and fun. Children of all ages learn through physical contact, and therapy sessions can provide a safe environment for this type of contact. Children may push each other playfully, and adults do not always need to intervene.

CLINICAL *Pearl*

Musical games are fun and playful ways to help a child become more attentive to verbal directions. The child must pay attention to the words of the song or beat of the music to follow along.

Playful environments take advantage of themes and are decorated for the occasion. Make sure that the play environment is not too stimulating. Use warm colors such as pinks, melons, and yellows.[2] The temperature of the room should be warm, not too hot or cold. Children enjoy being outdoors, so they should be able to play in outdoor settings as well. They should also have places for quiet time and concentration.

The best way to promote play and playfulness in children is to be a playful adult in a playful environment. Arranging the play environment helps OT practitioners become skillful at utilizing the environment therapeutically.

SUMMARY

OT practitioners view play as the major occupation of childhood and believe it is crucial to a child's development. They facilitate the development of play in children with special needs. Therefore, they must understand the characteristics of play if they wish to make significant changes in the play of the children they treat. OT practitioners play an important role in helping parents, teachers, and peers play with children with special needs. The OT practitioners may be able to make simple play adaptations that allow these children to be included with their peers in play.

Play is a fun, spontaneous, internally motivated, and self-directed activity that is free from rigid rules. *Playfulness* is defined as an individual's disposition to play. OT practitioners typically use play as a tool to improve a child's skills and as a goal for therapy.

OT practitioners should expand their use of play by exploring its characteristics and practicing these techniques in the treatment of children. They can have a tremendous impact on the lives of children and their families through fun, creative, enjoyable, and spontaneous activities, allowing children to develop play skills that will carry over to the home, school, and community settings and help prepare the children for adult roles.

References

1. Axline VM: Play therapy procedures and results. In Schaefer C, editor: *The therapeutic use of play*, New York, 1976, Jason Aronson.
2. Ayres AJ: *Sensory integration and learning disorders*, Los Angeles, 1972, Western Psychological Services.
3. Bantz DL, Siktberg L: Teaching families to evaluate age-appropriate toys. *J Pediatr Health Care* 7:111, 1993.
4. Barnett LA: Characterising playfulness: correlates with individual attributes and personality traits. *Play and Culture* 4:371–393, 1991.
5. Barnett LA: The adaptive powers of being playful. In Duncan MC, Chick G, Aycock A, editors: *Play and culture studies*, vol 1, Greenwich, CT, 1998, Ablex Publishing.
6. Berger KS: *The developing person through the lifespan*, ed 3, New York, 1994, Worth Publishers.
7. Brentnall J, Bundy AC, Kay F: The effect of the length of observation on test of playfulness scores. *OTJR* 28:133–140, 2008.
8. Bryze KC: Narrative contributions to the play history. In Parham LD, Fazio LS, editors: *Play in occupational therapy for children*, ed 2, St. Louis, 2010, Mosby.
9. Bundy AC: Assessment of play and leisure: delineation of the problem. *Am Occup Ther* 47:217, 1993.
10. Bundy AC: Play and playfulness: what to look for. In Parham LD, Fazio LS, editors: *Play in occupational therapy for children*, St. Louis, 1997, Mosby.
11. Bundy AC: Play theory and sensory integration. In Fisher AG, Murray EA, Bundy AC, editors: *Sensory integration: theory and practice*, Philadelphia, 1991, FA Davis.
12. Bundy AC: *Test of playfulness—4.0*, Sydney, Australia, 2003, University of Sydney.
13. Bundy AC et al: Playful interaction: occupational therapy for all children on the school playground. *Am J Occup Ther* 62:522–527, 2008.
14. Bundy AC et al: Reliability and validity of a test of playfulness. *Occup J Res* 21:276, 2001.
15. Bundy AC et al: How does sensory processing dysfunction affect play? *Am J Occup Ther* 61:201–208, 2007.
16. Bundy AC, Waugh K, Brentnall J: Developing assessments that account for the role of the environment: an example using the Test of Playfulness and Test of Environmental Supportiveness, *OTJR* 29:135–143, 2009.
17. Carlson BW, Ginglend DR: *Play activities for the retarded child: how to help him grow and learn through music, games,* handicrafts, and other play activities, New York, 1961, Abingdon Press.
18. Cass JE: *The significance of children's play*, London, 1971, Batsford.
19. Clifford JM, Bundy AC: Play preference and play performance in normal boys and boys with sensory integrative dysfunction. *Am J Occup Ther* 9:202, 1989.
20. Cohen D: *The development of play*, New York, 1987, New York University Press.
21. Cordier R et al: A model for play-based intervention for children with ADHD. *Austral Occup Ther J* 56:332–340, 2009.
22. Coster W: Occupation-centered assessment of children. *Am J Occup Ther* 52:337, 1998.
23. Csikszentmihalyi M: *Beyond boredom and anxiety*, San Francisco, 1975, Jossey-Bass.
24. Florey L: Development through play. In Schaefer C, editor: *The therapeutic use of play*, New York, 1976, Jason Aronson.
25. Greenstein DB: It's child's play. In Galvin J, editor: *Evaluating, selecting, and using appropriate assistive technology*, Gaithersburg, MD, 1996, Aspen.
26. Hart R: *Therapeutic play activities for hospitalized children*, St. Louis, 1992, Mosby.
27. Jernberg AM: *Theraplay: A new treatment using structured play for problem children and their families*, San Francisco, 1979, Jossey-Bass.
28. Kielhofner G, editor: *A model of human occupation*, Baltimore, 1985, Lippincott Williams & Wilkins.
29. Lane SJ, Mistrett SG: Play and assistive technology issues for infants and young children with disabilities: a preliminary examination. *Focus Autism Other Development Disabil* 11:96–104, 1996.
30. Linder TW, editor: *Transdisciplinary play based assessment*, Baltimore, 1990, Paul H. Brookes.
31. Llorens LA: *Application of a developmental theory for health and rehabilitation*, Bethesda, MD, 1976, American Occupational Therapy Association.
32. Marfo K, editor: *Parent-child interaction and developmental disabilities*, New York, 1988, Praeger.
33. Millar S: *The psychology of play*, New York, 1974, Aronson.
34. Moran JM, Kalakian LH: *Movement experiences for the mentally retarded or emotionally disturbed child*, Minneapolis, 1974, Burgess.
35. Morrison CD, Bundy AC, Fisher AG: The contribution of motor skills and playfulness to the play performance of preschoolers. *Am J Occup Ther* 45:687, 1991.
36. Morrison CD, Metzger P, Pratt P: Play. In Case-Smith J, Allen A, Pratt PN, editors: *Occupational therapy for children*, ed 3, St. Louis, 1996, Mosby.
37. Musselwhite CR: *Adaptive play for special needs children*, San Diego, 1986, College-Hill Press.
38. O'Brien JC et al: The impact of positioning equipment on play skills of physically impaired children. In Duncan MC, Chick G, Aycock A, editors: *Play and culture studies*, vol 1, Greenwich, CT, 1998, Ablex Publishing.
39. O'Brien JC et al: The impact of occupational therapy on a child's playfulness. *Occup Ther Healthcare* 12:39, 1999.

40. O'Brien JC, Shirley R: Does playfulness change over time: a preliminary look using the Test of Playfulness. *Occup Ther J Res* 21:132, 2001.

41. Okimoto AM, Bundy AC, Hanzlik J: Playfulness in children with and without disability: measurement and intervention. *Am J Occup Ther* 54:73, 2000.

42. Parham LD, Primeau L: Play and occupational therapy. In Parham LD, Fazio LS, editors: *Play in occupational therapy for children*, ed 2, St. Louis, 2010, Mosby.

43. Parten M: Social play among pre-school children. *J Abnorm Soc Psychol* 28:136, 1933.

44. Reed CN, Dunbar SB, Bundy AC: The effects of an inclusive preschool experience on the playfulness of children with and without autism. *Phys Occup Ther Pediatr* 19:73, 2000.

45. Reilly M, editor: *Play as exploratory learning: studies in curiosity behavior*, Beverly Hills, 1974, Sage.

46. Rubin K, Fein GG, Vandenberg B: Play. In Mussen PH, editor: *Handbook of child psychology*, ed 4, New York, 1983, Wiley.

47. Sipal R et al: Course of behaviour problems of children with cerebral palsy: the role of parental stress and support. *Child Care Health Develop* 36:74–84, 2010.

48. Skaines N, Rodger S, Bundy AC: Playfulness in children with autistic disorder and their typically developing peers. *Br J Occup Ther* 69:505–512, 2006.

49. Skard G, Bundy AC: The test of playfulness. In Parham LD, Fazio LS, editors: *Play in occupational therapy for children*, ed 2, St. Louis, Mosby, 71-94, 2008.

50. Sutton-Smith B: Play in cognitive development. In Schaefer C, editor: *The therapeutic use of play*, New York, 1976, Jason Aronson.

Recommended Reading

Hamm E: Playfulness and the environmental support of play in children with and without developmental disabilities. *OTJR* 26:88–96, 2006.

Linder T: *Transdisciplinary play based assessment*, ed 2, Baltimore, 2008, Paul H. Brookes.

Muys V, Rodger S, Bundy AC: Assessment of playfulness in children with autistic disorder: a comparison of the Children's Playfulness Scale and the Test of Playfulness. *OTJR* 26:159–170, 2006.

Parham LD, Fazio LS, editors: *Play in occupational therapy for children*, ed 2, St. Louis, 2010, Mosby.

Pierce D, Munier V, Myers C: Informing early intervention through an occupational science description of infant-toddler interactions with home space. *Am J Occup Ther* 63:273–287, 2009.

REVIEW *Questions*

1. Describe the characteristics of play and playfulness.
2. What is the difference between play and playfulness?
3. How would you facilitate play and playfulness in children with special needs?
4. What characteristics do you possess that would promote play and playfulness in children with special needs?
5. How is play used as a tool in the treatment of children?
6. Describe the way(s) that play can be the goal of therapy.
7. List three play assessments used by OT practitioners. Describe the ways they are administered and the information you gain from them.
8. How can the environment stimulate play and playfulness?

SUGGESTED *Activities*

1. Volunteer to babysit a child with special needs. Play with the child. Reflect on the experience by writing a one-page composition describing the way you felt about the time you spent with the child.
2. Plan and participate in an activity you enjoy with others. Describe the activity, materials needed, and environment. How did you feel during the activity?
3. In a small group, discuss your favorite childhood games and playmates. What types of skills did you learn as a child during play? What feelings do these memories bring to mind?
4. In a small group, role-play the characteristics of OT practitioners that promote playfulness in children.

Play Assessments

KNOX PRESCHOOL PLAY SCALE

The Knox Preschool Play Scale (PPS) provides a developmental description of play behavior in four domains: (1) space management, (2) materials management, (3) imitation, and (4) participation.[9] It is designed for children 0 to 6 years old. The Knox PPS is easy to administer and score. It requires two 30-minute observations of free play (indoors and outdoors). The revised scale provides age equivalencies to 6 months for children 0 to 3 years of age and yearly for children 3 to 5 years of age.[12]

TEST OF PLAYFULNESS

The Test of Playfulness (ToP) provides an objective measurement of playfulness.[2,3] Children are observed playing in familiar environments suitable for that purpose with peers for 15 minutes inside and 15 minutes outside. Administration of the scale requires training by viewing videotapes of children playing and scoring them according to ToP guidelines. Occupational therapy (OT) practitioners can use the information to systematically examine playfulness in children.[3] It has been found to be an accurate test for assessing typically developing children and those with disabilities.[5]

TRANSDISCIPLINARY PLAY-BASED ASSESSMENT

The Transdisciplinary Play-Based Assessment (TPBA) is a procedure for administering a comprehensive transdisciplinary assessment for children 0 to 3 years of age.[10] The TPBA provides structured guidelines for performing this assessment. OT clinicians can use this procedure to design intervention. The TPBA is an observational assessment that may take as long as 90 minutes to administer. All of the team members participate in the assessment. Information is gained in cognitive, social–emotional, communication and language, and motor skills.[10]

PLAY HISTORY

A play history is a semi-structured interview designed to obtain information about the child's behavior.[12,13] The play history is based on the developmental progression of play and examines behaviors in five developmental phases: (1) sensorimotor, (2) symbolic and simple constructive, (3) dramatic and complex constructive, (4) games, and (5) recreational. OT practitioners using this scale must have a firm knowledge of the normal progression of play. The scale provides a framework for gathering information on it.[13]

CHILDREN'S PLAYFULNESS SCALE

The Children's Playfulness Scale scale consists of 23 Likert-type format items and uses a five-point response/scoring system: (1) "sounds exactly like the child," (2) "sounds a lot like the child," (3) "sounds somewhat like the child," (4) "sounds a little like the child," and (5) "does not sound at all like the child."[1] Children receive a playfulness score. This scale is efficient and inexpensive and requires no direct observation of the child. Bundy and Clifton, however, questioned the use of this scale for children with disabilities.[4]

THE CHILD OCCUPATIONAL SELF ASSESSMENT

The Child Occupational Self Assessment (COSA) is a self-report evaluation most commonly given to children in school settings but is acceptable in numerous other contexts and alongside other assesments.[7,8] In schools, the COSA is often used to elicit the child's viewpoints and own goals when developing an individualized educational program (IEP). Children may complete the COSA as traditionally done, using pencil and paper; to accommodate children with special needs, a card-sort version is available.[7,8]

The COSA was developed using foundational components of the Model of Human Occupation (MOHO), which theorizes that performance is affected by an individual's motivation, habits, physical/cognitive abilities, interests, and environment. The assessment first asks children how they feel about their skills in communication, interaction, motor control, and processing. It then asks children to identify how important that activity is to them. For example, the COSA asks children how well they believe they "keep working on something even when it gets hard." Children then choose from four

CHAPTER 20 APPENDIX A—cont'd

Play Assessments

different options ranging from "I have a big problem doing this" to "I am really good at doing this" (p. 12).[7] For the same question, children are asked how important that ability is to them, and they may answer again from four choices, ranging from "not really important to me" to "most important of all to me."[7,8]

TEST OF ENVIRONMENTAL SUPPORTIVENESS

The Test of Environmental Supportiveness (TOES) follows the Person-Environment-Occupation (PEO) model. The TOES is a 17-item assessment administered to children between 15 months and 12 years of age.[5,6] Children are observed during 15 minutes of free play, as in the ToP, to evaluate what motivates and supports them at play. This assessment can be used to evaluate many different environments, such as daycare, home, and the outdoors.[5] Caregivers, playmates, spaces, and objects are four environmental domains that have been found to affect play. The TOES uses a four-point scaling system to identify the significance of each environmental component in supporting or inhibiting a child's playfulness. The TOES has been found to be a valid and reliable assessment tool that can be used for children with or without disabilities.[5,11]

References

1. Barnett LA: Playfulness: Definition, design, and measurement, *Play Culture* 3:319, 1990.
2. Bundy AC: Play and playfulness: What to look for. In Parham LD, Fazio LS, editors: *Play in occupational therapy for children*, ed 2, St Louis, 2010, Mosby.
3. Bundy AC: *Test of playfulness (ToP) version 3.5*, Fort Collins, CO, 2000, Colorado State University Press.
4. Bundy AC, Clifton JL: Construct validity of the children's playfulness scale. In Duncan MC, Chick G, Aycock A, editors: *Play and culture studies*, vol 1, Greenwich, CT, 1998, Ablex Publishing.
5. Bundy AC, Waugh K, Brentnall J: Developing assessments that account for the role of environment: An example using the Test of Playfulness and the Test of Environmental Supportiveness, *OTJR* 29(3):135–143, 2009.
6. Hamm E: Playfulness and the environmental support of play in children with and without developmental disabilities, *OTJR* 26(3):88–96, 2006.
7. Keller, J., Kafkes, A., & Kielhofner, G. (2005). Psychometric characteristics of the Child Occupational Self Assessment (COSA), part one: An initial examination of psychometric properties. Scandinavian Journal of Occupational Therapy, 12, 118-127
8. Keller, J., Kafkes, A., Basu, S., Federico, J., & Kielhofner, G. (2005). Child Occupational Self Assessment (COSA) Version 2.1, 2005, University of Illinois at Chicago, MOHO clearinghouse.
9. Knox S: Development and current use of the Knox preschool play scale. In Parham LD, Fazio LS, editors: *Play in occupational therapy*, ed 2, St. Louis, 2010, Mosby.
10. Linder TW, editor: *Transdisciplinary play-based assessment*, Baltimore, MD, 1990, Paul H Brookes.
11. Muys V, Rodger S, Bundy AC: Assessment of playfulness in children with autistic disorder: A comparison of the Children's Playfulness Scale and the Test of Playfulness, *OTJR* 26(4):159–170, 2006.
12. Reilly M, editor: *Play as exploratory learning*, Beverly Hills, CA, 1974, Sage.
13. Takata N: Play as a prescription. In Reilly M, editor: *Play as exploratory learning*, Beverly Hills, CA, 1974, Sage.

CHAPTER 20 APPENDIX B

Resources for Play Activity Ideas

PUBLICATIONS

Burkhart LJ: *More homemade battery devices for severely handicapped children with suggested activities,* College Park, MD, 1982, Linda J Burkhart.

Cole J, Tiergreen A, Calmenson S: *Eentsy, weentsy spider: Fingerplays and action rhymes,* New York, 1991, Mulberry Books.

Coleman K, McNairn P, Shioleno C: *Quick tech magic music-based literacy activities,* Solana, CA, 2004, Mayer-Johnson Company.

Dexter S: Joyful play with toddlers: *Recipes for fun with odds and ends (tool for everyday parenting series),* Seattle, WA, 1996, Parenting Press.

Hamilton L: *Child's play around the world: 170 crafts, games and projects for 2-6 year olds,* New York, 1996, Beverly.

Judith G, Ellison S: *365 days of creative play for children 2 years and up,* Trabuco Canyon, CA, 1995, Sourcebooks.

Kranowitz CS: *101 activities for kids in tight spaces: At the doctor's office; on car, train, and plane trips; and home sick in bed,* New York, 1995, St Martin's Press.

Miller K: *Things to do with toddlers and twos,* West Palm Beach, FL, 1984, Telshare.

Morris LR, Schultz L: *Creative play activities for children with disabilities: A resource book for teachers and parents,* ed 2, Champaign, IL, 1989, Human Kinetic Books.

Munger EM, Bowden SJ: *Beyond peek-a-boo and pat-a-cake: Activities for baby's first twenty-four months,* ed 3, Clinton, NJ, 1993, New Win Pub.

Nipp S, Beall PC: *Wee sing children's songs and fingerplays (audiocassette),* New York, 1994, Price Stern Sloan Audio.

Nolan A: *Great explorations: 100 creative play ideas for parents and preschoolers from playspace at the children's museum,* Boston, MA, 1997, Pocket Books.

Silberg J: *300 3-minute games: quick and easy activities for 2-5 year olds,* Beltsville, MD, 1997, Gryphon House.

Totline Staff: *1001 rhymes and fingerplays,* Pomona, CA, 1994, Warren Publishing House.

Ulene A, Shelov S: *Discovery play: Loving and learning with your baby,* Berkeley, CA, 1994, Ulysses Press.

Wright C, Nomura M: *From toys to computers: access for the physically disabled child,* San Jose, CA, 1990, C Wright.

WEBSITE GAMES, ACTIVITIES, AND PRINTABLES FOR CHILDREN

www.brighting.com
Activities, experiments with science explanations, coloring pages

www.childfun.com
Printables, crafts, themes

www.Disneyland.com
Games, printables

www.Kidwizard.com
Crafts, games

www.Learningplanet.com
Educational activities, printables, games

www.PrimaryGames.com
Online games, coloring pages, mazes

www.School.discovery.com
School activities, awards, certificates

Resources for Play Activity Ideas

www.Teachervision.com
Teacher lessons, certificates, behavior management forms, printables, articles

COMPANIES AND PUBLICATIONS HELPFUL IN ADAPTING PLAY FOR CHILDREN WITH SPECIAL NEEDS

Ablenet
1091 Tenth Avenue, Southeast
Minneapolis, MN 55414-1312
(800) 322-0956

Linda Burkhart
8503 Rhode Island Avenue
College Park, MD 20740
(301) 345-9152

Crestwood Company
6625 North Sidney Place
Milwaukee, WI 53209-3259
(414) 352-5678

Exceptional Parent Magazine
PO Box 5446
Pittsfield, MA 01203-9321
(800) 247-8080

CHAPTER 20 APPENDIX B—cont'd

Resources for Play Activity Ideas

Don Johnston
PO Box 639
Wauconda, IL 60084-0639
(800) 999-4660

National Therapeutic Recreation Society
2775 South Quincy Street, Suite 300
Arlington, VA 22206
(703) 820-4940

Toys for Special Children
385 Warburton Avenue
Hastings-on-Hudson, NY 10706

21

Functional Task at School: Handwriting

MONICA D. KEEN*

CHAPTER *Objectives*

After studying this chapter, the reader will be able to accomplish the following:

- Identify prewriting strokes, their developmental sequence, and at what age they emerge
- Explain how handwriting skills affect the ability of children to perform written assignments in the school setting
- Recognize the client factors required for handwriting
- Identify the reasons handwriting difficulties occur
- Suggest strategies to improve handwriting or written expression
- Describe direct intervention techniques
- Describe how visual perception affects handwriting
- Identify types of grasping patterns
- Describe types of handwriting assessments used in pediatrics

*The author would like to acknowledge Diana Bal, MS, OTR/L, for her contributions to the revision of this chapter.

The most frequent referral for occupational therapists in the school setting is for problems with handwriting.[4] As a result, handwriting remediation programs are often delivered on site at school, either individually or in small groups.[13] **Handwriting** is one of the functional tasks required of a child in his or her occupation as student. McHale and Cermak report that as much as 60% of a school day can be spent on fine motor tasks, including handwriting.[15] It is an important part of the educational process because handwriting is the most common means by which a student expresses knowledge of the material being taught. In addition, a student uses writing to summarize information taught in class, complete assignments, take tests, and interact with others for noneducational purposes.[21] Between 10% and 30% of elementary school children struggle with handwriting.[9] Likewise, experts claim that illegible handwriting has secondary effects on school achievement and self-esteem.[7,14]

Handwriting difficulties in children include illegible handwriting and speed-related issues; in addition, areas that affect the legibility of handwriting include letter formation, horizontal alignment, size, spacing, and slant.[13,15,18]

Handwriting is one of the tools teachers use to measure a student's academic comprehension. Handwriting allows children to express themselves, learn information, organize their work, and communicate with others. It is vital that occupational therapy (OT) practitioners working in schools address handwriting difficulties to improve students' performances in their occupation.[15,18]

The Appendix to this chapter provides an overview of commercially available handwriting programs that OT practitioners may find useful when providing interventions to children.

EVALUATION AND ASSESSMENT OF HANDWRITING SKILLS

CASE *Study*

Molly is a first grader at Lincoln Elementary. She sits at a table at the front of the class and loves to participate in most of the classroom activities. She is not able to draw most of her shapes; when encouraged to draw freely, her drawings appear very immature. When asked to write, she becomes nervous. She has trouble remembering the letters of the alphabet, and when called on to identify a letter, she is not always able to provide the correct answer. She has difficulty recalling the letters of the alphabet and then struggles with forming any letter on paper. She tends to write large letters, so the entire page is covered with very little writing. She is able to write her first name, but she

starts all of her letters from the bottom of the line and sometimes uses multiple strokes to form one letter.

Handwriting is a multifaceted developmental task. When a student is unable to put **prewriting strokes** together to form simple shapes, it is quite a challenge, if not impossible, for the student to form a letter. When evaluating a student's handwriting, the OT practitioner looks at myriad components that are needed to successfully perform this task. Visual, perceptual, and fine motor skills must be assessed. In addition, considering the child's developmental stage provides insight into where his or her handwriting abilities may fall. It is the job of the OT practitioner to analyze the task and determine what components are missing or weak. Lastly, considering how the student's sensory systems are being impacted by this task requires consideration.

Handwriting is an important occupational skill requiring motor, sensory, perceptual, and cognitive abilities.[13] Formal and informal assessments of the ability to imitate and copy lines and shapes, hold a pencil or tool, and complete perceptual motor tasks help identify the factors for intervention. Figures 21-1 and 21-2 are examples of checklists which may be used to identify a child's prerequisite skills for handwriting.

The OT practitioner is responsible for evaluating all aspects of handwriting; designing intervention or **compensatory strategies**; and consulting with children, teachers, and parents. The goal of OT in the school is to promote participation in the general educational curriculum. As such, teachers and parents benefit from recommendations to enhance handwriting skills. Compensations and accommodations allow the student to be successful in the classroom or home (refer to the section on classroom accommodations later in this chapter).

Standardized/Nonstandardized Assessments and Classroom Observation

A variety of standardized and nonstandardized assessments are available to determine the client factors interfering with handwriting. Classroom observation is yet another valuable means to assess handwriting. The following sections describe different types of assessments as well as classroom observation considerations that are used to assess areas that impact handwriting ability.

Developmental Assessments

Developmental assessments examine the developmental level of a child's handwriting abilities. They provide OT practitioners with information concerning the age level at which the child performs. For example, in Molly's situation, the assessment can answer the following question: Does Molly have the handwriting abilities required

Name : _____   Date: _____

---

1. Describe class work compared with the other students in class

2. Describe posture at the desk

Desk height 2" above bent elbow _____   Feet on floor _____   Wrist stable _____

Body symmetrical _____   Head aligned _____   Trunk upright _____

3. Imitation of whole body motions in a timely manner without touching:

Straighten arms over head _____

Stretch arms out to side _____

Cross arms in front of body _____

Right arm straight, bend left elbow _____   Left arm straight, bend right elbow _____

Shift arms and hands from one side of the body to the other _____

X midline of body with arms/hands _____

4. Imitation of hand and finger motions in a timely manner without prompts:

Rotate wrist _____

Open and shut fingers/thumb _____

Touch thumb to fingers _____   when told which finger to touch _____

Move each finger separately imitatively _____ when told which finger to move _____

Routine finger songs (Thumbkin, Itsy Spider) _____

5. Grasp on pencil: Static _____   Dynamic _____

fingers on pencil _____   Distal thumb _____   Pressure on paper _____

FIGURE 21-1   Handwriting checklist—manuscript.

Continued

Open web space _____   Distal control _____   Wrist stable _____

6. Hold down paper _____

7. Reversals _____

list

8. Hand dominance _____

R   L

9. Write the following sentence on paper with lines and evaluate the following:

"The dirty plane flies up high into the sky"

Curved lines	Rounded	Straight
Sentence begins with capital		Ends with punctuation
All other letters lower case		Start "d" with a "c"
% letters initiated at top		% letters and words going left to right
% letters on the line		% spaces between words

10. Visual perceptual test results:

FIGURE 21-1, cont'd

of a student in Grade 1? Box 21-1 provides sample developmental assessments.

Visual Perception Assessments

Visual perception is the ability to organize and interpret what is seen. Handwriting requires children to visually perceive the organization of letters and spacing between words. They must also determine the direction of letters (e.g., *b* compared with *d*). Visual perception is required to know where to start writing on the page, sequence the strokes of letters, and space words. When writing, children must recognize that the sizes of letters do not change the meanings of words. Molly may be experiencing poor visual perception. In this scenario, she is unable

Name: _____   Date: _____

---

1. Describe class work compared with the other students in class.

2. Describe posture at the desk.

Desk height 2" above bent elbow _____   Feet on floor _____   Wrist stable _____

Body symmetrical _____   Head aligned _____   Trunk upright _____

3. Imitation of whole body motions in a timely manner without touching:

Straighten arms over head _____

Stretch arms out to side _____

Cross arms in front of body _____

Right arm straight, bend left elbow _____   Left arm straight, bend right elbow _____

Shift arms and hands from one side of the body to the other _____

X midline of body with arms/hands _____

4. Imitation of hand and finger motions in a timely manner without prompts:

Rotate wrist _____

Open and shut fingers/thumb _____

Touch thumb to fingers _____   when told which finger to touch _____

Move each finger separately imitatively _____ when told which finger to move _____

Routine finger songs (Thumbkin, Itsy Spider) _____

5. Write the following sentence on paper with lines and evaluate the following:

"The brown dog wags his fat tail"

FIGURE 21-2 Handwriting checklist—cursive.

Continued

Curved lines	Smooth	On same slant	Rounded
Sentence begins with capital		End with punctuation	
All other letters lower case		All letters in word connect	
% letters starting at line		% letters and words going left to right	
% letters on the line		% spaces between words	

6. Grasp on pencil: Static _____   Dynamic _____

fingers on pencil _____   Distal thumb _____   Pressure on paper _____

  Open web space _____   Distal control _____   Wrist stable _____

7. Hold down paper _____

8. Reversals _____

list:

9. Hand dominance _____

      R   L

10. Visual perceptual test results:

FIGURE 21-2, cont'd

BOX 21-1

Developmental Assessments

- The *Peabody Developmental Motor Scale–2* (Folio & Fewell, 2000) evaluates copying and writing readiness skills and provides an age-equivalent score on grasp development, manual dexterity, and developmental writing skills.
- *The Hawaii Early Learning Profile (HELP)* (Furuno, O'Reilly, Hosaka, Zeisloft & Allman, 2004) can be used to examine prehandwriting skills in children 0 to 3 years of age. This developmental checklist is helpful in tracking the development of hand skills.
- The *Bayley Scale of Infant Development* (Bayley, 2005) assesses the motor development of children from 1 to 42 months of age.
- The *Erhardt Developmental Prehension Assessment* (Erhardt & Baune, 1994) measures the components of arm and hand development in children.
- The *Bruininks-Oseretsky Test of Motor Proficiency–2* (Bruininks & Bruininks, 2005) measures the gross and fine motor proficiencies of children 4.5 to 14.5 years old, testing such areas as response speed, upper limb speed, and visual motor control.

BOX 21-2

Visual Perceptual Assessments

- The *Test of Visual Motor Integration–Revised* (Gardner, 1995) combines both the developmental sequencing of geometric shapes and visual motor integration.
- The *Motor-Free Visual Perception Test–Revised* (Colarusso & Hammill, 2002) and the *Test of Visual Perceptual Skills* (nonmotor) (TVPS) (Martin, 2006) measure nonmotor visual perception in children by testing visual perception without requiring a motor response.

to make sense of how letters are formed. Molly may not recognize the differences among *b*, *p*, and *d* (Box 21-2).

Visual perceptual tests examine the following skills:

- *Discrimination*: The ability to detect a difference or distinction between one item or picture and another, for example, the ability to identify which picture is not like the others.
- *Visual Memory*: The ability to remember a shape or word and recall the information when necessary. With handwriting, children must remember how to form letters, numbers, and shapes. In later school years, this skill is used when remembering how to form the letters to spell words or form multidigit numbers.
- *Form Constancy*: The ability to realize and recognize that forms, letters, and numbers are the same or are constant whether they are moved, turned, or changed to a different size. This means that a square is always a square no matter what size or color. A daily example of this is when a person recalls the shape of the "yield" sign.
- *Sequential Memory*: The ability to remember a sequence or chain of letters to form a word. With handwriting, children need motor as well as cognitive sequencing. Therefore, they need the ability to remember how letters make words and sequence them according to their motor abilities to make those words. For example, when taking a spelling

test, the child needs to be able to recall what the word "dog" looks like and remember that it is *d – o – g* and not *g – d – o*.

- *Figure Ground*: The ability to identify the foreground from the background. When looking at pictures, people, or items, it is essential to separate important visual aspects from the background. When writing, children identify written words on lined paper. An example of this is the game of finding hidden objects in a drawing.
- *Visual Closure*: The ability to identify a form or object from its incomplete appearance. This enables a child to figure out objects, shapes, and forms by finishing the image mentally, for example, finding a jacket when it is partially covered by others. This ability is required when a letter may not be completely formed.

Handwriting Assessments

A variety of different handwriting assessments that can be used to evaluate a child's handwriting are available (Box 21-3). Assessments can be standardized or nonstandardized and include clinical observations. The evaluating OT practitioner needs to know the purpose of the evaluation. Do the results need to be standardized? Does the OT practitioner, parent, or teacher want to know where this child's handwriting abilities are in comparison with his or her peers, or is getting an example of the child's handwriting abilities the goal? Is the OT practitioner interested in learning how the child is writing or spacing letters and words? The nature of the evaluation will determine which type of assessment(s) is to be used.

CLASSROOM OBSERVATION

Most of a child's handwriting occurs in the classroom. Therefore, it makes sense that the student be observed doing this task in this environment. Classroom

---

BOX 21-3

Handwriting Assessments

- The *Children's Handwriting Evaluation Scales* (Stott et al., 1984) measures the speed and quality of the child's handwriting skills.
- The *Evaluation Tool of Children's Handwriting (ETCH)* (Amundson, 1995) evaluates legibility and speed in six areas of handwriting: (1) alphabet production of lower and uppercase letters from memory, (2) numeral writing of 1 to 12 from memory, (3) near-point copying, (4) far-point copying, (5) speed, and (6) sentence composition in both manuscript and cursive formation.[15] The ETCH provides legibility scores for the child's age level.
- *The Print Tool*™ is a nonstandardized assessment from Jan Olsen's Handwriting Without Tears curriculum. "The Print Tool focuses on the eight key components of handwriting: memory, orientation, placement, size, start, sequence, control, and spacing." In addition to being an assessment, The Print Tool also "helps pinpoint the cause of difficulty and provides guidance for a remediation plan specific to the child's needs."

---

observations allow OT practitioners to see how children work, how they organize their work/desk surface, and how they use their time. When evaluating a child's handwriting, observation of the child's performance in the classroom is beneficial.

Classroom observation allows the OT practitioner to view the functional task (e.g., handwriting) in the context in which it occurs. Understanding the child's performance within the context of the classroom guides the intervention plan. For example, examination of the *physical context* provides information on such things as classroom space, seating arrangements, the height of the desk, visual stimuli, and environmental supports. Molly may be sitting in a chair that is too high, and the classroom space may not be conducive to writing. In terms of *personal context*, classroom observation may reveal information about Molly's needs. Perhaps she is easily distracted by the noise outside the door or by the decorations on the walls or hanging from the ceiling of the classroom. OT practitioners will want to consider the writing demands of a Grade 1 classroom as well as Molly's temperament and attitude toward the writing task. From the case study presented earlier, it is apparent that Molly becomes nervous during writing assignments, which provides the OT practitioner a window into her feelings. *Temporal context* refers to the time of day in which the handwriting task is performed. If handwriting is performed in the afternoon, Molly may very well be

tired and restless; however, Molly produces her best work in the morning. Classroom observation may provide insight into how Molly is managing her time as well. *Cultural context* refers to expectations with regard to the classroom. How organized is the teacher? Are accommodations a natural part of the classroom? Is the classroom too busy for a child who requires a quiet environment for writing? Is the child able to interact easily with his or her peers?

Classroom observations provide valuable information on the factors that may be interfering with function in the classroom. Teachers are able to provide OT practitioners with information about the child's performance in the classroom, classroom expectations, and possible solutions. In addition, the teacher is able to provide the OT with handwriting samples done by the student at various times of the day.

CLINICAL *Pearl*

Visual or auditory distractions in the classroom may interfere with visual attention to handwriting tasks.

CLINICAL *Pearl*

Asking teachers and families what strategies they have used in the past and using those strategies in OT interventions may help children succeed. Matching strategies to the classroom is effective.

DEVELOPMENTAL SEQUENCE

Referrals to OT for handwriting are made based on children not performing at age-appropriate standards. Teachers notice that the child is not as fluent, clear, or legible as his or her classmates. OT practitioners are called in to determine the developmental level at which the child is functioning and the cause(s) for the handwriting difficulties so that an appropriate intervention can be designed. Development occurs through the learning, experiencing, and acquisition of the skills. The rate of development and the progression of skills vary in children but usually follow sequential patterns.

Prewriting

Prewriting strokes are the foundation for making shapes and letter formation. A child must understand and be able to stroke positional concepts such as *down* (vertical) and *across* (horizontal) before they can put them together to form letters For example, when providing verbal prompts for stroking the capital letter "L," the student would hear, " Big line down, little line across."

Motor, cognitive, and sensory systems must work together for success in pre-writing. Children start performing prewriting activities at a very early age. Consider the child putting open hands into the chocolate pudding and rubbing the pudding on the high-chair tray in circular motions. Then there is the toddler who takes Mom's marker and makes numerous marks on the kitchen wall. As their little hands strengthen, they take crayons and paper and scribble with abandon. As they are taught about circles and vertical and horizontal lines, they start to put them together to make shapes such as squares, rectangles, circles, and intersecting lines. Diagonals are the last prewriting strokes to develop. The child is then able to put them together to form triangles and diamonds. Prewriting strokes develop at the following ages:

* 2- to 3-year-olds: vertical and horizontal lines
* 3- to 4-year-olds: circles and intersecting lines
* 4- to 6-year-olds: diagonal lines and the ability to form shapes

Grasping Patterns

Children with handwriting difficulties show a less mature grasp, immature pencil grip, and inconsistent hand preference.[3] The most mature grasps are the dynamic tripod (Figure 21-3, A) and lateral tripod grasps. By definition, in a *tripod grasp* three fingers are used for holding the writing utensil. The thumb is bent, the index finger points to the top of the writing utensil, and the writing utensil rests on the side of the middle finger. The last two fingers are curled in the palm and stabilize the hand.[16] The lateral quadrupod and four-finger grip can be as functional as the dynamic tripod, lateral tripod, and dynamic quadrupod pencil grips in Grade 4 students.[10] A quadrupod grip (four fingers) is another way children may hold their writing utensil. The thumb is bent, the index and middle finger point to the top of the writing utensil, and the writing utensil rests on the ring finger.[16]

In the dynamic tripod grasp, finger movements are used rather than those of the whole hand or arm. When forming a letter, dynamic movements of the fingers create smooth curves. Awkward **grasping patterns** result in poor letter formation, fatigue, and poor handwriting. Hank holds the pencil tightly with minimum web space and a cross-thumb grasp (see Figure 21-3, B). The resulting strain and contraction of the wrist and finger muscles may cause pain, fatigue, and discomfort.

Preschool children have small hands. It is difficult for them to manipulate regular-sized pencils and markers. Some teachers have preschool children use large pencils and/or triangular pencils to promote functional grasps.

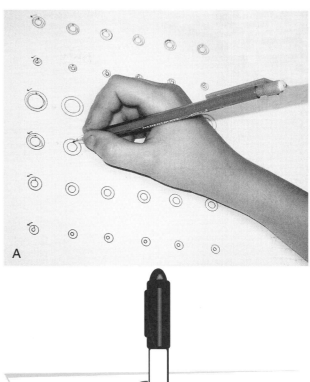

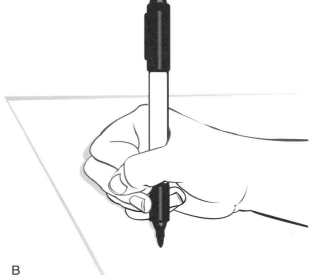

FIGURE 21-3 A, Dynamic tripod grasp. **B,** Cross-thumb grasp.

However, preschool children should use only short crayons and small pencils for writing/coloring. Crayons are made of colored wax, which provides resistance (and strengthening) when coloring. This also provides kinesthetic feedback to the user. Golf ball–sized pencils or regular pencils broken into two are perfect for children with small hands. Smaller pencils/crayons help prepare the child's hand for a good pencil grip and encourage the child to use a tripod grasp, which allows for better control of the pencil.

Knowledge of the progression of grasping patterns is useful to the OT practitioner in evaluating handwriting.[18] Cross-thumb (thumb wrap) or static tripod grasps can be fatiguing or painful but offer more stability and power. Tight grasps limit the variety of movements and make smooth, flowing motions difficult. Writers using tight grasps often press hard on the paper, which results in the formation of dark, sometimes smeared, letters.[18]

CLINICAL *Pearl*

Many adults use a variety of pencil grasps with minimum web space and a very tight grasping pattern. Look around and observe the variety of grasping patterns that are used.

Developmental Stages in Writing Readiness

As children grow and develop, so does their handwriting ability. Table 21-1 provides an outline of the sequence of writing development. The children's ability to manipulate writing/coloring utensils as well as their ability to use their "helper hand" improves. As they become more comfortable with the task of scribbling, coloring, and ultimately writing, their posture during this task changes and matures. A 2-year-old uses all of his or her fingers to hold a crayon in the palm of the hand. The helping hand is of no use, as the upper extremity is usually retracted at the shoulder, flexed at the elbow, adducted to the side, with semicontracted fingers. This is a position of stability for the child. In addition, the hand performing the scribbling is abducted at the shoulder and flexed at the elbow, and the wrist is pronated and does not make contact with the paper at all. The posture of the 3-year-old is more advanced in that the child starts to use the helping hand. The shoulders are still elevated but are not

TABLE 21-1

Prewriting Skill Development*

ITEM NAME	AGE (MONTHS)
Stirring spoon	12
Scribbling—I scribble I inch long	14
Imitating vertical line 2 inches long	23-24
Imitating horizontal line 2 inches long	27-28
Copying circle—end points within half inch of each other	33-34
Copying cross—intersecting lines within 20 degrees of perpendicular	39-40
Tracing line—deviates <2 times	41-42

*Based on *Peabody Developmental Motor Scale–2*.

as retracted. All of the fingers may still be used to hold the utensil, and the wrist of the dominant hand continues to be in the air. As the fourth year approaches, the utensil is being held with a more mature grasp. Shoulders are relaxing to a certain extent but continue to be elevated and somewhat retracted for stability. In addition, the child uses the helper hand to hold the paper in a more deliberate fashion. The elbow of the dominant hand is still elevated, and the writing hand still is not making contact with the surface of the table. By the fifth year, a mature grasp has evolved, and the dominant elbow, wrist, and hand all lie comfortably on the surface of the table. The shoulders are relaxed, and the child sits confidently at the table for handwriting and coloring activities.

In-hand Manipulation

In-hand manipulation refers to the precise and skilled finger movements made during fine motor tasks. In-hand manipulation is correlated with handwriting legibility.[21] In order to perform in-hand manipulation tasks, the child needs to be able to adjust objects within the hand while maintaining the grasp on the object. A general example of this skill is working coins from the palm of the hand to a pincer grasp to deposit the coins into a piggy bank. In-hand manipulation skills during writing are observed when a child rotates the pencil to use the eraser. Another example is manipulating the pencil to write dynamically with a tripod grasp while the ring and little fingers remain still to stabilize the hand. In-hand manipulation requires strength, timing, and coordination. Examples of exercises that can strengthen the intrinsic muscles of the hand for improved in-hand manipulation include the following:

- *Shifting*: working items from the palm of the hand to the tips of the fingers without dropping items
- *Translation*: using only the fingers, the student "walks" his or her hand from the lead end of the pencil to the eraser end without the aid of items for stabilization
- *Rotation*: turning the pencil from the lead end to the eraser end without putting the pencil down on the table or using the chest to stabilize the pencil while turning it.

CLINICAL *Pearl*

Children with Down syndrome tend to use their third finger and thumb to pick up small objects because their thumb does not curve, or oppose, enough to reach the index finger.

INTERVENTION USING A DEVELOPMENTAL FRAME OF REFERENCE

When using a developmental frame of reference to address handwriting issues, the OT practitioner must first determine the developmental level at which the student is performing. The goal of this approach is to improve the child's performance from his or her current developmental level to the next developmental one. An intervention session using this approach may take place as follows:

CASE *Study*

Henry, a kindergarten student, has just started coming to OT for assistance with handwriting. The Peabody Developmental Motor Scales assessment has shown that Henry is still having difficulty making the circular stroke. He tends to form the shape backward and then does not have a definite stopping point when making the circle. The first activity that the OT practitioner, Darby, has Henry do is to make a series of circles on the dry erase board. As Henry strokes, Darby provides hand-over-hand assistance as well as the verbal prompt, "Circle, STOP!" As they stop the formation of the circle, Darby intentionally raises Henry's hand from the board so that he can experience the literal "STOP" to the stroke. Then they add some small vertical strokes to the bottom of the circle and turn the series of circles into a caterpillar. Next, Darby takes Henry to the table where she has him spread out shaving cream. Darby then has Henry make circles in this shaving cream. They also play games of Tic-Tac-Toe, where Henry is always the circle. Darby draws large circles on construction paper for Henry to cut out. In doing this, the construction paper provides kinesthetic feedback while cutting, and Henry's motor planning is challenged while cutting the circular shape out. Throughout the session, they are identifying objects in the therapy room that are circular in shape. She rewards Henry with praise and small treats every time he strokes the circle correctly. The last activity they do is draw circles on a piece of paper. Darby

makes sure to consult with the classroom teacher about the day's session and to send a note home providing the parents with fun activities for the home setting.

Developmental Activities

- Follow the developmental sequence as outlined in a developmental assessment or checklist. Perform the listed developmental visual motor tasks such as cutting with scissors.
- Trace simple line drawings such as beginning shape designs. The lines of the shapes can be emphasized by highlighting them with a magic marker and then outlining with white glue. The glue will dry clear, making a raised border highlighted to call attention to the lines.
- Draw circles using a sticker, stamp, or other coloring objects to represent the starting point. Provide arrows that point in the direction the stroke should go. Fade the visual prompts over time.
- Have the student march to music in a circle around chairs. Play musical chairs if it is a group of children.
- Have the child roll out "snakes" using Play-Doh; then have the child form the snakes into shapes.
- Use special handwriting paper to emphasize and highlight the lines with embossed, raised lines. The top line could be green and the bottom line red to indicate the boundaries.
- Have the child color within a designated area; use a template to cover the area not to be colored, and put emphasis on that area.
- Have the child copy and imitate designs and body motions. He or she can imitate body motions while moving from one location to another.
- Provide a variety of tools such as screwdrivers, hammers, and tongs, encouraging working with one hand while the other hand stabilizes the object.
- Cut putty and paper with scissors to work on a one-handed task designed to strengthen the intrinsic muscles of the hand and further develop tool usage.

MOTOR SKILLS AND INTERVENTION

Motor skills include a variety of components that directly impact the child's ability to write. Examples of motor skills necessary for writing include upper extremity range of motion (ROM); trunk, upper body, and upper extremity stability; limb integrity; and muscle strength and endurance. All of these areas need to be properly functioning for optimal handwriting performance. The OT practitioner considers these factors when evaluating and providing interventions to improve handwriting.

CASE *Study*

Matthew, a Grade 2 student, has cerebral palsy. He has mild increased tone in his hip extensors and trunk muscles. He is able to sit in the classroom chairs that are scooped in the lower back and seat area. When sitting in this chair, Matthew's trunk tone increases significantly as he works hard to maintain his sitting balance. He is able to write, but the quality of his handwriting is shaky, and his print is large. However, when the OT practitioner provides Matthew with a chair with lateral sides that has a straight back and a flat seat, his posture improves significantly. In addition, a seat belt securely fastened across his hips reduces his hip extensor tone considerably, and he sits comfortably in the chair. Matthew is now able to access the paper on the table with ease from this sitting position. Because he is no longer using his upper body and upper extremity muscles for trunk stabilization, he is now able to write with improved legibility and with appropriate-sized letters.

This case illustrates the importance of examining the motor skills required for handwriting.

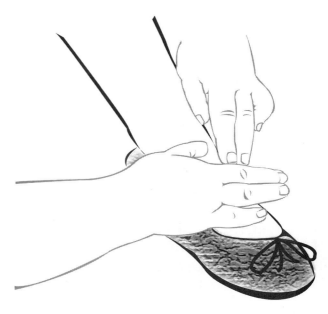

FIGURE 21-4 Child who is missing fingers practices tying her shoes.

Range of Motion

The OT practitioner evaluates the available ROM of the trunk, elbows, shoulders, wrist, and fingers. Contractures or limitations in ROM may interfere with the smooth, coordinated movements required for writing. For example, a student with rheumatoid arthritis may not be able to hold a writing utensil with the tripod grasp. However, when the utensil is placed between the index and long fingers, the child is able to manipulate the writing utensil more comfortably, as this position takes the pressure off of the joints.

Integrity and Structure of Arm, Hand, and Fingers

OT practitioners examine the integrity of the arm, hand, and fingers to determine whether deformities, edema, or open wounds are interfering with writing. Poor integrity of the upper extremity and the hand can cause a lot of pain. This must be taken into consideration, and the activity must be adapted to allow the student to participate with the rest of the class. A student with epidermis bulosa may have blistered, weeping, and peeling skin. In addition, the fingers may be severely contracted. The child may have to hold the writing utensil between the palms of both hands for optimal performance.

OT practitioners examine the child's hand, arm, and fingers to determine if any structural differences are interfering with the ability to write. For example, some children may be missing digits or have contractures that interfere with writing (see Figure 21-4). These

children may need to learn compensatory strategies or use adaptive techniques.

Posture: Trunk, Shoulder, Wrist, and Finger Stability

When evaluating posture, always start with the trunk. Trunk stability is the very foundation from which the rest of the body gains its stability. Children must call on strong abdominal and lateral muscles to maintain a strong core. Having a strong core enables the child to sustain an upright seating posture during writing. When the child leans or slouches in a chair, it is an indicator that his trunk lacks muscular strength or muscle tone (see Figure 21-5A and 21-5B). Interventions to improve posture (such as playing on a ball to improve trunk extension) may help the child write more efficiently (see Figure 21-5, B). When slouching or leaning, the child may compensate by placing the elbows on the writing surface to hold the body up. The child expends so much energy working to maintain an upright position and fatigues quickly, which interferes with coloring or writing. When the child leans on the forearms, the dominant hand cannot be used effectively for writing, and this also impedes the helper hand from stabilizing the paper.

Posture can be easily influenced by the height of the desk and chair. The best sitting position for a child is sitting with the hips and knees at 90 degrees, feet flat on

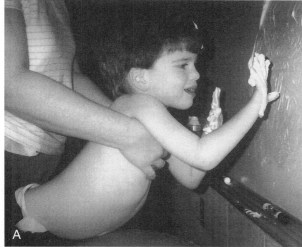

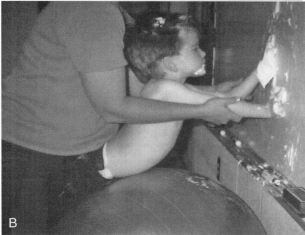

FIGURE 21-5   A, Low muscle tone in the trunk. **B,** Working on the ball in the prone position optimizes body alignment and trunk extension.

The sequence of the typical development of tool usage is provided below.
- Initially, children move the whole arm with shoulder movements while holding the utensil in a grasping pattern with the thumb and index finger toward the paper.
- Movement occurs at the forearm, with the shoulder more stable.
- The upper arm and forearm are more stable as movement occurs primarily at the wrist and with the whole hand.
- Movement occurs at the metacarpal joints of all the fingers or with a static tripod grasp.
- Finally, dynamic movement occurs at the thumb and index finger, with the middle finger stabilizing the writing utensil and the ring and little fingers stabilizing and maintaining the wrist angle.

The child must be able to hold the finger joints steady when writing. OT practitioners examine how much control the child has in keeping the fingers in position. The child who cannot stabilize the joints will have difficulty with fine motor movements. A variety of activities that increase finger strength and finger joint stability are available.

CLINICAL *Pearl*

Because children flex forward slightly while writing, those with poor trunk control may benefit from sitting at an angle of less than 90 degrees.

the floor, and the ankles at 90 degrees. The desk should be at a height of two inches above the flexed elbow.[1]

Children must be able to hold the shoulder steady to use the wrist and fingers for writing. Sometimes children retract or "fix" the shoulders to keep them steady. This makes it difficult to write effectively. The term *wrist stability* refers to the ability of the child to keep the wrist in one position. Wrist stability is important for the child to perform precise hand skills and to move the fingers more efficiently. The wrist should be straight or slightly extended while writing. Using a vertical surface rather than a horizontal one promotes the development of wrist extension and strengthens the arm and shoulder muscles.[22] For example, try to grasp a hammer with a flexed wrist. The hammer cannot be securely held or controlled because the hand is not in a power-grasping pattern. In a slightly extended posture, the wrist stabilizes the hand while using a tool.

Strength and Endurance

Hand strength and endurance are necessary for performing the complex tasks of writing. The arches of the hand are formed as the hand muscles develop. These muscles shape the hand for grasping objects of different sizes, enable skilled movements of the fingers, and control the power and force of prehension. This force is modulated to pick up fragile items, for example, a pencil, without breaking them. Children with poorly developed hand arches have flat, underdeveloped, weak hands. The lack of hand arching interferes with the strength and development of the hand because the intrinsic muscles are not adequately developed. When the arches are well developed, the hand is able to form a bowl in the palm, and distinct creases are seen in the palm. Children with poorly developed arches may compensate by holding the pencil tightly against the palm, showing no web space.

Hand strength that is adequate to hold objects and endurance to repeat motor patterns without fatiguing are important for writing tasks. The process of writing is a continuous one. Therefore, promoting optimal muscle strength and endurance for the task is an essential intervention for improving handwriting (Figure 21-6).

CLINICAL *Pearl*

To work at a table with a writing tool, the child's posture must be prepared and ready to work. Abnormal muscle tone interferes with body symmetry and positioning. Low muscle tone and tremors may interfere with writing.

INTERVENTION USING A BIOMECHANICAL FRAME OF REFERENCE

Children with ROM limitations, poor hand strength, and poor endurance benefit from OT with a biomechanical approach. The following is an example of an intervention session to increase handwriting skills by using a biomechanical approach: The OT practitioner performs a general ROM and manual muscle assessment. In addition, the length of time the child is able to perform handwriting tasks without fatiguing is determined. The OT practitioner examines the child's posture and makes the necessary adaptations to seating so that the child can sit in an upright position for writing. Next, the OT practitioner addresses the ROM limitations through

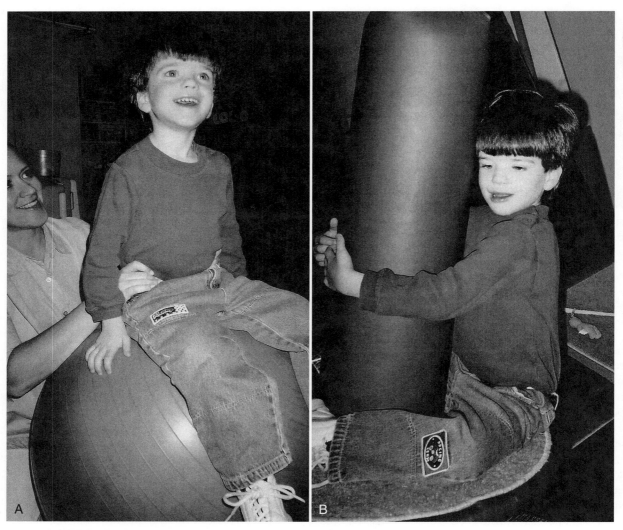

FIGURE 21-6   A, A ball makes the body ready for the occupational performance of sitting and writing. **B,** Being swung on a suspended piece of equipment provides vestibular stimulation to the child to promote muscle tone.

gentle stretching techniques, splinting, or serial casting if necessary. The session begins with warm-up and strengthening activities and ends with a "cool-down" period consisting of functional writing. Strengthening activities are designed to be fun for the child (see the following intervention activities) and are graded to challenge him or her. The OT practitioner works with the child to improve writing endurance by increasing the time for writing and decreasing the breaks.

Motor Activities

- Have the child lie on the stomach to strengthen the back and upper trunk. Mike has low muscle tone in the trunk. He also has very poor ability to sustain trunk and neck extension. Exercising on a ball in the prone position optimizes body alignment and trunk extension. Facilitated handling to provide support to the elbows and co-contraction to the shoulders strengthens Mike's upper trunk and shoulders (see Figure 21-5).

- Play with the child while the child is bouncing on a ball to provide vestibular stimulation and joint proprioception, increase muscle tone throughout, and make the body ready for the occupational performance of sitting and writing (see Figure 21-6, A)

- Swing the child on a suspended piece of equipment to provide vestibular stimulation and promote muscle tone. Playing on a bolster swing encourages Mike to hold on tight, strengthening his upper trunk and shoulder muscles (see Figure 21-6, B). Mike loves swinging, which makes it an excellent tool to start the session and a wonderful reinforcement when he has completed working.

- While providing gentle hand-over-hand assistance, have the child pick up items to promote a thumb–index finger grasping pattern and flexing of the ring and little fingers. Provide hand-over-hand assistance to place the pencil in the optimal, most dynamic position in the child's hand.

- Have the child pinch a zip-lock bag with the thumb and fingertips to promote finger strength and fingertip control. Put desired therapeutic items in these bags to promote opening and closing with each task.

- Have the child crumple and throw away waste paper. This activity works on hand movements and coordination.

- Programs to promote handwriting readiness are commercially available (e.g., Diana Henry's *Tool Chest: For Teachers, Parent's, Students, and Teens* provides activities to promote a child's sensory needs and alertness in the classroom, and Brain Gym provides techniques that encourage movement and the integration of both sides of the body and crossing the midline.[6,10])

- Use thread pegs or string beads on small eyehooks to encourage thumb and index finger prehension. Attaching the pegboard to the wall and vertically orienting it promote grasping and upper trunk strengthening (Figure 21-7).

- Arm strengthening and prone activities decrease arm tremors. Use wrist weights of varying heaviness, and remove them when writing is finished to prevent accommodation. These can also be made with fishing weights sewn onto neoprene. Another option is to glue magnets onto a wristband and place paper on a metal sheet (e.g., cookie sheet) to stabilize the wrist or use a commercially weighted pencil. (Commercially weighted pencils may, however, be too large and often difficult for children to grasp.)

- A pencil gripper or a small pencil encourages a tripod grasp.[15] Large bulb-shaped grippers facilitate open web space. This may also be accomplished by wrapping a rubber band around the pencil at the grip site.[5] Many classrooms have a common pencil basket and the individual child does not have his or her own storage place. Providing a bag that attaches to the back of the child's chair often helps with organization and keeping track of purchased pencil grippers.

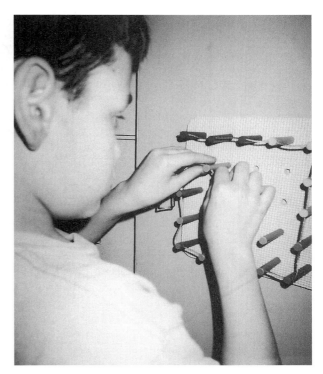

FIGURE 21-7 Grasping and upper trunk strengthening is promoted with the use of a pegboard.

- Have the child pinch the top of a medium-sized jack and with a snapping or twisting motion make the jack spin all over the table. See how many jacks the student can get spinning at one time.
- Loop a soft hair band over the eraser end of the pencil and over the student's wrist. This will pull the pencil back into the web space of the hand for easier control of the utensil.

SENSORY PROCESSING AND INTERVENTION
Midline Crossing

CASE *Study*

Melissa, a 5-year-old kindergartner, is right handed. When writing her name, she switches the pencil to the left hand when she gets to the first "s" in her name. She finishes writing her name and then switches the pencil back to her right hand. This is an example of not being able to cross the midline. Another example is using only the right hand to retrieve puzzle pieces on the right and the left hand to retrieve the pieces on the left.

A student should be able to smoothly cross the midline when writing. By definition, **midline crossing** is the ability to continue a motor act (e.g., writing) without switching hands at the point in front of a person's middle.[21] The inability to do so may be an indicator of an immature nervous system. Switching hands at the middle of the paper (hand dominance not established) instead of writing across the paper or moving the paper to the dominant side may indicate difficulty with midline crossing. OT practitioners must determine if the child is ambidextrous or is unable to cross the midline. A child who is ambidextrous is able to write efficiently with either hand and demonstrate the ability to cross the midline when writing.

Eye–Hand Coordination

The term *eye–hand coordination* (also called *hand–eye coordination*) refers to the control of eye movement coordinated with the control of hand movement, the processing of visual input to guide reaching and grasping, and the use of proprioception of the hands to guide the eyes. Children with poor handwriting skills score lower on eye–hand coordination tasks than those with adequate handwriting skills.[3] Examples of poor eye–hand coordination include the inability to pick up an object from a table or the inability to hit a ball with a bat or tennis racket. In terms of handwriting, a student with poor eye–hand coordination has difficulty staying within the lines when coloring or working on a maze.

Visual Perception Skills

Visual perception is not the same as visual acuity. While a student may *see* a sentence with 20/20 vision, his brain may not *interpret* it accurately. *Visual perception* refers to the way the child makes sense of the visual input. Signs and symptoms of poor visual perceptual skills may include the following:

- May have reversals (*b* for *d*, *p* for *q*) or inversions (*u* for *n*, *w* for *m*)
- Complains that eyes hurt and itch; rubs eyes; complains that print blurs while reading
- Has difficulty navigating the school campus
- Turns the head when reading across the page; holds the sheet of paper at odd angles
- Closes one eye while working; may yawn while reading
- Cannot copy accurately
- Loses the place on a page frequently
- Does not recognize an object or word if only part of it is shown
- Holds the pencil too tightly; often breaks the pencil point or the crayon
- Struggles to cut or paste
- Misaligns letters; may have messy papers, which can include letters colliding, irregular spacing, letters not on line

Children who have difficulty learning letters or recognizing words may have difficulty understanding the relationships between letters and words. In order to write, children need to recognize and perceive the letter forms and understand their differences and similarities. Children who do not perform well on visual perception tests in the areas of visual memory and visual-motor integration typically have poor handwriting skills.[20]

Directionality

The term *directionality* refers to the way print is tracked during reading and writing. Children must know to begin at the top of the page and work toward the bottom and to start on the left-hand side and move to the right. Directionality, or the understanding of which way to go or move the pencil, is essential for writing because writing is performed left to right and top to bottom, with some letters placed on the line and some under the line. Forming letters in the correct direction or sequence, orienting them on the page, and starting or stopping letters at the right location are essential for writing.

CASE *Study*

Johnny, a Grade 3 student, continues to start all the letters of his name from the bottom of the line. In addition, he strokes the letter "o" to the right versus to the left and tends to retrace the majority of his letters. He has been referred to the school OT for handwriting remediation. It is important that letters be formed in the correct manner and direction, as it will impact cursive writing later.

Motor Planning

Children with poor handwriting skills may have deficits in **motor planning** (i.e., figuring out how to move their bodies and then actually doing it) or motor memory (i.e., remembering the motor patterns and being able to repeat them).

Motor planning problems may be due to poor proprioception (poor awareness of muscle and joint positions). Children with motor planning difficulties are unable to maneuver around their school environment without bumping into other people or knocking things down. For example, when walking in line and when the line stops, the child unintentionally runs into the back of another student in front or is constantly feeling the walls. Feeling the walls is a means of information for the child about his or her position in space (close to the wall). If the child did not feel the wall, he or she may very well keep bumping into it and sometimes even fall. If even walking down the hall in a smooth, coordinated manner is difficult, then doing a refined task such as moving a pencil over a piece of paper and creating letters could be daunting. Smooth writing requires the ability to motor-plan on a much smaller scale and requires the separation and isolation of finger movements for dynamic grasping patterns.

A well-organized proprioceptive system provides an unconscious awareness of where the body is in space. It helps the child understand the touch and movement that he or she is experiencing. Therefore, difficulties with proprioception include not knowing where one's arms or hands are positioned in space with the eyes open or closed, finger identification, and finger isolation. Children with poor proprioceptive abilities do not "feel" the pressure they need to put on the pencil to hold it (so they may squeeze it tightly or hold it too loosely). In this instance, they may bear down too hard and write too darkly or not apply enough pressure and write too lightly. These children may need to visually monitor or observe where their hands are positioned on the paper.

The tactile system plays a key role in writing. This important skill requires the ability to feel the pencil and manipulate it without the aid of vision. Some children with handwriting deficits do not feel objects adequately. To fully understand this, try writing while wearing mittens. The lack of tactile sensation interferes with the ability to manipulate the pencil. To feel the pencil, the child with a poor tactile system may have to hold it more tightly, which interferes with refined movements and results in messy writing.

INTERVENTION USING A SENSORY APPROACH

Children are surrounded by different types of sensory information all day long. Most children take this information in, process it, and respond or act upon it by completing tasks. Other children may have difficulty doing this. They may become overloaded with the amount of sensory information and shut down, or they may actually require even more sensory information in order to complete an activity. Using a combination of tactile, visual, and auditory stimulation when teaching handwriting tasks helps children remember activities. Some children may benefit from a sensory integration approach to remediate their handwriting difficulties, while others require sensory activities. OT practitioners evaluate the sensory needs of children with the understanding that the inability to process sensory input may interfere with learning. Movement activities are helpful in stimulating tactile, proprioceptive, and vestibular processing and may help children perform in a variety of occupations (see Figures 21-6, *A*, and 21-6, *B*).

The following is a sample session in which a sensory integrative frame of reference is used to address handwriting abilities: The OT practitioner sets up the clinical environment in such a way that the child is able to choose activities that will help him or her modulate the senses (e.g., vestibular and movement activities) and prepare for postural control. This could include fast-moving vestibular activities such as swinging in a net or tire swing and wheelbarrow races. Once the child is ready, the OT practitioner engages in a variety of activities to improve the child's motor-planning abilities (e.g., obstacle course, climbing a rope swing). Next, the child is engaged in activities to promote hand strength, coordination, and tactile discrimination. Finally, he or she participates in writing tasks. The OT practitioner provides the child with opportunities for success throughout. (See Chapter 24 for a more detailed explanation of sensory integration intervention.)

Some handwriting sessions focus on the sensory aspects. In this case, the session may include preparatory tactile activity such as games in which the child has to find objects hidden in rice, water, or sand. These activities may be followed by in-hand manipulation activities using tactile media such as Play-Doh or Theraputty. The child may use a brushing technique to desensitize the hand. Other sensory activities may include participating in finger painting or writing over sandpaper for proprioceptive input. The Brain Gym program may provide activities to enhance the child's handwriting through sensory experiences. Finally, the child participates in handwriting activities.

Sensory Motor Activities

- Have the child play common children's games such as hopscotch or Simon Says for coordination and leisure. These may need to be done at a slower pace and rhythmically so that the child is able to perform the movement.
- Have the child squat on the floor to pick up small objects and place them in a container that has a small opening. This is an excellent activity for sorting objects, and the squatting will strengthen the trunk and lower extremities and also challenge motor planning.
- Create an obstacle course using classroom furniture. The child will learn important directional language skills such as in/out, over/under, and top/bottom.
- Give the child a job or task in the classroom, such as handing out papers. Let him or her figure out how to accomplish it with minimum prompting.
- Have the child imitate body movements in a mirror image. Vary the difficulty by going faster or slower or having the child perform the exact body movements while you both face each other.
- Have the child imitate isolated finger patterns in different spatial orientations. Do the finger movements above the head to eliminate visual input. To make the finger patterns easier, doing them to a song or rhythmic chant (e.g., singing the ABCs) is often helpful to make more automatic movements later.
- Have the child trace the letters that have been drawn with a marker and highlighted with dried glue.
- Have the child do the following: Write or draw on a vertical surface with different media, such as shaving cream or pudding; write letters or designs in zip lock bags filled with hair gel; form letters on a tray in water mixed with cornstarch. Change the standard writing tool or surface by using magic markers, slanted writing surfaces, or vibrating pens.
- Have the child practice writing using handwriting sheets or commercially available programs to facilitate fluid and automatic movements. Provide hand-over-hand assistance to promote directionality and correct letter configuration.

Visual Perception Intervention Activities

- Use worksheets and perceptual motor booklets that are commercially produced to promote proprioception, figure ground, and eye–hand coordination.
- Reproduce designs with variations so that the child can learn that a circle is a circle even when it is small or in different locations on the page.
- Use a chalkboard to encourage free movement patterns with resistance, and then allow a transition from the chalkboard (i.e., vertical surface) to paper.
- Have the child trace on a line or a drawing of a roadway with a toy car. This promotes directionality and eye–hand coordination. A hand-made mat that is easily transportable can be used to represent a roadway (Figure 21-8).
- Copy forms and designs (e.g., parquetry, block, pick-up-stick, and pegboard designs) to enhance form perception, matching, and figure completion.
- Construct simple puzzles obtained from pictures, which the child can glue on sturdy paper and then cut apart, or use a prepackaged puzzle. Locating the puzzle pieces on the table is a visual targeting task as well as a figure ground perceptual skill.
- Illustrate stories using crayons, chalk, a felt board, or finger puppets.
- Have the child draw a picture, label the items, and write a sentence about the picture.
- Have the child create a book about an event or a family member, or even write a play about his or her day.
- Use the Box and Dot 7 program, which encourages the child to form letters of the same size and place

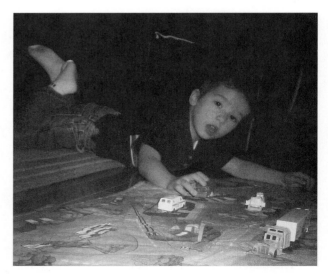

FIGURE 21-8 Tracing encourages directionality and eye–hand coordination.

the letters inside the box. The program is also helpful if a child reverses letters or needs an idea to establish a starting place for them.

CONSIDERATIONS FOR HANDWRITING INTERVENTION

Learning Styles

Children learn using various senses and learning styles. Consideration of the child's learning style is helpful in designing interventions and classroom strategies. Some children are tactile or kinesthetic learners, that is, they need to physically feel and act out the task to remember the sequence. These children learn or perform a task better when they are allowed to stand while writing or when given the opportunity to move the body through the act. Using proprioceptive input—such as practicing and feeling the letter formation in the air with or without hand-over-hand assistance for additional tactile sensation of the letter shape—supports their learning. They frequently respond well to physical rewards such as a pat on the back or being sent on errands to the school office.

Children who learn through auditory means write better if they hear or verbalize the letters or words while putting them on paper. These children may talk to themselves while writing, saying the letters and verbally describing the letter formation as they write. Using fun "sayings" for letter formations are also helpful in learning how to stroke a letter. For example, when writing the capital letter "B," the OT practitioner would say: "Big line down. Frog jump up. Now, little curve, and another little curve."

Visual learners rely on visual prompts to replicate shapes, letters, and words. Visual prompts can be something as simple as a dot to remind them where a letter starts or the drawing of a line or box to show where to set/place their letters; or it can be as involved as writing out the letter or word or drawing shapes for the student to trace. Using a variety of bright, neon marker colors is helpful in visually presenting and separating a handwriting task into its components. For example, if you want Buster to trace his name on a line, write his name in neon orange, with a neon green dot to represent the starting point of each letter. However, make the line on which he is to trace his name neon pink. This provides him with all the visual prompts he needs to succeed in the task; yet, it also breaks the activity up into line orientation, starting points for correct letter formation, and visual presentation of his name so that he can remember what the letters look like and how to correctly spell his name. When paired with auditory "sayings" of how to form the letters, Buster gets a sensory-rich explanation of how his name is formed. As Buster becomes more

independent in the writing of his first name, decrease the amount of visual prompts you provide.

> **CLINICAL** *Pearl*
>
> Children have preferred learning styles. For example, visual learners need to see examples, auditory learners need to hear the steps of the process, and kinesthetic learners need to feel and act out the steps of the process.

Organizational Skills

Having a neat and organized workstation is helpful to all students, especially to those with handwriting difficulties.

Improper placement and orientation of the letters on the line or improper spacing between words may indicate organizational difficulties. Children with poor organizational skills may use letters of varying sizes and wrongly mix uppercase (capital) and lowercase (small) letters in words. Some organizational problems are related to poor visual processing, while others are related to poor motor planning or attention. OT practitioners can help determine the root of the organizational problem. For example, visually figuring out how far apart letters should be placed is a perceptual skill, and moving the fingers to create a letter or form letters counterclockwise requires motor planning. Organization can be taught with frequent reminders and follow-up. Simple systems that the child initiates or helps design are effective.

> **CASE** *Study*
>
> Jerome cannot find anything in or on his desk. As a result, he spends too much time looking for papers, folders, or books and misses the lessons. Jerome turns in homework late or loses it in his desk. His papers are torn and wrinkled, which causes his getting lower grades. The teacher is sometimes unable to make sense of his writing. When he writes, Jerome does not know where to start on the paper or does not move to the next line, leading to the letters running together or being superimposed.

Organizational Intervention

- Help the child keep desk clean and organized so that only the important papers are kept.
- Have the child use folders of different colors for different subjects and cover the textbooks with paper or material of the same color.

- Verbally cue the student; remind the teacher to encourage the student to clear off the writing surface before starting handwriting assignments.
- Make a bag that can be hung on the back of the classroom chair in order to store pencils, scissors, and paper and thus make them readily available.
- Highlight the starting and stopping locations on the paper with dots or stickers, or highlight the lines on the paper.
- Work with the child, the parents, and the teachers to develop strategies.
- Have the child keep two sets of books (one at home and one in school) so that he or she does not have to remember to bring them.
- Have the child use a planner to record assignments, and have the teacher check to make sure that every item is correct.
- Ask the teacher to list homework assignments online (so that parents may follow up).
- Provide consequences for late work and bonuses for work on time.

Classroom Accommodations

OT practitioners may help students and teachers by providing classroom accommodations and strategies to encourage success in the classroom. Accommodations or strategies assist with the completion of writing assignments. Repetitive rote writing of words or multiplication tables does not improve the child's knowledge of the information, nor does it improve the handwriting. Children who fatigue easily may not pay attention to or learn from long writing assignments. Writing repetitively may also reinforce inappropriate letter formations. Accommodations that are appropriate for the individual child should be written on the individualized education program (IEP) or the 504 plan (See Chapter 4: Educational System) to be followed in the classroom.

Strategies for the Classroom

- Decrease the amount of written work expected, and reduce redundant written assignments (e.g., completion of 50% of the required work).
- Encourage a buddy system to help with journal keeping or other written assignments . The child can dictate the story to a peer with adequate handwriting, who can write down the story, and the child can then rewrite the story.
- Have the child use a tape recorder so that the child can dictate a story or tape the teacher's lecture.
- Allow preferential seating and optimal positioning of the student in the classroom. Some children need midline positioning because of decreased visual scanning from one side to the other or one-sided neglect. In addition, auditory learners and easily distracted students frequently need to sit close to the teacher so that they can be more attentive.
- Recommend a word processor as a supplemental aid to facilitate written expression. Be careful not to state the name of a specific computer or machine on the child's IEP because if it breaks suddenly or another one is tried, a new IEP would need to be developed immediately to document the change.
- A written list of homework assignments and a checklist of each book or folder that needs to go home can be provided to the child.
- Delegate a packing buddy to help the child pack up at the end of the day to make sure that all of the necessary papers and books are put in the bag.
- Allow the child more time to complete written assignments, or use an outline format for them.
- Grade and emphasize the content of assignments of written expression; separate the grade from the mechanics of writing.
- Modify testing procedures to maximize student learning (e.g., children with writing difficulties may score poorly on written spelling tests due to poor handwriting, so conduct oral spelling tests for them).

Left-Handed Writers

Children who are left handed may require special accommodations for writing. Writing in a notebook is more difficult for left-handed children because of the placement of the spirals or rings. When writing with the left hand, they find it difficult to see what they have just written because the left hand covers the writing.[2] Left-handed children place their notebooks at a right angle and hook the left wrist in an awkward posture because that is how they were taught to angle the paper (Figure 21-9). In the sitting posture, the body is frequently twisted to accommodate the angle of the paper. The left-handed writer tends to push the pencil rather than pull it from left to right.

Intervention for the Left-Handed

- Group left-handed children together or at the end of the row so that their hands do not hit the hands of right-handed writers.
- Develop left-to-right directionality. Do exercises on the blackboard to encourage full arm movements, and discourage excessive loops and flourishes in writing.

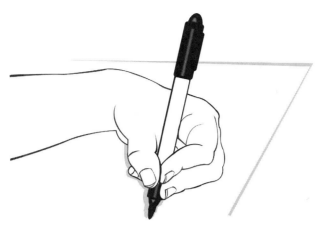

FIGURE 21-9 Left-handed writing is often awkward.

- Teach vertical writing. Do not insist on a right slant. Left-handed children should be allowed to write with a left-handed slant and with the paper at the midline and angled in the same direction as the forearm.
- Have the child cross the letter "t" from right to left so that the child is pulling the stroke toward the hand.

COMPENSATORY STRATEGIES
Keyboarding

In some circumstances, even after intervention, a student's writing may not be proficient enough to support his or her studies and communication. In such cases, other strategies and compensatory intervention models, such as using a computer (i.e., **keyboarding**) to support writing are considered.[21] A word processor is an accommodation or supplemental aid in the classroom for the child with handwriting difficulties. A student could write out his or her rough draft, or "sloppy copy," and then type the final draft. If the child is using a word processor, it should be presented to the child as early as possible in his or her educational career. The early provision of a word processor does not allow the handwriting difficulties to interfere with written expression skills. The keyboard would improve legibility and reduce spelling errors in written assignments.[8] Many school districts have computer keyboarding skills included in their curriculum; OT practitioners should review what is recommended. Box 21-4 shows the progression of keyboarding development recommended for schools in North Carolina.

Keyboarding requires memorization of where the keys are on the keyboard and how to access the keys and documents. On the one hand, to be a touch typist, timing, rhythm, and bilateral coordination are important. On the other hand, keyboarding does not require spatial organization and directionality as does handwriting.[17]

Few studies have been conducted on the use and benefits of word processors in comparison with teaching handwriting. Before recommending a word processor or a laptop computer, the OT practitioner considers the child's ability to organize his or her work area. Children who are unable to locate their materials may have further difficulty organizing themselves with an additional piece of equipment. The AlphaSmart keyboard may suffice if more than one child uses the computer. A stand-alone computer is beneficial, but computers are frequently located along the wall of the classroom, away from the teacher and classroom peers. Laptops have advantages, but the screen interferes with the visibility of the board or the teacher. The OT practitioner or assistive technology team should evaluate the use of a word processor in the classroom and in other settings.

Computer Keyboard Intervention

- Correct positioning and optimal seating should be provided to the student where the computer is located. Make sure that the screen and keyboard are not too high, the keyboard is aligned at the midline, and the seat is steady.

BOX 21-4

Summation of the North Carolina Keyboarding Curriculum

- Kindergarten: Identify all letters, numbers, and other commonly used keys on the keyboard. Know the parts of the computer and how to operate.
- Grade 1: Be familiar with the home keys. Fingers should reach keys, and correct finger positions should be used while typing spelling words. Explore multimedia, use word processing.
- Grade 2: Locate and use symbol keys such as %, ?, Caps Lock, Shift, and Esc. Collect, sort and display data, use drawing tools, use electronic database to locate information.
- Grade 3: Be familiar with punctuation marks, and practice spelling words and fast written expression. At this time, the child should return the hands to the home key promptly after typing. Explore information technologies, build on word processing, awareness of copyright law.

Adapted from: http://www.ncpublicschools.org/curriculum/computerskills/scos/06kindergarten Accessed July 9, 2010.

- Written instructions about how to use the programs should be placed near the computer so that the staff can refer to it if necessary.
- Have the child look across the room periodically to reduce eye strain; also have the child take breaks for stretching exercises.[19]
- Encourage the student to use the right hand on the right side of the computer keyboard and the left hand on the left side. Placing color-coded stickers on the fingernails can be a visual reminder. Have the child push the shift key with the little finger and the space bar with the thumb.
- A large mat in the QWERTY order rather than in the ABC order can be made for the children to sit on.
- Play keyboard Bingo on laminated copies of the keyboard with Bingo markers. Have the child mark out spelling words on the laminated keyboard.
- Use a commercially available child-sized keyboard with keys that are smaller and closer together.
- Use an AlphaSmart, Dreamwriter, Quickpad, or alternative keyboard, such as Intellikeys or Big Keys, to encourage word processor usage in the classroom. Computer keyboards can be altered with Sticky Keys, Filter Keys, or others from the accessibility options of the computer to meet the student's specific needs.
- The team should decide who is responsible for teaching and monitoring keyboarding skills.
- Recommend an assistive technology evaluation to help identify the best equipment or adaptive devices for the specific needs of the student.

Computer Mouse

Many of the computer programs used in the school computer labs are mouse driven; that is, the mouse controls most of the action. After the child types his or her name and identification number into the computer, the specific computer lesson comes up. Since many of these programs are mouse driven, the child is required to move the mouse and click on the correct answer. One way to evaluate the proficiency of students in preschool and upper elementary school in using a computer mouse is the Test of Mouse Proficiency (TOMP).[12] The TOMP looks at pointing, clicking, dragging, and pursuit tracking with the mouse. Preliminary reliability and validity studies indicate that the TOMP is a reliable and valid measure to see how fast and accurate a child is in using the mouse.[11]

ROLE OF THE OCCUPATIONAL THERAPY ASSISTANT

The OTA and the occupational therapist work together to assess and provide services to children with handwriting deficits. The OT is responsible for interpreting assessment results. The OTA may contribute to the evaluation process by completing a handwriting checklist or a standardized assessment to examine the child's skills. The OTA, under the supervision of the occupational therapist, may also contribute to the evaluation process by working directly with the student to promote motor planning, postural stability, visual–motor integration, grasping patterns, and letter formation for writing. The OTA provides handwriting interventions and may lead handwriting groups. OT practitioners assist children in gaining handwriting skills within the classroom curriculum. The OT practitioner is involved in consultation with caregivers and teachers to provide ideas on remediation and techniques to improve handwriting in the classroom and at home.

SUMMARY

Children's handwriting demonstrates their educational progression. Therefore, handwriting is an important component in children's occupational performance. OT practitioners help children by carefully analyzing the factors that may be interfering with a child's ability to write. These factors may include muscle tone, strength, endurance, posture, integrity of structures, visual perception, and sensory processing. OT practitioners then design appropriate interventions to help children succeed in the classroom.

References

1. Benbow M: Principles and practices of teaching handwriting. In Henderson A, Pehoski C, editors: *Hand function in the child: foundations for remediation*, St. Louis, 1995, Mosby.
2. Boardman C: Reasonable answers to commonly asked handwriting questions—the second in the series. *Occup Ther Forum* 19:14, 1994.
3. Case-Smith J: Effectiveness of school-based occupational therapy intervention on handwriting. *Am J Occup Ther* 56:17, 2002.
4. Chandler B: The power of information: school-based practice survey results. *OT Week* 18:24, 1994.
5. Clark-Wentz J: Improving student's handwriting. *OT Practice* 2:29, 1997.
6. Dennison PE, Dennison G: *Brain gym,* Ventura, CA, 1987, Edu Kinesthetic, Inc.
7. Engel-Yeger B, Nagauker-Yanuv L, Rosenblum S: Handwriting performance, self-reports, and perceived self-efficacy among children with dysgraphia. *Am J Occup Ther* 63: 182–192, 2009.
8. Handley-More D et al: Facilitating written work using computer word processing and word prediction. *Am J Occup Ther* 57:139, 2003.

9. Karlsdottir R, Stefansson T: Problems in developing functional handwriting. *Percept Mot Skills* 94:623–662, 2002.

10. Koziatek SM, Powell NJ: Pencil grips, legibility, and speed of fourth-graders' writing in cursive. *Am J Occup Ther* 57:284, 2003.

11. Lane A, Dennis S: *The test of mouse proficiency (TOMP)*, Brisbane, Australia, 2000, Spectronics.

12. Lane A, Ziviani J: Assessing children's competence in computer interactions: preliminary reliability and validity of the test of motor proficiency. *Occup Ther J Res* 23:18, 2003.

13. Mackay N, McCluskey A, Mayes R: The Log Handwriting Program improved children's writing legibility: a pre-test–post-test study. *Am J Occup Ther* 64:30–36, 2010.

14. Malloy-Miller T, Polatajko H, Anstett B: Handwriting error patterns of children with mild motor difficulties. *Can J Occup Ther* 62:258–267, 1995.

15. McHale K, Cermak S: Fine motor activities in elementary school: preliminary findings and provisional implications for children with fine motor problems. *Am J Occup Ther* 46:898, 1992.

16. Phelps J, Stempel L: *The children's handwriting evaluation scale: a new diagnostic tool*, Dallas, 1984, Texas Scottish Rite Hospital for Crippled Children.

17. Preminger F, Weiss P, Weintraub N: Predicting occupational performance: handwriting versus keyboarding. *Am J Occup Ther* 58:193, 2004.

18. Schneck CM, Henderson A: Descriptive analysis of the developmental progression of grip position for pencil and crayon in nondysfunctional children. *Am J Occup Ther* 44:893, 1990.

19. Strup J: Getting it right. *Adv Occup Ther Pract* 19:47, 2003.

20. Tseng MH, Murray EA: Differences in perceptual-motor measures in children with good and poor handwriting. *Occup Ther J Res* 14:19, 1994.

21. Weintraub N, Grill NG, Weiss PLT: Relationship between handwriting and keyboarding performance among fast and slow adult keyboarders. *Am J Occup Ther* 64:123–132, 2010.

22. Yakimishyn J, Magill-Evans J: Comparisons among tools, surface orientation, and pencil grasp for children 23 months of age. *Am J Occup Ther* 56:564, 2002.

REVIEW *Questions*

1. Name two ways that motor and sensorimotor factors, developmental delays, and visual perception can impede the ability to perform handwriting.

2. How should the wrist and hand be positioned for optimal handwriting performance?

3. How do motor planning difficulties interfere with the child's ability to learn and perform handwriting?

4. Identify two different learning styles, and describe the ways that OT intervention can be adjusted to meet the needs of children with these different learning styles.

5. Outline five different remediation techniques and what the benefits of each strategy are.

6. What are the benefits of using a word processor or computer as an accommodation for a child with handwriting difficulties?

7. How should a left-handed student angle the paper, and what other accommodations can be recommended?

8. In what ways does an OTA work with children to improve their handwriting skills?

SUGGESTED *Activities*

1. Observe the variety of pencil grasps that are used. Find out if a tight, nondynamic style of grasp is painful or fatiguing.
2. Try to write with your body in a variety of positions and postures to understand how an awkward posture greatly affects handwriting performance.
3. Use the movement of your shoulder to write instead of the movement of your hand to understand how smooth writing is very dynamic in nature. Evaluate your pencil grasp and writing method.
4. Perform handwriting with the nondominant hand to understand how difficult directionality and letter formation are for some children.
5. Most adults have one learning style that they prefer but are able to use a blend of different styles. Identify what kind of a learner you are.
6. Name the prewriting strokes in their developmental order.
7. In the classroom, what kind of accommodations would be helpful for you to learn?
8. Observe the grasping patterns of people who write with the left hand. How many left-handed writers angle the paper the same way that right-handed writers do rather than angle the paper in the same direction as the forearm?

CHAPTER 21 APPENDIX

Commercially Available Handwriting Programs

This list provides a brief overview of some commonly used handwriting programs.

1. A Reason for Handwriting
   A Reason For
   700 E Granite
   Siloam Springs, AR 72761
   800-447-4332
   www.areasonfor.com
   This program uses a simplified version of Zaner Bloser's handwriting program and is based on Scripture verses and Christian content. It gives students a practical reason for using their very best handwriting and can be highly motivating.

2. Callirobics
   Laufer
   PO Box 6634
   Charlottesville, VA 22906
   800-769-2891
   www.callirobics.com
   This program consists of exercises that are repetitive, simple writing patterns done to music. Callirobics can be beneficial to students who are auditory rather than visual learners.

3. D'Nealian Handwriting
   Thurber DN
   D'Nealian Handwriting
   1 Jacob Way
   Reading, MA 01867
   www.dnealian.com
   This program is developed to ease the transition from manuscript to cursive writing because most of the manuscript letters are the basic forms of the corresponding cursive letters. These letters are formed with one continuous stroke rather than the "ball and stick" method. In addition, many of the letters have a "monkey tail," so the letters are easily converted to cursive formation. The program can be confusing to children who have directionality and orientation difficulties because they do not know in which direction to put the "monkey tail."

4. First Strokes Multisensory Print Program
   The Handwriting Clinic
   3314 N Central Expressway, Suite A
   Plano, TX 75074
   972-412-4119
   www.firststrokeshandwriting.com
   This program was designed by an occupational therapist and provides a multisensory approach to teaching printing.

5. Getty-Dubay Handwriting
   Continuing Education Press
   Portland State University
   http://www.cep.pdx.edu/
   This program, developed by Barbara Getty and Inga Dubay, is an italicized handwriting program that promotes efficient, simple movements. Exercises to strengthen hand muscles and improve coordination are provided in the book *Write Now: The Comprehensive Guide to Better Handwriting.*

6. GUIDE-write Raised Line Paper
   601 SW 13th Terrace, Suite G
   Pompano Beach, FL 33069
   954-946-5756
   www.guide-write.com
   GUIDE–write provides products such as raised-line letters and raised-line paper that can be helpful when teaching a student to form letters.

7. Handwriting Without Tears
   Jan Olsen, 1990, 2000
   8801 MacArthur Blvd
   Cabin John, MD 20818
   301-263-2700
   www.hwtears.com
   This handwriting program uses a developmental approach toward prewriting through cursive writing. The letters are grouped by difficulty in formation of the letter. In addition, the letters are formed with a simple vertical line rather than a slanted line. In this program, there are only two writing lines, a baseline and a center line, which are visually less confusing for children with visual figure-ground deficits.[10] This program was created by an occupational therapist for her son and is very user-friendly.

CHAPTER 21 APPENDIX—cont'd

Commercially Available Handwriting Programs

8. Loops and Other Groups
   Mary Benbow, 1990, OT Ideas
   124 Morris Turnpike
   Randolph, NJ 07869
   877-768-4332
   www.otideas.com

   This handwriting curriculum is a kinesthetic program that combines cursive connectors with manuscript letters for a more efficient writing style. The letters are taught in groups that share a common movement pattern. These motor and memory cues are used to help the student visualize and verbalize while experiencing the "feel" of the letters. Mary Benbow is an occupational therapist and provides suggestions for handwriting remediation. Her program is very helpful to students in Grades 2 and higher, who have been taught cursive handwriting but have difficulty with letter formation.

9. Palmer Method
   Palmer, A.N. *The Palmer Method of Business Writing.* The A.N. Palmer Company: New York. 1935.
   Embridge, D. 2007. "The Palmer Method: Penmanship and the Tenor of Our Time" in *Southwest Review. Platinum Periodicals:* 92 (3): 327

   This handwriting program has been traditionally used in schools for many years and has been the foundation for handwriting styles. The program begins with the letter "A" and goes through to "Z." It uses a "ball and stick" method, causing the child to lift the pencil as the letters are created. This program is really not used anymore, but teachers tend to teach the "ball and stick" method anyway.

10. Zaner Bloser Handwriting
    2200 W Fifth Ave
    Columbus, OH 43215
    800-421-3018
    www.zaner-bloser.com

    This handwriting program is based on the Palmer method but has simplified the material. This program can be easily purchased by schools and has literature and easy-to-use materials to support the handwriting program.

## 22

Therapeutic Media: Activity With Purpose

NADINE K. HANNER

ANGELA CHINNERS MARSH

RANDI CARLSON NEIDEFFER

CHAPTER *Objectives*

After studying this chapter, the reader will be able to accomplish the following:

- Describe considerations necessary when selecting media
- Describe the role of the occupational therapy assistant in choosing therapeutic media
- Select developmentally appropriate therapeutic media for different age groups
- Describe gradation of therapeutic activities based on client factors and activity demands
- Explain the importance of the impact of context and environment (e.g., cultural, physical, social, personal, temporal, and virtual) conditions when choosing therapeutic media

KEY TERMS

Media

Method

Therapeutic media

Client factors

Context

Grading

Activity demands

Collaboration

Service competency

CHAPTER OUTLINE

Background and Rationale of Therapuetic Media

Selection of Therapeutic Media

OCCUPATION/INTERESTS

GOALS

CLIENT FACTORS AND PERFORMANCE SKILLS

CONTEXTS AND ENVIRONMENTS

GRADING AND ADAPTING

ACTIVITY DEMANDS

Role of the Occupational Therapy Assistant and Occupational Therapist in Selecting Therapeutic Media

Use of Therapuetic Media

Activities

INFANCY: BIRTH THROUGH 18 MONTHS

EARLY CHILDHOOD: 18 MONTHS TO 5 YEARS

MIDDLE CHILDHOOD: 6 YEARS UNTIL ONSET OF PUBERTY

ADOLESCENCE: PUBERTY UNTIL ONSET OF ADULTHOOD

Summary

This chapter serves to introduce the entry-level occupational therapy assistant (OTA) to the definition, background, and application of therapeutic media.

The term **media** (plural of *medium*) is defined as "an intervening substance through which something else is transmitted or carried on. An agency by which something is accomplished, conveyed or transferred."[1] **Method** refers to "a means or manner of procedure, especially a regular and systematic way of accomplishing something."[1]

To further clarify these terms in the context of the OT profession, a purposeful activity is chosen to produce desired outcomes for a client and carried out with the use of selected **therapeutic media**. The media and method are chosen for their therapeutic value and individualized for each client's specific needs.

BACKGROUND AND RATIONALE OF THERAPUETIC MEDIA

In the early days of OT, arts and crafts were the primary therapeutic activities utilized by occupational therapists and OTAs. As social and economic times changed and technology grew rapidly, the repertoire of media used in the OT profession expanded and evolved to meet the changing needs of clients. However, craft activities continue to be used in various practice settings and are of particular value in the treatment of the pediatric population. Children can acquire and practice skills necessary to function in their occupations through the use of crafts as therapeutic media. Furthermore, engagement in crafts is typically an occupation of childhood. This chapter describes the selection and use of traditional and nontraditional therapeutic media as an intervention for children.

SELECTION OF THERAPEUTIC MEDIA

OTAs use clinical reasoning skills when choosing therapeutic media for their clients. Specifically, activities that are meaningful and motivating to clients and address these client's goals are deemed therapeutic. The OTA considers the client's interests, therapy goals, **client factors**, performance skills, performance patterns, and contexts. For example, the OTA considers and respects the beliefs and traditions of the client's culture when planning activities. Gradability of the media as well as activity demands are important aspects to be reviewed before selecting media. Activities carried out in group settings must be easily graded and adapted to meet the "just right" challenge for individual members. The following will help facilitate the thought process necessary in successful media selection for intervention planning and implementation.

CLINICAL *Pearl*

As defined by the *Occupational Therapy Practice Framework, 2nd Edition*, activity demands are "the aspects of an activity, which include the objects and their properties, space, social demands, sequencing or timing, required actions and skills, and required underlying body functions and body structure needed to carry out the activity."[2]

Occupation/Interests

The following questions may help the OT practitioner select meaningful, motivating, and age-appropriate media for children and adolescents.

1. Are the media relevant to the client's age and occupational role (e.g., student, sibling, worker)?
2. Are the media related to the client's current interests and/or hobbies? Can they possibly spark their interest to pursue a new leisure activity (e.g., drawing, computers, photography, needlecraft)?

Goals

The OT practitioner selects activities and media based on the client's goals.

1. What specific goals will be addressed?
2. How will the activity (media and method) facilitate the client's goals?
3. Are these media the best choice to facilitate desired outcomes?

Client Factors and Performance Skills

The goal of OT intervention is to enable the client work toward his or her goals while feeling successful and safe. The OTA analyzes activities in terms of body functions (i.e., mental functions; sensory function and pain; neuromusculoskeletal, cardiovascular, hematologic, immunologic, and respiratory system functions; voice and speech functions; skin and skin-related functions; and structural functions of the body) to design interventions to meet the client's goals. The following questions may be useful in guiding the OT practitioner:

1. What physical requirements (e.g., neuromusculoskeletal and movement-related functions) are needed to complete the activity or use the media (e.g., range of motion [ROM], strength, bilateral integration)?
2. What global or specific mental functions (e.g., level of arousal, motivation, attention, awareness, memory, perception, emotional, experience of self and time)

must the client possess to successfully work with the selected media?

3. What performance skills (e.g., motor and praxis, communication and social skills) are required to successfully complete this activity?
4. What are the safety issues surrounding the use of the media? Does the client possess the safety awareness to handle the media or participate in the activity without risk (e.g., impulsivity, allergies)?
5. What sensory functions are required for the client to participate in the activity or with the media (i.e., vision, hearing, vestibular, taste, smell, proprioceptive, touch functions)?

Contexts and Environments

"The term **context** refers to a variety of interrelated conditions that are within and surrounding the client. Context includes cultural, personal, temporal, virtual, physical and social. The term *environment* refers to the external, physical, and social environments that surround the client and in which the client's daily life occupations occur" (p. 645).[2] OT practitioners consider the clients' contexts when selecting intervention activities. The OT practitioner should consider the following questions with regard to contextual and environmental influence in activity selection:

1. Is the therapeutic activity consistent with the client's cultural, social, and personal background?
2. What social conditions (e.g., expectations of significant others, relationships with systems such as economic and institutional) surround the activity?
3. What are the personal characteristics of the client, and how will these affect activity selection (e.g., age, gender, socioeconomic status, educational status)?
4. Does this activity have any spiritual aspects that must be considered?
5. What are the temporal aspects (e.g., stage of life, time of day, time of year, amount of time needed for the activity) of the activity? How will this influence the selection of media?
6. What are the physical characteristics of the activity? In what environment will it take place (e.g., classroom, home, playground)?

Grading and Adapting

OT practitioners may need to change therapeutic activities to promote success. The following questions may assist the OT practitioner in **grading** (i.e., changing the degree of difficulty of the activity) activities and

adapting (i.e., changing how the activity is performed) activities:

1. Can the level of complexity of the activity be increased or decreased according to the client's thought processing level (e.g., decreasing steps, taught by backward chaining, fading assistance)?
2. Can the provided media be modified, if necessary, for the client's physical skills (e.g., less or more resistance, larger or smaller objects)?
3. Can the media be changed for the client's sensory function requirements (e.g., placing media on bright background to increase contrast for a client with low vision or using a material with a different texture to accommodate a client's tactile needs)?
4. Are the media versatile enough to be individualized within a group activity?
5. Is adaptive equipment needed to enhance the client's performance? Is it available?

Activity Demands

Successful planning of an activity requires the OT practitioner analyze the aspects of the activity. **Activity demands** refers to the objects and their properties, space demands, social demands, sequence and timing, required actions and skills, and required underlying body functions and body structures.[2] Analyses of activity demands help the OT practitioner select appropriate activities and media. The following questions may guide the OT practitioner:

1. Are the tools and equipment necessary to use the media available and in good repair?
2. Are there adequate tools and materials for all of the clients?
3. Is there an adequate working surface, open space, and lighting for the activity?
4. What social and communication skills are needed to participate in the activity?
5. What are the steps, sequence, and timing of the activity? Will there be enough time to complete the activity?
6. What skills are required to successfully complete the activity?
7. What body structures are needed to complete the activity?
8. How can the activity be changed for clients who have deficits?
9. What are the safety precautions?
10. What is the cost of the activity?
11. Where can the activity take place?

ROLE OF THE OCCUPATIONAL THERAPY ASSISTANT AND THE OCCUPATIONAL THERAPIST IN SELECTING THERAPEUTIC MEDIA

Collaboration refers to "working cooperatively with others to achieve a mutual goal."[3] OTAs deliver OT services under the supervision of and in collaboration with occupational therapists. It is the legal and ethical responsibility of both the occupational therapist and the OTA to ensure that the OTA has the established service competency to choose media that are relevant to the client's occupational goals.

CLINICAL *Pearl*

Service competency ensures that one occupational therapist is able to obtain the same results from a procedure or activity as another. Some ways of establishing service competency are videotaping treatment techniques to be critiqued by an experienced occupational therapist and review of standardized test results to ensure correct administration procedures and accurate scoring. Another method is using competency check-offs for skills such as measuring range of motion with the goniometer, manual muscle testing, and safe transfer techniques.

OTAs who do not practice within close proximity to other therapists (such as those working in some school systems or home health care) can establish **service competency** and expand her or his skills by seeking an experienced mentor. Pediatric focus groups provide opportunities to collaborate with other OT practitioners and discuss intervention strategies. Furthermore, OTAs may discover new intervention strategies and use of media by attending professional conferences and continuing education. Commercial companies offer online resources for media projects and supplies which may prove helpful to OT practitioners.

USE OF THERAPUETIC MEDIA

The OT practitioner uses therapeutic media during the intervention process. The media may be used within the context of a purposeful activity; one that directly relates to the client's goals and occupational role or as a *preparatory* activity to address client factors and the underlying skills necessary to achieve the client's goal.

CASE *Study*

Kevin, a 7-year-old boy with juvenile rheumatoid arthritis, is in Grade 2. Kevin enjoys art class but has difficulty painting when his joints are inflamed. He also has difficulty holding the paint brush. The OTA has decided to work on Kevin's goal to improve fine motor skills for academic work by using a painting activity. As a preparatory activity, Kevin and the OTA complete some stretching exercises (both passive and active). The OTA sets up a painting activity, similar to the one that will be conducted in art class later that week. Since Kevin takes longer than the other children to complete his work, the art teacher is very pleased that the OTA is able to break down the steps and allow Kevin to get a head start. Furthermore, this allows the OTA to determine what types of adaptations work best for Kevin. She provides Kevin with a built-up handled paintbrush and an easel positioned close to him and at a lower level (so that he does not have to raise his arm as high as the other children). Kevin enjoys painting and is looking forward to finishing his project in art class later in the week.

In this scenario, painting is the goal (fine motor skills to participate in a school activity) and is also the medium (to work on increasing fine motor skills). The OTA is able to help Kevin achieve a meaningful activity, which is part of his occupational role as a student. The preparatory activity, in this case, is the stretching and exercising prior to beginning the painting. The OTA provides the child with adaptations (built-up paint brush) to ensure success in art class. The child is invested in the painting and motivated to continue the activity in art class later. The OTA recognizes the importance of utilizing media and activities that are occupation based and meaningful to the child.

ACTIVITIES

The following section provides examples of how the OTA chooses meaningful and therapeutic activities. Each scenario provides a client's occupational profile, a description of the chosen media and method, suggestions for grading and adapting the activity, and an overview of the required client factors specific to the case. Tables 22-1 through 22-4 provide commonly used therapeutic media for each age group.

Infancy: Birth Through 18 Months

CASE *Study*

MIGUEL'S WATER PLAY SESSION. Miguel is a 12-month-old boy with a diagnosis of Down syndrome. He receives outpatient occupational and physical therapy services once a week. The

TABLE 22-1

Examples of Activities for Infancy

ACTIVITY	BRIEF DESCRIPTION OF ACTIVITY OR PRODUCT
Handprint wreath	Arrange cut-out or painted handprints in wreath pattern
Body awareness dressing/bathing games	Use lotion, soap, powder, and movements while naming body parts during bathing and dressing.
Bubbles	Adult blows bubbles while cuing infant to visually track, reach, and pop.
Multi-texture mat	Can be purchased or homemade for infant to crawl over, walk on, or explore textures.
Cardboard box play	Push/pull infant across floor for vestibular input.
Hand/foot games	Examples are Peek-A-Boo, Patty Cake, and This Little Piggy.
Scooping/Pouring activities	Use various media: water, sand, dirt, rice.
Pots and pan music	Use various-sized pots, pans, plastic bowls, and wooden spoons.
Commercially available developmental toys	Examples are cause-and-effect, sequencing, push/pull toys, stuffed animals, and texture books. Examples are nesting toys, push lawnmower toy, and See and Say.

TABLE 22-2

Examples of Activities for Early Childhood

ACTIVITY	BRIEF DESCRIPTION OF ACTIVITY OR PRODUCT
Paper bag puppets	Use paper lunch bags. Cut, glue, or color puppet features onto bag.
Marshmallow people	Use pretzel stick to connect marshmallow body parts.
Birdfeeder	Roll pinecone in peanut butter and birdseed.
Sorting games	Use pincer grasp or tweezers/tongs to pick up small manipulatives for sorting.
Tissue paper collage	Have child crumple up with fingers precut squares of tissue paper and place on glue dots within a defined space.
Parachute	Great group activity! Incorporate with songs. Emphasize up, down, around. Toss items on parachute.
Loop cereal or noodle jewelry	String items on curling ribbon, plastic craft lace, pipe cleaners, etc.
Painting	Examples are finger painting, sponge painting
Body movement games	Examples are I'm a Little Teapot; Head and Shoulders, Knees and Toes; and Row, Row, Row Your Boat.
Commercial games/toys	Examples are Don't Spill the Beans, Barrel of Monkeys, Candy Land, Hi Ho Cheerio, Memory, Ants in the Pants, Don't Break the Ice, Mr. Potato Head, Shape Sorter, nesting items, and Counting Bears.

goals for OT include improving Miguel's physical endurance and hand skills for play. During the OT sessions, the OTA works on increasing postural stability for independent sitting as well as improving reaching and grasping skills. This week, the OTA and the physical therapy assistant (PTA) collaborate and plan activities to address Miguel's OT and PT goals in the clinic's pool. The OTA discusses this upcoming session with Miguel's parents who report that he loves to play in the water and that they would like him to develop preswimming skills. Miguel will wear a swimsuit with an attached floatation device for safety while in the pool. To prepare Miguel for the water and increase body awareness, the OTA will rub Miguel's arms, legs, and back with water while naming each body part.

TABLE 22-3

Examples of Activities for Middle Childhood

ACTIVITY	BRIEF DESCRIPTION OF ACTIVITY OR PRODUCT
Paper chains	Have child cut strips of paper or use precut strips and attach them with various means such as paperclip, staples, glue. Vary colors. Consider cultural differences.
Windsocks	Have child roll construction paper to form cylinder and secure with staples or tape; attach crepe paper streamers along bottom edge; punch holes and thread yarn for hanger; and use markers, stickers, etc. to decorate.
Gingerbread house	Buy a ready-made kit, or provide pint-sized milk carton, graham crackers, stiff icing, and candies to decorate.
Sun catchers	Melt crayon shavings between two pieces of wax paper using iron. Have child make a frame out of popsicle sticks, construction paper, etc.
Paper mache piñata	Provide a thin box. Have child dip tissue or newspaper strips into a flour-and-water mixture (consistency of thin white glue), lay them over box in layers, and allow them to dry completely. Adult slits a hole in the box to fill with candy. Child decorates with paint, stickers, etc.
Body movement games	Examples are Red Light/Green Light, Simon Says, Hopscotch, Animal walks, and Twister.
Commercial games/toys	Examples are Bop It, Hungry Hippo, Connect Four, Tidily Winks, Leggos, Mega Links, Uno, Go Fish, Barrel of Monkeys, and Pick-up-Sticks.

TABLE 22-4

Examples of Activities for Adolescence

ACTIVITY	BRIEF DESCRIPTION OF ACTIVITY OR PRODUCT
Origami	Fold paper to form 3-D shapes. May use purchased kits or craft book.
Flowerpot découpage	Cut out pictures in magazines, greeting cards, old books. Have child brush découpage glue on back of picture, apply picture to flowerpot, and apply additional découpage glue covering picture and surface completely until entire area is smooth and uniform.
Picture frame	Have child decorate an old picture frame using various media (seashells, puzzle pieces, twigs, gemstones)
T-shirt painting/tie-dye	Provide various fabric paints, stencils, sponges, or brushes to be used on T-shirt. Buy commercial tie-dye kits, or use instructions available in craft books (see references).
Collage	Have child cut out pictures from magazines or catalogs of interest to him or her and glue them onto poster board and add decorative accents as desired (glitter bows, stickers).
CD mobile	Have child decorate and hang promotional or unwanted CDs from fishing line, coat hanger, drift wood, etc.
Rubbings	Have child rub crayons, charcoal pencils, pastels, etc. on thin paper placed over embossed surfaces (building cornerstones, carved wood, coins).
Commercial games	Examples are Dominoes, Mancala, Pictionary, Jenga, card games, Backgammon, Simon, and Perfection.
Rubber stamping	Have child create cards, gift tags, and stationary by using commercial rubber stamps and stamp pads.

Media/Materials

The media/materials needed are as follows:

- Water
- Kickboard
- Small water toys that require hand skills (e.g., plastic fish, simple squirt toys, etc.)
- Sponge balls
- Beach ball

Method

The method used comprises the following components:

1. Set up the environment with all materials within reach.
2. Miguel is positioned on the edge of the pool with the PTA providing support at his trunk, as necessary, for safety. The OTA, positioned in front of Miguel, holds up pool toys in various planes to facilitate reaching up, down, and across midline. The OTA carefully monitors Miguel's facial expressions for any signs of fear and provides positive feedback while facilitating the "just right" challenge. Once the OTA has ensured his comfort level, she asks him to kick a large ball positioned in front of him.
3. Once Miguel becomes more comfortable, he is positioned prone on the kickboard in the pool, with the PTA facilitating trunk stability in the prone extension position. Miguel is working on head and trunk control in this position and is encouraged to kick through the water to move forward to reach toys placed in front of him. The OTA holds a sponge ball just below the surface of the water for Miguel to grasp and pull toward him. This movement simulates the dog paddle motion, which is needed for swimming. To improve hand strength, the OTA shows him how to squeeze the water out of the ball to sink a small toy boat.

CLINICAL *Pearl*

Working while in the prone position strengthens cervical, trunk, and scapular musculature. Strengthening these muscle groups will increase overall postural stability.

Client Factors
Mental Functions

Miguel's level of arousal was sufficient to follow verbal cues provided by the adults, and he was motivated by his enjoyment of water play.

Neuromusculoskeletal and Movement-Related Functions

Miguel reached in various planes with upper and lower extremities which required stability and mobility of the joints. Although Miguel has low muscle tone, the buoyancy of the water allowed efficient use of his strength and endurance as he moved his arms and legs against the resistance of the water. Miguel needed control of voluntary movement for reaching, grasping, eye–hand coordination, and eye–foot coordination to complete the activity. He also utilized bilateral integration while reaching across the midline for toys.

Skin and Related-Structure Functions

Miguel had skin integrity evidenced by no open wounds or abrasions. This was an important consideration when engaging in water play in a public pool.

Grading and Adapting

Suggestions for grading and adapting are as follows:

- Use a variety of positions and surfaces (e.g., edge of pool for stable surface versus kickboard/raft for unstable surface).
- If a pool is not available, these or similar activities can be carried out using a water table or a bathtub.
- Vary distance and height when presenting objects for reaching and grasping.
- The level of assistance can be increased or decreased according to the client's needs.
- Simulate swimming activities to help prepare children for the occupation of swimming. For example, blowing bubbles, kicking feet, reaching forward, and cupping water are all prerequisite skills for swimming.

The OTA selected water as a motivating medium based on the parent's report of Miguel's enjoyment of water play. Through collaboration, both the OT and PT practitioners were able to safely address Miguel's goals by working in the pool. Furthermore, swimming is an occupation of childhood in which the child and parents were interested.

CASE *Study*

JESSICA'S HANDPRINT/FOOTPRINT BUTTERFLY. Jessica, an 18-month-old child, receives early intervention OT services at her daycare center two times a week. She has a diagnosis of agenesis of the corpus colosum and hypotonia. Jessica's mother would like Jessica to be able to sit independently and tolerate sensory input during bath time. The OTA addresses these aspects of the individualized family service plan (IFSP) by providing controlled sensory input in order to decrease Jessica's tactile sensitivity and by working to improve trunk stability. The OTA and the preschool teacher collaborate and plan a group activity for Mother's Day that

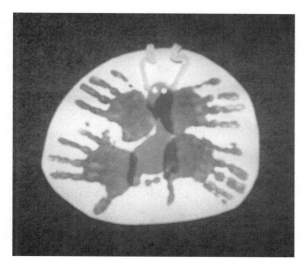

FIGURE 22-1   A butterfly print.

can be adapted to Jessica's needs—a footprint/handprint butterfly (Figure 22-1). As preparatory activities, the OTA brushes Jessica's hands on both sides as well as the soles of her feet with paint. She then facilitates transitional movements to various positions to maximize trunk stability and upper extremity weight bearing.

CLINICAL *Pearl*

Many OT practitioners utilize specific brushing/deep pressure protocols for decreasing tactile sensitivity with the pediatric population. This is a powerful tool and should only be used once training has been completed and service competency established.

Media/Materials

The media/materials needed are as follows:

- Several colors of nontoxic paints in pie tins
- Poster board
- Soft bristle paintbrush
- Pipe cleaner for antennae (preformed)
- Protective covering for floor
- Glue
- Paper towels

Method

The method used comprises the following elements:

1. Set the environment. Cover the floor, place all materials nearby, and position the poster board.
2. Sit on the floor behind Jessica to provide supported sitting.
3. Brush Jessica's foot with paint and press it on the poster board to form the body of the butterfly.

Rotate the paper a half turn, and brush Jessica's hand with paint. Press Jessica's hand onto one side of the body at the top and bottom. Repeat the procedure with the opposite hand to make the other side of the butterfly's body. This forms the wings. Add more paint with the paintbrush, as needed, for detail. Dab Jessica's index finger into the paint, and daub the top of the butterfly's body to form its eyes.
4. After the paint dries, glue on the antennae.

Grading and Adapting

Suggestions for grading and adaptations are as follows:

- Complete in more than one session.
- Provide adapted positioning for external trunk support (e.g., adaptive chair, adult assistance, environmental support).
- Add various media to paint in order to increase tactile input (e.g., sand, uncooked rice, cornmeal).
- Thin paint with water to change tactile input.
- Dip the child's hand into the paint instead of brushing paint onto the palm.
- Apply paint onto the hand with a cotton-ball.
- If tactile input is not tolerated, trace the shape of the child's hand, and have child use paintbrush to fill in the shape. Use hand-over-hand assistance as needed.

Client Factors

Client factors addressed and considered for Jessica during this activity are as follows:

Mental Functions

Jessica needed an appropriate level of arousal in order to participate in the activity. She was motivated by the playful way the activity was presented.

Sensory Functions

Proprioception was required for Jessica to sustain various positions such as the upright sitting position and upper extremity weight-bearing position. Jessica's visual functions were stimulated by the bright colors of the paint, and vestibular functions were necessary for her to sustain balance in upright sitting. Her touch functions were sufficient to accept the sensation of the OTA's hand and the texture of the paint.

Neuromusculoskeletal and Movement-Related Functions

Although Jessica had low muscle tone, she had sufficient strength and endurance to sustain the upright sitting position and the transitions to various postures with assistance.

Righting reactions were required to re-establish the midline after her painted palm was placed onto the surface of the paper. With minimal assistance, Jessica was able to initiate voluntary movement of her hands and fingers to press her painted palms onto the paper.

The OTA chose the activity based on Jessica's IFSP goals and integrated it into the classroom. Making Mother's Day projects is an important occupation for children of all ages. By considering the demands of the activity, the OTA was able to work on the IFSP goals, namely, trunk stability and decreasing tactile sensitivity, while working in the least restrictive environment. See Table 22-1 for other commonly used therapeutic media for infants.

Early Childhood: 18 Months to 5 Years

CASE *Study*

PUDDING PAINTING. Allie is a 36-month-old child with a diagnosis of autism. She receives OT services from a home health agency twice a week. OT interventions focus on improving self-feeding, manipulating objects with hands for play and dressing (fine motor skills), and improving visual motor skills through imitation of age-appropriate prewriting strokes. Allie demonstrates oral sensitivity. Allie's mother requested activities that she can do easily with her at home during play. The OTA will model a pudding painting activity that the mother can do with Allie. As a preparatory activity, Allie will squeeze and manipulate Play-Doh to prepare her for the tactile input of the pudding as well as to facilitate hand strengthening and digit isolation.

Media/Materials

The media/materials needed are as follows:

- One snack-size pudding cup (choose a flavor and color that the child will like)
- Flat surface such as a cookie sheet or paper plate
- Large pullover shirt that can get messy
- Spoon
- Napkin

Method

The method used comprises the following elements:

1. Set the environment. Since this activity is messy, cover the work surface, and gather all the materials.
2. Allie dons pullover shirt with help as needed.
3. With Allie, open the pudding cup. Allie scoops pudding onto cookie sheet with assistance to sustain grasp or reposition as needed. She spreads the pudding with her hand.

4. Assist Allie in establishing index finger isolation, and provide occasional assistance as needed during the activity. Allie imitates prewriting strokes in pudding (i.e., vertical line, horizontal line, circle, and cross) as demonstrated.
5. Once the prewriting activity is over and cleaned up, Allie's mother gives her a new pudding cup. With assistance, Allie eats the pudding with a spoon as a snack.

Client Factors
Mental Functions

On a global level, Allie was motivated by the new experience of completing prewriting strokes in the pudding. She showed an interest in the new activity. Allie turned when her name was called throughout the activity, showing orientation to person. Specifically, Allie needed sustained attention for 3-minute periods to complete both the visual motor and self-feeding tasks. Spatial perceptual skills were used throughout the prewriting activity to imitate the strokes.

Sensory Functions

Allie engaged in vestibular functions to sustain dynamic sitting balance while reaching to complete prewriting strokes. Proprioception was necessary to manipulate the pudding, to reach, and to move fingers through the pudding. Touch functions were required as Allie accepted the texture of the pudding both through her fingertips and in her mouth while eating the pudding.

Neuromusculoskeletal and Movement-Related Functions

Functional ROM of the upper extremity bones and joints was sufficient to don the pullover shirt. Allie needed control of voluntary movement, specifically eye–hand coordination for both the fine motor and self-care components.

Grading and Adapting

Suggestions for grading and adapting the activity are as follows:

- Use thicker/thinner food textures to change resistance.
- Use items such as pretzel sticks, carrot sticks, marshmallows, or similar items for the child to write with if he or she is tactile defensive.
- Increase/decrease difficulty by having the child imitate, copy, or write from memory.
- Use adaptive equipment such as a scoop bowl or adaptive spoon to increase independence with self-feeding.

- Use nonfood items to practice prewriting and writing skills (shaving cream, sand, lotion, fingerpaint).
- Vary the working positions (e.g., supported sitting, prone on floor, standing, etc.).

After the session is over, the OTA and the mother discussed the process and outcome of the activity. The OTA suggested similar activities using different food items and other prewriting activities so that the mother could participate fully in reaching Allie's goals.

CASE *Study*

CLOTHESPIN CATERPILLAR MAGNETS. Carrie is a 4-year-old child who attends a child development class in a public elementary school. This class includes children with and without special needs. She receives weekly OT services from the school-based OTA in this setting to support her educational goals in her individualized education program (IEP) (see Chapter 4). The goals of OT services include addressing difficulty with fine motor, visual perception, and sensory processing. The class thematic unit this week is "Insects." The OTA plans to have the children make clothespin caterpillar magnets. As a preparatory activity, the children participate in a music and movement group. In addition, Carrie will string large beads onto a pipe cleaner as a fine motor warm-up and search for small plastic items hidden in a rice bowl to decrease tactile sensitivity.

CLINICAL *Pearl*

Preparatory activities can be thought of as warm-up techniques to prepare the client for a specific desired action. Activities such as gross motor movements can increase motor planning for tasks such as handwriting. Hand musculature may be developed by upper extremity weight bearing that occurs during activities such as crawling through a tunnel. Similarly, bead stringing can be used to facilitate the pincer grasp needed to hold a pencil for writing.

Media/Materials
Each child will need the following:

- One standard-size wooden clothespin
- Craft glue or wood glue
- Six multicolored pompoms (about half inch)
- One chenille stick (pipe-cleaner) about four inches long
- Two small wiggle eyes

- A two-inch piece of magnet with adhesive backing
- Cotton swabs
- Small dish or paper plate
- Tweezers

Method
The method used comprises the following elements:

1. Set the environment. Make sure that the table and chair are the appropriate height. Have all the materials on the table within reach.

CLINICAL *Pearl*

Provide adequate supervision at all times when using small materials to ensure the safety of children. Many children have poor impulse control and safety awareness and may use materials inappropriately.

2. Follow the simple color pattern of a completed caterpillar model.
3. Carrie squeezes glue from the bottle onto a small dish, with assistance as needed.
4. Using a cotton swab to dip into the glue, Carrie spreads the glue onto one side of the clothespin. As tolerated, the child uses index finger to spread the glue evenly.
5. Following the model for color pattern, Carrie picks out the needed pompoms from a large assortment.
6. Carrie uses tweezers to pick up and place pompoms onto glue following the color pattern.
7. Carrie uses a cotton swab to apply two drops of glue to the caterpillar's head (first pompom) for the eyes and places two wiggle eyes onto the drops of glue.
8. With assistance, Carrie twists the pipe cleaner around the side of the clothespin, behind the head of the caterpillar, to form the antenna.
9. Carrie peels the adhesive backing from the magnet and places it onto the back of the clothespins, with assistance as needed.

Client Factors
Mental Functions
Spatial perceptual skills were needed to line pompoms on the clothespin as shown in the model. Interpretation of sensory stimuli (tactile) was required whenever Carrie spread the glue with her fingertips. Choosing pompom color and size required recognition and categorization skills to follow the given pattern of the model.

Sensory Functions and Pain

Proprioceptive functions provided feedback necessary for Carrie to sustain adequate pressure when using the tweezers to pick up, move, and place the pompoms without dropping them. Although Carrie's touch functions were hypersensitive, she tolerated a limited amount of input from the glue.

Neuromusculoskeletal and Movement-Related Functions

Control of voluntary movement functions were needed during aspects of the activity that required eye–hand coordination to place pompoms matching the given pattern.

Grading and Adapting

Suggestions for grading and adapting the activity are as follows:

- Use larger/smaller clothespins and pompoms.
- When decreased fine motor skills are present, use tongs instead of tweezers.
- Adult uses the glue when the child places pompoms.
- Give more or less assistance depending on child's abilities.
- Instead of twisting the pipe cleaner to make the antenna, the child can glue on a paper antenna.
- Adjust the complexity of the color pattern depending on the child's abilities.
- Adapt the environment. For example, increase or decrease the group size; reduce the amount of materials presented at a time; use a location in the classroom that offers the least visual stimulus.

The OTA conducted this activity in Carrie's least restrictive environment (classroom). By working with the teacher, the OTA was able to design, develop, and implement a therapeutic activity that related both the weekly classroom thematic unit and Carrie's goals. See Table 22-2 for other commonly used therapeutic media for the early childhood age group.

Middle Childhood: 6 Years Until Onset of Puberty

CASE *Study*

BIRTHDAY CROWN. David is a 6-year-old kindergartener with a diagnosis of attention-deficit hyperactivity disorder (ADHD). He has difficulty completing cutting and handwriting tasks, and the teacher notes that he struggles with puzzles and become frustrated easily. David receives school-based OT services once a week to address fine motor and visual perceptual difficulties that interfere with classroom activities. David's teacher has asked the OTA to help David make a "birthday crown" to celebrate his birthday. The OTA is excited to work with David on this activity because it addresses both of David's goal areas. As a preparatory activity, the OTA has David manipulate firm therapy putty to retrieve beads. The OTA also provides an air-filled cushion for David to sit on during this activity, which may help increase his attention.

CLINICAL *Pearl*

Various products are available on the market, such as air-filled cushions and ball chairs, to help clients attend to the tasks by providing them with vestibular input controlled by their movements.

Media/Materials

The media/materials needed are as follows:

- Poster board
- Small items for decoration (stickers, sequins, buttons, etc.)
- Scissors
- Glue
- Cotton swabs
- Stencils (letters and shapes)
- Markers, crayons
- Stapler
- Glitter

Method

The method used comprises the following elements:

1. Set the environment. Make sure that the chair and table are an appropriate height. Have the materials within reach. Reduce the amount of visual and auditory stimuli. Make sure that the lighting is adequate.
2. Draw a crown pattern onto the poster board, and David cuts the pattern.
3. Measure David's head, and mark the crown that he will staple later.
4. David decorates the crown (Figure 22-2). He uses letter stencils to write his name with correct formation, with verbal cues for direction. He practices in-hand manipulation with buttons and sequins that are placed on the crown. David also works on his pincer grasp by using a cotton swab to spread the glue.
5. David staples the crown in the previously marked spot, and he places the crown on his head.
6. David cleans up the area with assistance.

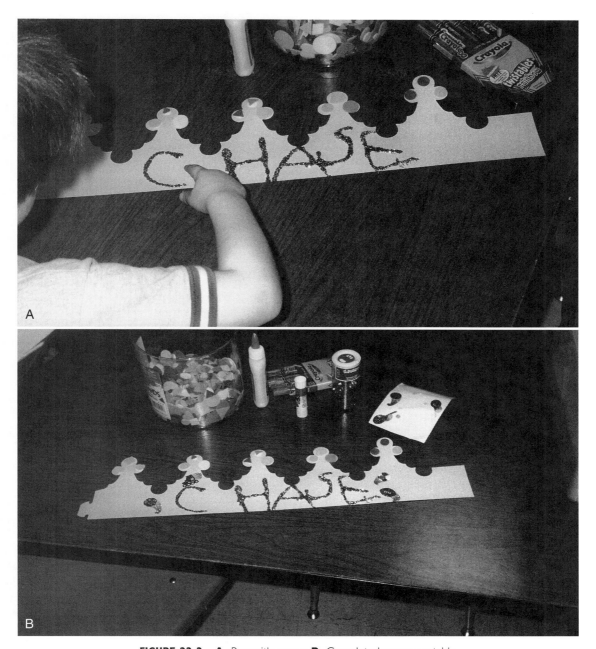

FIGURE 22-2   A, Boy with crown. **B,** Completed crown on table.

Client Factors
Mental Functions
David was motivated to make the crown for his birthday. He, as most children do, valued the celebration of personal holidays. He was able to modulate his level of arousal to carry the task through to its completion. David was able to sustain attention to complete the multistep task with adaptations (e.g., cushion, one-on-one assistance, simple directions). He used perceptual functions to place the stencils neatly in a line and in the correct sequence to write his name. He was able to implement problem-solving skills to identify and correct errors in the project. David had to regulate his emotional functions to control his impulsivity. He experienced a positive sense of self by completing and wearing the crown in celebration of his special day.

Neuromusculoskeletal and Movement-Related Functions

David's muscle tone and strength allowed him to sustain a grasp on the scissors, hold the pencil correctly, and depress the stapler. Control of voluntary movement for bilateral integration and eye–hand coordination allowed David to stabilize the stencil with the non-dominant hand as he wrote with his dominant hand.

Sensory Functions and Pain

Proprioceptive functions were required for David to gradate his movements to use the stapler without tearing the paper. These functions also allowed him to move the scissors forward through the paper in a smooth and controlled fashion.

Grading and Adapting

Suggestions for grading and adapting the activity are as follows:

- Provide a model.
- Have the child use tape rather than a stapler if safety is a concern or if strength is poor.
- Have the child use glue sticks, squeeze glue bottle, or use other items to spread glue (paintbrush, cotton ball).
- Give wider/thinner lines to cut.
- Increase or decrease difficulty of crown pattern for cutting.
- Divide the activity over several intervention sessions depending on the child's attentiveness or needs.

The OTA made the activity meaningful by centering it on David's birthday. She chose preparatory activities that would increase his success in making the birthday crown. The OTA considered David's difficulty attending to tasks and adapted the environment by providing the air-filled cushion.

CASE *Study*

CRISPY RICE CEREAL TREATS. Casey, a 13-year-old with moderate intellectual disability, is a student in a self-contained class at the local middle school. His class often engages in cooking activities to work on their independent living and transitional job training skills. Casey has a short attention span, and the teacher and the OTA have often discussed his inability to carry out multistep tasks to completion. The OTA targets these areas during OT sessions. The class is planning to host a fall luncheon for parents. The students have compiled a shopping list and purchased the ingredients during a community-based outing. The classroom has a full kitchen, and the students will be preparing side dishes for the meal. Casey is making the dessert, a pumpkin-shaped crispy rice cereal treat. After a discussion about the various cultures within the classroom, the teacher and the OTA have decided that it would be most appropriate to make a generic pumpkin motif rather than a jack-o-lantern. The OTA has decided to incorporate the activity within the OT session. She prepares Casey for the activity by carefully reviewing the rules of the session and showing him a sample of the finished product.

Media/Materials

The media/materials needed are as follows:

- 6 cups of crispy rice cereal
- 1 bag of marshmallows
- 2 tablespoons of margarine
- Orange decorative sprinkles
- Raisins, chocolate chips, chocolate-covered candies
- Spearmint gumdrop leaves
- Pretzel sticks
- Large mixing bowl (microwave-safe)
- Large spoon
- Wax paper

Method

The method used comprises the following:

1. Set the environment. Gather all the ingredients, and place the cooking utensils within reach. Casey washes and dries his hands.
2. Casey opens the bag of marshmallows with supervision. He empties the contents into the bowl along with the margarine. He puts the bowl in the microwave for 1 minute; he then stirs the mixture and microwaves it for an additional minute. (Verbal cues may be provided to assist Casey in setting and attending to the microwave timer).
3. Using potholders, Casey removes the bowl from the microwave oven.
4. Casey measures 6 cups of cereal.
5. He then pours the cereal into the bowl and mixes it thoroughly with the melted marshmallow and margarine mixture using a large spoon.
6. Casey washes and dries his hands before handling the food.
7. Demonstrate how to obtain an adequate amount of cereal mixture to form a ball. Have Casey roll the cereal ball in orange sprinkles and place each one on a sheet of wax paper.

8. Casey adds features to the pumpkins using raisins, chocolate chips, and chocolate-covered candies. He pushes a pretzel stick into the top and places spearmint candy leaves on each side to make the stem of a pumpkin.

9. Casey finally washes all the items used in warm soapy water; rinses and dries them; and cleans the countertops.

Client Factors
Mental Functions

Casey was motivated to complete this activity because his parents were going to be guests.

Casey demonstrated 30 minutes of sustained attention with frequent cueing and verbal directions. He used higher-level cognitive functions to adhere to safety precautions when using scissors and handling hot cooking utensils. Casey had to interpret sensory stimuli visually and use calculation functions to measure the ingredients. He had to plan and execute movements to carry out steps such as pouring ingredients into the measuring containers and emptying them into a bowl. Sequencing skills were needed to follow the recipe and to clean up.

Neuromusculoskeletal and Movement-Related Functions

Casey used asymmetrical bilateral hand skills to stabilize a mixing bowl while stirring ingredients and forming the rice crispy mixture into a ball. He used symmetrical bilateral hand skills to remove the bowl from the microwave oven.

Grading and Adapting

Suggestions for grading and adapting the activity are as follows:

- If tactile sensitivity or defensiveness is a concern, have Casey insert his hands into sandwich bags to decrease sensitivity to the texture of the mixture or have him pour the mixture into a flat container and pat it down with a nonstick spatula.
- Complete more of the activity (i.e., touching mixture) yourself, and Casey does the pouring and stirring.
- Place dycem under the bowl to increase its stability on the flat surface.
- Adapt the spoon as needed.
- Provide thicker pretzel rods that will not break as easily.
- Provide tongs or tweezers to place items.
- Use visual aids to describe the sequence of activity.

CLINICAL *Pearl*

Many children who have difficulty following verbally issued directions for multistep tasks benefit from visual sequence cards or a visual schedule.

- Substitute another dry cereal to change the consistency of the mixture and change the input to Casey's hands.
- Use large visual timers (available from adapted equipment catalogs or educational stores) to provide temporal cues.

The OTA adapted the activity taking into consideration Casey's short attention span by providing verbal cueing and redirection as needed. The OTA coordinated Casey's treatment around the classroom activity so that he could remain in the least restrictive environment and fulfill his role as a student. After discussing the activity with the teacher, the OTA decided to make a pumpkin-shaped dessert for the fall season versus a Halloween jack-o-lantern. Some children in the class did not celebrate Halloween, and thus cultural preferences were respected.

CLINICAL *Pearl*

Before working with food products, ensure that the client has no allergies to items such as wheat or peanuts. Also, consider religious or other dietary restrictions (e.g., gluten-free diets, lactose intolerance).

Adolescence: Puberty Until Onset of Adulthood

CASE *Study*

SARAH'S SCRAPBOOKING SESSION. Sarah, a 13-year-old girl with a diagnosis of spastic–hemiplegic cerebral palsy, receives OT services in an outpatient clinic once a week to address difficulties with self-care and leisure due to limited use of her right arm. In a previous session, Sarah and the OTA had talked about making a scrapbook containing photographs of what she did over the recent winter holidays. Sarah had agreed that she would like to work on such a project. For the current session, Sarah brought in selected photos of a family get-together during their Hanukah celebration. Sarah began the session with preparatory activities to increase sensory awareness and active range of motion (AROM) of her right arm so that she could use it as an assist during the scrapbooking activity.

Media/Materials

The media/materials needed are as follows:

- Cardstock (culturally appropriate colors and varying thicknesses)
- Scrapbook pages
- Glue
- Adapted cutting equipment
- Stamps and stamp pads
- Hole punch
- String
- Scissors with varied cutting designs
- Stickers, cropping stencils, markers/colored pencils

Method

The method used comprises the following elements:

1. Set the environment. Gather all the materials, adjust the chair and table to appropriate height to provide support for postural control; position the materials to facilitate reaching and crossing the midline.

CLINICAL *Pearl*

Optimal seating posture for completing fine motor activities is obtained by sitting with hips, knees, and ankles at or slightly less than 90 degrees of flexion. Feet should be flat on the floor or stable surface. The tabletop height should be no more than two inches above the bent elbow.

2. Sarah organizes the pictures onto the desired pages, cuts the cardstock to frame pictures with the use of adaptive equipment if needed, stamps phrases or motifs onto background of scrapbook pages, places stickers on background of pages, and uses cropping stencils.
3. Sarah decorates a cover for the book with cardstock, stickers, and drawings, punches holes with a hole punch, and secures the book by tying it with string.
4. Sarah cleans up the work area with assistance. Sarah discusses family activities shown in the pictures.

Client Factors
Mental Functions

Sarah was motivated to complete the project, since she had positive memories of this important family event that represented her family's values and religious traditions. She was aware of person, place, time, self, and others as observed in her description of the events.

Thought processes such as recognition were needed to choose the appropriate tools to complete the project. Sarah applied categorization skills as well as perceptual skills to complete tasks such as sorting and placing pictures on the pages, decorating the pages with the stamps, and cutting the borders to frame the pictures. Higher-level cognitive functions such as judgment were used to safely use scissors and cropping tools.

Sensory Functions and Pain

Acuity and visual functions were necessary for Sarah to visually locate and distinguish between the materials on the table. Preparatory activities of weight bearing and AROM and PROM helped Sarah retrieve tools and materials with her affected arm.

Neuromusculoskeletal and Movement-Related Functions

Sarah needed to sustain postural alignment while working at and crossing through the midline. ROM was needed for reaching and grasping. The OT practitioner began the session by inhibiting muscle tone (spasticity) in Sarah's right upper extremity to help her use the arm as an assist. Muscle power functions were employed for her to sustain a sufficient grasp on the scissors, hole punch, and stamp. The asymmetrical tonic neck reflex was integrated well enough to allow her to turn toward needed materials without abnormal movement patterns impeding the use of her bilateral upper extremities. Eye–hand coordination was required for cropping pictures, arranging photos, and designing the album.

Grading and Adapting

Suggestions for grading and adapting this activity are as follows:

- Vary the thickness of the paper (e.g., thicker paper/cardstock is easier to hold and gives more sensory feedback during cutting).
- Vary the type of scissors.
- Provide adaptive equipment for stabilizing paper.
- Provide a completed scrapbook to use as a model.
- Provide assistance and fade assistance as appropriate.
- Increase/decrease time constraints (e.g., two sessions versus one).

The OTA addressed Sarah's goals to increase the functional use of her right arm and considered areas of occupation and Sarah's personal, cultural, and temporal contexts when choosing an activity that she would be able to continue at home. The OTA adapted the activity to ensure a "just right" challenge for her client.

CASE *Study*

HARRY'S WOODWORKING PROJECT. Harry, an 18-year-old who is moderately intellectually disabled, is getting ready to transition from a self-contained classroom in high school to a sheltered workshop. The team feels that Harry could complete simple woodworking projects successfully in a supervised workshop setting. The OTA has been treating Harry once weekly for 30 minutes by consulting with his teacher and working toward goals such as improving motor planning to complete multistep activities. The OTA also monitors and supplies adapted equipment to help Harry complete fine motor activities more efficiently. Harry's interdisciplinary team (school psychologist, job coach, teacher, OTA speech therapist, parents, and Harry) agree that it is in Harry's interests that he should become familiar with the materials he will be using at the sheltered workshop. The team will examine Harry's adapted equipment needs. The OTA first speaks to personnel involved in the workshop to better understand Harry's needs. Later, the OTA consults with them regarding Harry's abilities and needs. Harry decides to make a small wooden jewelry box as an "end of the year" present for his teacher. The OTA requests sequencing cards from the speech therapist to increase Harry's independence in completing the task. Since Harry has a weak grasp, the OTA gathers supplies such as a paintbrush with a built-up handle and a sanding block. The shop environment is safe, conducive to woodworking, and free from distractions. Harry may work with one-on-one assistance. The OTA and Harry review the plans of the project and decide that Harry will need two sessions to complete it.

Media/Materials

The media/materials needed are as follows:

- Small wooden box obtained from craft supply store
- Paints and paintbrush (with built-up handle, if necessary)
- Sandpaper and sanding block
- Facemasks to wear during sanding
- Decorations (e.g., faux jewels, shells, colored tiles, stencils)
- Glue
- Cloth
- Picture sequence cards

Method

The method used comprises the following elements:

1. Set up the environment, considering lighting, seating, height of work surface, and positioning of materials. Position Harry to avoid visual and auditory distractions. Protect the work surface with newspaper or drop cloth.
2. Set up the sequence cards on the working surface.
3. Harry dons the mask in preparation of sanding and uses the sanding block to smooth out the small wooden box.
4. Harry cleans all of the surfaces of the wooden box with a soft cloth.
5. Harry applies the paint and lets it dry.
6. Harry chooses decorations and applies them with glue.

CLINICAL *Pearl*

When working with pediatric clients, use low-odor paints and finishes in a well-ventilated area. Also, consider any skin allergies that may be present, and take necessary precautions such as using gloves. When using tools and potentially hazardous materials, ensure that the client has good safety awareness, and provide proper supervision.

7. Harry cleans up the work area.

Client Factors
Mental Functions

Harry sustained attention for 30 minutes to complete the multistep process and safely worked with the materials. His memory was sufficient to remember the procedures, follow the sequence, and use objects for their intended use. Harry relied on perceptual functions to interpret tactile and visual information when sanding and painting the box. Harry smelled the odors of the paint and the freshly sanded wood. He used good judgment and problem-solving skills to determine when and where to sand. Visual cards were useful to Harry. A positive sense of self was reinforced in Harry as he carried out the process of choosing the project, constructing it, and presenting it to his teacher.

Neuromusculoskeletal and Movement-Related Functions

Harry initiated and sustained sufficient grasp on the surface of the sanding block and the adapted paint brush despite the decreased strength in his hands. Harry showed control of voluntary movement functions when keeping the paint in the correct areas, applying the small objects used to decorate the jewelry box, as well as opening, closing, and manipulating the containers.

Skin and Related-Structure Functions

Integrity of the skin was required as protection against sawdust or paint residue getting into open wounds or abrasions.

Grading and Adapting

Suggestions for grading and adapting this activity are as follows:

- Adaptive equipment can be used to increase the client's independence, for example, the sanding block in Harry's case. Another example would be dycem or a jig for stabilizing materials.
- Divide the task into several sessions.
- Use written or pictorial sequencing cards as needed.
- Allow the client to gather, clean, and put away supplies.
- Nonlatex gloves can be worn for skin sensitivities or in the presence of small cuts or abrasions.

The OTA considered Harry's client factors as well as his social and occupational issues while choosing and setting up the activity. Harry felt invested in the project; he was given choices and successfully performed the work with little intervention because of the OTA's careful consideration of activity demands.

SUMMARY

Use of therapeutic media, which is an important component in OT intervention, has changed with time and technology varies according to culture. Media are used within functional activities as well as preparatory tools to enhance skills in order to reach OT goals. The collaboration between the occupational therapist and the OTA is best served once the OTA has established service competency and sound clinical reasoning skills such as those required to choose media that facilitate accomplishment of OT goals and are meaningful to clients. Other important considerations include selection of media that are developmentally relevant to clients and are graded on the basis of client factors and activity demands. This chapter provides examples of how the OTA uses media to design, develop, and implement intervention activities that present the "just right" challenge for each client.

References

1. *American heritage dictionary of the English language*, ed 4, New York, 2000, Houghton Mifflin.
2. American Occupational Therapy Association: Occupational therapy practice framework: domain and process, ed 2. *Am J Occup Ther* 62:625–703, 2008.
3. Punwar AJ, Peloquin SM: *Occupational therapy principles and practice*, ed 2, Baltimore, 2000, Lippincott Williams & Wilkins.

Recommended Reading

Drake M: *Crafts in therapy and rehabilitation*, ed 2, 1992, Slack Inc. New Jersey.

Johnson C et al: *Therapeutic crafts: a practical approach*, 1996, Slack Inc. New Jersey.

Kranowitz C: *The out-of-sync child has fun: activities for kids with sensory processing disorder*, 2003, Perigee Books. New York.

Kuffner T: *The busy books series*, 1999, Meadowbrook Press. Minnesota.

Resources For Supplies and Materials s For Media

Catalogs

S & S Worldwide
Southpaw
Integrations
Childcraft
Lakeshore

Retail

Michael's
AC Moore
Wal-Mart
Hobby Lobby

Internet

www.craftsforkids.com
www.creativekidsathome.com
www.kidsdomain.com
www.crayola.com
www.theideabox.com
www.abcteach.com

REVIEW *Questions*

1. What should you consider when selecting media?
2. What is the role of the OTA in selecting therapeutic media?
3. Describe why choosing appropriate therapeutic media for different age groups is important.
4. Give some examples of cultural considerations a practitioner makes when selecting therapeutic media.
5. Explain the principle of gradation of therapeutic activities.
6. What purpose do craft activities serve in pediatric OT?
7. Distinguish between preparatory activities and functional activities.

SUGGESTED *Activities*

1. Visit a daycare center or a preschool during a group craft activity. Observe the media used, activity demands, and methods used. Did you notice the staff using any sort of preparatory activities? Considering the results of the activities you observed, do you think preparatory activities would have made a difference in these results? Would the results have been different with OT interventions?
2. Choose a medium and formulate five different activities using the same medium.
3. Consider one of the five activities, and adapt/grade it for various client factors (refer to *Occupational Therapy Practice Framework, 2nd edition*), age groups, and culture as outlined by this chapter.
4. Plan a craft activity or game considering the following:

   - What materials do you need?
   - How much time will it take to prepare the materials?
   - Can you use the items on hand, or do you have to buy specific items (i.e., playground ball and empty water bottles versus a purchased bowling game)?
   - Which is more cost effective?

   List the activity demands required to complete your planned craft activity or game for the above question. (Refer to activity demands section of *Occupational Therapy Practice Framework, 2nd edition*)

5. Choose a culture other than your own and find a therapeutic media activity related to it. Describe its significance to the culture. Teach classmates how to do the activity.

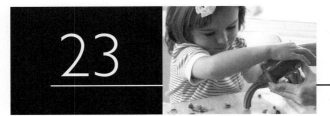

23

Motor Control: Fine Motor Skills

HARRIET G. WILLIAMS

CHAPTER *Objectives*

After studying this chapter, the reader will be able to accomplish the following:

- Describe fine motor development in typically developing children
- Identify common problems of children with fine motor control deficiencies
- Describe techniques to promote fine motor functioning in children
- Understand basic motor learning principles
- Describe how basic motor learning principles relate to occupational therapy intervention

KEY TERMS

Fine motor development
Construction activities
In-hand manipulation activities
Tool use
Bilateral motor control
Eye movement control
Saccadic eye movements
Pursuit tracking movements
Object manipulation
Power grasp
Precision grasp
Grip reflex

CHAPTER OUTLINE

Foundations of Fine Motor Skill Development
BILATERAL MOTOR CONTROL: LARGE MUSCLE
BILATERAL MOTOR CONTROL, SMALL MUSCLE CONTROL, AND OBJECT MANIPULATION
REACHING, GRASPING, RELEASING, AND FINE MOTOR DEVELOPMENT
EYE MOVEMENT CONTROL

Development of Object Manipulation Skills
PICKING UP AN OBJECT
GRASPING AN OBJECT
MANIPULATING AN OBJECT

Force Production and Object Manipulation Skills
ACTIVITIES TO PROMOTE STRENGTH DEVELOPMENT

Developmental Progression for Object Manipulation

Development of Implement Usage Skills
CUTTING
PENCIL USAGE

Developmental Progression of Implement Usage
SCRIBBLING
SIMPLE LINE DRAWING
TRACING
FREEHAND DRAWING

Prerequisite Experiences for Writing
DEVELOPMENTAL READINESS
BALANCE
STABILITY
OBJECT MANIPULATION
FUNCTIONAL ASYMMETRY: LEAD-ASSIST HAND USAGE
GRASP OF WRITING TOOL
GENERAL PREWRITING
COLORING ACTIVITIES

Important Motor Learning Concepts
TRANSFER OF LEARNING
FEEDBACK
VERBAL INSTRUCTION
KNOWLEDGE OF RESULTS
KNOWLEDGE OF PERFORMANCE
DISTRIBUTION AND VARIABILITY OF SKILL PRACTICE
WHOLE VERSUS PART PRACTICE
MENTAL PRACTICE

Summary

This chapter addresses two major topics in fine motor development: (1) the nature of fine motor development in typically developing children, and (2) common problems of children with fine motor control deficiencies. In the first part, we address the following issues: what fine motor development is, why it is important, what the important foundations for developing fine motor skills are, how object manipulation and implement usage skills develop, and some comments and recommendations for the development of writing skills. In the final part of the chapter, we discuss some basic motor learning principles that are important for planning and conducting occupational therapy (OT) sessions to improve fine motor control and facilitate skill acquisition.

Fine motor development is generally defined as the ability to use the eyes, hands, and fingers together in carrying out precise movements that are necessary for performing a variety of daily activities. These movements range from those involved in coloring, drawing, and writing to pasting, cutting, and the manipulation of small objects and implements. Other terms commonly used interchangeably with fine motor development include *eye–hand coordination*, *visuomotor coordination*, and *distal extremity control*.[39-41]

Fine motor control does not just happen but rather develops in an orderly, organized fashion and is built on a number of underlying or foundational processes. The development of fine motor skills is an integral part of the overall development of the young child and reflects the increasing capacity of the nervous system to pick up and process visual and proprioceptive information and translate that information into skillful and refined movements. The optimal development of fine motor skills is important, as they are critical components of most of our self-help skills (e.g., eating, dressing, buttoning, zipping), the child's learning environment (e.g., writing, coloring, drawing, cutting, pasting), and other activities of daily living (ADLs; e.g., typing, turning the pages in a book, threading a needle). They are also integral to successful performance of a number of professionals (e.g., surgeons, dentists, musicians, artists, mechanics). Since hand skills are essential to a child's engagement in academics, ADLs, and play, OT practitioners routinely evaluate fine motor skills.

CLINICAL *Pearl*

Children with poor fine motor skills may exhibit the following performance problems:
- Difficulty in cutting and pasting
- Difficulty in manipulating objects
- Lack of smoothness in clapping or tapping rhythmically
- Tendency to hold a pencil awkwardly
- Tenseness in writing and drawing
- Producing strokes that are too heavy or too light

FOUNDATIONS OF FINE MOTOR SKILL DEVELOPMENT

In understanding and working with the development of fine motor skills, it is important to be aware of several elements that make up the foundation of fine motor skill development; these include bilateral motor control, reaching/grasping, object manipulation, and implement usage.[7,18,20,21,28,32,35,39,40,42] Bilateral motor control includes large and small (proximal and distal) muscle control; reaching/grasping is, in part, an extension of proximal and distal control and is the key component in grasping and in the manipulation of objects. Refined object manipulation that follows is built on the foregoing elements and involves construction and in-hand manipulation activities. **Construction activities** include stacking blocks, putting simple puzzle pieces together, and putting pegs into a pegboard, among others (Figure 23-1). **In-hand manipulation activities** involve moving objects within the hand (translation) and include adjusting a toy or object in the hand (shift), rotating an object in the hand (rotation), or picking up multiple objects. Precision grasping and releasing are critical to all of these activities. Finally, **tool use**, or the use of implements, evolves with and, in part, from earlier experiences with object manipulation skills. Overall, the development of fine motor skills is an ongoing, integrated, and complex process. A schema that depicts the relationships among the various elements involved in fine motor development is shown in Figure 23-2 and discussed in more detail below.

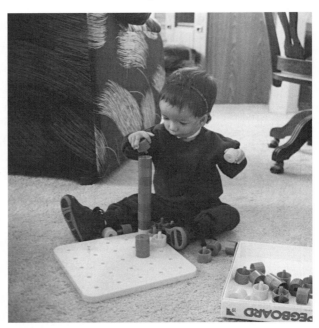

FIGURE 23-1 Construction activities require fine motor skills. (From Parham, L. Diane. *Play in Occupational Therapy for Children.* 2nd Edition, Mosby, 2007.)

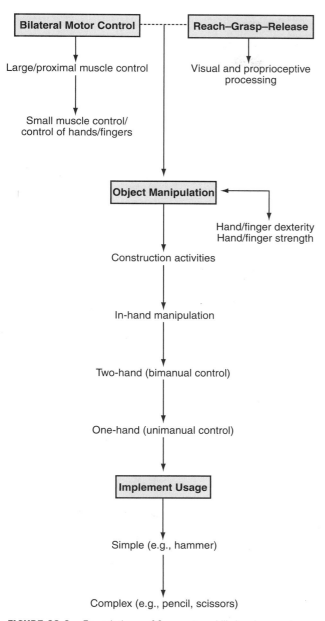

FIGURE 23-2 Foundations of fine motor skill development.

Bilateral Motor Control: Large Muscle

Most manipulative activities require both arms and both hands to work together in various ways; this is referred to as **bilateral motor control**. For example, in cutting, one hand holds and controls the scissors while the other hand is holding and positioning the paper. Therefore, to cut with precision, both hands must move skillfully and in an appropriate relationship to each other.

An initial step in the process of fine motor skills development is the development of control of the large, or proximal, muscles of the trunk and arms. Control of the proximal muscles frees the arms and allows them to move independent of the trunk, which ultimately provides the hands and fingers with the support needed for independent, intricate, and delicate movements.

There appears to be a general developmental sequence in acquiring large, or proximal, muscle control. First, control of the muscles of the trunk develops; the arms and legs can then be moved independently. This is followed by the ability to move an arm and a leg on one side of the body independent of the opposite side. This action appears to occur initially on the side of the dominant hand and then on the side of the nondominant one. Finally, control extends to the movement of an arm and a leg on opposite sides of the body, first on the side of the dominant hand and then on the side of the nondominant one. The former movement is known as *ipsilateral* and the latter as *contralateral*. Contralateral movements are the forerunner of the arm/foot opposition inherent in most locomotor skills. Control of these large, proximal muscles is typically present by 6 years of age; the major developmental changes occur between 4 and 6 years. The examination of bilateral large muscle control can be accomplished at three different levels: (1) by touching the body parts to be moved (concrete, touch-based level), (2) by pointing to the body parts to be moved (less concrete, more visually based level), and (3) by using verbal labels for the body parts to be observed (abstract, language-based level).

The bilateral motor control involved in fine motor development also progresses from crude two-hand (bimanual) movements to one-hand (unimanual) control to refined use of both hands in lead and assist roles in activities such as buttoning and cutting. Crude bilateral movements represent an initial, possibly inherent, linkage between the hands and typically involve the hands working together as one unit, each performing the same action. The processes involved in unimanual control and refined bimanual control (functional asymmetry) are discussed in greater detail below.

> ### CLINICAL *Pearl*
>
> An infant first transfers objects from one hand to another in two steps. The hands first come into contact with each other; then the object is released from the holding hand to the receiving hand. As unimanual control or dissociation of the hands develop, the infant is able to transfer objects from one hand to another in one step.

Bilateral Motor Control, Small Muscle Control, and Object Manipulation

The term *small muscle control* refers to the control or use of the small muscle masses of the wrist, hands, and fingers to grasp, hold, and manipulate objects. Small muscle, or distal, control typically follows and builds on the development of a minimum of control of the large, more proximal muscles of the trunk, shoulders, and arms. The development of proximal stability of the large muscles supports the mobility of the distal muscles of the wrist, hand, and fingers. Small muscle, distal control allows the child to carry out more precise, adaptive movements that involve intricate manipulation and/or the use of objects and implements. Small muscle control requires adequate hand and finger strength and dexterity; these aspects of hand function are assessed and included in fine motor OT interventions (Figure 23-3).

The development of unimanual control is associated with the establishment of hand preference or hand dominance. Bimanual control is also intricately linked to small muscle control and hand preference because both optimal unimanual control and hand dominance are integral to the development of lead and assist hands, or *bimanual functional asymmetry*. All of the foregoing factors are important in acquiring the capacity to manipulate objects and use implements skillfully. The terms *lead and assist hands* and *bimanual functional asymmetry* refer to the use of hands individually in performing different actions involved in a single activity. For example, in the activity of buttoning, one hand manipulates the button, and the other manipulates the fabric where the button is to be placed. Two different actions are performed, one by each hand, to accomplish a single goal or task.

The greatest developmental changes in unimanual distal control appear to take place between 4 and 6 years of age, with lesser improvements between 6 and 8 years. Distal control is often assessed through the performance of such actions as repetitive hand patting, alternating wrist flexion/extension, alternating arm and hand supination/pronation, and repetitive and successive finger tapping. Hand patting requires the child to tap the whole hand against a surface as quickly as possible, while alternating hand flexion/extension requires the child to move the wrist into and out of flexion/extension as rapidly as possible. Alternating supination/pronation involves moving the hands and forearms in alternating rotatory movements (hand palm up to hand palm down repeatedly) as rapidly as possible. Finger movement tasks involve either tapping one finger repeatedly or touching each finger to the thumb in sequence, starting with the index finger; both of these tasks are performed as rapidly as possible. The capacity to perform such movements rapidly and easily is one way to establish the possible presence or absence of deficits in underlying fine motor control processes.

> ### CLINICAL *Pearl*
>
> Whole-hand and finger puppets can be used to encourage repetitive hand and finger movements to make the intervention session more fun and playful.

Reaching, Grasping, Releasing, and Fine Motor Development

Reaching, grasping, and releasing are other important components of the development of fine motor skills (both object manipulation and implement or tool usage). For example, to manipulate an object, the child must first obtain it; this requires the child to reach for and grasp the object and then use the fingers to move or manipulate it in appropriate ways. *Reaching* for an object and grasping it successfully involve locating the hand in space, locating the object in space, and then acting to bring the two together. It is important that the child both see and feel the hand in relation to the

Fine Motor Evaluation

Child's Name: _____

DOB: _____ DOE: _____

Diagnosis: _____

Therapist: _____ COTA: _____

Reason for Referral:

Background Information (Include the child's grade, developmental history, medications, home situation.):

Physical Structure of the Hand (Note any deformities, contractures, edema, structural integrity of the muscles and joints.):

Muscle Tone (Describe the development of the arches of the hand; very young children and those with low muscle tone exhibit flat hand arches.):

Range of Motion (Examine the wrist, supination/pronation, and all finger and thumb movements.):

Strength (grip strength, pincer strength):

Posture/Balance (Can the child sit, stand, walk independently? What is the quality of his or her movement?):

Postural Adjustments during Fine Motor Tasks (Observe how the child adjusts to changes during fine motor tasks. Does the child move his or her hand/fingers, or whole body?):

Coordination (Are tremors, over reaching, under reaching, or associated reactions noted during activities?):

Attention to Task (Is the child interested in task? Does the child visually attend to task?):

Emotional Reactions to Fine Motor Tasks (Does the child become frustrated easily? Has the child developed compensatory strategies? Does the child attempt to avoid tasks?):

Vision (Does the child get very close to work? Does the child appear to be looking at task? Does the child rely heavily on vision?):

Sensory Reactions to Fine Motor Tasks (Does the child avoid manipulating objects? Does the child under or overreact to touch? Does the child explore objects?):

Development of Fine Motor Skills (Is the child able to grasp, release, manipulate? Use both hands together? Cut? Write? Developmental assessments such as the Hawaii Early Learning Profile provide age ranges.):

Timing and Sequencing:

Quality of Movement (Is the child able to alternate supination/pronation? Release objects precisely?):

Finger Individuation (Is the child able to use one or two fingers alone? Or do all fingers move in the same pattern?):

Pencil Grasp:

Assessment:

FIGURE 23-3   Occupational therapist conducts fine motor assessment with input from the occupational therapy assistant (OTA). *DOB,* Date of birth; *DOE,* date of evaluation.

object to be grasped. In other words, it is important for the person to see and feel the hand and arm as they move toward and grasp the object. The child must effectively process visual, proprioceptive, and tactile information (seeing and feeling the hand and arm move) and then create and carry out a movement that gets the hand to the object for grasping and manipulation. This process is known as *intersensory integration* or *sensory-motor integration*. These processes tend to happen naturally and spontaneously during development. When or if they do not, fine motor development is often difficult.

Overall, infants tend to reach out spontaneously for objects that move across their visual fields; this reaching tendency is present at birth and is initially visually evoked; that is, the response appears to be a spontaneous reaction to seeing an object in the environment. Although this early reaching action is crude, it is directed toward the object and will later become a voluntary act that is more precise and better controlled. At this point in his or her development, the child decides when, where, how, and whether to reach for an object and does so skillfully.

Grasping an object is the second step in its manipulation. The early grasping response is reflexive or instinctive in nature and is based largely on proprioceptive and tactile input; later it evolves into a voluntary grasp that relies more on visual information. Vision allows the young child to examine the object (determine its size, shape, location, and other factors) more precisely and then shape the hand and create the force necessary for holding and manipulating the object. Of course, this process is repeated multiple times in many different ways for objects of different sizes, shapes, weights, and uses. Therefore, vision and visual perception become integral factors in the development of fine motor skills. *Releasing* an object, or letting it go, is another part of fine motor development and object manipulation. It requires some inhibition of the earlier grasp reflex response because manipulating an object actually involves skillful grasping and releasing of the object in a variety of ways, which allow the child to explore and/or use the object for a particular purpose (in-hand manipulation).

Eye Movement Control

Visual perception and thus **eye movement control** (how the child moves the eyes to focus on or follow objects in the environment) play an important role in fine motor control and development. Some evidence has shown that a significant number of children (approximately 78%) with fine motor control problems also exhibit poor saccadic eye movements along with less well-developed pursuit eye movements. In **saccadic eye movements**, the eyes move rapidly and accurately from item to item (e.g., from point to point in a picture or letter to letter or word to word in reading). In **pursuit tracking movements**, the eyes move to follow slow-moving objects, among other things. These eye movements allow the eyes and the brain to get the information needed to make appropriate decisions about phenomena such as movement, objects, and the content of the written word. Both types of eye movement can be improved with practice and may be worth considering as part of the enrichment activities for improving fine motor control.

CLINICAL *Pearl*

Using black-and-white infant toys (created to stimulate infants) may improve the eye muscles of children with eye tracking difficulties. OT practitioners may encourage children to follow the slow-moving (for pursuit tracking movements) or fast-moving (for saccadic movements) object. For older children, black-and-white pictures or computer games in which the child must point to the object on the screen may be more appropriate.

CLINICAL *Pearl*

If a child has eye movement control deficits, the OT practitioner may work closely with an optometrist who specializes in vision therapy. Optometrists who specialize in vision therapy have special lenses and other visual tools that enhance eye movement control interventions.

DEVELOPMENT OF OBJECT MANIPULATION SKILLS

Object manipulation may be thought of as the manual control of objects (i.e., the ability to manipulate or use an object in a variety of desired ways). Object manipulation may involve what some refer to as construction activities and in-hand manipulation activities; both can be bimanual or unimanual. Examples of *construction activities* include putting puzzles together, building towers out of building blocks, making shapes with Lego, and putting pegs into a pegboard. Examples of *in-hand manipulation activities* include turning the lid of a jar, picking up multiple objects, and others in which

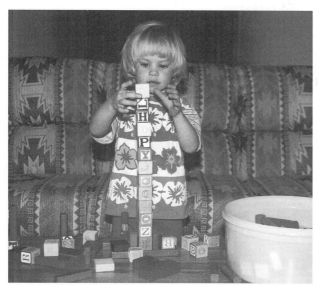

FIGURE 23-4 Table top activities such as constructing block structures require fine motor skills, concentration, and the ability to problem solve and sequence. (From Hockenberry, *Marilyn J. Wong's Essentials of Pediatric Nursing*, 7th Edition. Mosby, 2005.)

the thumb plays a prominent role (Figure 23-4). The skillful manipulation of objects involves, in particular, the ability to control the actions of individual fingers and groups of fingers (manual dexterity). It also requires that the arm and hand work together to control or use the object (bimanual control); this is often referred to as the *arm–hand linkage system* and is the basic foundation for the subsequent development of implement usage skills.[5,6,11-15,19,22,28,29,39,40]

The arm and the hand each play different roles in the successful manipulation of objects, the nature of which changes in relation to the goal of the task and the age and developmental level of the child. For example, in placing pegs into a pegboard (construction activity), the arm provides support for the hands and fingers to hold the pegs and also positions the hand in such a way that the pegs can be put into the board. In eating with a spoon (implement or tool usage), the arm positions the hand to hold the spoon; and the hand and fingers control the position and movement of the spoon.

Generally, the arm and the hand each have three independent functions that are used in different ways to accomplish different tasks. The three functions of the arm are (1) positioning the hand (i.e., getting the hand in an appropriate location or position for grasping the object of interest); (2) supporting the hand (i.e., keeping the arm/hand combination relatively immobile so that the necessary hand and finger movements can be executed properly); and (3) on some occasions, producing force such as that required in pounding a peg or turning a doorknob. The functions of the hand are to pick up the object, hold or grasp the object, and execute the movements needed to manipulate the object or implement. Developmental progressions have been loosely defined for each of these hand functions.

Picking up an Object

In picking up an object, the child may initially scoop it up with the whole hand, often on the ulnar (little finger) side. Later, the person uses individual fingers and finger actions to pick up the object. A pincer grasp that involves finger–thumb opposition, for example, is the use of the thumb and the index finger. A pincer grasp is usually effective in picking up very small objects such as a Cheerio or a piece of pinestraw. A three-jaw chuck or pince involves the thumb opposing with the index and middle fingers, which is usually the most effective way to pick up slightly larger object such as a one-inch block.

CLINICAL *Pearl*

A child first develops a pad-to-pad pincer grasp, in which the small object is held between the pads of the thumb and the index finger. As motor control is refined, a tip-to-tip pincer grasp evolves such that the small object is held between the tip of the thumb and the tip of the index finger.

Grasping an Object

Two types of grasps are used in holding objects or implements. One is the **power grasp**, in which the handle or object is held tight against the palm, and the arm and shoulder produce the movement. A good example of this type of grasp is the use of a hammer in pounding a nail or a peg; the hammer is held in a kind of cylindrical grasp (type of palmar grasp), and the arm and shoulder create the force needed to pound the peg. The other is the **precision grasp**, in which the thumb and fingertips are used to change the object's position or move the implement. In contrast to the power grasp, the precision grasp involves a wrist-and-finger action (distal control) to perform the task. More accurate movement is possible with the precision grasp.

Manipulating an Object

As with grasping an object, in manipulating an object, the palm or the whole hand is used initially; later, the fingers and the thumb are used to explore, examine, or move the object or implement in intricate ways.

FORCE PRODUCTION AND OBJECT MANIPULATION SKILLS

Generally, adults and children with typical development or function exhibit patterns of *force production* and modification that allow them to create and apply the force needed to manipulate objects effectively. Therefore, adequate strength, along with the ability to produce appropriate force and apply that force when it is needed, is integral to fine motor control and development. If the amount of force is inadequate or the application or use of that force is poorly timed, the object may slip or slide, and the skillful and efficient use or manipulation of the object may be hindered. Producing force involves, among other things, the activation of appropriate muscles and the proper timing of the contraction of those muscles to produce the force needed for effective object manipulation. Force production and modification of that force are integral to all types and forms of object manipulation. For example, appropriate levels and timing of force are needed to lift an object; here, the amount of force produced should be equal to the weight of the object to be lifted. This requires accurate anticipation of the weight of the object and the ability to plan the movement to produce that force. Another example is the *transport*, or movement, of an object from one place to another (e.g., picking up pegs and putting them into a pegboard). This involves upward, downward, and horizontal movements and varying the force as needed. Another important component is the ability to respond appropriately to variables such as changes in object position and slippage of the object; this is referred to as **grip reflex**, or the timing and application of appropriate force to adapt to changes in object position.[16,17,23,38,41]

In typical development, the force aspects of fine motor control evolve naturally and spontaneously; however, with a number of developmental delays, after trauma, or with certain neurologic disorders, these processes are disrupted. In other words, the child is unable to produce or modify the force needed to meet the changing demands inherent in the use of objects. For example, children with fine motor problems begin to initiate force for lifting objects prematurely (i.e., before that force is really needed). Often, a delay occurs in increasing the force as needed once the object is lifted or moved; therefore, control of the object may become problematic. In addition, the response to slippage or some unexpected change in the position or orientation of the object is slower and more variable than that seen in typically developing children. In other words, the initiation

of the grip reflex takes significantly longer and is extremely inconsistent. As a result, for the child who has difficulties with fine motor development, the grip reflex is at times rapid and appropriate; at other times, it is slow and maladaptive. This frequently results in fumbling, dropping, or awkward handling of objects.

CLINICAL *Pearl*

Children who have force production deficits often will crush a styrofoam cup because the force of their grasp is too much. A plastic cup is recommended to prevent dropping and spillage.

ACTIVITIES TO PROMOTE STRENGTH DEVELOPMENT

Adequate muscular strength of the hands and fingers is important to produce the force needed to carry out fine motor tasks with skill and efficiency.[40] The following are some examples of activities that may be helpful in strength development:

- Pinch putty between the thumb and individual fingers in sequence from the index to the little finger, and vice versa.
- Push slowly into a putty ball; hold each finger extended.
- Press cookie cutter into Play-Doh or another similar substance.
- Hold putty or soft ball in the palm of the hand and squeeze.
- Squeeze a turkey baster or other plastic item.
- Crumble sheets of paper into a ball.
- Twist or wring putty or other material with palm toward and away from the body.
- Squeeze water out of a sponge or other soft material.
- Hold playing cards between two fingers; try to knock the cards out of the finger grasp
- Holding a weight in one hand, with the palm down and forearm supported, flex and extend the wrist.
- Use rubber bands as resistance to finger and wrist movements.

One way to assess the ability of the child to consistently produce an appropriate amount of force is the use of tapping activities. Can the child tap consistently for a designated period? Variation in tapping can be easily observed, and it becomes readily evident when a metronome is used in the assessment. The metronome can be used to help the child improve the consistency of the timing of force production. Children with coordination difficulties generally exhibit an inability to maintain a consistent tapping rate; this is especially true if the tapping has to be performed for a long period. The performance of these children becomes more variable as the time involved in tapping increases. Their performance is most consistent in the initial 10 seconds of such an activity and becomes much more variable as the duration increases to 20 or 30 seconds. It is a good idea to use short durations initially and gradually increase them as the child improves.

CLINICAL *Pearl*

For older children, computer typing programs that use musical rhythms to teach keyboarding skills are available.

DEVELOPMENTAL PROGRESSION FOR OBJECT MANIPULATION

Several overlapping trends or dimensions of behavior need to be considered in assessing the development of fine motor object manipulation skills.[6,14,39,40] The manipulation skill indicators include the development of hand control (how and for what purpose the child uses the hands), spatial–temporal accuracy (skills that require judging the space and timing of the action of the hands), and self-help skills. Examples of the general developmental sequence of some of these behaviors are given in Box 23-1.

DEVELOPMENT OF IMPLEMENT USAGE SKILLS

Implement usage skills involve the use of tools to accomplish specific goals.[6,8,40] Tools can be used to act on oneself or the environment. Development begins with the use of simple implements, for example, a hammer, a brush, or another object, and proceeds to the use of more complex and specialized tools such as pencils and scissors. Using an implement involves functional asymmetry, or the use of lead and assist hands. To use a tool or implement properly, the child must hold it correctly and maintain the appropriate relationship between the tool and the object on which it is used. For example, in using a hammer, it is important to maintain an appropriate relationship between the hammer and the nail to make successful contact. The same is true in using scissors for cutting, a pencil

---

BOX 23-1

Examples of General Developmental Sequences for Object Manipulation

HAND CONTROL
- Hands fisted: flexion dominates
- Hands open: more opportunity for use
- Fingers used in play
- Picks up cube: uses the whole hand (left and right)
- Transfers cube hand to hand: whole hand involved
- Transfers cube hand to hand: thumb/finger opposition involved
- Reaches unilaterally (one arm)
- Builds tower of cubes
- Unwraps cube
- Turns pages
- Holds crayon adaptively
- Scribbles spontaneously
- Imitates vertical and horizontal strokes

SPATIAL–TEMPORAL ACCURACY
- Visually tracks object across midline
- Reaches for objects
- Plays pat-a-cake
- Puts three cubes in a cup
- Puts several beads in a box
- Puts one peg into pegboard (repeated)
- Puts nine cubes in cup
- Places round, square, and triangular shapes in form board

SELF-HELP SKILLS
- Drinks from cup
- Uses spoon; spills a little
- Removes clothes
- Washes/dries hands
- Puts on shoes (does not tie)

---

for writing, and a wrench for turning a screw. Developmental steps in acquiring the skills of cutting and writing are addressed below.

CLINICAL *Pearl*

OT practitioners often use cobbler toys to promote effective use of implements (toy hammer) and to increase a child's arm strength (Figure 23-5).

Cutting

The development of cutting skills involves several components, including how the scissors are held (the grasp or prehension of the scissors), the use of the assist

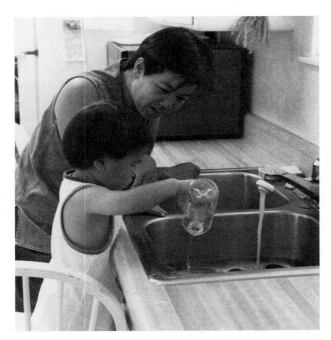

FIGURE 23-5 Gross motor and fine motor abilities are important in manipulating objects such as pouring from a container. (From Parham, L. Diane. *Play in Occupational Therapy for Children.* 2nd Edition. Mosby, 2007.)

hand (lead and assist usage), the relationship between the paper and scissors, and the cutting action.[31,39,40] Cutting skills are often assessed by observing and evaluating the child as he or she cuts a straight line, a square, and a circle. Of the three, the circle is reported to be the most difficult.

Holding the Scissors

The mature and preferred grasp of the scissors is with the thumb on the upper handle and the index finger or the index and middle fingers on the other, with the other fingers gently flexed. Another early grasp that is also biomechanically efficient for the young child is with the thumb on one handle, the middle finger on the other, and the index finger extended along the scissors for stability. Most children with fine motor difficulties use immature prehension or grasp patterns (82% in cutting a line, 69% in cutting a square, and 77% in cutting a circle). About 73% to 83% of children with typical development use the mature grasp for cutting shapes and lines.

In developing cutting skills, the scissors are initially held with both hands; each hand holds one handle that moves the blade to cut. A second person holds and moves the paper to assist in cutting. This is usually followed by the child holding the scissors with one hand and using the thumb and fingers to move the scissors, which frees the opposite hand to hold or move

the paper to accommodate the cutting. At this point, the mouth also often moves in concert with the action of the scissors. Ultimately, the thumb primarily controls the action of the scissors. When the scissors are grasped with one hand, the thumb is usually placed on the upper handle and the index finger or the index and middle fingers on the lower handle.

> ### CLINICAL *Pearl*
>
> When a child is learning a new skill and concentrating on performing a task, associated reactions may occur in different parts of the body (e.g., the mouth moving in concert with the scissors).

Using the Assist Hand

Use of the assist hand, or *lead and assist usage* (also known as *paper strategy*), refers to how the child holds the paper and uses the assist hand. The mature manner of holding the paper involves the thumb being placed on top and the fingers underneath. Children with fine motor difficulties use immature lead and assist patterns for cutting tasks (59% for the line, 50% for the square, and 65% for the circle, which are significant percentages). In terms of development, the assist hand is not used initially because the child holds the scissors with both hands while a second person has to hold the paper. The next stage involves the use of the assist hand; when it is used, the paper is often held with the fingers on top and the arm in a pronated position. This is a less efficient position for ease and flexibility in cutting. At this time, the assist hand is used inconsistently, and many different combinations of fingers or thumb on top are seen. The mature stage involves using the assist hand with the thumb on top and the arm in a more supinated position. This position allows for greater freedom in orienting the paper to the action of the scissors and makes for increased ease and efficiency in cutting.

Paper–Scissors Relationship

The *paper–scissors relationship* involves (1) how the paper is maintained in relation to the scissors, and (2) where the child holds the paper in relation to the blades of the scissors. With regard to how the paper is maintained in relation to the scissors, the paper is initially held against the table for support. This is usually related to inadequate stability of the trunk and shoulder girdle. In the next stage, the paper is held in place (the paper is not moved), and the scissors are moved to accomplish the cutting task. The biomechanically more efficient approach is seen in the subsequent development of cutting skills and involves the scissors being maintained in a relatively stationary position, and the paper is moved to accommodate the cutting action.

With regard to where the child holds the paper in relation to the blades of the scissors, typical patterns include holding the paper in front of the blade, holding it behind the blade, holding it so that it crosses over the scissors, and holding it in multiple positions in relation to the blade. Holding the paper in inappropriate positions in relation to the paper makes it difficult to cut accurately, smoothly, and in an efficient, coordinated fashion. Children with coordination difficulties often use immature patterns in executing the appropriate paper–scissors relationships (41% for the line, 75% for the square, and 65% for the circle).

CLINICAL *Pearl*

> For a child who has the use of only one arm, the OT practitioner can adapt the cutting activity by having the child use a jig to hold the paper.

Cutting Action

Cutting action is sometimes referred to as *cutting strategy* and involves the type of cutting motion and the selection of the appropriate place to initiate cutting (i.e., where to start to cut). Two major types of cutting action are possible: (1) The first is the short, segmented cutting action, or what is referred to as *snipping*. This type of action appears to be easier to control and therefore is usually seen in the initial steps of cutting. (2) The second is a longer gliding action that is more continuous in nature. This action is seen in more skillful cutters. Depending on the nature of the item to be cut, the ultimate skill in cutting requires an appropriate combination of short, segmented cuts integrated with longer gliding actions.

With regard to where to start to cut, 65% to 69% of children with fine motor control difficulties use inappropriate starting positions; they have to snip, return to the edge of the paper, and restart the cutting task multiple times. Many children with fine motor problems do not use a continuous motion in cutting.

Pencil Usage

Handwriting is one of the most important skills that adults and children alike acquire and use throughout life; for children, handwriting is a skill that is critical during the school years. Between 10% and 20% of school-aged children have difficulties with handwriting. Handwriting problems are the most frequent reason that children are

referred to OT practitioners working in schools. When handwriting is deficient or problematic, often consequences related to academic performance as well as social interaction can limit participation in basic school and social activities.[2-4,6,9,10,25,30,31,33,34,36,37,42] What is involved in handwriting? What are some of the major foundational skills that are prerequisites to developing skillful handwriting? The skills in Box 23-2 have been shown to contribute in different ways to speed and/or accuracy in handwriting.

The important elements to consider in examining skill in the use of a pencil can and should include all of the items listed in Box 23-2. The major motor control issues are related to the grasp of the pencil and the locus of control for the action of moving it. Examples of the steps in grasping and controlling the pencil are described below.

BOX 23-2

Foundational Skills Contributing to Handwriting Speed and Accuracy

FINGER FUNCTIONS
Intricate and skillful use of the fingers:
- Finger lifting: accuracy in lifting fingers pointed to (related to speed and accuracy)
- Finger recognition: accuracy in lifting fingers touched when vision is not available (related to speed)
- Complex finger opposition: speed and accuracy of touching fingers to thumb rapidly/consistently (related to speed)

VISUOMOTOR INTEGRATION
Appropriate use of visual information and ability to integrate vision with movement responses:
- Copying forms: design copying (related to speed and accuracy)
- Identifying forms: visual recognition of forms (related to speed)
- General eye–motor coordination: drawing lines accurately (related to speed)

LEFT–RIGHT DISCRIMINATION
Awareness of left–right parts of the body (related to accuracy)

PENCIL EXCURSION
Accuracy of figures drawn without vision (related to speed)

EYE MOVEMENT CONTROL
Appropriate saccadic and pursuit tracking movements (related to speed)

Palmar Grasp

The palmar grasp appears earliest in development. Two types of palmar grasp have been described: (1) the radial cross-palmar and (2) the palmar supinated, with the former preceding the latter developmentally. With the palmar grasp, the writing implement is usually held tightly in the palm, as in a power grip. The hand holds the pencil, and the arm and shoulder move it through proximal muscle action. The arm is usually held in the air; neither the wrist nor the elbow touches the writing surface. Approximately 31% of young children with handwriting difficulties tend to use variations of the palmar grasp. These children often move the hand as a single unit, with little or no finger involvement.

CLINICAL *Pearl*

Radial cross-palmar grasp. The pencil tip extends out from the thumb (radial) side of the hand and crosses the thumb.
Palmar supinated grasp. The pencil tip extends out from the little finger (ulnar) side of the hand, with the hand fully fisted in a power grasp.

Prestatic Tripod: Transitional Grasps

A variety of transitional grasps occur before the more consistent use of the static tripod. These include the digital pronated, brush, and cross-thumb grasps.

CLINICAL *Pearl*

Digital pronated grasp. This grasp is essentially the same as a palmar supinated grasp, with the index finger extended along the pencil; the arm and the shoulder move the pencil.
Brush grasp. The pencil is held with the fingers but is positioned against the palm; the palm is pronated; and the wrist and the shoulder move the pencil, with the forearm held in the air.
Cross-thumb grasp. The fingers are tucked loosely in the palm, the pencil is held against the index finger; and the thumb is crossed over the pencil and against the index finger. Both the wrist and the fingers move the pencil, and the forearm is supported against the table.

Static Tripod Grasp

The static tripod grasp is an important and integral step toward the development of the dynamic tripod. In this grasp, the implement is held with the thumb and the index and middle fingers. For the first time, the thumb is in full opposition to the index finger. The pencil rests in the open web space between the thumb and the index finger. The forearm is supported by the table or other support surface. The arm and the shoulder control the action of the implement, with occasional wrist action. The hand moves as a whole unit, with very little or no finger action. Approximately 19% of young children with writing difficulties use this type of grasp.

Predynamic Tripod: Transitional and Frequently Observed Grasps

Several transitional grasps are observed as the child moves toward the consistent use of the dynamic tripod grasp. They include the four-finger grasp, lateral tripod grasp, locked grip with thumb wrap, locked grip with thumb tuck, and quadrupod grip.

CLINICAL *Pearl*

Four-finger grasp. The implement is held with the four fingers and the thumb in opposition. The wrist and the fingers move the pencil, while the forearm is being supported by the table or other writing or drawing surface.
Lateral tripod grasp. The implement is stabilized against the radial side of the middle finger; the thumb is abducted and braced along the lateral border of the index finger. The wrist is slightly extended, with the ring and little fingers flexed to stabilize the grasp. Some finger and wrist action is seen in making vertical and horizontal strokes. The forearm rests on the table.
Locked grip with thumb wrap. This grasp is also commonly called the *white-knuckle grip.* The pencil is pressed against the radial side of the middle finger, with the index finger against the pencil; the thumb is wrapped over the index finger and presses it downward. The ring and little fingers flex to support the pencil. Little or no digital action is seen in moving the implement.
Locked grip with thumb tuck. This grasp is similar to the thumb wrap except that the thumb is tucked under the index and/or middle fingers. Little or no use of the fingers is seen in moving the pencil.
Quadrupod grasp. The pencil is held against the ring, or fourth, finger by the thumb. The little finger is flexed to support and stabilize the pencil. The thumb and the index and middle fingers hold the pencil securely. The pencil is essentially held in the open web space between the index finger and the thumb. This grasp can be either static or dynamic.

Dynamic Tripod Grasp

The dynamic tripod grasp is the preferred mature grasp. The pencil is held between the thumb and the index and middle fingers; the index finger is placed on top of the pencil, with the thumb in full opposition. The ring and little fingers are flexed to stabilize the grasp. The wrist and fingers are used to move the pencil with greater digital control. The arm simply positions the hand for the appropriate manipulation of the pencil by the fingers. The dynamic tripod grasp is typically present by 6 to 7 years of age. Approximately 19% of young children with fine motor problems use this mature grasp. Overall, most children, typically developing or otherwise, use the same hand for cutting and writing. Some of them may use an adapted tripod grasp. The pencil is held between the index and middle fingers, with the thumb pressed against it for stability. The ring and little fingers are flexed to assist in supporting the implement. The action of moving the pencil is similar to that in the dynamic tripod grasp.

DEVELOPMENTAL PROGRESSION OF IMPLEMENT USAGE

The following are simple descriptions of some aspects of the development of pencil usage.[14,39,40] (They may or may not resemble the recovery of similar functions after injury or trauma.)

Scribbling

If given a figure to copy, the young child's reaction is often a spontaneous scribble that bears no resemblance to the figure or model. In other words, the response does not seem to be influenced by the visual configuration. Later, the figure to be copied is given more attention, even though the product may not closely resemble the target figure and is often not reproduced in any detail. Looping is also a common response in scribbling.

Simple Line Drawing

In simple line drawing, the child draws vertical, horizontal, diagonal, and curved lines. Initially, the lines are copied in a large space and in response to a line drawn by another person. With increasing experience and further growth, the child draws lines independently (i.e., without an example) and can do so in structured areas with more narrow boundaries. Drawing vertical, horizontal, and diagonal lines with increasingly greater precision is an important forerunner of skill in writing letters, numbers, and other conventional symbols.

Tracing

The child completes simple dot-to-dot line grids that involve vertical, horizontal, diagonal, and curved lines in various combinations and different degrees of complexity.

Freehand Drawing

Freehand drawing involves both copying (i.e., the item is drawn from a model that is provided) and sketching (the figure is drawn from memory). Various types of configurations, ranging from simple geometric figures to more complex, abstract designs, are used. With regard to geometric shapes, the circle is typically the first one to be mastered (3 years); the cross and square are next (4 years). The progression continues to mastery of the triangle and rectangle; the diamond and the star are the last to be mastered. These latter shapes primarily involve the production of diagonal lines and angles and are typically mastered by 6 to 7 years of age. More complex, abstract designs are accomplished later. The ability to draw or copy shapes accurately is strongly related to copying letters legibly in early childhood.

PREREQUISITE EXPERIENCES FOR WRITING

Experience and practice are important ingredients in mastering pencil skills; a number of foundational experiences are integral to the effective mastery of pencil usage.[2,3,40,42] They include developmental readiness; balance; shoulder, forearm, and wrist stability; object manipulation; functional asymmetry; grasp of the implement; general prewriting; and coloring activities. Each of these experiences is described briefly below.

Developmental Readiness

The child must be ready to write!

Balance

At a minimum, the child must be able to sit independently with good trunk control; this is necessary to free the arms for writing or using an implement. If the balance is poor, the ability to concentrate on writing may be compromised. Therefore, the child should be placed in the most stable position possible. Different positions should be considered, such as prone, sitting in a chair with support, standing at a board, and kneeling at a low table.

Stability

Stability can and should be addressed in many ways. Positions in which the child leans forward and rests the elbows on the table, holds the upper arms at the sides of the body, and performs the activity in a prone position are techniques for improving shoulder and elbow stability. For forearm and wrist stability, weights on the wrists;

placing the weight of the body on the forearms; or writing, drawing, or copying on a board that is slanted are possible techniques.

Object Manipulation

A wide variety of experiences in using and manipulating objects of various sizes, weights, and shapes are important. Incorporating the gross motor eye–hand coordination skills of throwing, catching, and striking are also helpful.

Functional Asymmetry: Lead-Assist Hand Usage

To develop functional asymmetry, incorporate a variety of bimanual tasks that involve manipulation of objects and implements. If the opposite hand cannot be used, the paper can be attached to the writing surface in different ways (e.g., taped or placed on a clipboard). The assist hand may also be used to hold an object or squeeze a ball, Play-Doh, or other object.

Grasp of Writing Tool

To develop a comfortable and efficient grasp, a wide variety of different implements should be used. Pencil grips, triangular-shaped pens, easy-grip crayons, and talking pens are among other possibilities. The child should be involved initially in activities that do not require fine or precise control.

General Prewriting

A broad base of prewriting experiences is important in preparing the child for writing. Writing on different kinds of surfaces (e.g., aluminum foil, waxed paper, sandpaper, paper bags) is important and fun. Tracing around stencils with the finger(s) and around different two- and three-dimensional shapes and using a crayon or other implement (e.g., scented markers, weighted paintbrushes, chalk, toothpick, small stick, thimble on the finger) to trace around different shapes, figures, or objects can be done as well. Writing in the sand, mud, pudding, gelatin, and soap suds are also fun ways to engage the child in prewriting. Using scarves, paper towels, or magic wands to make lines or shapes in the air adds another dimension that challenges the child. Remember that the sequence to follow is from the imitation of the adult's drawing to tracing prepared figures to copying lines, shapes, and letters to writing freehand.

Coloring Activities

In developing or recovering implement usage skills, coloring is an important technique for providing experience. The following are some suggestions that may be used to promote progress. Initially, use a large space or area for coloring; often, the child who is coloring has no real pattern or pays no attention to lines. Proceed to using gradually smaller spaces (e.g., 8.5 × 11 inch paper) and then a circle, a square, or another shape with a ≤6 inches diameter, then a ≤2 inches diameter, and finally smaller designs that are more complex. Each of these steps requires increasingly greater control. The initial response is usually to color with random strokes and go outside the boundaries because of lack of control. This is followed by a more controlled use of unidirectional strokes and moving the paper to fit the stroke direction. Finally, multidirectional strokes are used to fit the design to be colored; the strokes are more controlled and remain within the boundaries of the figure. For additional information on handwriting see Chapter 21.

IMPORTANT MOTOR LEARNING CONCEPTS

Several motor learning concepts, if understood and followed by practitioners, can help facilitate the skill learning/acquisition process.[1,24,26,27] Some of the more common and scientifically sound concepts related to skill acquisition are discussed below. They include transfer of learning, selected aspects of feedback, distribution and variability of practice, whole-part practice, and mental practice. See Table 23-1. OT practitioners are urged to practice using these concepts in practice.

Transfer of Learning

Transfer of learning refers to the influence of the previous practice of, or exposure to, a skill on the learning or acquisition of a new skill. This concept is important because it helps direct the OT clinician in determining the protocol(s) to be used with clients; it can and should be used to determine the sequence in which the skills are practiced. Since the goal of OT is to assist the child in developing the ability to use the skill(s) acquired in the clinical setting in everyday activities, awareness and use of the concept of transfer of learning is important. The following are basic guidelines for applying this concept.

- Skill experiences need to be presented in a logical progression.
- Simple foundational skills should be practiced before more complex skills.
- Skill practice should include practice in real life and simulated real-life settings to enhance transfer.
- Skills with similar components are more likely to show the transfer effect.

TABLE 23-1

William's Motor Learning Principles

TRANSFER OF LEARNING

- Skill experiences need to be presented in logical progression.
- Simple, foundational skills should be practiced before more complex skills.
- Skill practice should include "real" life and simulated settings.
- Skills with similar components are more likely to show transfer effect.

FEEDBACK
Modeling or Demonstration

- Demonstration is best if it is given to the individual prior to practicing the skill and the early stages of skill acquisition.
- Demonstration should be given throughout practice and as frequently as deemed helpful.
- Demonstrations should not be accompanied by verbal commentary as this can reduce attention paid to important aspects of the skill being demonstrated.
- It is important to direct the individual's attention to the critical cues immediately before the skill is demonstrated.

Verbal Instructions

- Verbal cues should be brief, to the point, and involve 1–3 words.
- Verbal cues should be limited in terms of numbers of cues given during or after performance.
- Only the major aspect of the skill that is being concentrated on should be cued.
- Verbal cues should be carefully timed, so they do not interfere with performance.
- Verbal cues can and should be initially repeated by the performer.

Knowledge of Results and Knowledge of Performance

- A variety of different combinations of both KR and KP typically helps to facilitate learning.
- KP error information may help performer change important performance characteristics and thus may help facilitate skill acquisition.
- Information about "appropriate" or "correct" aspects of performance helps to motivate the person to continue practicing.
- It is important to balance between feedback that is error-based and that which is based on "appropriate" or "correct" characteristics of the performance.
- KP feedback can also be descriptive or prescriptive; prescriptive KP is more helpful than just descriptive KP in early or beginning stages of learning.
- KP and KR should be given close in time to but after completion of the task.
- KP and KR typically should not necessarily be given 100% of the time.
- Learning is enhanced if KP/KR are given at least 50% of the time.
- A frequently used procedure for KR/KP is to practice a skill several times and then provide the appropriate feedback.

DISTRIBUTION AND VARIABILITY OF SKILL PRACTICE

- Shorter, more frequent practice sessions are preferable to longer, less frequent practice.
- If a skill or task is complex and/or requires a relatively long time to perform or if it requires repetitive movements, relatively short practice trials/sessions with frequent rest periods are preferable.
- If the skill is relatively simple and takes only a brief time to complete, longer practice trials/sessions with less frequent rest periods are preferable.
- It can enhance skill acquisition to practice several tasks in the same session.

Continued

TABLE 23-1

William's Motor Learning Principles—cont'd

- If several tasks are to be practiced, divide the time spent on each and either randomly repeat practice on each or use a sequence that aids the overall practice.
- Providing a number of different environmental contexts in which the skill is practiced appears to facilitate learning.
- With regard to the amount of practice, more is not necessarily always better.
- Clinical judgment should be used to recognize when practice is no longer producing changes; at this time a new or different task could and probably should be introduced.

WHOLE VERSUS PART PRACTICE

- Whole practice is better when the skill or task to be performed is simple.
- Part practice may be preferable when the skill is more complex.
- If part practice is used, be sure that the parts practiced are "natural units" or "go together" so to speak.
- To simplify a task, reduce the nature and/or complexity of the objects to be manipulated, e.g. use a balloon for catching instead of a ball, etc.
- To simplify a task, provide assistance to the learner that helps to reduce attention demands, e.g. provide trunk support during practice of different eye-hand coordination tasks.
- To simplify a task, provide auditory or rhythmic accompaniment; this may help to facilitate learning through assisting the learner in getting the appropriate "rhythm" of the movement.

MENTAL PRACTICE

- Mental practice can help to facilitate acquisition of new skills as well as the relearning of old skills.
- Mental practice can help the person to prepare to perform a task.
- Mental practice combined with physical practice works best.
- For mental practice to be effective, the individual should have some basic imagery ability.
- Mental practice should be relatively short, not prolonged.

CASE *Study*

Kevin, a 5-year-old boy in kindergarten, has developmental delays. His teacher is concerned that he holds the crayon awkwardly. Kevin scribbles spontaneously but does not imitate horizontal or vertical strokes. His mother is concerned that he is not developing the necessary skills for school and also states that Kevin refuses to practice.

The occupational therapist evaluated Kevin and identified his grasp pattern as a brush grasp. The team decided that Kevin would receive OT services twice weekly in school to work on improving handwriting skills.

Natasha, the occupational therapy assistant (OTA), designed an intervention using the principles of motor learning. She began her treatment session by working on some gross motor activities to ready his posture and attention to fine motor tasks; she presented Kevin with some Lego pieces to build trucks and move them along so that he could work on his hand strength. Finally, Natasha worked with large crayons and allowed Kevin to scribble at first. She showed him how to hold the crayon with a static tripod grasp and allowed him to scribble this way. She then made a road for the Lego truck by drawing a line and asked Kevin to make another one next to it. Kevin was intrigued with the idea of the line; he asked Natasha how to do it. Natasha showed him using a hand-over-hand approach. They drew many roads until he could do it on his own. At the end of the session, Natasha played teacher and asked Kevin to draw vertical lines on a sheet of school paper. She decided to ask the teacher to allow Kevin to use the large crayon and that they would continue to work on his grasp until he was able to hold a regular crayon with a tripod grasp.

Following motor learning principles, Natasha used a logical progression of activities. They practiced simple foundational skills (e.g., posture, hand strength, grasping a large crayon) before the more complex skills. Finally, Natasha simulated school by playing teacher and using school paper. She also asked the teacher to follow through with the work they had done in the session.

Feedback

The use of feedback to inform the learner about his or her progress and about issues that still need to be addressed is integral to developing a skill. Many forms or types of feedback exist. Our focus is on some guidelines for using augmented feedback to promote skill development. The term *augmented* refers to the fact that the feedback information is provided by some external source, either a person or the environment. The goal of augmented feedback is twofold: (1) to help the learner achieve the goal of developing a skill, and (2) to motivate the client to continue to work toward achieving that goal. Several important concepts related to augmented feedback and their roles in improving skill performance are described below.

Modeling or Demonstration

This type of feedback involves providing visual information about how to perform a skill or task. It is a common approach to facilitating skill acquisition and has been shown to be an effective technique. The following are principles that have been shown to hold true in using demonstrations to enhance skill learning:

- Demonstrations are best if they are given to the individual before practicing the skill and in the early stages of skill acquisition.
- Demonstrations should be given throughout practice and as frequently as deemed helpful.
- Demonstrations should not be accompanied by verbal commentary because this can reduce attention devoted to the important aspects of the skill being demonstrated.
- It is important to direct the individual's attention to the critical cues immediately before the skill is demonstrated.

The case study above illustrates these principles; Natasha demonstrated how to hold the pencil and draw the two lines to make a road. During her demonstration, she did not provide verbal commentary but did direct Kevin's attention to the critical cues. "See, I started at the top and went to the bottom; nice, straight roads. I will draw one side; you draw the other." Natasha demonstrated one side; Kevin made the other. Natasha did not say anything while they were making the lines. She would periodically stop and look at the roads and say, "Start at the top and go to the bottom; nice, straight roads."

Verbal Instruction

The practice of a skill is often preceded or accompanied by verbal instruction or cues. These cues can affect the learning or skill acquisition process in positive ways if organized and used appropriately (Box 23-3).

BOX 23-3

Verbal Cues

- Verbal cues should be brief, to the point, and involve one to three words.
- Verbal cues should be limited in terms of the number of cues given during or after the performance.
- Only the major aspect(s) of the skill that is being concentrated on should be cued.
- Verbal cues should be carefully timed so that they do not interfere with the performance.
- Verbal cues can and should be initially repeated by the performer.

During Kevin's session, Natasha provided brief verbal cues such as "nice, straight roads." She did not correct him on holding the crayon but only on the quality of his lines. She repeated these verbal cues throughout the session until Kevin was also saying them.

Knowledge of Results

Knowledge of results (KR) involves information provided from an external source about the outcome, or end result, of the performance of a skill or task. It answers the question: Was the goal achieved? KR is usually provided by the OT clinician; however, at other times, the OT clinician may structure the environment or task such that KR can be a natural part of it. For example, when the OT practitioner says that a client completed the task in 45 seconds, the practitioner is providing information about the outcome of the performance. If the OT practitioner provides a target to throw at, whether the ball or beanbag hits or misses the target, immediate KR is provided about the outcome of the performance (i.e., the performer knows if the goal was achieved). This is a result of structuring the environment to provide information about the outcome of the performance.

Natasha provided Kevin with KR by saying that he had made a road.

Knowledge of Performance

Knowledge of performance (KP) involves providing information about the nature or characteristics of the movement used to perform the task. In other words, the OT clinician provides information about how the task is performed; it answers the question: "What did the individual actually do?" or "How did he or she move to carry out the task?" For example, an OT practitioner might say, "I need you to sit up straight with your back against the chair when you place the pegs"; or he or she might say, "You should use the thumb, index, and middle fingers to grasp the pegs." Both of these suggestions/directions involve providing information about the movement or performance characteristics of KP. If the OT practitioner also said that a client placed 10 pegs in 20 seconds, he or she has provided KR as well. KP can be provided nonverbally as well, for example, with the use of videotapes of actual performance.

A variety of different combinations of both KR and KP typically help facilitate learning. KP error information (information about what the client did incorrectly) may help the performer change important performance characteristics and thus may help facilitate skill acquisition. Information about the appropriate or correct aspects of performance helps motivate the person to continue practicing. It is important to provide a balance between feedback that is error based and that which is based on appropriate or correct characteristics of the performance.

- KP feedback can be descriptive (i.e., describing only the error observed in the performance) or prescriptive (both describing the performance errors and indicating what needs to be done to correct them); prescriptive KP is more helpful than descriptive KP alone in the early or beginning stages of learning.
- KP and KR should be given close in time to but after completion of the task.
- KP and KR should not necessarily be given 100% of the time.
- Learning is enhanced if KR and KP are given at least 50% of the time.
- A frequently used procedure for giving KR and KP is to have the child practice a skill several times and then provide the appropriate feedback.

Natasha asked Kevin which road he liked best, and they drove the truck on that road. This provided him with KP because he was able to see that the road was wide and straight enough for the truck to fit. She emphasized how straight and long the road was, which provides information about the correct aspects of performance. Since they practiced the skill many times, Kevin was provided with plenty of KR and KP feedback.

Another approach to providing feedback is to ask for comments and thoughts from the child. For example, the OT practitioner might ask the child, "Do you understand what you have to do?" Or the OT practitioner may say, "What are two things that you need to think about as you do this?" After completion of the task, it is also appropriate to ask the child for his or her opinion(s) about how he or she performed the task and whether he or she thought the goals had been reached. These

comments can, and probably should, be discussed in preparation for the next practice. This type of interaction with the child also provides a way for the OT practitioner to determine if the child understood the task and how he or she is feeling about how he or she is doing.

Distribution and Variability of Skill Practice

Skills may be practiced in a variety of ways, which include *massed practice* (a practice schedule in which the rest intervals between practice sessions or trials are very short), *distributed practice* (a practice schedule in which the rest intervals are longer), and *variable practice* (practice experiences in which there are a variety of tasks in different environmental contexts).

- Shorter, more frequent practice sessions are preferable to longer, less frequent practice sessions.
- Relatively short practice trials or sessions with frequent rest periods are preferable if a skill or task is complex and/or requires a relatively long time to perform or it requires repetitive movements.
- Longer practice trials or sessions with less frequent rest periods are preferable if the skill is relatively simple and takes only a brief time to complete.
- Practicing several tasks in the same session can enhance skill acquisition.
- If several tasks are to be practiced, divide the time spent on each, and either randomly repeat them or use a sequence that aids the overall practice.
- Providing a number of different environmental contexts in which the skill is practiced appears to facilitate learning.
- With regard to the amount of practice, more is not necessarily always better.
- Clinical judgment should be used to recognize when practice is no longer producing changes; at this time, a new or different task could and probably should be introduced.

CASE *Study*

Delia, a 9-year-old girl, has developmental coordination disorder. She exhibits poor hand strength, poor quality of movement, and poor coordination. The team decided that Delia must learn to type efficiently so that she can eventually use a laptop for course work. Shauna, the OTA, has developed a plan for Delia to use a computer typing program daily for 10 minutes at school and two nights at home. The typing program is designed for children, and frequent rest breaks are embedded in the program. Delia is allowed to repeat the same session if she wishes to. She is also encouraged to use the computer in the classroom for assignments. The teacher is aware that it may take her longer at the start.

This plan takes into account the principles and the variability of skill practice outlined above. Specifically, Delia will engage in shorter, more frequent sessions (10 minutes 5 days a week and two nights at home). Since typing is a complex task, the program has frequent rest breaks. Furthermore, Delia will be practicing several typing tasks during the session (e.g., hand position, accuracy, timing, copying). The tasks are set to be practiced at the child's level so that Delia will not get frustrated or overwhelmed. The OTA has designed the session such that Delia practices in school and at home to provide different environmental contexts. Since more practice is not always better, the OTA will be careful to recognize when Delia needs a new or different task. The computer program also allows for some variability in the tasks.

Whole versus Part Practice

How a skill is practiced is important. In general, skills may be practiced as a whole or in parts. The three major approaches to part practice are: (1) fractionalization, which is an approach to part practice that is often used with bimanual skills; each arm/hand is practiced separately before the two are put together to perform the task; (2) the progressive part method, which is an approach that involves dividing the skill into its component parts; one part is practiced initially, and then another one is added to the first until the whole skill is completed; and (3) simplification, which is a part approach that involves simplifying the task in a variety of ways. The critical ingredient in any approach to part practice is identifying the appropriate parts.

- Whole practice is better when the skill or task to be performed is simple.
- Part practice may be preferable when the skill is more complex.
- If part practice is used, be sure that the parts practiced are natural units or go together.
- To simplify a task, reduce the nature and/or complexity of the objects to be manipulated (e.g., use a balloon, instead of a ball, for catching).
- To simplify a task, provide assistance that helps reduce attention demands (e.g., provide trunk support during the practice of different eye–hand coordination tasks).
- To simplify a task, provide auditory or rhythmic accompaniment; this may help facilitate learning through assisting the learner to get the appropriate rhythm of the movement.

CASE *Study*

Corey, the OTA, is working on improving the ability of 3-year-old Donovan to feed himself with the use of a spoon. Before practicing the task, Corey works with Donovan to be sure that he can sit independently in a supportive chair and can hold a spoon (part practice). Once Donovan is positioned in a supportive high chair, Corey provides finger foods to Donovan, who quickly picks up the food and brings it to his mouth. This is a natural unit for spoon-feeding. Corey then brings out Donovan's favorite pudding. He holds the spoon but has difficulty keeping it upright once it is full of pudding. Corey allows Donovan to spill the pudding and helps him correct his grasp of the spoon. Later, Corey builds up the tray so that Donovan does not have to bring up the spoon so far to his mouth (i.e., reducing the demands of the task).

Corey structured the session such that Donovan could complete the task. It is not desirable to bring a spoon halfway to the mouth; this is not functional. Therefore, Corey adapted the environment such that Corey could achieve the task, which would promote more practice of this skill. Corey may be able to move the tray closer to the original position in the next session.

Mental Practice

Mental practice involves cognitive or mental rehearsal of a skill; it is done without actually moving, and typically involves mental imagery (i.e., mentally picturing oneself practicing the skill).

- Mental practice can help facilitate the acquisition of new skills as well as the relearning of old ones.
- Mental practice can help the person prepare to perform a task.
- Mental practice combined with physical practice works best.
- For mental practice to be effective, the individual should have some basic ability to use imagery.
- Mental practice should be relatively short, not prolonged.

Children with developmental coordination disorders have at least average intelligence quotients (IQs) and are therefore able to practice the skills mentally. Clinicians can encourage older children to picture themselves completing motor tasks. After the child completes the task, it may be beneficial to review the performance to help him or her develop mental imaging strategies.

SUMMARY

This chapter provides a brief look at the foundations of fine motor development and the intricacies of a number of components contributing to, and critical in, the development of fine motor skills. The description of the steps involved in the development of object manipulation and implement usage skills provides a simple guideline that can be used in organizing and planning appropriate sequences for therapeutic activity. Last, but not the least, a number of simplified motor learning concepts along with some behavioral examples are presented; they are designed to help support the planning of practice for the learning and/or relearning of a wide variety of fine motor skills and should be helpful to the thoughtful and caring OT clinician.

References

1. Bass-Haugen J, Mathiowetz V, Flinn N: Optimizing motor behavior using the occupational therapy task-oriented approach. In Trombly C, Radomski M, editors: *Occupational therapy for physical dysfunction*, Philadelphia, 2002, Lippincott Williams and Wilkins.

2. Benbow M: Principles and practices of teaching handwriting. In Henderson A, Pehoski C, editors: *Hand function in the child: Foundations for remediation*, St Louis, 1995, Mosby.

3. Benbow M, Hanft B, Marsh D: Handwriting in the classroom: Improving written communication. In Royeen CB, editor: *AOTA self-study series: Classroom applications for school-based practice*, Rockville, MD, 1992, American Occupational Therapy Association.

4. Berninger V, Rutber J: Relationship of finer function to beginning writing: Application to diagnosis of writing disabilities, *Dev Med Child Neurol* 34:198, 1992.

5. Case-Smith J: Comparison of in-hand manipulation skills in children with and without fine motor delays, *Occup Ther J Res* 13:87, 1993.

6. Case-Smith J: Hand function and developmental coordination disorder. In Cermak S, Larkin D, editors: *Developmental coordination disorder*, Albany, NY, 2002, Delmar Thomson Learning.

7. Cermak S: Somatodyspraxia. In Fisher A, Murray E, Bundy A, editors: *Sensory integration: Theory and practice*, Philadelphia, 1991, FA Davis.

8. Connolly J, Dalgleish M: The emergence of a tool-using skill in infancy, *Dev Psychol* 25:894, 1989.

9. Daly J, Kelley G, Krauss A: Relationship between visual-motor integration and handwriting skills of children in kindergarten: A modified replication study, *Am J Occup Ther* 57:459, 2003.

10. Deuel R: Developmental dysgraphia and motor skill disorders, *J Child Neurol* 10:57, 1995.

11. Eliasson A: Sensorimotor integration of normal and impaired development of precision movement of the hand. In Henderson A, Pehoski C, editors: *Hand function in the child: Foundations for remediation*, St. Louis, 1995, Mosby.

12. Exner C: Development of hand skills. In Case-Smith J, O'Brien J, editor: *Occupational therapy for children*, ed 6, St Louis, 2010, Mosby.

13. Exner C: In-hand manipulation skills. In Case-Smith J, Pehoski C, editors: *Development of hand skills in the child*, Rockville, MD, 1992, American Occupational Therapy Association.

14. Folio R, Fewell R: *Peabody developmental motor scales*, Allen, TX, 1983, DLM Teaching Resources.

15. Hill E, Wing A: A dyspraxic deficit in specific language impairment and developmental coordination disorder? Evidence from hand and arm movements, *Dev Med Child Neurol* 40:388, 1998.

16. Hill E, Wing A: Coordination of grip force and load force in developmental coordination disorder: A case study, *Neurocase* 5:537, 1999.

17. Hill E, Wing A: Developmental disorders and the use of grip force to compensate for inertial forces during voluntary movement. In Connolly KJ, editor: *Psychobiology of the hand*, London, UK, 1998, Mac Keith Press.

18. Hulme C, Smart A, Moran G, et al: Visual, kinaesthetic and cross-modal development: Relationship to motor skill development, *Perception* 12:477, 1983.

19. Jucaite A, Fernell E, Forssberg H, et al: Deficient coordination of associated postural adjustments during a lifting task in children with neurodevelopmental disorders, *Dev Med Child Neurol* 45:731, 2003.

20. Kuhtz-Buschbeck J, Hoppe B, Golge M, et al: Sensorimotor recovery in children after traumatic brain injury: Analyses of gait, gross motor, and fine motor skills, *Dev Med Child Neurol* 45:821, 2003.

21. Langaas, T., Mon-Williams, M., P. Wann, J., Pascal, E., & Thompson, C. (1998). Eye movements, prematurity and developmental co-ordination disorder. *Vision Research*, 38(12), 1817-1826.

22. Lederman S, Klatzky R: The hand as a perceptual system. In Connolly KJ, editor: *Psychobiology of the hand*, London, UK, 1998, Mac Keith Press.

23. Lundy-Ekman L, Ivery R, Keele S, et al: Timing and force control deficits in clumsy children, *J Cogn Neurosci* 3:367, 1991.

24. Magill R: *Motor learning: Concepts and applications*, New York, 2001, McGraw-Hill.

25. Meulenbroek R, van Galen G: Perceptual-motor complexity of printed and cursive letters, *J Exp Educ* 58:95, 1990.

26. Missiuna C, Mandich A: Integrating motor learning theories into practice. In Cermak S, Larkin D, editors: *Developmental coordination disorder*, Albany, NY, 2002, Delmar Thomson Learning.

27. Niemeijer A, Smits-Engelsman B, Reynders K, et al: Verbal actions of physiotherapists to enhance motor learning in children with DCD, *Hum Movement Sci* 22:567, 2003.

28. Pehoski C: Object manipulation in infants and children. In Henderson A, Pehoski C, editors: *Hand function in the child: Foundations for remediation*, St Louis, 1995, Mosby.

29. Pitcher T, Piek J, Hay D: Fine and gross motor ability in males with ADHD, *Dev Med Child Neurol* 45:525, 2003.

30. Preminger F, Weiss P, Weintraub N: Predicting occupational performance: Handwriting versus keyboarding, *Am J Occup Ther* 58:193, 2004.

31. Rodger S, Ziviani J, Watter P, et al: Motor and functional skills of children with developmental coordination disorder: A pilot investigation of measurement issues, *Hum Movement Sci* 22:461, 2003.

32. Rosblad B, van Hofsten C: Repetitive goal-directed arm movements in children with developmental coordination disorders: Role of visual information, *Adapt Phys Activ Quart* 11:190, 1994.

33. Schneck C: Comparison of pencil-grip patterns in first graders with good and poor writing skills, *Am J Occup Ther* 45:701, 1991.

34. Schneck M, Henderson A: Descriptive analysis of the developmental progression of grip position for pencil and crayon control in nondysfunctional children, *Am J Occup Ther* 44:893, 1990.

35. Smits-Engelsman B, Wilson P, Westenberg Y, et al: Fine motor deficiencies in children with developmental coordination disorder and learning disabilities: An underlying open-loop control deficit, *Hum Movement Sci* 2:495, 2003.

36. Thomassen A, Teulings H: The development of handwriting. In Martlew M, editor: *The psychology of written language*, New York, 1983, John Wiley & Sons, Inc.

37. Weil M, Cunningham Amundson S: Relationship between visual motor and handwriting skills of children in kindergarten, *Am J Occup Ther* 48:982, 1994.

38. Williams H: Motor control in children with developmental coordination disorder. In Cermak S, Larkin D, editors: *Developmental coordination disorder*, Albany, NY, 2002, Delmar Thomson Learning.

39. Williams H: *Perceptual and motor development*, Englewood Cliffs, NJ, 1983, Prentice-Hall, Inc.

40. Williams H: *Smart text: Fine motor control and development*, Columbia, SC, 2004, University of South Carolina.

41. Williams H, Woollacott M, Ivry R: Timing and motor control in clumsy children, *J Mot Behav* 24:165, 1992.

42. Ziviani J: The development of graphomotor skills. In Henderson A, Pehoski C, editors: *Hand function in the child: foundations for remediation*, St Louis, 1995, Mosby.

Recommended Reading

Benbow M: Hand skills and handwriting. In Cermak S, Larkin D, editors: *Developmental coordination disorder*, Albany, NY, 2001, Delmar Thomson Learning.

Schmidt R: *Motor control and learning: A behavioral emphasis*, ed 4, Chicago, IL, 2005, Human Kinetics Publishers, Inc.

REVIEW *Questions*

1. Define and differentiate between the following terms: *motor adaptation*, *motor control*, *motor learning*, and *occupation*.

2. Describe an OT session that teaches a child to use both hands together using random practice.

3. Describe how you would provide a child feedback and demonstration using motor learning principles.

4. Describe how the principles of motor control would be applied to teach a child to button a shirt. Be sure to discuss demonstration, feedback, practice, adaptations, and so on.

5. Describe the progression of fine motor skill development.

SUGGESTED *Activities*

1. Demonstrate an OT activity to improve fine motor skills using massed, distributive, and variable practice, and distributed practice. Discuss the benefits of one type of practice over the other.

2. List five principles of motor learning, and describe how you would use these to teach a child a new skill.

3. Bring in an item that could be used as an activity in a fine motor or gross motor kit. Discuss how this item could be used in the clinic, with special emphasis on the client factor it addresses. All of you can share your items so that everyone leaves with a variety of items that may be useful in the clinic.

4. Visit a Web site to find activities that would improve fine or gross motor skills in children. Share the activities and Web sites with your classmates so that they may be used as a resource.

5. Observe typical children learning a new fine motor or gross motor skill. Which teaching techniques were helpful, and why? How could these techniques be used in OT practice?

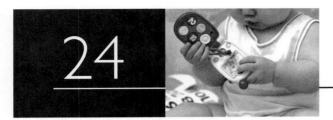

Sensory Processing/
Integration
and Occupation

RICARDO C. CARRASCO

SUSAN STALLINGS-SAHLER

CHAPTER *Objectives*

After studying this chapter, the reader will be able to accomplish the following:

- Define the basic principles underlying sensory integration theory, assessment, and treatment
- Review sensorimotor, perceptual motor, environmental adaptations, and other approaches used in alleviating sensory processing disorders
- Understand the role of the certified occupational therapy assistant in working with children who have sensory processing disorders
- Define sensory modulation disorder
- Describe sensory modulation observational assessment and intervention strategies
- Describe sensory discrimination intervention strategies
- Understand the types of sensory-based movement disorder and intervention strategies
- Identify/describe intervention methods for children who have postural–ocular and bilateral integration dysfunction
- Identify/describe intervention techniques to work with children who have developmental dyspraxia

KEY TERMS

CHAPTER OUTLINE

Dr. A. Jean Ayres, the originator of sensory integration (SI) theory, assessment, and treatment, strongly believed and advocated that the practice of SI by an occupational therapist should take place only at the postgraduate level. SI theory, assessment, and treatment are extremely complex, although the activities appear deceptively easy because they are very playful when effectively implemented by a skilled therapist. However, in settings with close supervision by an appropriately SI-trained and experienced pediatric occupational therapist, the occupational therapy assistant (OTA) can contribute effectively to the intervention program for **sensory integration dysfunction**.

The term *sensory processing* refers to the means by which the brain receives, detects, and integrates incoming sensory information for use in producing adaptive responses to one's environment. Children who have sensory integrative dysfunction have a cluster of symptoms that are believed to reflect dysfunction in central nervous system (CNS) processing of sensory input rather than a primary sensory deficit such as hearing or visual impairment; a frank CNS insult such as *cerebrovascular accident* (CVA, or stroke) or *traumatic brain injury* (TBI); or even deficits that come from chromosomal or genetic abnormalities such as Down syndrome. The disorder leads to disorganized, maladaptive interactions with people and objects in the environment. Such interaction, in turn, produces distorted internal sensory feedback, which reinforces the problem.[5]

However, there are several subtypes of **sensory processing dysfunction**. Whereas individuals with SI dysfunction (or those with sensory processing dysfunction) share many similarities, they do not all appear alike. Children with the disorder often have a primary diagnosis such as autism, learning disability, or attention deficit disorder; or *psychogenic comorbidities* related to anxiety, panic, or attachment disorder. Also, a range of levels of severity, from mild to quite severe, exist. In some children, sensory processing dysfunction may lead to disabling learning problems, causing academic failure.[5] In others, it may be reflected in clumsiness and the struggle of the child to perform everyday occupations that others take for granted. Whereas some children may exhibit impairment in the ability to regulate incoming sensations, others may fail to detect and orient to novel or important sensory information, which is called **sensory modulation disorder**.[5,6,12,62,68]

Some types of sensory processing impairment may lead to poor social adaptation; the inability to form close, intimate relationships; and difficulty in expressing and interpreting socioemotional cues.[44] Led by the pioneering work of Jean Ayres, occupational therapists have examined and developed treatment strategies for sensory integrative dysfunction in the early intervention and school-age populations since the early 1970s.[2,4,5,8,10,12,33,42,59,62,58,71]

The early signs of sensory processing problems can be observed even in infancy (Figure 24-1).[63] Parents often report that they have noticed subtle differences—such as lack of cuddling behavior, failure to make eye contact, oversensitivity to sounds or touch, difficulty with the oral–motor demands of suckling, and chewing food—as early as in the perinatal period (Figure 24-2).[45,70] Poor *self-regulation* of arousal states, irritability, and colic are frequently reported.[1,46,67,70] In the toddler period, the motor, social, and self-care milestones may be delayed. The child may lack normal curiosity about the environment. On the other hand, he or she may explore the world in a disorganized and destructive manner, which does not lead to learning and mastery. Figuring out basic whole body movements, for example, climbing downstairs backwards or climbing onto a riding toy, are bewildering and frightening tasks.[61,63]

The preschooler with sensory-based motor planning problems may be unable to organize the body postures and gestures that are appropriate for nonverbal communication, such as the need for affection, to use the toilet, or for a favorite snack.[63] Typically developing preschoolers can seem almost mesmerized with learning the process of dressing and will attempt the donning and doffing of clothes, shoes, and coats seemingly for hours at a time. However, the child with sensory-based motor planning deficits (called *dyspraxia*) may be dependent on caregivers for assistance and often avoids dressing and hygiene activities altogether. He or she may handle toys and objects ineptly, constantly damaging or breaking them.

As the child attains school age, the heightened challenges of the elementary grades—sitting at a desk, paying attention in class, reading, listening, using writing and art tools, and interacting with peers—bring sensory processing dysfunction to light even more. During leisure time, the child may avoid fine manipulative activities or skilled gross motor play, instead preferring more sedentary activities such as watching television, playing video games, looking at books (Figure 24-3). Highly creative and intelligent children may conceal their motor control inadequacies by engaging in verbal make-believe play, which emphasizes imagination and social interaction (with a lot of aimless running around) over toy manipulation and body coordination.

Occupational therapy (OT) practitioners need to consider observations such as the above behaviors within the context of the child's family system, cultural expectations and norms, and socioeconomic advantages and limitations. As members of a team of professionals, they also utilize multiple sources of information from co-workers about the child's cognitive, language, and social development because these areas of function will

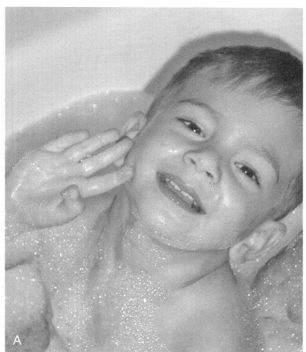

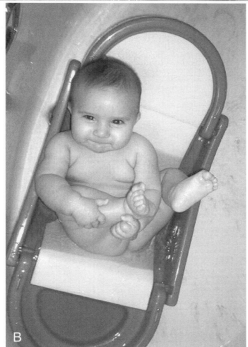

FIGURE 24-1 A, Typically developing children enjoy sensory experiences such as bath time. **B,** Typically developing infants enjoy the sensory experience of finding their feet and playing in the bath.

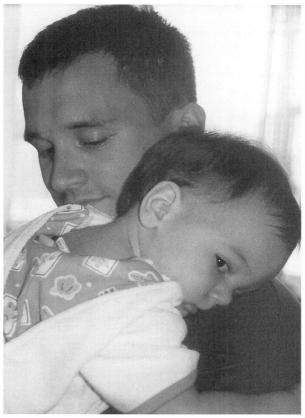

FIGURE 24-2 Whereas typically developing children gain comfort in being held closely by their fathers, those with sensory processing difficulties may find it discomforting.

have significant effects on the quality of the child's adaptive behavior.[29] A child whose sociocultural and socioeconomic environments do not provide adequate opportunities for movement, exploration, and object play may need environmental enrichment to facilitate the emergence of motor planning skills.

SCREENING AND ASSESSMENT OF SENSORY PROCESSING

Initial OT evaluation typically employs a *top-down approach*, the first tier of focus being the child's daily occupational and role performance.[31,65] However, it may become apparent during the evaluation of occupational performance that sensory processing deficits are major contributors to the child's functional difficulties, although the specific nature of the deficits cannot be delineated without further assessment. The OTA may be trained to physically administer a number of sensorimotor screening tests and other structured assessments of sensory processing and/or motor performance. However,

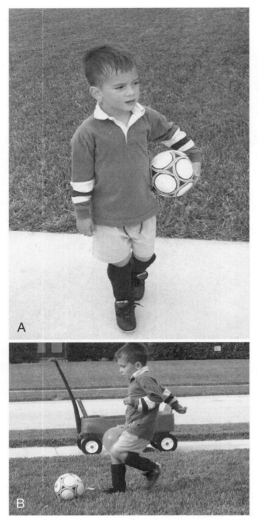

FIGURE 24-3 A, A child's ability to participate successfully in leisure/play activities such as soccer requires coordination, motor planning, sequencing, timing, and body awareness. **B,** The child shows adequate coordination, motor planning, sequencing, timing, and body awareness as he kicks the soccer ball in the desired direction.

the *interpretation* of the results should be performed by the occupational therapist, with the OTA providing important insights about the child. The OT practitioner will often collect this type of information on the children referred for OT because sensory processing dysfunction frequently contributes to the occupational performance difficulties for which children are referred, such as poor fine motor/handwriting skills, trouble with self-care tasks, social–emotional problems, or inability to participate in gross motor play activities with peers.

A very important part of the assessment process includes getting initial data from observations of the child by his or her caregivers, teachers, and/or other therapists. If the existence of a sensorimotor processing issue cannot be ascertained, the OTA and his or her supervisor may then decide to administer a standardized screening test. Based on the results of those two sources, an experienced team of OT practitioners may have enough data to formulate an intervention plan. Otherwise, a decision may be made to pursue more comprehensive evaluation of the child's capacities for sensory processing.[22]

A complete sensory processing evaluation typically covers five major areas: (1) sensory modulation across each sensory system (i.e., tactile, vestibular, visual, auditory, olfactory, and taste); (2) perceptual discrimination ability in most of these areas; (3) postural–ocular function; (4) bilateral motor coordination (including organization at and across the midline of the body); and (5) **praxis** (the ability to internally visualize and plan skilled or unfamiliar movement actions).[6,18] However, the OT supervisor may elect to focus on fewer areas if the initial OT assessment and SI screening indicate that certain areas are not problematic.

Observational and History-Taking Assessment

Observation of the child in his or her *natural environments* is essential because not only can it identify areas in which sensory issues may be present, but it should also demonstrate how those issues affect the child's performance during daily occupational roles and tasks. The main concerns of the child, family, and others usually relate to difficulties with vital age-expected play skills, social activities, capacity for self-regulation, and academic learning that the child must master to grow up successfully. It is to these concerns that attention must be paid, and then, like peeling away the layers of an onion, the "why?" underlying those occupational challenges must be probed.

CASE *Study*

Jason's teacher may report that his letter formation is acceptable, but his handwriting movements are slow and laborious, and he presses down so hard that he tears his paper or breaks the pencil lead. He stops frequently to shake or stretch his fingers and complains of pain in his hand. Consequently, Jason fails to complete both classroom and homework written assignments on time, and his grades are suffering. His parents complain that it is a struggle each night at home to get Jason to begin and complete his written homework.

In this case, the inability to complete handwritten assignments is the occupational activity that initially brought about the referral. However, assuming that other causes have been ruled out, sensory processing theory and research evidence can be used to analyze the qualitative nature of Jason's handwriting. From this, it can be hypothesized that Jason is receiving insufficient *proprioceptive* feedback from the joints and muscles in his fingers; so he must bear down harder on his pencil to obtain it, and this assists him in controlling and guiding the pencil. This attempt to respond adaptively to his impairment slows Jason's progress and creates exceptional fatigue and discomfort in his hand and finger joints. This hypothesis must then be tested by means of a sensory processing evaluation of Jason's *somatosensory* (tactile-pressure sense) *system*.

The hypothesis about the contribution of sensory processing dysfunction will help shape one aspect of the intervention approach, which will probably include activation of Jason's proprioceptive system before handwriting activities. Therefore, when relating the SI assessment results to caregivers and other members of the team and in planning a course of intervention, the OT team must bring their interpretation of sensory processing issues full circle to explain their concern about the child's occupational performance, which was the original source of the referral. Furthermore, either classroom or direct service interventions to address the underlying sensory processing issues will be recommended (Figure 24-4).

Multiple observation checklists are available for use.[24] Some can be found in pediatric OT textbooks, whereas others are available for purchase from test publishers. Some checklists are informal and based on SI problem

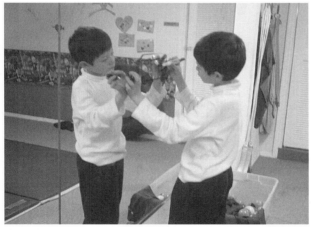

FIGURE 24-4   Children with sensory processing difficulties may experience poor body awareness. Standing while writing may help them become more aware of their bodies and movements. This child writes on a mirror, which also provides visual cues to help him.

behaviors cited in the clinical literature rather than on norms derived from children of various ages. They can be used to gain informative data from teachers as well as caregivers. Such tools can be helpful if used with the age range intended.[19] Two examples of such tools are *The Sensorimotor History Questionnaire* and *The Teacher Questionnaire of Sensory Behavior* (see Appendices A and B at the end of this chapter).[25, 27,28]

Formal Assessment Tools

> **CLINICAL** *Pearl*
>
> Informal checklists, as in the examples given in the text above, should never form the entire basis of the conclusions made about a child's sensorimotor functioning.

Formal rating scales are based on knowledge of a child's developmental history and direct observation and are administered by trained professionals who know the child's behaviors, abilities, and preferences well. Such scales are often well researched and standardized on normative groups and fit into the class of SI screening instruments. A summary of them can be found in the literature, and some are described in Table 24-1.[21]

Comprehensive Evaluation of Sensory Processing/Integration

The most comprehensive standardized test battery of sensory integrative functioning for children ages 4 years and 0 months through 8 years and 11 months is the *Sensory Integration and Praxis Test (SIPT)*.[3] These tests include measures of vestibular, proprioceptive, and somatosensory processing; visual perceptual and *visuomotor integration*; integration between the two sides of the body; and many of the components of the complex set of abilities known as *praxis*. The praxis tests include measures of postural imitation, motor planning in response to a verbal request, motor sequencing ability, imitation of oral movements, graphic reproduction, and three-dimensional block construction.[2,3,11]

Because of its complexity, only certain licensed rehabilitation professionals with a baccalaureate or graduate degree who have undergone documented rigorous training may administer the SIPT. To become more familiar with the various components of SI evaluation, pediatric OTAs should have a qualified SIPT examiner administer this instrument to them and engage in a reflective discussion of their experiences. This will provide valuable insights about both the process of SI and its assessment.

TABLE 24-1

Summary of Screening or Structured Assessments of Sensory Processing and Sensory-Based Motor Dysfunction

NAME OF SCREENING TOOL	STATED PURPOSE	INTENDED AGE RANGE
Test of Sensory Function in Infants[33]	Designed to measure an infant's sensory reactivity and processing to determine the presence and extent of the deficit	4–18 months
The Infant/Toddler Sensory Profile[36]	By means of the parents' report, measures infant and toddler reactions to everyday sensory events across all modalities	Birth–36 months
The Sensory Profile[35]	Measures child's responses to sensory experiences as well as perceived movement competence by means of the parents' report	3–10 years
The Short Sensory Profile[51]	A one-page questionnaire with 38 items divided into 7 sections; answers based on a 5-point scale	3–10 years
The Adolescent/Adult Sensory Profile[40]	Self-report; measures responses of teens through mature adults to sensory events in everyday life	11–90 years
The First STEP Screening Test for the Evaluation of Preschoolers (Parent Checklists)[52]	General screening of major developmental areas, including several creative items of bilateral integration and praxis	2 years, 9 months– 6 years, 2 months
The DeGangi-Berk Test of Sensory Integration[34]	A total of 36 items that measure overall sensory integration as well as postural control, bilateral motor integration, and reflex integration	3–5 years
The Miller Assessment for Preschoolers[53]	Broad overview of a child's developmental status; several indices assessing key areas of sensory integration performance	2 years, 9 months– 5 years, 8 months
Clinical Observations of Sensory Integration[2] Clinical Observations Based on Sensory Integration Theory[14]	Informal floor assessment primarily assessing a child's postural reactions and oculomotor responses that are included in most neurologic screenings of soft neurologic signs	Various ages; recommended for approx. ages 5–10 years
Bruininks-Oseretsky Test of Motor Proficiency[17]	Both short screening and long evaluation forms included; measures a variety of gross and fine motor skills; includes many items for assessing bilateral coordination	4.6–14.5 years

One of the most challenging aspects of the interpretation of SI and praxis evaluation data is the lack of a concrete one-to-one correspondence between a low score on a particular test and the meaning of that score. Invariably, the SI assessment is about discovering the underlying sensory disorganization that leads to poor performance in one or more functional "end products." In the typically developing child, these end products can come in the form of functional motor skills such as riding a bicycle or using tools, academic learning skills such as reading and computation, cognitive abilities such as language and abstract thinking, or psychosocial capacities such as emotional attachment and self-esteem. It is the end products of sensory integration which enable children to participate in age-appropriate occupational tasks and roles. However, between sensory organization and these end products there are also intermediate abilities termed *functional support capacities* by Kimball.[47] **Functional support capacities** represent secondary neurobehavioral, motor, social–emotional, and cognitive proficiencies that are not functional in the occupational sense but are considered precursors for end products to develop normally. A number of these are measured by the SIPT and other tests and include components such as self-regulatory mechanisms, *postural tone*, *bilateral motor coordination*, ability to cross the midline of the body, various subtypes of praxis, *cognitive sequencing*, and other intermediate-level capacities. Therefore, numerous patterns of underlying dysfunction are possible; end product impairments are interpreted according to the way in which the SI and praxis test scores cluster.

CASE *Study*

Two 7-year-old children, Emma and Brian, present with severe handwriting problems along with other fine motor difficulties. However, their SIPT results are distinctly different. Emma's profile displays a low score on copying designs along with many low scores on visual and tactile space perception and low postrotary nystagmus (a vestibular marker), but her scores on the motor accuracy and praxis tests fall within normal limits. By comparison, Brian's SIPT profile also shows a low score on copying designs, but the postrotary nystagmus and visual and tactile space perception scores are in the normal range. However, his motor accuracy performance is poor, the scores on a number of praxis tests are low, and he has low scores on finger identification, touch localization, and kinesthetic perception.

Both these children had similar end product outcomes, yet their SI and praxis evaluations demonstrated significantly different sensory processing and functional support pathways. Emma's pattern of scores suggests that her poor handwriting and design reproduction skills are probably attributable to impaired *visual space perception* resulting from poor integration of vestibular, somatosensory, and visual sensory input. On the other hand, disorganized *motor planning*, which is attributable to the inefficient processing of upper extremity proprioceptive input and a poor body scheme, is the hypothesized source of Brian's impaired handwriting.

Herein lies the difference between a sensory processing evaluation approach and a direct occupation-based assessment model. The former is based on an attempt to measure the underlying neuromotor and sensory mechanisms that support the function and occupation (in our example, poor handwriting). The latter approach documents and describes the nature of the occupational outcomes. Accordingly, OT interventions based on a *top-down teaching* strategy to address handwriting issues might look very similar for these two children. However, an SI approach would take the differences in underlying sensorimotor organization into consideration, and the SI treatment program for these two children would look quite different. It should also be noted that these two approaches are not mutually exclusive and probably should be used in tandem, with sensory integration strategies applied first in order to prepare the CNS for the direct teaching of the desired occupational skill.

In summary, research using the SIPT as well as Ayres's earlier tests has demonstrated that (1) various aspects of the components of sensory discrimination, bilateral motor organization, and motor planning tend to group together statistically to form predictable clusters; (2) developmental trends can be identified in most SI constructs; and (3) certain sensory systems integrate with one another to give rise to higher-order capacities in behavior and ability.[3,5,7,9] With regard to the role of the additional neurobehavioral construct of sensory modulation, although Ayres originally identified the phenomenon of *sensory registration disorders*, which are now called sensory modulation disorders, she died before she was able to pursue a more objective method of measurement of these disorders. Fortunately, others have taken up this area of work.[35,36,39,40,55,56,57,58,68,69] Research on psychophysiologic measurement has contributed significantly to our understanding in this area.[36,38-40,49-51,54,55,57,58,69,70]

SENSORY MODULATION DISORDER

When an OT practitioner hears terms such as *tactile defensiveness*, *gravitational insecurity*, sensory-seeking, and sensory hypersensitivity, he or she is exposed to some of the clinical language that refers to behaviors representing the class of sensory processing impairments termed *sensory modulation disorder*. Normal sensory modulation is a regulatory process of the nervous system that controls the perceived intensity of incoming sensations through the raising or lowering of neuronal thresholds to that sensory input. This is achieved by means of adaptive balancing of inhibition and excitation at many levels of the CNS. Excitation of a neuron tends to lower its threshold to stimulation, thereby allowing more of the sensory input to be experienced in the nervous system. In contrast, if there is more inhibition, the neuronal threshold tends to rise, in effect partially or fully blocking the sensory input from being registered in a person's awareness. Your CNS is regulating sensations in this way as you read this chapter. If it did not, on the one hand, your brain might be so flooded with sensory messages that you would not be able to focus your attention, control your posture, or think about what you are reading. On the other hand, you might have such high sensory thresholds that you overfocus, being unable to hear someone calling you from another room, feel a tap on your shoulder, or sense that your body is about to fall out of a chair.

This is only an imaginary taste of what life is like for people with sensory modulation dysfunction. However, some have sensory experiences that are so distorted that everyday sensations are uncomfortable, painful, frightening, or surreal in nature. A woman with *agoraphobia* and sensory modulation disorder reported to one of the authors that at times she would be walking on a concrete floor in a department store and suddenly feel as if the floor were soft and her feet were going through it, rather than striking the hard surface. At other times, she had trouble falling asleep because she felt as if bugs were crawling on her, or she was unable to habituate to the sound of a clock ticking in another room. Children commonly manifest sensory modulation irregularities by their intolerance of such stimuli as clothing, food textures, imposed touch, and household noises (e.g., a phone ringing or an appliance running) or, conversely, by not noticing salient stimuli in their environment. Probably the earliest harbinger of SI dysfunction in infancy is unusual over-reactivity to touch, taste, or smell. Some forms of *gastric reflux* in infancy appear to be precipitated not by gastroesophageal abnormalities but by olfactory hypersensitivity, which causes the infant to become nauseous.[64]

Examples of hyper- and hypo-reactivity can be identified as you look through *The Sensory History Questionnaire* (SHQ) shared previously. Research in which *The Sensory Profile* and *The Adolescent and Adult Sensory Profile* were used revealed that children and adults develop behavioral patterns of dealing with their modulation problems, which have been described by Dunn in her model of sensory processing.[15,16,37,39] These patterns tend to divide into four quadrants that are bounded by (1) a continuum of sensory avoidance to sensory seeking, and (2) a continuum of acting *in accordance with threshold*, to acting *to counteract threshold*. We all fall within one of these quadrants, but dysfunction lies more at the extreme ends of the continua, where a person's daily life and relationships are more apt to be disrupted by modulatory irregularities. These patterns of sensory modulation are also associated with various types of *temperament*, as identified by Thomas and Chess.[32,66] For more information on this, the reader is referred to the work of Dunn, Miller, Wilbarger, and associates.[35,37,52,58,59,60,62,70,71]

SENSORY-BASED MOVEMENT DISORDER

Sensory-based movement disorder refers to both (1) postural system disorganization due to poor vestibular and proprioceptive processing, and (2) impairments of complex midbrain or cortically controlled internal visualization and motor planning. Children who are found to have sensory integrative problems leading to **postural-ocular and bilateral integration dysfunction** typically manifest poor vestibular–proprioceptive processing, mild *hypotonia*, a delay in the development of postural and equilibrium reactions, and problems with midline integration. A more motorically involved child will usually exhibit a similar picture of immaturity in *postural mechanism* development but be compounded by a motor control condition Ayres and others have termed **developmental dyspraxia**. Of these two conditions, the child with dyspraxia is usually identified more readily because of his or her obvious

awkwardness and tendency to have more difficulties with play and acquisition of functional skills.

Postural–Ocular and Bilateral Integration Dysfunction

Of the two broad patterns of sensory-based motor dysfunction, this one is milder in severity. It may be identified by a cluster of several sensory, behavioral, and motor characteristics, including irregularities in sensory modulation; atypical ocular pursuits, convergence, and visual fixation; low duration of postrotary nystagmus; slow or irregular vestibular response to tilt; sluggish postural preferences for inactive positions and sedentary activities; impairments in midline crossing, and delayed establishment of lateral dominance after age 4 (Figure 24-5).[3,48,63]

Other related concerns frequently noted include poor protective, righting, and equilibrium responses during functional movement or clinical assessment; and immature gait patterns such as the use of a wide base, with *lateral weight shifting* of the lower extremities. To compensate for low extensor muscle tone in the upper body, shoulder girdle positioning may be marked by *scapular retraction*, *scapular elevation*, and high-guard arm posturing. (These postural patterns are typical in normal toddler and early preschool development but usually give way to mature postural organization, smooth bilateral–reciprocal movements, and normal lateral dominance during the period between the ages of 4 and 6 years.[41,65])

Assessment of Posture, Ocular Functioning, and Bilateral Integration

Potential problems with postural adaptation can be observed during the performance of certain items from standardized child development or motor proficiency tests. In infancy, the items from tests such as *The Miller Assessment for Preschoolers*, *The Bayley Scales of Infant Development–II*, *The Peabody Developmental Motor Scales-II*, and others help OT practitioners understand the child's performance (see Box 24-1 for a list of selected items).[13,43]

For example, the preschooler with low muscle tone and/or difficulties with balance, postural mechanisms, and bilateral coordination as well as symmetry of left/right function may be identified from the items of *The Miller Assessment for Pre-Schoolers* listed in Box 24-2.[51] Three-year-olds who are at risk for postural and bilateral integration deficits will experience difficulty with many items on *The DeGangi-Berk Test of Sensory Integration*, which are listed in Box 24-3.[34] *The Bruininks-Oseretsky Test of Motor Proficiency*-II contains many good postural–ocular and bilateral coordination items, which are listed in Box 24-4.[17]

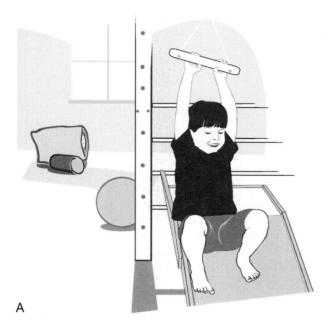

A

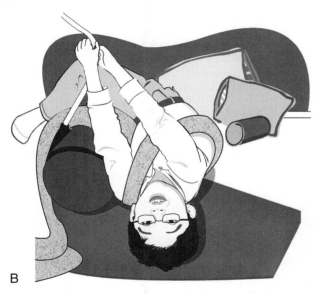

B

FIGURE 24-5 Children with postural–ocular and bilateral integration dysfunction have difficulty maintaining postures and using both hands together. **A,** The child uses both hands and plans how he is going to lift his legs, hold on, and move down the ramp. This requires processing of postural, vestibular, and proprioceptive information as well as timing and sequencing. **B,** A bolster swing requires postural control and bilateral integration.

Developmental Dyspraxia

This disorder represents the second broad category of sensory-based motor dysfunctions. It is important to realize that children with cognitive impairments will usually

BOX 24-1

Test Items to Observe Postural Adaptation in Infants

- Postural responses while being picked up, held, and handled
- In late toddlers/young preschoolers, more mature postural responses such as shifting weight in preparation for kicking a ball; positioning the upper body for catching a ball
- Observations of protective, righting, and equilibrium reactions
- Observations of organization of two-sided body/leg movements: early crawling movements, crawling/creeping patterns; stair-climbing patterns; jumping with both feet; hopping; arm thrusts
- Observations of organization of two-sided upper extremity movements: test items examining symmetry/asymmetry; the ability to use the hands together at midline; catching a ball with two hands; hand-to-hand object transfer; all items requiring one hand to hold or stabilize one object while the other hand is moving or placing objects into or on it

BOX 24-2

Test Items to Observe Postural Adaptation in Preschoolers

- Tower
- Sequencing
- Stereognosis
- Finger localization
- Maze
- Romberg
- Stepping
- Kneel/stand
- Walk line
- Rapid alternating movements, depending on the age of the child and normative expectations

have some degree of motor planning difficulty, which is part of the diagnosis of severe developmental delay and is consistent with their development across the board. However, in some cases, sensory processing deficits may also play a role along with the inborn condition. Three major processes are involved in praxis, and impairment in any of them can lead to dyspraxia. (1) The first and most fundamental process is the ability to register and

BOX 24-3

Test Items to Observe Postural Adaptation in 3-Year-Olds

- Airplane
- Diadokokinesis
- Drumming
- Jump and turn
- Monkey task
- Prone on elbows; neck co-contraction
- Rolling-pin activity
- Scooter board co-contraction
- Side-sitting co-contraction
- Upper extremity control
- Wheelbarrow walk

BOX 24-4

Test Items to Observe Postural Adaptation for Postural–Ocular and Bilateral Coordination

- Balance items
- Bilateral coordination items
- Visuomotor control items
- Upper limb speed and dexterity items
- Strength (e.g., observations of postural tone during writing or manipulation tests, play)

organize tactile, proprioceptive, vestibular, and visual input in order to assemble accurate internal cognitive maps of the body and the environment with which the body typically interacts. (2) The second process, which is based on these constructions, requires the ability to conceptualize internal images of purposeful actions, termed **ideation** in the neuropsychological and rehabilitation literature. (3) The third process is the planning of sequences of movements within the demands of the task and environmental context, including the ability to program anticipatory actions within the next few seconds.[2]

Impairment in praxis ability can occur anywhere within this neurodevelopmental chain of events. On the one hand, children who are most severely impaired lack even that internal visualization of what could be done with many objects. They typically also demonstrate poor registration of (i.e., failure to notice) sensory events. On the other hand, children who have only a planning problem know what could be done, but they cannot program the aspect of "how to do it." These children typically do not have poor registration (sensory hypo-reactivity); in fact, they may have a sensory modulation disorder in the direction of hyper-reactivity or defensiveness. Furthermore, they tend to have poor *somatosensory* perception of the body for use in motor planning (Figure 24-6). Ayres named the subtypes of developmental dyspraxia based on the hypothesized underlying sensory processing dysfunction associated with each one, in research conducted

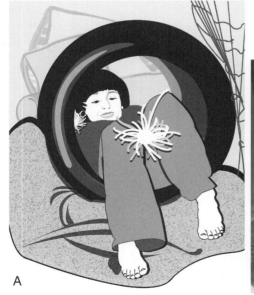
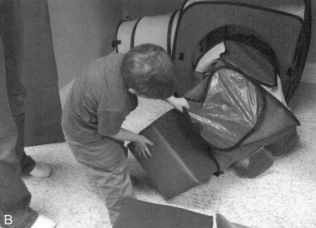

FIGURE 24-6 A, A child with developmental dyspraxia may benefit from understanding the concepts of "in and out" while rocking in a barrel. **B,** This child is trying to figure out how to arrange the materials in the tunnel so that he can move through it.

with the use of the *SIPT*, building on previous research with the *Southern California Sensory Integration Tests*.[3,9]

Ayres termed the most common subtype of dyspraxia *somatodyspraxia*. This disorder refers to praxis deficits that result from the inefficient processing of tactile–kinesthetic, proprioceptive, and/or vestibular sensory input within the body. A second type was termed *visuodyspraxia*, which reflects deficits in praxis that result from the poor processing of visuospatial cues, and affects one's ability to program movements in performing a visual construction task such as drawing designs, directing a pen along a line accurately, or building a three-dimensional structure with blocks. In some cases the child may have a combination of these two clusters; this condition is termed *visuosomatodyspraxia*. A third type is called *dyspraxia on verbal command* and is the result of difficulty translating a verbal command into a motor plan; therefore, it is more language related. For this reason, Ayres proposed that this category of praxis dysfunction is the result of cortical-level left hemisphere dysfunction and is consequently not a true SI disorder, which is by definition subcortical in origin.[3,30,60]

Assessment of Praxis

Praxis difficulties can be observed during many exploratory, play, self-care, school, and physical education activities. Infants may display problems and frustration with simple adaptive movement responses that challenge their problem-solving abilities within the environment (i.e., "What do I do?"). Some examples might include the inability to figure out how to climb onto a riding toy; to remove an irritating clothing item on the head; to imitate simple gestures; and to lead grownups to something the child wants done (e.g., opening a door). Children ages 4 to 7 with dyspraxia may struggle to use tools and materials at school properly (e.g., during cutting, pasting, or coloring). They may actively avoid challenging motor planning tasks such as self-dressing, using eating utensils, and playing with manipulative toys; or they may avoid participating in gross motor activities and games requiring praxis ability.[60,63]

Besides the praxis tests of the SIPT, other developmental and motor tests have items that directly test praxis, or the child's quality of execution can be observed. However, as stated earlier, most other tests cannot provide information on underlying sensory processing. In infants, *The Bayley Scales of Infant Development–II* has the following relevant items:[13]

- Imitates hand movements
- Imitates postures
- Pats toy in imitation

Items on *The Miller Assessment for Preschoolers*, which are used to observe praxis qualities, include the following:[52]

- Imitation of postures
- Items that require the child to follow the demonstration of the examiner (rapid alternating movements, kneel/stand, walk line, stepping)
- Maze
- Tower and block designs (constructional praxis)
- Block tapping (motor sequencing)
- Puzzle (visuoconstructional praxis)

As Ayres says, "The child must organize his own brain; the therapist can only provide the milieu conducive in [sic] evoking the drive to do so. Structuring that therapeutic environment demands considerable professional skill."[5]

INTERVENTION
General Principles of Sensory Integration Intervention

The central principle of this intervention approach is the provision of controlled sensory input, through activities presented by the therapist, to elicit adaptive responses from the child, thereby bringing about more efficient brain organization (Figure 24-7).[6] This latter result becomes observable in the increased organization of behavior, movement, and affective expression that is seen in the child. Perhaps the most difficult aspect for new or untrained OT practitioners to comprehend is the absence of an SI "protocol" or "curriculum." (This aspect also needs to be explained carefully to both parents and teachers.) Nor is there a set protocol for treating each of the various types of SI dysfunction, although each type has its unique guiding principles. However, the results of the evaluation should provide the sensorimotor developmental road map that shapes the treatment plan.

SI treatment is centered on the child and guided by the OT practitioner; it is *freedom within structure* (Figure 24-8). The OT practitioner follows the child's lead but at the same time does not allow the child to run wildly around the treatment space. Nor does the OT practitioner present the child with a predetermined list of "what we are going to do today." How can this be? How do we reconcile these seemingly opposite concepts?

For example, let us begin with the challenge of a child who is running aimlessly around a room or area of a clinic, stopping briefly to look at or touch toys and equipment and then charging on to the next room or area. We might ask ourselves, "Is that a 'lead' I should be

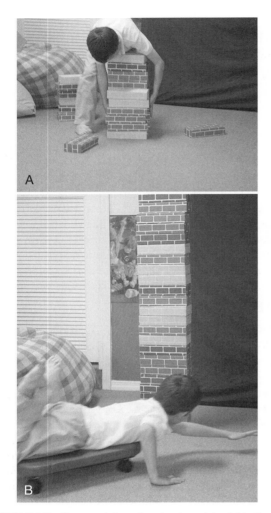

FIGURE 24-7 Sensory integration treatment is child directed and initiated. **A,** This child decides to build a block tower. **B,** The child chooses to knock the blocks down while riding a scooter. This activity provides proprioceptive and vestibular input to the child; it is child directed and fun.

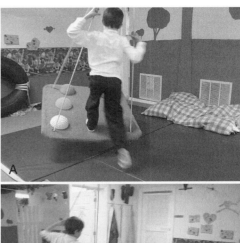

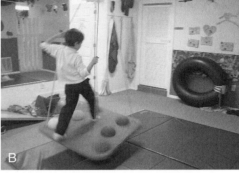

FIGURE 24-8 **A,** This child uses the platform swing to challenge his balance and timing. He pretends that he is on a spaceship and must deflect the meteors by hitting them with a "scientific deflector." Children with sensory integration dysfunction may be very creative. Occupational therapy (OT) practitioners can use this creativity to make intervention sessions fun and interesting. **B,** The OT practitioner is able to provide the "just right" challenge to this activity by controlling the speed of the spaceship (platform swing) and the location of the deflectors (objects to be thrown) and meteors (targets).

following?" The answer is yes and no. In this situation, the client is leading his therapist—or at least trying to communicate to him or her. The child is telling the therapist, "I am overstimulated, disorganized, and out of control. I don't know how to modulate and organize all of these novel sensations coming into my nervous system. I need you to help me self-regulate." The OT practitioner must then think critically (and quickly) about how to do this. The questions to consider would be: "What is overstimulating this child? Is the child seeking additional input? What types of sensory input would be calming and organizing to his nervous system? How can I get him to arrest this random running around,

and instead channel that poorly directed drive into meaningful exploration and interaction?"

The treatment of sensory processing disorders appears deceptively easy and playful because the OT practitioner is skilled in directing therapy procedures that are *child-directed*, active, and result in meaningful *adaptive responses* which promote better brain organization. This ability to "go with the client's flow" derives from the OT practitioner's knowledge of *neurobiology*; capacity to observe when the child is attempting to make an adaptive response to a challenge; and skill in knowing when to introduce novelty, equipment adjustments, or changes in task difficulty to make the challenges "just right." This therapeutic artistry prevents the child from becoming frustrated if the activity is too difficult or bored if the activity is not sufficiently challenging.

These strategies stand in contrast to the more structured "sensory-motor" or "perceptual–motor" programs often used in adaptive physical education. That type of intervention is typically technique oriented and repetitive, places emphasis on end-product physical skills, and many times requires a more cognitive orientation on the part of the client. However, if utilized properly, these specially selected activities may still provide experiences that are rich in helpful sensory input and can be implemented in a variety of settings. Examples of these strategies and treatment activities are shown in Table 24-2, adapted from Carrasco, as well as the ages and stages of typical development and the corresponding sensory processing levels proposed by Kimball.[23,47]

PROMOTING DIFFERENT LEVELS OF SENSORY PROCESSING AND MOTOR CONTROL

Facilitating Sensory Modulation

Just like intervention for other types of sensory processing disorder, the treatment of sensory modulation dysfunction follows similar guiding principles. Here are some suggestions from Carrasco, which are outlined in Box 24-5.[23]

As the child walks into the room, his or her arousal level can be determined by observing behaviors that provide clues about whether the child is alert, tired, agitated, sleepy, wired, or some other state. This can help decide whether the planned intervention is appropriate. If the child needs excitation, then it would be appropriate to provide arousing activities that incorporate jumping; fast movements on various swings, rotational or linear. Perhaps vigorous music of the child's choice might be selected, and energy and enthusiasm might be conveyed through the OT practitioner's own voice. Awareness of the child's arousal level tells the OT practitioner where to start, when to adjust, and whether to discontinue a certain activity or type of equipment.

However, if the child seems overaroused, engaging in random, disorganized, poorly directed activity, sensory input that will promote healthy *inhibition* and nervous system organization is called for. This might include rhythmic linear vestibular input on a swing or physioball, while the child engages in an oral–motor activity such as using a "chewie," sucking on a lollipop, or blowing bubbles. Generally, activities that promote midline orientation of trunk, upper extremities, oral structures, and eyes are calming and organizing. Sometimes, disorganized behavior can occur during a session and is usually the result of overstimulation and poor monitoring on the part of the OT practitioner. This requires a rebalancing of the child's nervous system by the OT practitioner prior to end of the session.

If necessary, initial sensory preparation for the session may include methods such as the *Wilbarger protocol* if the OT practitioner is correctly trained. If not, the OT practitioner should obtain appropriate training and supervision and emphasize to the family that the protocol needs to be followed consistently at home according to instructions. Occupational therapists are increasingly incorporating one of the several auditory integration programs that are now available into their vestibular swing-based treatment. Otherwise, simply being aware of the relative excitatory or calming properties of sound and music, and utilizing them appropriately in a session supports adaptive arousal levels. For example, children often enjoy hearing calming "nature sounds" and receiving total-body deep pressure while lying between two large crash pillows.

The focus of sensory processing intervention is aimed toward the organization of multiple sources of sensory input. The focus is also on the lower brain processing of vestibular input integrated with proprioceptive and visual inputs, making it important to identify the target sensory system(s). Pumping a platform swing to move forward and backward while in a circle/ring-sitting position not only provides vestibular input but also integrates proprioception in the neck, trunk, and eyes. This integration of sensations paves the way for postural integration as well as conjugate eye movements that are necessary for fine and visuomotor activities. However, some behaviors that suggest sensory modulation dysfunction are system specific, such as sensitivity to touch, taste, sights, movement, and smells.

Although movement is a commonly observed end product of efficient sensory processing, the OT practitioner should also monitor cognitive, affective, and physiologic responses to sensory processing demands on an ongoing basis. Sweating, paleness, and other autonomic signs of distress indicate that the sensations being introduced are overwhelming, and the activity should be discontinued. This is always the risk when OT practitioners provide too much passive stimulation to the child without appropriately eliciting adaptive responses that would help the child organize the sensory input.

TABLE 24-2

Intervention Strategies to Promote Sensory Processing and Related Developmental and Occupational Information*

LEVEL OF SENSORY PROCESSING	AGE/STAGE	DEVELOPMENTAL TASK	OCCUPATIONAL CHALLENGES	TREATMENT STRATEGIES FOR CLASSIC TREATMENT OF SENSORY PROCESSING DISORDER
Sensory modulation	First 2 years of life	Physiologic homeostasis; self-regulation of arousal and attention Attachment based on self-regulation Primary sensorimotor stage of learning, or learning through sensory input Adaptive reflex behavior to purposeful action Exploratory play	Irritability Poor sleep cycles Intolerance to being held or cuddled or exploring objects and people Poor tolerance to positional changes Frequent startling Slow development but usually within normal limits	Use inhibitory* techniques to decrease heightened sensitivity down to levels of functional modulation, with activities rich in one of the following: slow, rhythmical movements; deep proprioceptive input; low-spectrum sounds; dim lighting; minimized environmental sensory input; low-pitched voice and tone. Employ excitatory* techniques to alert the central nervous system, such as fast movements; higher and louder pitch of voice; fast, rhythmical sounds or music; light touch; and different textures and consistency of toys and walking surfaces. *Many individuals with sensory modulation disorder exhibit paradoxical behaviors and responses to treatment. Paradoxical behaviors are manifested when they show hyper-responsiveness to tactile input but hypo-responsiveness to vestibular input; their responses to inhibitory and excitatory strategies may also show such paradoxical behavior, so they respond with excitation when the occupational therapist's intention is for the input to be inhibitory. In such cases, close observation of a pattern of behavior is necessary so that appropriate changes in the strategies can be made as they happen. In such cases, consultation with a supervising occupational therapist trained in sensory integration is warranted.
Continuous sensory modulation	Preschool	Automatic self-regulation Integration of both sides of the body Crossing the midline of the body balance reactions Development of body scheme Development of gross motor planning Imagination expressed through pretend play	Short attention span Clumsiness Poor articulation Over-reaction or under-reaction to slight injury Fear of playground equipment and some walking surfaces (e.g., sand or plush carpet) Very messy and picky eater No awareness of danger and avoidance of novelty Avoidance of peers; a tendency to play with much older or younger children	While conducting activities that promote sensory modulation (i.e., inhibition and facilitation), include those that promote the foundation for the ocular and bilateral integration, balance reactions, and body scheme. Helpful strategies include the use of controlled sensory input that taps the proximal senses (vestibular and somatosensory, especially deep proprioceptive input that includes those of neck proprioceptors and extraocular muscles), which form the foundation for the work of the more distal senses, such as vision and hearing. These strategies should involve the active participation of the child in gross and fine motor activities that require the use of the entire body or parts thereof while moving through space and playing with a variety of objects that he or she can move, manipulate with the fingers, inspect with the eyes, make sounds with, or use some other sense.

Sensory discrimination	Early school age, 5–7 years	Increased skill in differentiating the qualities and characteristics of sensations, such as the intensity, degree, volume, and direction of sensory input Increased fine motor planning Establishment of dominance (lateralization) Flexible social and peer play	Fine motor problems Hyperactivity (often associated with sensory seeking) Impulsiveness Dislike or avoidance of textures in food (lumps), activities (finger painting), and clothing (labels or seams, softness) Difficulty in gross motor activities, with falling or avoidance Accidentally breaks toys or is rough playing with objects or peers	While system-specific sensory input is useful, a strategy that also provides multisensory input is helpful. The novelty and variety of sensory input provide challenges in differentiating and remembering such qualities as sound, distance, texture, color, movement, and taste but also in categorizing and organizing as well as other challenges. Use activities that promote sensory discrimination during but especially at the end of the treatment session.
Sensory-based movement disorder—postural–ocular and bilateral integration disorder	School age and up (7 years and older) Continued in next age/stage level	Increased abstract thinking Academics More sophisticated tool use Competence in complex skills dependent on previous phases Games with rules and competition	Increased academic problems frequently associated with attention and frustration Poorly or compulsively organized Reversals in writing Continued clumsiness with poor sequencing of tasks Self-esteem problems "Splintered" skills (i.e., lack of generalization ability) Trouble keeping up with peers in activities (especially motor based—slower)	Observe in order to monitor sensory modulation and behavior regulation that may be expressed as inattention or diminished frustration tolerance and endurance. Provide a balance of movement challenges that incorporate flexional, extensional, and rotational components, preferably during activities that require the child to move the whole body or, when seated at a table or the floor, the arms through space. Infuse the session with experiences that require the crossing of one arm across the midline. Also include activities that require the use of both sides of the body, especially but not only the hands with guidance by the eyes and with one side of the body performing independently or in collaboration with the other.
Sensory-based movement disorder Developmental dyspraxia	Starts with previous level and continues into adolescence and adulthood	Continuation of previous level Concern with physical relationships Team sports Establishing identity Career choice Leisure preferences	Organizational problems (e.g., time management) Trouble finishing homework or tasks started Immature physical skills and social relationships Increased dependence Loses or forgets things May be socially isolated Avoids team sports or chooses heavy contact sports	Observe in order to monitor sensory modulation. Provide challenges that require active participation in following verbal, written, or other types of directions for task performance and participation such as the construction of two-dimensional end products (e.g., drawings, written work) or three-dimensional constructions (e.g., block towers, obstacle courses). Provide multiple experiences that require the execution of gross, fine, oral, and visuomotor tasks with projected action sequences or those tasks that require planning of movement to hit targets.

*See level-specific treatment guidelines in the following sections.

Adapted from Kimball JG: Sensory integration frame of reference. In Kramer P, Hinojosa J, editors: *Frames of reference for pediatric occupational therapy*, Baltimore, MD, 1993, Lippincott Williams and Wilkins; Carrasco RC, Sahler SS: *Sensorimotor history questionnaire—research edition*, Winter Park, FL 2005, Fiestajoy Foundation, Inc.

BOX 24-5

Tips for Facilitating Sensory Modulation

- Determine arousal level.
- If necessary, use stimulation protocols.
- Identify the target sensory system(s).
- Monitor cognitive, affective, and physiologic responses to sensory processing demands.
- Compare the consistency of observed behaviors.
- Employ novelty.
- Influence the threshold level.
- Monitor signs of sensory overload or shut-down behaviors.
- Facilitate a balance between seeking and avoiding behaviors and contextual reality.
- Facilitate behavior regulation.
- Prescribe a sensory diet.

Cognitive and emotional responses are also helpful windows through which the child indicates whether or not the sensory experience is meaningful. Holding on tightly for comfort when placed on moving therapeutic equipment is an indication that the child is afraid—of the equipment, the rocking, perhaps the OT practitioner, or simply being away from the caregiver. Frustration and anger in the child can be the result of the inability to figure out what has to be done because the task is too difficult; boredom and lethargy can result if the task is too easy.

Behaviors related to hypersensitivity as well as hypo-sensitivity to sensory input can vary between what is observed at home and in other settings, such as the school or the clinic. These patterns of responsivity can also fluctuate within the same day or from day to day. Ideally, the response would be similar in all settings; so, for example, sensitivity to food textures would be similar at home and in school during snack time. Compare the consistency of observed behaviors; if they are not consistent, consider giving the parents and teachers some tips on how to handle the child who may be manipulative. Sometimes, while observing family dynamics, sleeping and eating patterns may provide information on how to manage sensory modulation disorder. For example, the parents might be able to distinguish between intolerance of certain foods and their child's attempts at controlling the situation or seeking attention, especially if such behaviors are not evident in other contexts such as the school or with grandparents. In these cases, consistency of behavior management together with sensory processing interventions is appropriate.

The introduction of new toys, sounds, smells, and even movement on a swing provides novelty to the interaction and elicits vigilance to new incoming sensations. Employing novelty does not necessarily mean changing the equipment (the toy) or, in the case of a writing activity, the size, shape, and color of the pen or the smell of the ink or the sound that the pen makes with pressure. For some children, too much novelty can be overwhelming, so it is helpful to introduce novelty in measured ways, embedded in familiar activities to make it more readily acceptable by the child.

Whether the thresholds to sensation are too high or too low, the goal of intervention is to influence and bring them into a range of adaptive *homeostasis*. Monitor the child's behaviors that suggest the need to raise or lower thresholds, depending on whether he or she withdraws from, seeks, or responds slowly to sensations. Provide activities which provide repetition of similar tasks requiring or producing similar sensations, for example, swinging a ball or throwing it at a target and sliding down outdoor equipment and ending up in a circle on the sandbox.

While engaging in the above activities, introduce changes in the sequence and other components of the activity to detect signs of sensory overload or shutdown behaviors such as purposeless running around, losing track of the end goal of an activity, a glassy-eyed expression, or simply suddenly becoming quiet, retreating to a corner, or even seemingly falling asleep. Introducing the changes can result in sustained interest and maintained vigilance, thereby influencing attention and purposeful interaction with the environment.

Seeking and avoiding behaviors are often considered "normal" at home but negative in school. Communication with teachers, family members, and OT practitioners is essential, especially when recommending environmental adaptations such as movable seating cushions, wedges, or ball chairs; "fidget" toys; a mini-trampoline in the classroom; or frequent movement breaks for the child. This communication will help facilitate a balance between seeking and avoiding behaviors and contextual reality. Rather than depriving the child of recess as punishment for "disruptive" behaviors, urge teachers to allow the child to go outside to engage in a structured physical activity, such as doing calisthenics or running a lap around the playground (adjusted for age and maturity of the child, of course). This way, the child gets the movement or the vestibular *sensory diet* he or she needs in order to stay organized for the remainder of the day but still receives a reasonable consequence for the disruptive behavior.

The OT practitioner facilitates behavior regulation by providing different levels of emotional engagement within a session, offering rewards as needed and progressing from immediate to delayed gratification. The OT clinician provides experiences in detecting not only changes in verbal expression of emotion but also nonverbal communication through body language and facial expressions. This may be through imaginative play experiences or indirectly through role playing with toys or other technology. The OT practitioner infuses sessions with experiences in detecting changes in feelings about what is going on during the session and the ability to label such feelings.

The OT clinician prescribes a program of activities that provides sensory experiences on a regular basis (i.e., a sensory diet). It may come in the form of a schedule that includes engaging in activities upon awakening in the morning or modulating the nervous system to a more adaptive level when returning home from the daycare center or the school. The sensory diet can include activities designed with and/or provided to the school or family. The activities consider the child's sensory needs on the basis of a comprehensive assessment and diagnosis of sensory modulation disorder but should include a variety of experiences to give the child the opportunity to participate as fully as possible without being threatened by the activities.

Suggestions for Promoting Sensory Discrimination

A summary of suggestions for promoting sensory discrimination for children who have sensory discrimination dysfunction can be found in Box 24-6.

It is important to observe the child for indicators or behaviors that suggest difficulty with sensory modulation or indicate current or residual modulation disorder, such as dyspraxia or postural–ocular and bilateral integration dysfunction. Even when the goals and activities are designed to promote sensory discrimination, it is likely that unresolved or residual sensory modulation disorder will come to the surface; this may be due to several factors, such as the novelty of the activity, stress, the event(s) that happened the previous night or on the way to the clinic, and due to health problems. When this happens, aim for functional modulation and proceed with caution toward your sensory discrimination goal.

Allow the child to be aware of his or her need to seek sensory input (e.g., the reason for the pencil grip, the purpose of the "fidget" toy, the wedge on the chair) as appropriate for age. By raising the modulation level to awareness, the child will hopefully understand and become an active participant in the therapy process.

Although the OT program may be very specific, identify the sensory "on ramp," such as visual versus tactile discrimination goals. The *sensory on ramp*, or the sensory system that you access to introduce activities, may differ from the goals prescribed by the OT program. For example, the child may be in a vestibular seeking mode when your goal is visual. In this case, activities

---

BOX 24-6

Tips for Promoting Sensory Discrimination

- Look out for indicators of current or residual modulation disorder.
- Raise modulation level to awareness.
- Identify the sensory "on ramp."
- Infuse activities with controlled novelty.
- Use a variety of materials to infuse novelty.
- Grade complexity of sensory input and adaptive responses.
- Be alert to affective responses.
- Intervene when difficulty comes with diminished visual inspection.
- Keep track of visual dependence, and intervene when its presence or absence is observed.
- Select activities that challenge visual discrimination.
- Provide challenging, age-appropriate, fun activities with intrinsic recognition, matching, and categorization of textures, shapes, sizes, or other characteristics of the object.
- Provide opportunities for auditory localization, sequencing, and figure–ground.
- Challenge localization of sensations.
- Provide opportunities for discrimination abilities.

---

that provide vestibular input such as running or swinging on the playground may be used as a starting point of the therapy session, but at the same time, visual activities that may in themselves have discrimination components to them may be provided as well.

With new sensory input introduced into the sensory experiences, the detection of new sensations and vigilance for new experiences to come can be promoted by the OT practitioner. Infusing activities with controlled novelty is similar to the way in which novelty is effective in managing sensory modulation disorder, only this time it is infused with opportunities to refocus on the variety of the qualities and characteristics of sensations. Additionally, novel activities should be approached with a variety of materials but not at the expense of needed continuation as expressed or observed.

The OT practitioner grades the complexity of sensory input and adaptive responses by matching the child's baseline arousal and processing levels with the sensory components of selected activities and the complexity of the responses expected. As necessary, the demands of the activity should be lowered or raised in relation to the equipment used (e.g., a platform, rather than a bolster or dual-sling swing) or the complexity of the toys used (e.g., limiting the Jenga game pieces to 20 instead of 45) (Figure 24-9).

It is important to observe the child for changes in affect, which serve as indicators of emotional responses

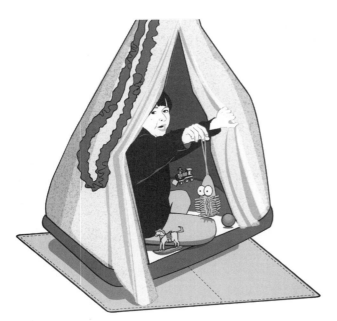

FIGURE 24-9 Swinging on a platform swing provides vestibular and proprioceptive feedback to children. This game requires that the child make adaptive responses in order to pick up tactile toys and place them in a container while moving. The covering over the swing helps calm the child so he is more able to tolerate tactile items. This activity requires timing; sequencing; motor planning; extension through the trunk, shoulder, and elbow; and visual attention.

to the sensory environment and include reactions to interaction and task demands, and be alert to other affective responses. Observation of the endurance level as well as frustration tolerance, problem solving, and creativity is critical to guiding the intervention session. The OT practitioner adjusts the bar as necessary, raising or lowering it for challenges accordingly. It is recommended the reader refer to the BRAINS (Behavior Regulation through Activities for the Integration of Novel Sensations) approach for infusing sensory processing treatment with socioemotional strategies for additional information.[20,26]

When difficulty comes with diminished visual inspection, especially of items that are manipulated, smelled, tasted, or some other sensation, intervention should be provided with reminders, for example, when manipulating zippers, guiding a spoon to the mouth, perceiving when clothing is twisted, finding items such as coins in pockets, or manipulating small objects and tools without vision (e.g., a pencil, spoon, screwdriver). In addition to observing diminished visual inspection, keep track of and intervene when you observe visual dependence, or a lack thereof as in the above situations, or when identifying which body part has been touched when vision is occluded, differentiating smells and tastes

without visual cues, or being alert to what certain smells mean, such as burning or gas leaks.

Activities in which letters can be easily reversed or inverted—as in the case of *p*, *b*, and *q*—can be used as selective activities that challenge visual discrimination. Other activities include those that challenge the child to match, recognize, and categorize items according to their qualities such as color, texture, shape, and size and to quickly scan visual images in sequence and those that provide challenges to connect dots, write between lines, and play hopscotch, all of which demand visual guidance of fine and gross motor movements.

It is recommended that the OT practitioner provide challenging, age-appropriate, fun activities with intrinsic recognition, matching, and categorization of textures, shapes, sizes, and/or other object characteristics, as well as experiences that are rich not only in recognizing symbols and gestures and perceiving depth, distance, the location of borders, boundaries, and spaces between objects but also in differentiating foreground from background images, closure of shapes, and pictures.

Challenge the child to localize sounds, sights, smells, and other sensations by differentiating and remembering similar words and sounds, for example, *pat/pack* and *mitt/meat*. Other suggested activities include following instructions with multiple steps and judging the source of a sound, such as turning in the direction of the person calling as well as recognizing the sound of a drum when it competes with the background noise of a toy flute. These activities provide opportunities for auditory localization, sequencing, and figure–ground.

The OT practitioner offers opportunities during and after the session to apply discrimination abilities to ensure their translation into occupations, for example, maintaining balance while taking a shower with the eyes closed or drying the feet with a towel while standing up, maneuvering the body through tight spaces such as in an obstacle course, and writing with appropriate pressure on the paper or chalkboard.

Intervention for Sensory-Based Movement Disorder

Many children referred for the treatment of sensory-based movement disorder are also referred for such reasons as fine motor evaluation, writing problems, and delayed development, but rarely for the underlying sensory processing problems. It is therefore important to identify the presenting problem by linking it to the underlying sensory processing deficit through assessment and historical review. By doing so, foundational intervention, sensorimotor treatment, and environmental adaptation can be designed.

For sensory-based movement disorder, promote improved somatosensory body scheme organization with activities such as whole-body playing in a plastic ball bath; rubbing cream/lotion on different parts of the body while discussing each one; brushing oneself with a paintbrush or other type of brush; drawing the silhouette of a body on a long sheet of paper; crawling through a lycra fabric "tube" while discussing which parts are passing through it; learning to hop-scotch to different patterns on the floor; putting on a new article of clothing; and positioning and adjusting the body on a scooter board, a swing, or even a chair. A summary of remediation for sensory-based movement disorder can be found in Box 24-7.

If the child is hesitant or unable to self-propel a selected swing, the OT practitioner may direct the swing in a direction, speed, or rhythm that would bring about the child's excitation, inhibition, or participation in a purposeful activity as desired. When initial activation of the swing by the OT practitioner is necessary, he or she should nevertheless use clinical procedural reasoning to ask, "How can I facilitate the child's active engagement in this activity?" Sometimes the answer is to sit with, or behind, the child on the swing, assist the child to place and maintain the hands on the ropes or handles, and enable the child to propel the swing with increasing independence.

Tasks that require bimanual manipulation promote symmetry as well as asymmetry by means of the efficient use of a preferred versus nonpreferred extremity. Bimanual or bipedal manipulation encourages the independent as well as cooperative use of two hands or two feet, respectively, such as clapping games, card games, drawing, and sewing. Likewise, watch out for overflow movements in the oral area as well as on the opposite side of the body.

Provide challenges to determine the difficulty and/or strength of the praxis component(s) by asking: "Can you show me a different position to move this swing?" "Can you show me a different way to ride on this scooter board?" or "Can you go through the obstacle course backward?" Such challenges indicate whether the praxis components are cognitive or motor. Include manual motor planning activities such as making an origami crane, which requires deciding what to do, what sequence to follow, and how to position and move the fingers and paper to accomplish the task.

Infuse the program with both two-dimensional and three-dimensional constructional activities such as writing, drawing, and block construction, in order to challenge visuopraxis, creativity, and problem solving. Ask the child to creatively determine how to put together objects and materials for play/leisure activities and school/work projects. "Construction" also implies the ability to organize one's belongings and objects in one's environment. "Clean-up time" should be an integral part of the close of every treatment session, as this activity engenders not only organizational ability in the child but also a sense of responsibility and respect for others' belongings that are enjoyed by the child. Challenge the 7-year-old clients to design their own obstacle courses during OT. They may first draw a map of the course on a sheet of paper (two-dimensional construction), then build it (three-dimensional construction), with Socratic questioning and cueing from the OT practitioner. Also, encourage parents to help the child organize his or her own spaces at home, such as the bedroom and/or playroom. Assist the child with developing language and reading/labeling skills and self-organization by having him or her label shelves, drawers, baskets, or room areas with appropriately worded cards or stickers, for example, "Books," "Movies," "Dolls," "Cars and Trucks," "Games," and so on.

Prepare activities with projected action sequences of different types; for example, have the child hit or "latch onto" a target with the force of his or her whole body, with something that is thrown, or have the child draw lines to a target while being aware of cognitive, motor, and affective abilities. Actively engage the child in organizing a series of actions to produce an intentional movement or in figuring out how to do something familiar yet different, such as writing his or her name with the nondominant hand or (more difficult) writing the word "Saskatchewan" spelled backward.

BOX 24-7

Tips for Remediating Sensory-Based Movement Disorder

- Identify presenting problem(s).
- Promote improved organization of somatosensory body scheme.
- Promote symmetry as well as asymmetry by means of the efficient use of a preferred versus nonpreferred extremity.
- Determine the difficulties and strengths of the practice component(s).
- Infuse the program with constructional activities.
- Infuse the activities with projected action sequences of different types.
- Challenge actions from ideas and images.
- Challenge the ability to learn and smoothly execute new movements.
- Include activities that challenge mouth and tongue movements in coordination with respiration.

To encourage the development of ideational praxis, design activities that challenge the formulation of actions from ideas and images. Ask the child to perform or translate ideas or images into verbal descriptions, interactions, or products, during play, at school, or at home (e.g., making a kite from a list of materials). Ask the following question: "How would you 'drive' a bolster swing if it were a school bus, spaceship, race car, fishing boat, or some other mode of transportation?" Assist the child to figure out how to play new games or put things together by organizing a series of actions as needed, by asking, "How can we use these big blocks to build things like a fort, a spaceship docking station, an igloo, and a Polly Pocket house?"

Fine motor planning can challenge the ability to learn and smoothly execute new movements. Ask the child questions such as: "Can you swing, let go, and land in the big pillow?" "Can you ride your elephant over here and roll over into the hay?" Some activities to challenge fine motor planning include movements required in making Mexican "Ojos de Dios" ("God's Eyes"), holiday-themed dream catchers out of colored pipe cleaners; yarn-and-stick projects; origami; simple knots of macramé; or cutting pictures for a scrapbook. Simple cooking projects also promote motor process sequencing, constructional praxis, and acceptance of sensory experiences inherent in many cooking tasks.

Include activities that challenge mouth and tongue movements in coordination with respiration, such as those required when eating foods of different textures; when sucking sour candy or popsicles, blowing bubbles, or blowing cotton balls or ping pong balls across the floor while lying prone on a scooter board; playing wind instruments such as a toy flute; blowing special whistles; and making appropriate facial gestures during interaction.

SUMMARY

This chapter presents a basic review of sensory integration theory, assessment, and intervention strategies. OT practitioners first assess the child's sensory processing abilities and determine the underlying causes for occupational performance deficits. Intervention techniques include following the child's lead and introducing vestibular, proprioceptive, and tactile activities so that the child is challenged to make an adaptive response. The art of OT includes designing interventions that look like play and in which the child is engaged, whereas the science of OT involves understanding the neurobehavioral basis of the interventions and outcomes. Explanations of the child's behavioral responses to processing of sensory information to family members and teachers help them understand and help the child participate in daily activities. The chapter provides clinical questionnaires and tips to help OT practitioners design interventions that will be meaningful and fulfilling for the child.

References

1. Als H: A synactive model of neonatal behavioral organization: Framework for the assessment of neurobehavioral development in the premature infant and for support of infants and parents in the neonatal intensive care environment, *Phys Occup Ther Pediatr* 6:3, 1986.
2. Ayres AJ: *Developmental dyspraxia and adult-onset apraxia*, Torrance, CA, 1985, Sensory Integration International.
3. Ayres AJ: *Manual: Sensory integration and praxis tests*, Los Angeles, 1989, Western Psychological Services.
4. Ayres AJ: Reading—a product of sensory integrative processes. In Henderson A et al, editors: *The development of sensory integrative theory and practice: A collection of the work of A. Jean Ayres*, Dubuque, IA, 1974, Kendall/Hunt.
5. Ayres AJ: *Sensory integration and learning disorders*, Los Angeles, 1972, Western Psychological Services.
6. Ayres AJ: *Sensory integration and the child*, Los Angeles, 1979, Western Psychological Services.
7. Ayres AJ: Sensory integrative processes in neuropsychological learning disability. In Henderson A, et al, editors: *The development of sensory integrative theory and practice: A collection of the work of A. Jean Ayres*, Dubuque, IA, 1974, Kendall/Hunt.
8. Ayres AJ: *Southern California Tests of Sensory Integration manual*, rev, Los Angeles, 1980, Western Psychological Services.
9. Ayres AJ: *The effect of sensory integrative theory on learning disabled children: The final report of a research project*, Los Angeles, 1976, University of Southern California.
10. Ayres AJ, Mailloux ZK: Influence of sensory integration procedures on language development, *Am J Occup Ther* 35:383, 1981.
11. Ayres AJ, Mailloux ZK, Wendler CLW: Developmental dyspraxia: Is it a unitary function? *Occup Ther J Res* 7:93, 1987.
12. Ayres AJ, Tickle LS: Hyper-responsivity to touch and vestibular stimuli as a predictor of positive response to sensory integration procedures by autistic children, *Am J Occup Ther* 34:375, 1980.
13. Bayley N: *Bayley scales of infant development*, ed 2, San Antonio, TX, 1993, The Psychological Corporation.
14. Blanche E: *Observations based on sensory integration theory*, Torrance, CA, 2002, Pediatric Therapy Network.
15. Brown C, Tollefson N, Dunn W, et al: The adult sensory profile: Measuring patterns of sensory processing, *Am J Occup Ther* 55:75, 2001.
16. Brown D: *Adolescent/adult sensory profile*, San Antonio, TX, 2002, The Psychological Corporation.
17. Bruininks RH: *Examiner's manual: Bruininks-Oseretsky test of motor proficiency*, Circle Pines, MN, 1978, American Guidance Services.

18. Bundy AC, Lane SJ, Murray EA: *Sensory integration: Theory and practice*, Philadelphia, 2002, FA Davis.
19. Cammisa KM: Testing difficult children, *Sensory Integration Special Interest Section Newsletter* 14:1, 1991.
20. Carrasco RC: Building brains with sensory integration, *Adv Occup Ther* 19:47, 2003.
21. Carrasco RC: Common test instruments, *Sensory Integration Special Interest Section Newsletter* 14:3, 1991.
22. Carrasco RC: Key components of sensory integration evaluation, *Sensory Integration Special Interest Section Newsletter* 16:5, 1993.
23. Carrasco RC: *Making sense: Classical and practical sensory integration testing and treatment for diverse populations and settings—course manuals*, Marietta, GA, 2005, Advanced Rehabilitation Services.
24. Carrasco RC: *Practical information and useful assessments in sensory integration*, Marietta, GA, 2001, Advanced Rehabilitation Services.
25. Carrasco RC: Reliability of the Knickerbocker sensorimotor history questionnaire, *Occup Ther J Res* 10:280, 1990.
26. Carrasco RC et al: *BRAINS (Behavior Regulation through Activities for the Integration of Novel Sensations): Linking sensory integration and emotions with human performance—infusing sensory integration assessment and treatment with socioemotional intervention*, Marietta, GA, 2002, Advanced Rehabilitation Services.
27. Carrasco RC, Lee CE: Development of the teacher questionnaire on sensorimotor behavior, *Sensory Integration Special Interest Section Newsletter* 16:1, 1993.
28. Carrasco RC, Sahler SS: *Sensorimotor history questionnaire – research edition*, Winter Park, FL, 2005, FiestaJoy Foundation, Inc.
29. Case-Smith J, O'Brien J: *Occupational therapy for children*, ed 6, St Louis, 2010, Mosby.
30. Cermak SA: Somatodyspraxia. In Fisher A, Murray EA, Bundy AC, editors: *Sensory integration: Theory and practice*, Philadelphia, 1991, FA Davis.
31. Coster WJ: Occupation-centered assessment of children, *Am J Occup Ther* 52:337, 1998.
32. Daniels D: *The relationship between sensory processing and temperament in young children* [doctoral dissertation], 2003, University of Kansas.
33. DeGangi GA: *Greenspan SI: Test of sensory function in infants*, Los Angeles, 1990, Western Psychological Services.
34. DeGangi GA, Berk RA: *DeGangi-Berk test of sensory integration*, Los Angeles, 1983, Western Psychological Services.
35. Dunn WW: *Sensory profile: User's manual*, San Antonio, TX, 1999, The Psychological Corporation.
36. Dunn WW: *The infant/toddler sensory profile manual*, San Antonio, TX, 2002, The Psychological Corporation.
37. Dunn WW: The sensations of everyday life: Empirical, theoretical and pragmatic considerations, *Am J Occup Ther* 55:608, 2001.
38. Dunn WW: *The sensory profile*, San Antonio, TX, 1995, The Psychological Corporation.
39. Dunn WW: *The sensory profile: Examiner's manual*, San Antonio, TX, 1999, The Psychological Corporation.
40. Dunn WW, Brown CE: *The adolescent and adult sensory profile*, San Antonio, TX, 2003, The Psychological Corporation.
41. Fisher AG, Bundy AC: The interpretation process. In Fisher AG, Murray EA, Bundy AC, editors: *Sensory integration: Theory and practice*, Philadelphia, 1991, FA Davis.
42. Fisher AG, Murray EA, Bundy AC: *Sensory integration: Theory and practice*, Philadelphia, 1991, FA Davis.
43. Folio MR, Fewell RR: *Peabody developmental motor scales*, ed 2, Chicago, 1984, Riverside Publishing Company.
44. Greenspan SI, Weider S: *The child with special needs*, Reading, PA, 1998, Addison-Wesley.
45. Harris MB: Oral-motor management of the high-risk neonate, *Phys Occup Ther Pediatr* 6:231, 1986.
46. Jirgal D, Bouma K: Sensory integration interview guide for infants, *Sensory Integration Special Interest Section Newsletter* 12:5, 1989.
47. Kimball JG: Sensory integration frame of reference. In Kramer P, Hinojosa J, editors: *Frames of reference for pediatric occupational therapy*, ed 2, Baltimore, MD, 1999, Lippincott Williams and Wilkins.
48. Mailloux Z, Parham LD: Sensory integration. In Case-Smith J, O'Brien, J editor: *Occupational therapy for children*, ed 6, St Louis, 2010, Mosby.
49. Mangeot SD, Miller LJ, McIntosh DN, et al: Sensory modulation dysfunction in children with attention deficit hyperactivity disorder, *Dev Med Child Neurol* 43:399, 2001.
50. McIntosh DN, Miller LJ, Shyu V, Dunn W: Overview of the Short Sensory Profile (SSP). In Dunn W, editor: *The sensory profile: Examiner's manual*, San Antonio, TX, 1999, The Psychological Corporation.
51. McIntosh DN, Miller LJ, Shyu V, et al: Sensory-modulation disruption, electrodermal responses, and functional behaviors, *Dev Med Child Neurol* 41:608, 1999.
52. Miller LJ: *Manual: The FirstSTEP screening test for evaluating preschoolers*, San Antonio, TX, 1993, The Psychological Corporation.
53. Miller LJ: *Manual: The Miller assessment for preschoolers*, San Antonio, TX, 1982, The Psychological Corporation.
54. Miller LJ, Brett-Green B, Dickinson M, James K: *Effectiveness of occupational therapy for children with sensory processing impairments: a pilot study*, (in process).
55. Miller LJ, Lane SJ: Toward a consensus in terminology in sensory integration and practice: Part I: Taxonomy of neurophysiological processes, *Sensory Integration Special Interest Section Quarterly* 23:1, 2000.
56. Miller LJ, Lane AE, James K: *Defining the behavioral phenotype of sensory processing dysfunction* [Paper presented at the University of Colorado Health Sciences Center Developmental Psychobiology Research Group 12th Biennial Retreat, "Behavioral phenotypes in developmental disabilities."], Estes Park, CO, 2002, University of Colorado Health Sciences Center Developmental Psychobiology Research Group.
57. Miller LJ, McIntosh DN, McGrath J, et al: Electrodermal responses to sensory stimuli in individuals with fragile X syndrome: A preliminary report, *Am J Med Genet* 83:268, 1999.

58. Miller LJ, Reisman J, McIntosh DN, et al: An ecological model of sensory modulation: Performance of children with fragile X syndrome, autism, attention deficit/hyperactivity disorder, and sensory modulation dysfunction. In Roley SS, Blanche EI, Schaaf RC, editors: *Understanding the nature of sensory integration with diverse populations*, San Antonio, TX, 2001, Therapy Skill Builders.

59. Parham DL: Evaluation of praxis in preschoolers, *Occup Ther Health Care* 4:28, 1987.

60. Reeves G, Cermak S: Disorders of praxis. In Bundy AC, Lane S, Murray EA, editors: *Sensory integration: Theory and practice*, ed 2, Philadelphia, 2002, FA Davis.

61. Stallings-Sahler S: Case presentation: Child with gastro-esophageal reflux and severe sensory modulation disorder, *Sensory Integration Special Interest Section Quarterly* spring/summer, 2000.

62. Stallings-Sahler S: Case report: Report of an occupational therapy evaluation of sensory integration and praxis, *Am J Occup Ther* 44:650, 1990.

63. Stallings-Sahler S: Sensory integration assessment and intervention. In Case-Smith J, editor: *Pediatric occupational therapy and early intervention*, ed 2, St Louis, 1998, Elsevier/Butterworth-Heinemann.

64. Stallings-Sahler S: Sensory integration: Creating a challenging environment, *Occup Ther Week* 5:10, 16, 1991.

65. Stewart S: *The relationship between children's intellectual abilities and their socio-emotional presentation in a clinically referred sample* [Paper presented at the Society for Research in Child Development], Atlanta, GA, April 2004, Society for Research in Child Development.

66. Thomas A, Chess S, Birch, HG, Hertzig M, Korn S: *Temperament and behavior disorders in children*, New York, 1968, New York University Press.

67. Turkewitz G, Kenny PA: The role of developmental limitations of sensory input on sensory/perceptual organization, *Dev Behav Pediatr* 6:302, 1985.

68. Wilbarger J, Stackhouse TM: *Sensory modulation: A review of the literature*, May 1989: September 12, 1998; http://www.ot-innovations.com/content/view/29/58/ Accessed October 3, 2010.

69. Wilbarger P: Planning an adequate sensory diet: Application of sensory processing theory during the first year of life, *Zero to Three* 5:7, 1984.

70. Wilbarger P, Wilbarger J: *Sensory defensiveness in children aged 2-12: An intervention guide for parents and other caregivers*, Denver, CO, 1991, Avanti Educational Programs.

71. Williamson GG, Anzalone ME: *Sensory integration and self-regulation in infants and toddlers: Helping very young children interact with their environment*, Washington, DC, 2001, Zero to Three National Center for Clinical Infant Programs.

REVIEW *Questions*

1. What is sensory integration?
2. Define and describe sensory modulation disorder.
3. Define developmental dyspraxia, and describe intervention techniques.
4. What are functional support capacities?
5. How does sensory processing affect movement in children?
6. Describe the principles of sensory integration intervention.
7. Identify intervention techniques to work with children who have postural–ocular and bilateral integration dysfunction.

SUGGESTED *Activities*

1. Administer a sensory integration (SI) questionnaire to parents of typically developing children. Discuss the results in class.
2. Go to a specialized SI clinic, and observe typically developing children playing on equipment. Describe the motor planning and activity levels of the children.
3. Go to a specialized SI clinic and use the equipment for play activities. Note the intensity levels of the experience. How did the activity feel to you?
4. Go through a catalog, such as that of Southpaw Enterprises, Inc., and develop a list of games and activities for each piece of equipment. Make a notebook of these activities for future use.
5. Observe an SI session with a child and take notes of examples of how the OT practitioner used the principles of SI treatment (e.g., child initiated, use of suspended equipment, adaptive responses, controlled sensory input).
6. Observe an SI session with a child either in person or by means of videotape. Describe the type of sensory input and the adaptive responses required. How would you modify the activity?

CHAPTER 24 APPENDIX A

Example of Informal Checklist for Parent/Caregiver

Sensorimotor History Questionnaire
Adapted by Ricardo C. Carrasco and Susan Stallings-Sahler, 2005

Child's Name: _____
Completed by _____

Birthdate: ___ , ___ , ___ Today's Date: ___ , ___ , ___
Chronological Age: _____

Please respond to the following statements concerning your child's past and present behaviors and abilities. What do you recall as being different from other children? Were there times when his or her behavior was difficult for the family to cope with? What solutions have you found for any of these behavior issues?

These questions are asked to help us assemble a more complete picture of your child's development across time. Some questions may apply to children who are older than your child. In these cases, you may cross out the verb tense that does not apply. Check the choice that applies: **Yes, No,** or **N/A** (i.e., not old enough yet, not applicable). Add any comments that provide information you feel would be important for us to know about.

1.0 RESPONSES TO VISUAL AND LIGHT STIMULI IN THE ENVIRONMENT

#	Which of the following statements describes your child either currently or in the past?	Yes: Currently	Yes: In the past	Seldom or never	Further explanation or N/A
1.1	Is highly distracted; stressed by too many surrounding visual stimuli				
1.2	Does not visually orient to people and objects in environment				
1.3	Avoids making eye contact; looks away from face				
1.4	Seems overly sensitive to light; prefers to sit in dark room				
1.5	Seems driven to visually inspect the details of objects closely				

2.0 RESPONSES TO SOUNDS IN THE ENVIRONMENT (AUDITORY)

#	Which of the following statements describes your child either currently or in the past?	Yes: Currently	Yes: In the past	Seldom or never	Further explanation or N/A
2.1	Has an actual hearing loss (please explain if mild, moderate, severe, or profound)				
2.2	Has been diagnosed with childhood auditory processing disorder				
2.3	Often fails to listen or pay attention to what is said				
2.4	Often fails to follow through or act on verbal requests to do something; forgets or misunderstands instructions				
2.5	Is very distracted by sounds; seems to hear faint sounds that go unnoticed by others				
2.6	Talks excessively, almost compulsively				
2.7	Is stimulated to be overly verbal when others talk				
2.8	Puts hands over ears even when others are speaking only at a conversational level				
2.9	Has difficulty understanding the teacher when there is background noise in the classroom				
2.10	Sounds such as vacuum cleaner and blender perceived as noxious and painful to hear				
2.11	Is distracted by environmental sounds such as air conditioner, fan, refrigerator, and fluorescent light bulbs				
2.12	Speech difficult to understand; contains sound reversals and substitutions (e.g., "callerpitter," "W" instead of "L" or "R")				
2.13	Responds with "Huh?" when spoken to, but after a delay of 1 to 3 seconds displays comprehension of what was said				

3.0 RESPONSES TO MOVEMENT SENSATIONS (VESTIBULAR)

#	Which of the following statements describes your child either currently or in the past?	Yes: Currently	Yes: In the past	Seldom or never	Further explanation or N/A
3.1	Late in pregnancy or at birth, infant presented in the breech position (feet first)				
3.2	Placed on back for sleeping 75% to 100% of the time after age 3 months				
3.3	Placed on back for awake play time for 75% to 100% of the time after 4 months				
3.4	Very low tolerance for being placed on stomach for awake play time after 4 months				
3.5	Not motivated to move from one spot, even toward a new toy or family member				
3.6	Seemed to have ability to stand and walk at normal age but was fearful and hesitant about doing so				
3.7	Dislike of being moved in space or tossed up in the air during play				
3.8	Unable to fall asleep without rhythmic movement (e.g., rocking, riding in car, putting infant seat on running washing machine)				
3.9	Seems more active than most infants of same age				
3.10	Becomes anxious and fearful when feet are not touching the floor				
3.11	Becomes car-sick frequently/easily.				
3.12	Becomes dizzy or nauseous easily from circling movements on rides or playground				
3.13	Craves being in high places; climbs up to unusual heights but without fear				
3.14	Extremely afraid of heights (e.g., going up a ladder, walking down a flight of stairs)				
3.15	Seems to crave substantial or intense movement (e.g., being swung through the air, whirling/spinning)				
3.16	History of chronic middle ear infections				Since age ____ Tubes? ____

4.0 RESPONSES TO SMELLS AND TASTES (OLFACTORY/GUSTATORY)

#	Which of the following statements describes your child either currently or in the past?	Yes: Currently	Yes: In the past	Seldom or never	Further explanation or N/A
4.1	Wants to smell almost everything; explores new environments by smelling				
4.2	Seems unaware of smells or tastes; uninterested in food				
4.3	Becomes nauseous when exposed to many common food smells				
4.4	Craves ingesting unusual or non-nutritive tastes and substances (e.g., glue, dirt, soap)				
4.5	Tolerates only very bland foods (e.g., vanilla pudding, white bread, mashed potatoes)				
4.6	Has a history of chronic gastric reflux				
4.7	Prefers extremely spicy, hot, sour, or sweet tastes (circle those that apply)				
4.8	Has a history of food allergies and/or lactose intolerance				

5.0 RESPONSES TO TOUCH, PRESSURE, TEMPERATURE, AND PAIN (SOMATOSENSORY)

#	Which of the following statements describes your child either currently or in the past?	Yes: Currently	Yes: In the past	Seldom or never	Further explanation or N/A
5.1	Was picky about shape of bottle or pacifier nipples as an infant				
5.2	Dislikes being fed or eating with metal utensils; prefers to finger-feed				
5.3	Rejects food that has too much texture, lumps, or different-sized pieces in it				
5.4	Seems overly sensitive to certain textures of clothing, bedding, or other material in contact with skin				
5.5	Seemed to dislike being cuddled or held as an infant				
5.6	During toilet training seemed not to notice when bladder was full, causing "accidents."				

5.7	Seems excessively ticklish; panics or becomes combative when tickled				
5.8	Seems easily irritated or enraged when touched by siblings or playmates				
5.9	Gets into fights at school, such as standing in line at water fountain or engaged in activities on the playground				
5.10	Has strong need to touch objects and people				
5.11	Unusually afraid of dogs and pets that move quickly and/or jump up				
5.12	Seems to lack normal awareness of cold outdoor temperatures; goes out in winter without appropriate clothing				
5.13	Overdresses; seems to be unaware of excessive summer outdoor heat				
5.14	Seems to feel room temperature in marked contrast to what others find comfortable ("too hot" or "too cold")				
5.15	Seems overly sensitive to warm water temperature for a bath, wants it to be noticeably cool				
5.16	Overly sensitive to food temperature; wants it to be cool				
5.17	Strong dislike for taking showers or placing hands under a spray faucet to wash				
5.18	Seems almost unaware of painful experiences such as falling on hard surfaces; doesn't cry or complain				
5.19	Has/Had difficulty learning to put clothes on the correct parts of the body; needs to be able to see own body in order to dress				
5.20	Stomps feet very hard on steps when going up stairs				
5.21	Likes roughhouse play on the floor, such as being thrown down or "crashing" play				
5.22	Bears down extremely hard on crayons or pencils to the point of breaking them				

5.23	Cried as a toddler with normal weight bearing during creeping or standing				
5.24	Dislikes being handled or held in a firm manner				
5.25	Interprets deep pressure on skin (e.g., rubbing and massaging) as ticklish				
5.26	Resists having hair washed or cut or having fingernails trimmed				

6.0 SELF-REGULATORY CAPACITIES (AROUSAL, ATTENTION, AFFECT, ACTION)

#	Which of the following statements describes your child either currently or in the past?	Yes: Currently	Yes: In the past	Seldom or never	Further explanation or N/A
6.1	Seldom sleeps through the night				
6.2	Other sleep "issues" (explain)				
6.3	Is an early riser; wakes easily and becomes alert fairly quickly				
6.4	Very difficult to wake up in the morning; takes a long time to "get going"				
6.5	Rapidly went from sleeping, to awake, to frantic crying during infancy				
6.6	Has difficulty experiencing the transition from one activity or environment to another				
6.7	Gets "wound up" easily and then is very difficult to calm down				
6.8	Uses a favorite self-regulatory strategy to calm down or go to sleep (e.g., sucking thumb, holding blanket)				
6.9	Has "meltdowns" in late afternoon (overwhelmed by day at school or day care)				
6.10	Seeks out enclosed spaces to play in at home or school (e.g., under table, in bed under canopy, in a corner)				
6.11	Struggles to pay attention at school, at music or dance lessons, in church, or in other environments				

6.12	Takes medication to improve attention or reduce hyperactivity				
6.13	Seems unusually shy or clinging; anxious around strangers				
6.14	Seldom smiles or laughs; has a limited range of emotions; seems "flat"				
6.15	Loses control of laughter and becomes overly silly if laughed at or someone says something funny				
6.16	Does things impulsively; blurts out comments in class; has difficulty waiting turn				
6.17	Overattends to activities to the exclusion of other stimuli (e.g., teacher calling name, activity of others signaling a change, bell ringing at school)				
6.18	Seems hyperactive; unable to stop random running around; squirms in seat at school				

7.0 GROSS MOTOR (LARGE MUSCLE) MOVEMENTS AND SKILLS

#	Which of the following statements describes your child either currently or in the past?	Yes: Currently	Yes: In the past	Seldom or never	Further explanation or N/A
7.1	As an infant or toddler, was difficult to hold and carry because of being "floppy"				
7.2	As an infant/toddler, was difficult to hold and carry because of stiffness and arching				
7.3	As an infant, was difficult to hold for feeding; needed to use infant carrier to feed				
7.4	Stage of crawling on stomach was brief or skipped				
7.5	Stage of creeping on all fours was brief or skipped				
7.6	Sat up, stood, or walked independently earlier than others of same age				
7.7	Sat up, stood, or walked later than others of same age				
7.8	Could creep up stairs but was unable to come back down				
7.9	Engages in unusual movements such as walking on toes, flapping arms, and repeated rocking				

7.10	Late in learning how to hop and skip				
7.11	Late in learning to ride a bicycle				
7.12	Movement appears slow, plodding, or sluggish				
7.13	Seems hyperactive; in constant motion for most of the day				
7.14	Prefers sedentary activities (TV, reading, video games) and positions (lying down, partially reclined) instead of active play at >4 years of age				
7.15	More frequent falls and other accidents than other kids of same age				
7.16	Trouble with learning new movement skills such as those involved in skating, dancing, and sports				
7.17	Seems clumsier than others of same age				
7.18	Runs into other people, furniture, or side of door for unknown reasons				
7.19	Misunderstands verbal instructions to move a certain way				
7.20	Plays with toys and/or other children immature for his age				
7.21	Dislikes playing with manipulative toys (e.g., blocks, puzzles, Legos, transformers)				
7.22	Undresses dolls or stuffed animals but is unable to put clothes back on				
7.23	Has difficulty engaging in any prolonged play activity at home; constantly complains of being bored even though toys are available and there are activities to participate in				
7.24	Seems overly destructive with toys; breaks things a lot				
7.25	Has trouble with handling clothing fasteners (e.g., zippers, buttons, shoelaces)				
7.26	Experiences difficulty with handling school, art, or construction tools and materials correctly (e.g., scissors, paintbrush, stapler, glue, tape, hammer)				

8.0 SCHOOL PERFORMANCE QUESTIONS (Omit items that are not age appropriate; teachers' reports and conferences from previous years would be helpful as well as discussions with the teachers about some of the following.)

#	Which of the following statements describes your child either currently or in the past?	Yes: Currently	Yes: In the past	Seldom or never	Further explanation or N/A
8.1	Does significantly better one on one for school assignments than in a group				
8.2	Frequently slouches, props head on hand, or lies down on arm while reading or writing at desk				
8.3	Hand dominance still unclear after age 4; switches hands frequently				
8.4	Gets confused when putting on shoes (which one goes on which foot)				
8.5	Makes top-bottom inversions when writing numbers or letters (they appear upside down)				
8.6	Prints letters or numbers backward				
8.7	Confuses similar letters when reading, such as *b* and *d* and *m* and *w*				
8.8	Reverses sequential order when reading or writing "teens" (e.g., "41" instead of "14")				
8.9	Confuses reversible words, such as *dog* and *god* and *saw* and *was*				
8.10	Has great difficulty writing and looking at and listening to the teacher simultaneously				
8.11	(For children studying Hebrew) The problem of reversal in letters and words in English reappears after having been mastered earlier				
8.12	Shows an unusual amount of confusion in recognizing letters in Hebrew that are very similar in form				
8.13	Experiences significant problems in coping with written instructions during laboratory sessions, cooking class, or shop work				
8.14	Regards gym and participation in sports in general as distasteful or too hard				
8.15	Please cite any additional information about performances that teachers indicate are problems at school, either academically or behaviorally.				

9.0 SOCIAL ADJUSTMENT

#	Which of the following statements describes your child either currently or in the past?	Yes: Currently	Yes: In the past	Seldom or never	Further explanation or N/A
9.1	Finds it hard to make friends with peers				
9.2	Prefers the company of adults or older children, who allow more room for mistakes				
9.3	Has difficulty reading body language and other nonverbal social cues from others				
9.4	Tends to play with children who are a year or two younger.				
9.5	Is picked on by other children; tends to be a "loner"				
9.6	Expresses feelings of low self-esteem				
9.7	Tends to be bossy and dominating in play with peers				
9.8	Frequently expresses feelings of failure and frustration				
9.9	Seems discouraged and depressed				

OTHER PROFESSIONAL REPORTS: Evaluations from the following sources are available and will be forwarded.

Physician

Psychologist

Other Physical or Occupational Therapists

Teacher(s)

ADDITIONAL COMMENTS:

Adapted from Knickerbocker BM: *A holistic approach to the treatment of learning disorders*, Thorofare, NJ, 1980, CB Slack.

CHAPTER 24 APPENDIX B

Example of Informal Checklist for a Child's Teacher: Teacher Questionnaire on Sensorimotor Behavior

RICARDO C. CARRASCO

The Teacher Questionnaire on Sensorimotor Behavior (TQSB) was designed as a screening tool for either the occupational therapy (OT) practitioner or the teacher so that children with behaviors that are suspect or at risk for learning and relational behaviors can be referred for further OT screening or a more comprehensive evaluation. The results are useful in refuting or supporting historical, contextual, and other data in an impression or sensory integration dysfunction (DSI). Information on internal, concurrent, and construct validity and reliability is published in the literature and available through the author.

ADMINISTRATION AND SCORING INSTRUCTIONS

The item behaviors in this questionnaire were selected to investigate your student's performance at school. They are divided into sections, namely Motor Organization, Somatosensory System, Form/Space Perception and Visuoconstruction, Auditory/Language, Olfactory and Gustatory Systems, and Social Adjustment. Most of the items address behaviors that can be readily observed in the classroom. However, there are some that may require additional observations during library or lunch time, recess, or outdoor equipment use or on arrival at school from either the bus or private transportation. Completing the questionnaire will assist in compiling a comprehensive and descriptive picture of the child's Sensorimotor function but more importantly in determining how such function affects the daily activities that comprise his or her daily occupations.

1. Put a check or an X mark under the Yes or No column as appropriate. If the behavior does not apply, please put N/A under Yes.
2. Use the column under Comments or Sample Behaviors to describe or give examples of behaviors for that particular item (e.g., for item 1.63—especially when printing letters but not when drawing figures).
3. After completing the questionnaire, total the number of Yes responses in each section and record the total at the bottom of that section.
4. Convert the section total score to Normal, Suspect, or High based on the ranges of scores specified in the conversion table below.

Conversion Table

SECTION	NORMAL	SUSPECT	HIGH
Motor Organization	0 to 4	5 to 15	15 or higher
Somatosensory System	0 to 3	4 to 11	12 or higher
Form/Space Perception and Visuoconstruction	0 to 2	3 to 10	11 or higher
Auditory/Language	0 to 1	2 to 5	6 or higher
Olfactory and Gustatory	0	1	2 or higher
Social Adjustment	0	1 to 2	3 or higher

A predominance of Suspect scores suggests further screening at the discretion of the professional; Predominantly High scores warrant further professional evaluation. The Interpretation Key can be used by the OT practitioner or other qualified professional and is available from the author.

Child's Name: _____ Date of Birth: ___ , ___ , ___
DOT: ___ , ___ , ___ Chronological Age: ___ ___ ___

1.00 Motor Organization: Vestibular, Proprioceptive, and Visual Senses

ITEM #	YES	NO	ITEM BEHAVIORS	COMMENTS OR SAMPLE BEHAVIORS
1.00			Performs school tasks with slow, deliberate movements	
1.20			Falls when attempting to hop on one foot	
1.21			Falls when attempting to skip	
1.30			Finds gym or outdoor play equipment distasteful	
1.31			Often feels sick on disembarking from school bus or car	
1.32			Gets sick and vomits from movement experiences, e.g., games, turning around	
1.33			Does not adequately inform others of these feelings	
1.34			Twirls on piano stools, swivel chairs, or similar equipment more than other children	
1.35			Seeks stimulation on school playground equipment, e.g., seesaw, merry-go-round, more than other children	
1.36			Hangs upside down on jungle gym	
1.37			Dislikes climbing on playground equipment	
1.38			Hesitates when going up or down stairs or stepping on or off curbs	
1.39			Avoids balancing activities	
1.40			Tires easily	
1.41			Stands with shoulders forward or swayed back	
1.42			Muscles seem tight	
1.43			Muscles seem flabby	
1.50			Poor rhythm walking	
1.51			Shuffles feet when walking	
1.52			Drops toes when walking	
1.63			Needs reminders to hold paper for writing	
1.70			Persistently gets confused over which hand or foot is left or right	

1.71			Gets confused easily about crossover patterns to find the right side of a person facing him	
1.72			Prints numbers or letters backwards	
1.80			Appears to be accident prone, e.g., spills milk, drops pencils or books, trips over or bumps into furniture	
1.90			Continues movements or mannerisms after it is time to stop	
1.91			While writing or working with dominant hand, other hand looks tense or mirrors dominant hand	
1.92			Inconsistent use of left or right hand	
1.93			Complains of hand or back fatigue or pain during pencil tasks	
1.94			Makes holes in paper while trying to erase or write	
1.95			Shakes or stretches hand during long periods of writing	

Motor Organization: Total ___   Conversion: Normal ___ Suspect ___ High ___

2.00 Somatosensory System: Touch and Proprioception

ITEZM #	YES	NO	ITEM BEHAVIORS	COMMENTS OR SAMPLE BEHAVIORS
2.10			Dislikes being held or cuddled	
2.11			Dislikes being barefoot	
2.12			Has changed from disliking to liking being held or cuddled	
2.13			Seems excessively ticklish	
2.14			Pulls away or is easily irritated when touched by classmates or school staff	
2.15			Picks fights at school, e.g., standing in line on the playground, in the lunchroom, in the library	
2.20			Fidgets, pushes or pulls fingers with other hand, repeatedly touches various parts of the body, or puts hands or objects in mouth	
2.21			Has a strong need to touch objects and people	
2.30			Lacks typical awareness of being touched by classmates or school staff	

2.31			Lacks awareness of cold outdoor temperature	
2.32			Overdresses, seemingly unaware of excessive summer heat	
2.33			Underdresses, seemingly unaware of excessive winter cold	
2.34			Feels room temperature in marked or some contrast to what others feel comfortable	
2.35			Often seems unaware of bruises, cuts, and bleeding gashes until informed by others	
2.40			Clumsy when playing with toys	
2.41			Volitionally engages in prolonged manipulative tasks, e.g., puzzles, mazes	
2.42			Engages but needs prompting in prolonged manipulative tasks given by teacher or aide	
2.43			Has trouble paying attention to classroom task at hand	
2.44			Overly destructive with classroom desk or materials, e.g., books, workbooks, toys	
2.50			Difficulty in manipulating tools with hands, e.g., spoons, pencils	
2.51			Cannot push blades of scissors together	
2.52			Holds pencil too tight	
2.53			Holds pencil too loose	
2.54			Grasps pencil without use of thumb and index and middle fingers	
2.56			Constantly changes pencil grasp while writing	
2.57			Pencil pressure on paper too heavy	
2.58			Pencil pressure on paper too light	

Somatosensory System: Total___   Conversion: Normal ___ Suspect ___ High ___

3.00 Form/Space Perception and Visuoconstruction

ITEM #	YES	NO	ITEM BEHAVIORS	COMMENTS OR SAMPLE BEHAVIORS
3.10			Highly distracted by visual stimuli	
3.11			Concentrates better when desk is not cluttered	
3.12			Functions significantly better in a one-on-one relationship in class	
3.19			Reads letters or numbers backward	
3.21			Reverses sequential order of "teen" numbers e.g., forming a 4 and then placing the 1 in front of it	
3.22			Gets confused when reading reversible letters such as *b* and *d*	
3.23			Gets confused when reading reversible words such as *dog* and *god* and *saw* and *was*	
3.30			Moves head rather than eyes only when reading sentences from a book	
3.31			Uses fingers or a line guide to prevent losing place while reading	
3.40			Blinks eyes, places hands over face, or ducks while playing ball	
3.50			Has trouble finding way from one place to another and gets lost easily	
3.60			Has trouble recognizing similarities and differences in patterns or designs	
3.70			Cannot make letters and numbers stay between lines or spaces	
3.71			Often overshoots or undershoots targets, e.g., placing pencils or crayons in a box	
3.80			Has difficulty putting parts of a toy or puzzle together	
3.81			Frequently supports head with hand while reading or writing at desk	
3.90			Difficulty copying from blackboard or chalkboard	
3.91			Cannot adequately draw forms or shapes	
3.92			Holds head close to paper while writing	
3.93			Rotates paper more than 45 degrees when writing	
3.94			Does not leave adequate space between words or letters	
3.95			Tips head to one side during activities, as if using only one eye	

Form/Space Perception and Visuoconstruction: Total ___   Conversion: Normal ___ Suspect ___ High ___

4.00 Auditory/Language

ITEM #	YES	NO	ITEM BEHAVIORS	COMMENTS OR SAMPLE BEHAVIORS
4.10			Gets distracted by sounds; hears sounds that go unnoticed by others	
4.12			Gets distracted by sounds in the classroom, e.g., music, classmates talking	
4.13			Gets distracted by sounds, e.g., fluorescent light bulbs, heaters, refrigerators	
4.20			Often fails to listen or pay attention to what is said	
4.21			Often fails to follow through or act on requests to do something	
4.22			Is unable to function if two or three steps of instructions are given at once	
4.23			Talks excessively	
4.24			Talking by others becomes stimulus to be overly verbal	
4.25			Talking interferes with ability to listen	
4.26			Has difficulty remembering sequence of numbers heard	
4.27			Has difficulty remembering sequence of words heard	
4.30			Reverses sequence of words or numbers heard	
4.31			Misunderstands the meanings of words used in relation to movement, e.g., push/pull, go left/right, up/down	

Auditory/Language: Total ___ Conversion: Normal ___ Suspect ___ High ___

5.00 Olfactory and Gustatory Systems

ITEM #	YES	NO	ITEM BEHAVIORS	COMMENTS OR SAMPLE BEHAVIORS
5.10			Highly sensitive to scents and odors	
5.20			Seems to lack typical awareness of odors easily perceived by others	
5.30			Expresses strong like or dislike of food smells (explain)	
5.40			Expresses strong dislike of other scents (explain)	

| 5.50 | | | Shows strong reaction to otherwise common food tastes, e.g., salty, sweet, sour | |
| 5.51 | | | Desires excessive flavor in or condiments for food, e.g., salt, ketchup, mustard | |

Olfactory and Gustatory: Total___   Conversion: Normal ___ Suspect ___ High ___

6.00 Social Adjustment

ITEM #	YES	NO	ITEM BEHAVIORS	COMMENTS OR SAMPLE BEHAVIORS
6.10			Finds it hard to make friends with peers	
6.11			Prefers company of adults or older children	
6.12			Tends to play with children a year or two younger	
6.20			Is a loner	
6.30			Expresses feelings of low self-esteem	
6.40			Expresses feelings of failure	
6.50			Gets frustrated easily	
6.51			Seems discouraged or depressed	
6.60			Is more emotionally sensitive; feelings get easily hurt	
6.70			Cannot tolerate changes in plans or expectations	

Social Adjustment: Total ___   Conversion: Normal ___ Suspect ___ High ___

Additional Information

_____
Teacher's Name and Signature

Adapted from the Sensorimotor History Questionnaire and other unpublished sensorimotor behavior questionnaires by Ricardo C. Carrasco.

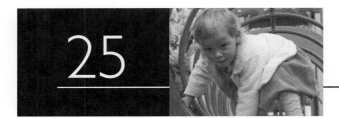

25

Applying the Model of Human Occupation*
to Pediatric Practice

JESSICA M. KRAMER

PATRICIA BOWYER

CHAPTER *Objectives*

After studying this chapter, the reader will be able to accomplish the following:

- Describe the meaning of MOHO concepts of volition, habituation, performance capacity, the environment, and skill
- Identify ways to address a client's volition, habituation, performance capacity, environment, and skill in therapy through the use of therapeutic strategies
- Practice using MOHO concepts to describe and analyze a clinical scenario

---

*Dr. Gary Kielhofner crafted the MOHO over 30 years ago. He inspired and supported researchers and practioners to use these concepts to enhance practice in order to help clients engage in daily occupations. His vision and scholarship has made a difference in the lives of children and their families. The authors acknowledge Dr. Kielhofner's work and contributions to the occupational therapy profession and are grateful for his role in mentoring them.

Shaun, an 11-year-old boy, has cerebral palsy. His handwriting did not improve this year, and he does not try very hard during his biweekly therapy sessions, so he continues to fall behind his classmates. Maria is a 2-year old girl receiving early intervention services after a medically complicated birth. She is just beginning to learn how to dress herself, and giggles with delight after her mother helps her put on her princess costume. Lizzy, a young woman with autism, is beginning vocational training as part of her transition plan and needs to identify the type of job that will enable her to be successful, given her interests, abilities, and support needs. Sessions with a client—whether an infant, child, or adolescent—can either represent a challenge or be an opportunity to make progress toward the achievement of an intervention goal.

As an occupational therapy assistant (OTA), you have the opportunity to create a therapeutic environment that is individualized to each client's preferences and challenges and as a result, more likely to enable young clients to reach their occupational therapy goals. So how do you motivate Shaun to practice handwriting so that he does not have to struggle in class? How do you ensure that Maria will learn to successfully perform self-care activities? While working with Lizzy on prevocational skills, what can you do to help her identify the employment setting that is most appropriate for her? The Model of Human Occupation (MOHO) is one way to systematically analyze clients' current occupational situations, understand their strengths and challenges, and identify the optimal therapeutic environment that enables children and adolescents to achieve their goals.

WHAT IS THE MODEL OF HUMAN OCCUPATION?

Dr. Gary Kielhofner crafted the MOHO over 30 years ago and inspired others to develop concepts in practice. Dr. Kielhofner was passionate about scholarship and dedicated to making a difference in clients' lives. The MOHO is an occupation focused, evidence-based, and client-centered way of thinking about your practice with children and youth. MOHO is concerned with a child's or adolescent's motivation for engaging in occupations, the pattern and organization of occupations, the ability to perform occupations, and the influence of the environment on occupations. The main concepts in MOHO are *volition, habituation, performance capacity,* and *environment.* We will define and explain these concepts later in this chapter. When first learning about these concepts, all the different definitions can sometimes be overwhelming. Rather than worrying about memorizing these definitions, it is helpful to keep in mind that the purpose of the concepts is to enable you to think, in a systematic way, about your clients, their strengths, and the challenges they encounter when

participatng in occupations. As you practice using these concepts to analyze your clients' occupational participation, you will find that it will become easier to remember the different MOHO concepts and their meanings.

MOHO is *occupation focused* because its concepts are focused on understanding the extent to which children or adolescents are able to participate in the occupations of taking care of self, playing, learning, and working. Further, MOHO does not just focus on children's or adolescent's impairments such as lack of strength or poor visual-motor integration, but the model also considers what motivates them to participate in occupations, how their participation in different occupations is organized and patterned on a daily basis, and how the environment supports or interferes with participation in occupations.

MOHO is also *evidence based,* and the associated concepts and tools have undergone almost 30 years of research and development. At the time this chapter was written, more than 250 MOHO-related publications of studies, case examples, and theoretical discussions were available to support practice. This research and development has occurred through the collaboration of a network of international researchers and OT practitioners. Today, MOHO has become the most widely used occupation-focused model in occupational therapy.[1,3,4] This large body of evidence cannot be incorporated into one chapter; the most recent evidence for practice can be easily accessed at the model of human occupation Web site at www.moho.uic.edu. The most recent text on MOHO, *Model of Human Occupation: Theory and application* (4th edition) also includes a chapter reviewing the evidence supporting the use of MOHO in practice.[2]

Finally, MOHO is *client centered* because the concepts are focused on identifying the unique occupational strengths and needs of each client. While these concepts can be applied to children of any age and with a range of abilities, the understanding gained about each child or adolescent will be unique and will enable you to individualize your OT interventions. MOHO also stresses the importance of incorporating the client's perspective into the therapy process. When working with children and adolescents, the family's perspective is also included. Some of the therapeutic strategies introduced in this chapter require the OT practitioner to first obtain the perspective of the child or adolescent and the family. Observations, informal interviews, and review of records and assessments are just some ways of obtaining information about the perspectives of the child or adolescent and the family. For more information, refer to the previously mentioned text, which includes several chapters on gathering information from children, adolescents, and families using observations, interviews, and self reports.[2]

The remainder of the chapter will introduce you to MOHO concepts and illustrate ways of systematically using these concepts to enhance OT interventions. As you practice applying these concepts, remember that MOHO is an occupation-focused, evidence-based, and client-centered way of thinking, in a systematic way, about the clients you encounter in therapy.

MOHO THERAPEUTIC STRATEGIES

Therapeutic strategies are specific actions that can facilitate client change by influencing the way a child or an adolescent feels, thinks, or does something in the context of therapy. OT practitioners use therapeutic strategies to engage a child or adolescent in therapy and to help create an optimal therapeutic environment. Nine therapeutic strategies have been listed in Table 25-1. Each therapeutic strategy can be applied in several different ways to address a range of client needs or therapeutic challenges. This chapter will demonstrate how OT practitioners use specific therapeutic strategies to address a particular aspect of a child's or adolescent's volition, habituation, skill, or his or her environment.

MOHO CONCEPTS: CLIENT FACTORS

Each child or adolescent brings a unique set of personal factors that influence his or her engagement in occupations. The MOHO concepts that help us to think about these personal factors, or *client factors*, are volition, habituation, and performance capacity.

Volition

Volition, or a child's or adolescent's motivation for occupations, is influenced by (1) those activities that the child or adolescent finds most enjoyable (interests), (2) his or her beliefs about what is important (values), and (3) beliefs about his or her ability to effectively perform occupations (personal causation). In combination, these three aspects of volition create a unique pattern of thoughts and feelings that influence how a child or adolescent anticipates, chooses, experiences, and interprets what he or she does.

Consider Shaun's lack of interest in practicing handwriting. Perhaps Shaun does not find handwriting activities fun and so is not interested in practicing with his OTA. It is also possible that Shaun considers it more important to conserve his energy to perform fine motor tasks other than handwriting, such as eating or using a computer. Another possibility is that Shaun is frustrated by his poor handwriting and believes that further practice will not improve his handwriting, and so he stops trying. By gathering more information, the OT practitioner can determine which of these aspects of volition is influencing Shaun's participation in therapy. The OT practitioner will then be better able to provide an individualized therapeutic environment that is based on Shaun's interests, values, and personal causation.

TABLE 25-1

Therapeutic Strategies and Definitions

THERAPEUTIC STRATEGY	DEFINITION
Advise	Recommend intervention goals and strategies to the child, adolescent, and family.
Coach	Instruct, demonstrate, guide, verbally prompt, and/or physically assist the child or adolescent while he or she is performing an occupation.
Encourage	Provide emotional support and reassurance to the child or adolescent during or after an activity.
Give feedback	Share an overall conceptualization of the child's or adolescent's situation or an understanding of the ongoing participation in occupations.
Identify	Locate and share a range of personal, procedural, and/or environmental factors that can facilitate the child's or adolescent's occupational participation.
Negotiate	Engage in give-and-take with the child or adolescent, parents, and other professionals to achieve a common perspective or agreement about something that the child or adolescent will or should do in the future.
Physical support	Have the child or adolescent use the body to support the completion of an occupational task when he or she cannot or will not use motor skills.
Structure	Establish parameters for choice and performance by offering alternatives to the child or adolescent, setting limits, and establishing ground rules.
Validate	Convey respect for the experience or perspective of the child or adolescent and the parents.

Adapted from Kielhofner G: (2008). *Model of human occupation: Theory and application*, ed 4, Baltimore, MD, 2008, Lippincott Williams and Wilkins.

Interests

Interests are things that a child or an adolescent finds enjoyable and satisfying to do. Usually, children and adolescents are interested in activities in which they are most likely to be successful and engage without possibility of failure, pain, or difficulty. Therefore, interests are inherently motivating and thus are quite likely to encourage participation in specific activities; children usually feel good about themselves when engaging in a preferred activity. Often, a child or an adolescent may have a pattern of interests that represents a primary interest in one area such as sports, arts and crafts, or animals. OT practitioners can incorporate a child's or adolescent's interests into therapy activities as a means to facilitate desired change.

CLINICAL *Pearl*

The therapeutic strategy of "encouraging" can be enhanced when it is incorporated along with a child's or adolescent's interests. If a child or adolescent is unsure, worried, or scared, the impact of encouragement strategies such as verbal assurance ("You can do it") can be strengthened by referring to his or her interests.

CASE *Study*

Maria's OTA decided to use Maria's interest in dressing up as a princess to encourage her to practice dressing herself. The OTA had Maria decorate a plain shirt with glitter and markers to make it a "princess shirt." The therapist then asked Maria to try putting on her shirt herself so they could pretend to be princesses. However, Maria became frustrated when she was unable to push her arm through the sleeve. The OT practitioner encouraged Maria and, drawing upon Maria's interest in dress-up, said, "You can do it, keep trying! I can't wait to play princess with you once you get your princess shirt on!"

Values

Values are those things that a child or an adolescent finds important and meaningful and which are influenced by his or her culture and context. Values result from internalized convictions and are associated with a sense of obligation. These internalized personal convictions define what matters to children and adolescents and may also be a reflection of what matters to other important people in their lives such as their families or communities. The resulting sense of obligation influences their decision to engage in

certain occupations. Understanding the values of clients and their families can help ensure provision of client-centered therapy.

CLINICAL *Pearl*

Sometimes other professionals, parents, and the child or adolescent place different levels of importance on certain activities, skills, or outcomes. As a result, they may not place equal value on the therapy goals or the activities presented during OT. The therapeutic strategy "negotiation" can help you identify intervention activities that are valued by all members of the child's or adolescent's support team or can enable you to reach a compromise that recognizes differences in values.

CASE *Study*

Shaun's teacher thinks that it is important for Shaun to complete the handwritten class notes to demonstrate that he is participating in class. However, Shaun's family feels that it is more important for Shaun to attend to the teacher and share his ideas during class discussions. Shaun cares most about conserving his energy so that he can complete the full school day. The occupational therapist meets with the teacher, Shaun, and his parents to discuss these conflicting values and negotiates an alternative solution. The teacher will provide Shaun with an outline for each class lecture, and Shaun will add his typed notes to the outline at home each evening. Shaun will receive class participation points by turning in his typed notes from the previous day and by participating in class discussions. The OT practitioner will stop working on Shaun's handwriting and instead help him learn how to type and use voice dictation software. Negotiation enabled the OT practitioner to identify a solution that recognized the values of the teacher, Shaun, and his parents with regard to learning and class participation.

Personal Causation

Personal causation is a child's or adolescent's sense of competence (sense of capacity) and effectiveness (self-efficacy) for doing different occupations. A child's or adolescent's personal causation is related to his or her awareness of the ability to engage in an occupation. When a child or adolescent believes he or she can achieve a desired outcome in an occupation, a sense of self-efficacy is developed. Self-perceptions of capacity and efficacy guide activity choices. A child who may believe she excels in ball sports is willing to play all ball-related games, another who may consider himself "musical" will try to learn how to play a new instrument, and another child who may think she is good at making new friends is willing to join a new club that meets at the community park. Personal causation is gradually built through continued accomplishments and increases the motivation to engage in other occupations. For example, a child who is comfortable walking across the room will be more motivated to explore the environment. A child who enjoys playing games with a brother or sister may feel comfortable initiating interactions with a same-aged peer.

Children and adolescents do not need to express their personal causation in words for occupational therapists to understand how they feel about their capacities and effectiveness. A child who has a good sense of personal causation in an occupation will seek out new challenges, while a child who feels a low sense of capacity will avoid new activities. For example, students, such as Shaun, who are unable to write at high speeds may not feel a sense of personal capacity for taking notes in class and therefore may begin to avoid participation in class. By observing this pattern of behavior, an OT practitioner can determine a child's sense of personal causation.

Volitional Process

Now that you have been introduced to the three aspects of volition—interests, values, and personal causation—they will help you understand why certain activities are motivating to some children, whereas other children are unmotivated or unwilling to engage in them. However, how can you change a child's or adolescent's sense of personal causation so that he or she believes that he or she has the capacity to try a new occupation? How can you help a child or adolescent identify a new interest? How can you help a child or adolescent evaluate values and make choices based on those values? An OT practitioner can influence a child's or adolescent's interests, values, or personal causation using the volitional process.

The *volitional process* is the way children or adolescents experience their participation in occupations and includes four steps: (1) anticipation, (2) making choices, (3) experience, and (4) interpretation. A child's or adolescent's interests, values, and personal causation influence each step of this volitional process, as illustrated in Figure 25-1. For example, if a child enjoys movement and swinging, he will most likely anticipate that rocking on a hammock will be enjoyable. As a result, he will be more likely to choose to do the activity of rocking on a hammock in therapy. He is likely to enjoy the experience of rocking in the hammock and will interpret the activity as enjoyable. Based on this positive interpretation, whenever encountering this activity in the future, the child is more likely to have a positive anticipation of playing in the hammock and choose the activity again.

OT practitioners can try to influence a child's or adolescent's volition by changing the way he or she anticipates, chooses, experiences, or interprets an activity. For example, consider Shaun and his poor sense of personal causation with regard to handwriting. When Shaun is asked to complete a handwriting activity in therapy, he anticipates that he does not have the ability to successfully complete the activity. The OT practitioner can try to change the way Shaun anticipates this activity by making the activity easier, by making the activity similar to an activity Shaun knows that he is able to complete, or by aligning the activity with one of Shaun's interests. The OT practitioner knows that Shaun enjoys collecting baseball cards and so asks Shaun to write a list of his 10 most valuable baseball cards. Making a list is easier than writing full sentences, and Shaun enjoys talking about his baseball card collection. As a result, he has a more positive anticipation of the activity and chooses to complete this activity with his OT practitioner. Although Shaun has some difficulty writing this list, he experiences the activity as more enjoyable because he is thinking about his card collection and sharing his ideas with the OT practitioner. When the list is complete, the OT practitioner then asks Shaun to type the list into the computer. It takes Shaun a long time to type the list, but he is pleased when he produces a typed list that is easy to read. Although he had some difficulty writing and typing the list, overall, Shaun believes he was able to successfully complete this activity and interprets his experience as positive. The OT practitioner believes that the next time this type of activity is introduced, Shaun will be more likely to anticipate a positive experience and therefore will be more willing to engage in such activities during therapy. By using the steps of the volitional process and thinking about Shaun's interests, values, and personal causation, the OT practitioner can help Shaun reach the desired goal of learning to type.

Habituation

Habituation explains the pattern and organization of a child's or adolescent's participation in different occupations. **Habituation** is the internalized readiness to engage in consistent patterns of behavior during certain times of day and certain days of the week, as determined by one's habits and roles. Habits and roles help children and adolescents organize their lives and participate in everyday occupations more easily.

Habits

When children or adolescents respond to familiar situations in consistent ways, they are demonstrating a habit. A **habit** is an acquired tendency to respond

Anticipation

When I think about doing this activity…

Does this activity seem to be fun and enjoyable? (interests)
Does this activity appear to be meaningful? (values)
Do I believe that I can successfully engage in and complete this activity?

Making Choices

I am more likely to choose this activity if….

I think it is fun and enjoyable (interests).
I think it is meaningful and if it is aligned with my sense of obligation (values).
I believe I can successfully engage in and complete the activity (personal causation).

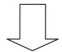

Experience

While I am doing this activity….

Is this activity fun and enjoyable? (interests)
Is this activity meaningful? (values)
Am I able to successfully engage in and complete this activity? (personal causation)

Interpretation

I am more likely to have a positive interpretation if….

I thought the activity was fun and enjoyable (interests).
I thought the activity was meaningful and aligned with my sense of obligation (values).
I thought I was able to successfully complete the activity (personal causation).

I am more likely to have a negative interpretation if….

I thought the activity was scary, unpleasant, or uncomfortable (interests).
I thought the activity was not meaningful and not aligned with my sense of obligation (values).
I thought I did not have the ability to successfully complete the activity or the activity was too difficult (personal causation).

FIGURE 25-1   How the volitional process is influenced by a child's or adolescent's interests, values, and personal causation.

automatically to a specific circumstance or environment. Habits help children to be efficient and effective when doing familiar, everyday activities. For example, a child who has an organized routine when entering his classroom (hang up the backpack, get the homework folder out, and place it in the desk) will be able to quickly put his belongings in the proper place and prepare for the school day. OT practitioners can help children develop new habits or routines to optimize the performance of occupations such as brushing the teeth, cleaning the room, or learning a new task at work.

Roles

When a child or an adolescent identifies himself or herself as a son or daughter, brother or sister, student, soccer player, band member, or worker, he or she is internalizing a role. **Roles** are a set of related actions and attitudes that, in combination, define a culturally and socially familiar status. For example, the role of a student is associated with the actions of attending school, listening to the teacher, participating in classroom activities, playing with classmates, and taking tests. Children and adolescents are expected to be able to perform the actions associated with their roles, and OT can be a time for children to learn and practice these role-related activities.

Roles also help children, adolescents, and families define their relationships and actions with others; a child is expected to act in different ways when interacting with his teacher, mother, and best friend. A child who does not identify with any roles will have difficulty interacting with others and participating in activities. In this instance, the OT practitioner may use therapy as an opportunity to identify potential roles for the child, such as pet owner, class helper, or community volunteer.

CLINICAL *Pearl*

OT practitioners can use the therapeutic strategy "advise" to help children take on and participate in new roles. For example, parents may not expect children to have a role in completing chores around the house because of concerns about accessibility, safety, or task completion. However, learning to complete chores can be an important part of children's development and enables them to hold a valuable role in their homes. OT practitioners can advise parents about chores that may be appropriate based on children's abilities and identify ways to incorporate those chores into the children's daily routines. For example, a child could take on the chore of "putting away dirty laundry." Laundry baskets could be labeled with different color blocks to help the child sort dirty laundry by color. This type of advice can enable parents to support their child's engagement in new roles.

Performance Capacity

Performance capacity is the third and final MOHO concept addressing client or personal factors. **Performance capacity** is a child's ability to do things as supported by the status of his or her physical and mental components as well as the subjective experience of living within his or her body.

OT practitioners can measure the status of physical and mental components, and therefore this aspect of a child's performance capacity is known as the *objective aspect of performance capacity.* Some examples of physical and mental components that can be measured objectively are strength, intelligence, and proprioception. OT practitioners use other theories to measure, classify, and describe the status of the physical and mental components of a child or adolescent. Therefore, MOHO acknowledges the importance of a child's or adolescent's physical and mental components but relies on the OT practitioner's use of other frames of reference (biomechanical, sensory integration) to evaluate and explain those components.

CLINICAL *Pearl*

If a child's physical and mental components make it difficult to complete certain tasks, an OT practitioner can use the therapeutic strategy "provide physical support" to help the child successfully complete a task or learn a new skill. This can also help OT practitioners ensure children's success while doing occupations and can influence the volitional process!

A child's or adolescent's own experience of using and living in his or her body is the *subjective aspect of performance capacity,* also referred to as the *"lived body" experience.* This aspect is subjective because it is based on a child's unique experience and cannot be measured by another person. However, OT practitioners can try to gather information to understand a child's or adolescent's subjective experience of using his or her body. For example, a child with sensory integration difficulties and gravitational insecurity may describe the experience of going down a slide as "falling into a black hole." This subjective experience influences a child's sense of capacity and experience of doing occupations as much as the status of his or her physical and mental components. Awareness of a child's subjective experience helps the OT practitioner provide a safe and comfortable therapeutic environment.

CLINICAL *Pearl*

Although there is no formal way to assess or measure a child's subjective experience of using his or her body, an OT practitioner can acknowledge a child's experience using the therapeutic strategy of "validation." OT practitioners should acknowledge when a child may be scared, unsure, uncomfortable, or in pain when completing therapy activities. For example, the OT practitioner may say, "I know this is really scary, but I won't let you fall" or "If this hurts too much, please tell me to stop." The use of this strategy demonstrates respect for the child's lived body experience.

MOHO CONCEPTS: ENVIRONMENTAL FACTORS

The MOHO concepts of volition, habituation, and performance capacity address personal client factors that influence participation in occupation. However, MOHO recognizes that the **environment** also influences children's participation in occupation. The MOHO concepts that help us think of the environmental factors that directly influence participation are *spaces, objects, social groups,* and *occupational tasks.* Other environmental factors, including economic conditions, culture, and political conditions, indirectly influence participation and the opportunities available to, and demands placed upon, children and adolescents.

Spaces

Spaces are physical places, or contexts, that are arranged in ways that influence what children do within those spaces. The unique features of natural or built spaces, such as a grassy hill, a staircase, the current weather, a row of chairs, or the length of a hallway, all influence the extent to which children or adolescents can participate in different occupations. Some settings influence the types of occupations that take place; for example, a library encourages quiet reading and hunting for books, a playground encourages running and climbing, and a kitchen encourages cooking and eating. OT practitioners can modify and rearrange spaces to ensure accessibility and to encourage participation in specific occupations. One example is rearranging desks so that a child who uses a wheelchair can more easily move about the classroom to obtain materials and interact with classmates.

Objects

Objects are natural or man-made things that children and adolescents interact with and use during occupations. Objects are used in play (blocks), self-care (shoes), mobility (wheelchair), and learning (books). Like spaces, objects also influence the types of occupations children engage in and the way they perform those occupations. Students such as Shaun in our case study can take notes using paper and pencil or a computer; the availability of these objects determines how they will take notes in class. OT practitioners may modify existing objects or provide different objects in order to facilitate a child's participation in different occupations. For example, since Maria had a weak grip and difficulty with her fine motor skills, the OT practitioner added a foam handle to her spoon so that she could hold her spoon more easily to feed herself. Finally, objects can signify children's special interests or roles that are important to them. Lizzy takes pride in her role of checking books into the school library and always carries the clipboard she uses to complete this job. Shaun always carries baseball cards in his backpack, and Maria's room is full of princess toys. OT practitioners can incorporate such objects of interest into therapy sessions to motivate and engage children.

Social Groups

Social groups are collections of people who come together for a variety of formal or informal purposes. Social groups include play groups, classrooms, worship communities, Internet social networking groups, families, and a neighborhood. In the neighborhood, play with other children may be informally organized by a group of children, but play at school during recess may be formally structured into the daily schedule and may involve specific types of games and activities.

Social groups also influence the types of occupations available to children or adolescents as well as the behaviors that the members of the social group expect from the children. The child's teacher may expect him or her to pay attention, work quietly, and follow classroom rules, while parents may expect the child to play nicely with siblings and eat dinner with the family. The OT practitioner can support the child's engagement in occupations by identifying the different social groups the child belongs to, determining the occupations and expectations of each social group, and either modifying those expectations according to the child's ability or helping the child practice those occupations.

Occupational Forms/Tasks

In any culture, one often finds common and typical ways of doing specific occupations, for example, playing a game of football, taking a test, or baking a cake. It is likely that each reader thinks of a similar sequence of actions that is required to do these occupations. **Occupational forms**, or **tasks**, are these conventional sequences of actions that are oriented to a specific purpose and are understood by and recognizable to members of a shared culture.[5] For some children or adolescents, these conventionalized ways of doing occupations are not accessible or possible, given their impairments and abilities. OT practitioners can modify the steps in a task or propose an alternative way of doing tasks to enable children to actively participate in occupations.

CLINICAL *Pearl*

Using the strategy "structure" to modify the social environment and occupational task helps create a therapeutic environment in which the child is most likely to be successful. One way to structure occupational tasks to ensure success is to limit the choices available to a child or ensure that the child has access to an activity that he or she will be able to successfully complete. Similarly, the OT practitioner structures the social environment when clear rules and expectations are set for the child's behavior.

THE INTERACTION BETWEEN CLIENT AND ENVIRONMENTAL FACTORS DURING PARTICIPATION

Environmental Impact

Each child or adolescent is unique; therefore, the impact that environmental factors have on his or her participation varies with the uniqueness of the child's impairments and abilities. The extent to which spaces, objects, social groups, and occupational tasks provide opportunities, supports/resources, demands, or constraints on participation constitutes the **environmental impact** on a child. Consider two children with mobility impairments; one child crawls to get around her house, and the other child uses a wheelchair. For the child who crawls, stairs demand the ability to climb, but if that child is able to crawl up the stairs, the stairs do not constrain her participation in that environment. However, for the child who uses the wheelchair, if he or she is unable to meet the environmental demand to climb, the stairs will constrain participation.

Whether and how different environmental opportunities, supports/resources, demands, and constraints are perceived by a child depends on his or her volition, habituation, and performance capacity. For example, low environmental demands may bore one child but calm another; similarly, high environmental demands may engage one child with a variety of interests and strong sense of personal causation but overwhelm another child who has a low sense of efficacy and capacity. OT practitioners should carefully consider how an environment uniquely impacts each child's participation in occupations and attempt to provide spaces, objects, tasks, and social expectations that match the child's abilities and interests and meet their needs.

CLINICAL *Pearl*

OT practitioners can use the therapeutic strategy "identify" to locate and share a range of environmental factors that provide the appropriate opportunities, supports/resources, and demands.

CASE *Study*

The OT practitioner working with Lizzy on her prevocational skills determined that she enjoyed interacting with people, felt capable of successfully completing three-step repetitive tasks, and was able to organize materials numerically and alphabetically when in a quiet environment. Using this knowledge of Lizzy's interests, personal causation, and skills, the OT practitioner determined that she could process simple customer requests and tickets in such places as a snack stand, a library, or a small movie theater; all these potential places of employment would provide Lizzy with the right balance of opportunities, resources, and demands.

Skill

This chapter already introduced the concept of performance capacity: the child's or adolescent's underlying physical and mental capacities. When a child uses those abilities in the context of a specific environment in order to engage in a task such as dressing, completing a puzzle, or working on homework, we observe skill. **Skills** are observable, goal-directed actions that the child uses to perform occupations. Skills are influenced by many things: both the environment and the child's personal characteristics. A child's underlying strength may certainly impact the level of skill observed, but the level of skill a child demonstrates while completing a task is equally influenced by other factors such as the child's level of interest in the task, the objects used to complete the task, and the other people doing the activity with the child. It is important to remember that we cannot "see" performance capacity. However, skills are always actions that we can "see" when a child is working to complete a task or activity.

CLINICAL *Pearl*

Therapists can "give feedback" during treatment sessions to help a child understand how she is doing with a selected activity. The child can then incorporate the information received and, by doing so, alter levels of participation. "Giving feedback" is a valuable way for OT practitioners to help a child have immediate insight into skill performance. The OT practitioner can provide verbal, physical, or both types of feedback, depending on the activity the child is performing.

Three types of skills exist. (1) *Motor skills* refer to moving one's body or moving objects used to complete tasks. When a child uses his or her underlying muscle strength and balance to pick a toy off the floor, we observe the motor skill of "lifting." (2) *Process skills* refer to the logical sequence of actions, the selection and use of appropriate tools and materials, and the ability to adapt one's performance and actions when encountering problems. When a child decides on the steps he or she will take and the materials needed to complete a homework assignment, we observe the process skills of sequencing and gathering. (3) *Communication and interaction skills* refer to the child's ability to convey intentions and needs and to coordinate social action with other people. When an adolescent approaches a teacher to ask a question, we can observe the verbal skills of articulation and speech, and nonverbal skills such as gestures and eye gaze.

CLINICAL *Pearl*

When the OT practitioner "coaches" a child, the child is receiving support to complete a task. For example, a child is working on copper tooling to improve fine motor skills and hand strength as well as tracking and eye–hand coordination. The OT practitioner notices that the child is missing spots when rubbing the copper with the etching tool to attain the shape of the mold. The OT practitioner "coaches" the child by encouraging the child to go back over the parts that were missed during earlier efforts. This helps the child to see what needs to be done and also provides encouragement to the child to keep working during what may be a period of frustration at not having enough hand strength or fine motor skills.

SUMMARY

This chapter examines the concepts of MOHO and reviews therapeutic strategies for implementing the model. This information provides OT practitioners with a way to explore, understand, and address issues

that impact a child's or adolescent's abilities. MOHO helps OT practitioners identify areas in a child's life that are supportive of participation in occupations as well as those that create challenges. MOHO highlights the importance of personal/client factors, including volition, habituation, and performance capacity. MOHO also stresses the importance of different physical and social environmental factors that enhance or impede a child's or adolescent's capacity for participation. Use of MOHO to methodically and systematically address areas of challenge and to identify the strengths of a child or adolescent supports best practice by focusing on the client. When an OT practitioner uses MOHO to guide intervention, he or she is using an occupation-focused, evidence-based, and client-centered thought process to guide practice.

References

1. Haglund, L., Ekbladh, E., Thorell, L. H., & Hallberg, I. R. (2000). Practice models in Swedish psychiatric occupational therapy. *Scandinavian Journal of Occupational Therapy*, 7, 107–113.
2. Kielhofner G: (2008). *Model of Human Occupation: Theory and Application*, ed 4, Baltimore, MD, 2008, Lippincott, Williams and Wilkins.
3. Lee, S., Taylor, R., Kielhofner, G., & Fisher, G. (2008). Theory use in practice: A national survey of therapists who use the Model of Human Occupation. *American Journal of Occupational Therapy*, 62, 106-117.
4. National Board for Certification in Occupational Therapy. (2004). A practice analysis study of entry-level occupational therapist registered and certified occupational therapy assistant practice. *Occupational Therapy Journal of Research: Occupation, Participation, and Health*, 24 (Suppl. 1), S1–S31.
5. Nelson D: Occupation: Form and performance, *Am J Occup Ther* 42:633–641, 1988.

REVIEW *Questions*

1. Define the three personal client factors and four environmental factors that influence a child's participation in occupations.
2. Explain the difference between an *interest* and a *value*. How may these two concepts be related?
3. Explain the difference between the concepts of *performance capacity* and *skill*.
4. In your own words, explain the meaning of *environmental impact*.

SUGGESTED *Activities*

1. Imagine a clinical challenge you have encountered either through observation or experience. Use the volitional process to think of a way that you could address the child's volition and encourage him or her to engage in the therapeutic activity.
2. Think of one setting such as a bedroom or a classroom and discuss with your classmates all the environmental factors within that setting (spaces, objects, social groups, and tasks). Now think of two different clients with two different types of impairments. How might the same setting and environmental factors impact each child differently?
3. Think of a client you have worked with in the past. How could you have used MOHO to address this client's issue with participation? What conceptual area of MOHO would have helped you develop an intervention to positively impact this client? How would that concept have helped?

26

Assistive Technology

GILSON J. CAPILOUTO

CHAPTER *Objectives*

After studying this chapter, the reader will be able to accomplish the following:

- Describe terms, concepts, legislation, and trends in the use of assistive technology in pediatric occupational therapy
- Demonstrate understanding of specific classes of assistive technology available to children with disabilities
- Discuss the role of the occupational therapy assistant as it relates to successful evaluation and implementation of assistive technology services
- Describe best practice strategies required for successful evaluation and implementation of assistive technology services
- Demonstrate understanding of the characteristics of assistive technology and its relative importance in making assistive technology decisions
- Compare and contrast assistive, rehabilitative, educational, and medical technologies
- Provide examples of switch technology and the ways it might be used to assist a child in achieving a goal
- Describe the characteristics of switches and specific considerations when selecting a switch for an individual user
- Describe the ways environmental control units operate and how ECU (environmental control unit) technology might be used for a child with a disability
- Discuss the role of simple communication technologies for children unable to communicate verbally

Technology continues to influence our lives considerably. We now have a daily dependence on a variety of technologies that include computers, cell phones, and personal digital assistant (PDAs). Each of these technologies has the potential to make our lives a little easier and more comfortable by helping us be more productive and efficient. For people with disabilities, technology is especially important as it can mean the difference between being able to accomplish a task alone and being forced to depend on someone else. In fact, technology has been described as the "great equalizer" for people with disabilities, since it provides an important vehicle for maximizing capability.[6,10] The U.S. Congress acknowledged the crucial role of technology in the lives of people with disabilities when, in 1988, it passed Public Law 100-407, titled the Technology-Related Assistance for Individuals with Disabilities Act of 1988.[11] In the preamble to PL 100-407, Congress described four major benefits of assistive technology (AT) for individuals with disabilities: (1) greater control over their individual lives, (2) increased participation in their daily lives, (3) more widespread interaction with nondisabled individuals, and (4) the capacity to benefit from opportunities that most people frequently take for granted.

The Tech Act, as it is commonly referred to, allocated a considerable amount of dollars to support the efforts of the states to increase the awareness of the benefits of technology for people with disabilities, funding for the provision of AT devices and AT services, the number of personnel trained to provide such services, and coordination among state agencies and public and private entities to deliver AT devices and AT services.[7]

DEFINITIONS

The formal definition of **assistive technology** (AT), according to the federal government, is as follows: "Any item, piece of equipment, or product system, whether acquired commercially off the shelf, modified, or customized, that is used to increase or improve functional capabilities of individuals with disabilities."* The important thing to remember about this definition is the fact that *anything* that helps a person be more functional is considered AT. The term *assistive technology* naturally makes one think that AT has to be commercially manufactured and expensive; however, this is not always the case. Also formally defined in the law is the term **assistive technology services** (AT services). This term includes "any service that directly assists an individual with a disability in the selection, acquisition, or use of an assistive technology device."** The inclusion of a

---

* From Public Law 100-407, 25 January, 1988
**From Public Law 100-407, 25 January, 1988

service component is particularly important to occupational therapy (OT) practitioners, and this suggests that those who framed this legislation realized an important truth: Eequipment alone is not enough; professional services are also required for the evaluation of AT and the training for its use.

Why should we consider the use of AT in the care of individuals with disabilities? A brief look at the World Health Organization's distinction of the terms *health condition, activity limitations,* and *participation restrictions* illustrate the importance of AT. Let us say that a child is born without his upper extremities (health condition), and so he is unable to perform basic activities of daily living (activity limitation) (the World Health Organization Web site: http://apps.who.int/classifications/icfbrowser/, accessed September 23, 2009). If this child is prevented from participating in a local drawing class because of this health condition or activity limitation, then his participation has been restricted. AT addresses the *health condition* aspect of the individual and minimizes *activity limitations* because when an aid or device that will allow the individual to meet the goal of drawing is identified, he or she can assume his or her role in society (e.g., a young child who wants to draw) and the *health condition* is thereby minimized.

> **CLINICAL *Pearl***
>
> Assistive technology refers to *anything* that helps a person be more functional in daily life.

> **CLINICAL *Pearl***
>
> Assistive technology *services* refer to *any* service that assists an individual with a disability in selecting, acquiring, and using an assistive aid or device.

ASSISTIVE TECHNOLOGY TEAM

Interdisciplinary teamwork is considered the cornerstone of effective rehabilitation.[2] The need for teamwork is particularly crucial as it relates to the use of AT. The disciplines represented as part of the **assistive technology team** (AT team) may vary according to the needs of the client and health condition or body functions (Box 26-1). For example, a physical therapist provides important information about gross motor strength and function as well as positioning for function and mobility. The occupational therapist gives valuable input relative to fine motor function, participation in

BOX 26-1

Potential Members of the Pediatric Assistive Technology Team

- Child
- Family/caregivers/guardians
- Regular and/or special educator
- Classroom assistants
- Daycare workers
- Physical therapist
- Occupational therapist
- Speech-language pathologist
- Vision specialist
- Audiologist (hearing specialist)
- Physician
- Case worker and/or social worker
- Rehabilitation engineer
- Vendor (assistive technology supplier)

activities of daily living (ADLs) and positioning for access. The speech–language pathologist is concerned with overall communication ability as well as specific strengths and abilities related to language comprehension and language expression. The user, and his or her parents, guardians, or caregivers, are always the central members of the team and should be involved in all aspects of equipment decision making and/or implementation. Additional team members could include a rehabilitation engineer charged with designing or fabricating aids or devices, an equipment vendor who provides medical equipment supplies and a teacher concerned with using technology to assist a student in meeting his or her educational potential and achieving educational goals. Regardless of which professionals make up an individual team, it is the responsibility of each AT team to work together to decide what technology will be of benefit to an individual user, how it will be used, how equipment will be maintained, and how the impact of the technology will be measured.[4]

CLINICAL *Pearl*

A team approach is necessary for successful assistive technology service delivery.

ROLE OF THE COTA

AT services vary depending on the setting and the experience of the individuals comprising the AT team. As such, the role of the certified occupational therapist (COTA) will also vary according to setting and experience. The registered occupational therapist (OTR) and the COTA are important members of the AT evaluation and service provision team.

At one time or another, the OTR and the COTA may be involved in securing necessary funding for AT, supervising the use of equipment, measuring outcomes related to equipment use, and equipment fabrication and/or adaptation. Additional roles of the COTA could include client and family education and instruction in the use of AT as well as education and instruction for other team members such as regular and special educators and classroom assistants.

CHARACTERISTICS OF ASSISTIVE TECHNOLOGY

The term *assistive technology* is used to describe a broad array of assistive aids and devices that include, but are not limited to, aids for daily living, seating and positioning aids, communication aids and devices, environmental control units, aids for persons with visual impairments, and assistive listening devices. As a group, these technologies share common characteristics, which are important to understand in delivering quality AT services (Table 26-1). First, and *most* important, is a solid understanding of the distinction between "assistive technology" and rehabilitative, educational, or medical technology.[5] The term *assistive technology* should only be used to refer to aids and devices that are used *daily* to complete a given task. The terms **rehabilitative** or **educational technology** should be used when referring to the use of technology as only *one* aspect of an overall rehabilitation or education program. **Medical technology** refers to the use of technology to support or improve life functions. The following case study illustrates why this distinction is so important.

CASE *Study*

Tyronne has chronic Gillian-Barré syndrome and, as a result, he is unable to use his upper extremities and is nonambulatory. He uses an electric wheelchair for mobility and operates it using a series of switches mounted to his headrest. Because of his upper extremity impairment, Tyronne cannot independently interact with age-appropriate toys. To eliminate this handicap and minimize Tyronne's disability, his OTA has adapted a commercially available, battery-operated toy so that it turns "on" when a switch is activated. The OTA wants Tyronne to use the switch so that he can play independently. To use the switch and adapted toy as AT, the switch would be placed in a location that matched Tyronne's current abilities. This might mean mounting the switch on the headrest of his wheelchair, since his

TABLE 26-1

Characteristics of Assistive Technology With Definitions and Examples

CHARACTERISTIC	DEFINITION	EXAMPLE
Assistive technology	Technology used daily to improve function	Communication aid
Rehabilitative or educational technology	Technology is only one aspect of rehabilitation or educational program	Software program for teaching ABCs
Medical technology	Technology used to sustain life	Respirator
Low technology	Technology that is easy to obtain and use	Reacher
High technology	Technology that is difficult to obtain and use	Electric feeding machine
Assistive appliance	Aid/device that is beneficial without development of skill	Foot orthotics
Assistive tool	Aid/device that requires development of skill to be useful	Switch-adapted toy

head appears to be his fastest, most energy efficient control site.

Now, let us consider another scenario. Marissa has a developmental disability characterized by gross and fine motor delays. Currently, she does not maintain her head in an upright position for any length of time. Her OTA is trying to devise activities that will encourage Marissa to maintain head control, thereby strengthening the muscles required to develop this skill. The OTA has decided that introducing a switch-operated toy may motivate Marissa to maintain an upright head position for increasingly longer periods of time. In this case, the strategy may be mounting the switch so that it is activated only when the head is upright. The same technology that was used for Tyronne *assistively* is now being used for Marissa *rehabilitatively*.

Recall that our definition of AT emphasizes *function*, not disability. Since Marissa has to work very hard to activate the toy and this is only one of many activities she is engaged in to increase independent head control, the use of the toy and switch would be considered rehabilitative technology.

CLINICAL *Pearl*

Assistive technology targets function, while rehabilitative and educational technologies target dysfunction.

You might still be confused as to why this distinction is so important. Consider that in the scenario with Tyronne, our goal is to make technology *easy* to access. But, in the second scenario, with Marissa, the technology is actually *hard* to access, since we are challenging her to move in ways that are not easy for her. We would certainly *not* want an individual to work as hard as Marissa if our goal was daily, independent play! This distinction is important for more practical reasons as

well. For example, the use of AT daily (as in the case of Tyronne) or temporarily (as in the case of Marissa) has a direct impact on considerations of durability, cost, and operational difficulty. If we are going to use a device for the development of a particular skill, we would not want to spend large amounts of money or consider an option that would require a significant amount of lead time to achieve operational competence. Instead, we would limit our options to an aid or device that was relatively inexpensive and easy to learn. This distinction between assistive and rehabilitative or educational technology is also very important for setting technology-related goals as well as gauging our expectations for technology use (i.e., whether we expect AT to be used daily or over a long period of time).

Another characteristic of AT is that it can be categorized as *low technology* or *high technology*.[5] This distinction is somewhat self-explanatory. **Low technology** is easy to obtain, easy to use, and of relatively low cost. In contrast, **high technology** is more difficult to obtain, requires greater skill to use, and is frequently more costly. We consider these factors when weighing options for individual users. For example, if we are working with an individual who we know to be "technophobic," then we would probably want to keep our AT options toward the low technology end. At the same time, we do not want to make AT decisions simply based on the fact that someone enjoys and is comfortable with technology. This author's motto is simple: Never buy a Jaguar when a Volkswagen will do! To be safe, we should always make sure that our decisions about technology are based on the goals and abilities of the client.[7]

The final characteristic of AT that we need to discuss is the distinction between assistive technology *tools* and assistive technology *appliances*.[5] The term **assistive appliance** includes any aid or device that provides benefit to the user with little to no training or development of skill. This could include items such as eyeglasses or orthotics. An **assistive tool**, on the other hand, requires the development of skill in order for it to be of value to the user. Examples of assistive tools include feeding machines, communication aids and devices, and mobility aids. This distinction is especially important when speaking with users and caregivers about their expectations of AT. A good example is the selection of a communication aid or device. Too often, there are misconceptions that if we "just find the right thing," the user will be able to communicate instantaneously. It is important for everyone to be clear about the fact that any communication aid or device is an assistive tool and, as such, requires a certain degree of training before it can be of benefit to the user.

> **CLINICAL** *Pearl*
>
> Assistive appliances such as eye glasses provide benefit to the user without the development of skill.

> **CLINICAL** *Pearl*
>
> Assistive tools, such as communication technologies, require the development of skill in order to be of benefit to the user.

ASSISTIVE TECHNOLOGY MYTHS AND REALITIES

In their book on assistive technology, Jan Galvin and Marcia Scherer describe a number of myths and realities with respect to AT, many of which are important to share before moving forward.[7] As already mentioned, AT does not need to be expensive or complicated. A simple pad and pencil can be the perfect communication aid. Moreover, keep in mind that people with the same disability do not necessarily require the same devices. For example, the same wheelchair is not recommended for every person needing one! It is especially important to keep in mind that "assessment," as it relates to AT, is an ongoing process. It is simply not possible to know everything about an individual user in the course of three or even four encounters. Additionally, as users develop and improve their skills as a result of intervention, reassessment of AT needs is warranted. We will discuss this further when we talk about the assessment process. Lastly, it is important to be open to multiple sources of information when it comes to AT. The field of AT is changing at a remarkably rapid pace, and it is very difficult for any single professional to be familiar with everything that is available. Consequently, consumers,

family members and even vendors can provide us with valuable input about appropriate technology for individual users.

ASSISTIVE TECHNOLOGY ASSESSMENT

Like so many aspects of rehabilitation, AT assessment is a team endeavor. Although COTAs do not conduct evaluations, it is critical to understand the process of evaluation so that the clinical information that is shared with the occupational therapist is valuable in making adjustments to AT goals and treatment procedures for individual users. Numerous approaches to decision-making for assistive technology exist. The one discussed here is adapted from a model rooted in the field of human factors engineering.[5] *Human factors engineering* is a field of study devoted to the interface between man and machines; its application to the field of AT is well suited. As you read this section, it will be helpful to refer to the schematic of the assessment process shown in Figure 26-1.

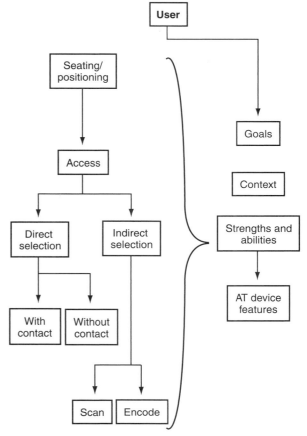

FIGURE 26-1 A schematic model of the assessment process for assistive technology adapted from human factors engineering.

In rehabilitation, the assessment process is frequently started by administering standardized tests and criteria-referenced measures in an attempt to answer the question: "What *can't* the individual do?" However, it must be remembered that AT targets function rather than dysfunction, so knowing what an individual *cannot do* is not very helpful when trying to determine whether technology would be of benefit. Instead, when considering technology, the rehabilitation specialist asks: "What is it the user wants to do?" and/or "What is it the user needs to be able to do?" With these questions as the focus, the AT assessment process begins where it should, with the *goals for the user.*

When establishing goals for individual users, OT practitioners consider the following: (1) Is this goal rehabilitative or functional? (2) Is this goal shared by the student/user, the family, and other members of the team? (3) Does the goal make sense; is it logical? You will recall that the distinction between goals that are assistive and those that are rehabilitative impacts how equipment is set up (i.e., conserving effort and energy as much as possible [assistive] *or* as a motor challenge [rehabilitative]) and the type of equipment that is considered (i.e., learning time and cost). Also, when equipment is being considered, intervention goals should be discussed with everyone who has a vested interest in the user, since assistive devices frequently require the support of caregivers and other team members for training and maintenance. For example, the OT practitioner, along with the physical therapist, may want to increase a student's exposure to powered mobility as part of a goal focused on independence. However, the student's family is committed to emphasizing the use of a walker and so does not want to consider a power wheelchair. Since the caregivers do not share the goal of powered mobility, it may not be wise to pursue that goal at this time.

Lastly, when establishing goals, it is important to consider whether we are asking the user to do something you and I could/would do. For example, if we have a goal that states the user will attend to an activity for 30 minutes, we have to ask ourselves whether or not *we* would attend to the same activity for that length of time! Once we have established goals, we can begin to explore whether or not the client's ability to achieve those goals would be enhanced by the use of assistive equipment.

Following the establishment of goals, the next question is: "Where and with whom will the goal(s) be addressed?" This question focuses on the settings for each of the client's goals such as home, school, and/or the community. Each of these has the potential of impacting decisions with regard to devices. For example, one of the user's goals might be to initiate interaction using a communication aid or device. Naturally, we would hope this goal would be addressed across all of the user's physical settings, so one important aspect of any aid or device we will consider would be its portability. The idea of context also includes a social component. For example, will the goal be addressed with familiar or unfamiliar peers, familiar or unfamiliar adults, strangers, or all of the above? Finally, context takes into account the physical contexts of a goal, including temperature (impact of excessive heat or cold), sound (ambient noise), and light (ambient light). The impact of these factors is fairly obvious. For example, any goal that includes the playground as a setting would need to account for the weather as well as changes in light (natural versus artificial).

The third primary component of assessment involves the specific strengths and abilities of the user. This is where information from specific team members becomes critical. The areas of strength and ability include family, gross motor, fine motor, cognitive, communication, and sensory strengths and abilities. The following case study provides examples in each of these performance skills.

CASE *Study*

Westin is a 9-year-old with cerebral palsy. He is also legally blind. He is believed to have mild intellectual disability. The goal for Westin is functional communication in all settings (home, school, church, community). Currently, he uses multiple nonsymbolic forms of communication, including gestures, facial expressions, vocalizations, and simple signs. He has experience using a switch for computer access that includes scanning. The social context for the goal includes familiar peers and nonpeers, family, community workers, and strangers. The physical contexts for his goal are inside, outside, school bus, and family van.

Family strengths and abilities include parents who are supportive and involved, insurance coverage for durable medical equipment, and parents who are technology literate. His gross motor abilities include being able to operate a manual wheelchair with customized seating systems and lap tray for upright support. No plans have been made to alter his system in the next 2 years. With respect to fine motor abilities Westin uses a gross swipe toward objects with fisted hands. Moreover, he uses a head-mounted switch to scan items on a computer screen. Cognitively, he appears to understand much of what is said to him, smiles and laughs when spoken to, makes choices between objects and pictures (groupings of four), and follows two- and three-step commands when they are within his physical capabilities. He uses multiple forms of nonsymbolic communication (vocalizations, facial expressions, body language) as well as simple, adapted manual signs. Information regarding sensory systems indicates his vision is limited to objects and pictures about 4 in. × 4 in., and auditory acuity is within normal limits. Other noteworthy strengths include a good sense of humor, mischievousness, and a friendly and outgoing personality.

The above case illustrates a number of key points with respect to assessment. First, note the emphasis on *ability*. In each domain, we have listed what Westin *can* do. By taking such an approach, we narrow our equipment options considerably; and with the plethora of equipment available to us, anything we can do to narrow our options is probably good! In this case, communication technologies, we already know we can capitalize on the use of his existing ability to use a head switch for scanning, so we need a device that accepts scanning. In addition, we know he can distinguish as many as four items and can follow three-step directions; this permits us to consider more operationally complex devices.

As information is gathered by various team members, the skills and abilities of the user translate into the necessary features of any aid or device that is considered. For example, if, in the course of team conferencing, it was learned that a client had decreased visual acuity, then any aid or device considered would include features that account for that, for example, bright colors, tactile features, auditory feedback, and/or magnification options.

Returning to our discussion on assessment, a fundamental aspect is determining how a potential user will interface with an assistive aid or device. This is referred to as *access*. **Access** is the point of contact between the user and the aid or device that he or she needs to control. For example, you and I "access" the computer via a keyboard and/or mouse. Initially, we work as a team on the identification of a particular "**control site**" or location on the body that can be used to operate a device.[5] Potential sites for controlling aids or devices include hands and fingers, arms, the head, eyes, legs, or feet. Ultimately, the site and movement chosen should represent the fastest, most energy efficient, and most reliable. Following the identification of a control site, the team begins the task of determining the most appropriate form of access for a given user.

One form of access is referred to as **direct selection**. Direct selection is a straightforward method for making a choice or selection.[3,5,7] The keyboard and the mouse are considered direct selection forms of access. For example, when we want to type an "*e*" we go directly to it and make that selection (by using a finger). Using your hands to operate the joystick on a computer game console is another example of direct selection; when you want to go left, you move the joystick to the left with no intermediate steps involved. Touching a picture to request a drink, using a head pointer or a mouth stick are also considered direct selection techniques.

Each of these examples illustrates direct selection *with physical contact*. However, for some individuals, physical contact with a control interface is not possible. In such cases, we might consider options that allow for direct selection *without physical contact*. For example, a person using the eyes to indicate a letter on an alphabet board is using direct selection in the absence of physical contact. A straightforward method of indicating a choice is still used but doing so without physically touching the choice. Another example of direct selection without physical contact would be using a laser pointer to make selections on a display.

As shown in the above examples, being able to select choices directly is fast and efficient; whether they be letters on a keyboard, directions for a wheelchair, or messages on a communication aid or device. Yet for many individuals with disabilities, direct forms of access are not possible. For these clients, we turn to *indirect selection* access options. **Indirect selection** requires intermediate steps in order to make a selection. Now, rather than going directly to the letter on a keyboard, the user might have to *scan* through the letters of the alphabet via rows and then columns using a switch. To drive a wheelchair, the user might use a switch array corresponding to each direction he or she wants to go (e.g., a switch for "right" and another one for "left"). Alternatively, he or she might use a single switch connected to a directional panel, scanning through the options (i.e., left, right, back, forward). Scanning is one form of indirect selection; another is referred to as *encoding*.[5] With encoding, the user relies on multiple signals together to specify response. For example, in the case of a person who cannot use his or her hands to operate a wheelchair, a "sip and puff" signal may be used to control the direction of the chair. In this example, varying combinations of signals serve as an encoded language for directional commands, such as soft sip + soft puff = forward, and hard sip + soft sip = left. Another example of multiple signal encoding is the Morse code, in which dots and dashes are combined to specify specific letters of the alphabet.

In summary, one important aspect of AT assessment is determining access or how the user will operate or interface with a given device or aid. Two primary forms of access are (1) indirect selection, and (2) indirect selection. Direct selection is a straightforward method of indicating a choice or selection. It can be accomplished with or without physical contact. In contrast, indirect selection requires intermediate steps in order to indicate a response. Indirect selection may be accomplished in one of two ways: scanning or encoding.

Clinically important distinctions exist between direct and indirect selection techniques, and it is important to keep these distinctions in mind. Physically, direct selection is considered more difficult than indirect selection because it requires more refined, controlled movements.[5] However, because all of the elements in the selection set are equally available and do not need to be scanned, direct selection is considered the faster form of device control.[3] Direct selection is also considered less cognitively complex than indirect selection because it is more intuitive.[1] For these reasons, direct selection forms of device control are considered a better option than indirect forms of control. Therefore, it is important to thoroughly examine the potential for direct selection forms of access before considering indirect selection techniques.[3,7]

> **CLINICAL *Pearl***
>
> Because indirect selection is slower and more cognitively complex than direct selection, direct selection forms of device control are considered a better option than indirect forms of control.

Returning to our model in Figure 26-1, one can see that seating and positioning issues, as well as issues of access, are superimposed on the assessment model aspect of skills and abilities. It is important for us to keep in mind that muscle tone (e.g., hypertonia and/or hypotonia), the presence of primitive reflexes, skeletal deformities, or movement disorders will all influence access to equipment. Therefore, seating and positioning become critical in minimizing the influence of these characteristics on functional device operation. The reader is referred to Chapter 13 for specific information regarding best practice principles of seating and positioning.

ASSISTIVE TECHNOLOGY FOR PEDIATRICS

A number of classes of assistive technology tools should be considered when working with pediatric clients. For the purposes of this chapter, we will focus on technology for leisure activities and environmental control and simple communication technologies. Although the focus here is primarily on simple technology solutions, high technology approaches are also equally important to consider for pediatric populations.

Technology for Leisure Activities

For very young children, "leisure activities" translates to "play." It is important to keep the definition of *play* in mind, since it is easy for us to turn play into therapy. Play is an intrinsic activity engaged in for its own sake, rather than a means of achieving a specific end.[9] Play should be fun, spontaneous, and voluntary. *Adapted play* refers to the fact that toys are modified to enable children with disabilities to participate and that learning is intentionally incorporated into play activities.[9]

Greenstein suggested that simply observing a child with a particular toy can tell us much about what we need to know before considering adapted toys.[9] First, we should ask ourselves whether a child is playing with a toy because he or she wants to (intrinsic motivation) or because someone else wants him or her to (extrinsic motivation). This is important, since research suggests that using rewards to encourage children to engage in an activity will decrease a child's subsequent interest in that activity. It reminds us that children should be playing because *they* want to. Angelo suggested three possible reasons to explain why children with disabilities do *not* engage with toys: (1) they are not interested in the toys (amotivated), (2) frequent failures interacting with toys have reduced their motivation to try (learned helplessness), or (3) they want to play but are physically unable to play with the toys.[9] Adapting toys is helpful to children who are physically unable to play with toys.

The first consideration in adapting play materials for children with disabilities is deciding whether materials simply need to be stabilized.[8] Frequently, children with physical disabilities need a stable surface on which to play so that objects will not move out of their reach. For example, lining a tray with indoor–outdoor carpet and then attaching male Velcro to the base of books, baby dolls, and trucks can serve to hold objects in a stable position and encourage play. A second strategy, suggested by Glennen and Church, is to enlarge materials, which serves to enhance visual perception and decrease reliance on fine motor skills.[8] Simple solutions include attaching handles to puzzle pieces and pop-up boxes and placing foam strips around brushes, markers, and utensils to make them easier to hold. Finally, toys can be attached to trays and/or to the children by using elastic bands so that if the toys fall out of reach they can be easily retrieved.

A third strategy, suggested by Musselwhite, is ensuring that all play materials are accessible; as much as possible, children should be able to physically select their own toys and activities.[11] For example, for children in wheelchairs, toys should be attached at chair height on a wall with Velcro or in nets hung from the ceiling. For children physically unable to retrieve their own toys, items should be arranged so that they are easy to select by a gross reach or by pointing. An alternative would be to develop simple picture or object displays that allow children to indicate the toy they want or the game they want to play. For example, attaching actual objects or large photographs to a strip of hard-backed poster board allows children to choose. Choices should be spaced far enough apart to allow children to select a picture of the activity or toy using either a gross upper extremity movement or their eyes (Figure 26-2).

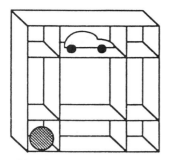

Plexiglass eye gaze object box

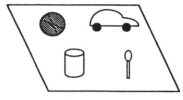

Object Choice Board

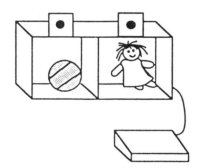

Scanning choice board with switch

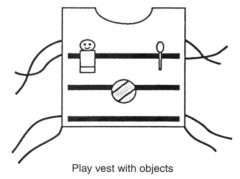

Play vest with objects

FIGURE 26-2   Play activity choice boards. (From Glennen S, Church G: Adaptive toys and environmental controls. In Church G, Glennen S, editors: *The handbook of assistive technology*, San Diego, 1992, Singular Publishing Group.)

Switch-Activated Toys

Using switches to interact with toys and appliances is another form of adapted play. Such adaptations allow children with physical limitations to engage in

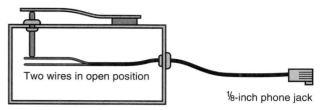

Plates that when pressed bring two wires into contact

Two wires in open position

⅛-inch phone jack

FIGURE 26-3   Anatomy of a switch.

independent exploration and interaction with the environment. Moreover, using switches with toys can be considered a preliminary activity that serves to develop the skills needed to control a wheelchair or operate a communication device. **Switches** open and close a circuit, so they operate in the same way as many of the appliances operated on a daily basis, such as televisions, light switches, CD players, and toasters (Figure 26-3).[1] Switches give a person with physical limitations the option to control toys and appliances that he or she otherwise would be physically unable to manage.

Switches come in all shapes and sizes with varying visual, auditory, and sensory features. When selecting a switch for an individual, consider the following questions:

1. What are the potential control sites for a switch (i.e., head, hand, arm, foot)?
2. What are the functional ranges of motion (ROM) of potential sites?
3. Does the user have any unique sensory needs that need to be considered?
4. What mounting issues need to be considered?

In fact, just looking at a given switch provides information about its intended user. Keep in mind that manufacturers design switches for very specific reasons—it is not a random process! For instance, OT practitioners ask such questions as: Does the size of the activation surface suggest a person who uses more gross movements or fine movements? Is the switch intended for foot and/or hand activation, cheek/chin activation, or head/thumb activation? Would the physical characteristics of the switch appeal to a child or to an adult? Do the physical characteristics of the switch suggest anything about vision or cognition? What about the strength requirements of the switch? Remember, the task is to match a user's skills and abilities to the features of a switch. The following case scenario provides an example of this process.

CASE *Study*

Jayden is a 12-year-old boy with a diagnosis of spastic-quadriplegic cerebral palsy. He has also been diagnosed as having visual impairment, although the degree of his visual loss is not known. He uses a manual wheelchair for mobility, but he is not independent in its use. Although it is difficult to ascertain his precise abilities using standardized tests, his teachers feel that he is responsive to communication and laughs and smiles appropriately when others direct attention to him. He uses multiple nonsymbolic forms of communication, including postural changes associated with excitement and anticipation, swiping at unwanted items with his right upper extremity, and vocalizing to express pleasure and displeasure. His professional team thinks he is a good candidate for an appliance operated by a switch.

Using the Switch Analysis Worksheet shown in Figure 26-4, note the descriptions of each of the pictured switches. Of those presented, which offers features that best match Jayden's described strengths and abilities? If you picked switch number one, congratulations! You are correct. The Lighted Signal Switch offers a relatively large surface area which complements Jayden's gross motor approach to tasks. It addition, it offers sensory features well suited to accommodate his visual impairment, including the fact that it lights up on activation and presents an audible click on activation. Finally, its ribbed surface offers Jayden tactile stimulation as well.

The preceding case reiterates the importance of selecting switches based on individual needs. A worksheet, such as the one provided in Figure 26-4, can help you analyze the options for various clients. If the appropriate switch is not selected, OT practitioners run the risk of drawing conclusions about a student's ability to use a switch that may or may not be incorrect. For example, if switch #2 is the only one available for use, Jayden would most likely be unsuccessful because of its small size and minimal feedback. As a result of his performance with this switch, the team might deduce that he is not capable of using a switch, when, in fact, the switch presented did not accommodate his specific strengths and abilities.

Once a specific switch is selected for trial use, we turn our attention to developing an activity for introducing the switch. The activity should be age appropriate and motivating to the user. It is also important to be precise in the placement of the switch and the appliance or toy, in relation to the user, and to make sure that we repeat that correct placement each time the user engages in switch-activated play. Moreover, trial use of a switch should be carefully monitored before altering the switch or its placement. Users need the opportunity to practice using switches across a variety of activities before changes are considered because switches are considered assistive

tools, so some development of skill is required before the switches can be of benefit *and* before conclusions are made about intervention success or the need for program adjustments.

As stated previously, a number of potential adapted play options are available, depending on the goals for an individual user. Adaptive switches can be used to operate a variety of battery-run or electronic toys and appliances.[8] Switches attach to toys or appliances via cables. More often than not, switches will come with cable attachments. At the end of the cable will be a miniature plug (Figure 26-5, A). Toys or appliances that have already been developed with switches will come equipped with cable receptors in the form of switch interface jacks (Figure 26-5, B). Alternatively, one can use a battery adapter specifically designed for use with commercially available battery-operated toys and appliances. *Battery adapters* have a cable receptor with a female phone jack at one end and a copper plate at the other end. The copper plate is sized to fit the specific battery type (e.g., AAA, C, D) and is placed between the battery and one of the metal battery contacts, thus interrupting the on/off circuitry (Figure 26-5, C).[8] Now, when the toy or appliance is placed in the "on" position, it will not operate until the switch is activated. The trick with using both adapted toys and/or battery adapters is that different manufacturers use different-sized cable jacks and receptors, so it is frequently necessary to use adapters to convert between female- and male-type jacks. Resources for battery adapters and cable adapters are included at the end of this chapter.

Finally, it is important to understand the three modes of operation available when using switch technology with individual users. In "momentary" or "continuous" mode, the user must maintain pressure on the switch in order to keep the toy or appliance operating.[1] This is also referred to as the *direct mode*. Unfortunately, this is not particularly functional. Think about how often you would watch TV or listen to music if you had to continually press the "on" button to do it! *Switch-latch timers* are devices designed to eliminate this need.[1] To work, the switch is plugged into one part of the switch-latch timer, and the device to be operated is plugged into another part (Figure 26-6). When set in the *latched mode*, activation of the switch turns the device on, and reactivation of the switch turns the device off. This is a very functional setting for activities such as making milkshakes using a blender or listening to the radio and watching TV. In the *timed mode*, activation of the switch turns the device on, and it stays on for the amount of time specified; this could be seconds, minutes, or hours. This mode is particularly helpful to determine whether an individual understands that the switch is being used to operate something. For example, using a tape recorder and a

Switch	Picture	Access	Control Site(s)	Sensory Features	Other
1. Lighted Signal Switch ($62.95) Enabling Devices 385 Warburton Avenue Hastings-on-Hudson, NY 10706 http://enablingdevices.com/	5" diameter	Gross access	Upper extremities; fisted or open hand; foot	Ribbed surface for tactile stimulation; activation feedback; lighted	Angled presentation; suction cup feet
2. Specs Switch ($49.00) AbleNet, Inc. 2808 Fairview Avenue Roseville, MN 55113-1308 http://enablingdevices.com/	1 3/8" diameter	Fine access	Single digit; head; cheek	Activation feedback; bright colors	Various mounting options-velcro strap
3. Pal Pad ($27.00) Adaptivation, Inc. 2225 W. 50th Street, Suite 100 Sioux Falls, SD 57105 http://www.adaptivation.com/	2.5 x 4 x .1 "	Gross access	Open hand; foot; elbow	Bright color	Completely flat
4. Plate Switch ($32.95) Enabling Devices 385 Warburton Avenue Hastings-on-Hudson, NY http://enablingdevices.com/	5" x 8"	Gross access	Open hand; foot	Activation feedback; bright color	Angled presentation; suction cup feet

FIGURE 26-4 Sample switch analysis worksheet.

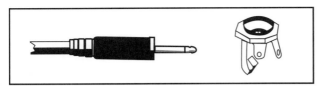

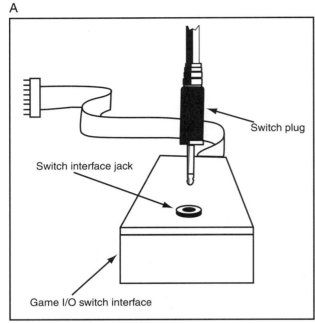

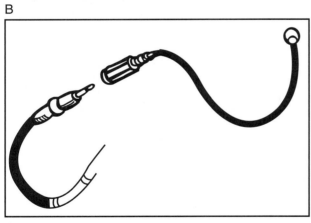

FIGURE 26-5 **A,** Miniature plug: typical sizes ⅛, ¼, and ½ inch. **B,** Switch plug and switch interface jack. **C,** Sample battery adaptor. (*B,* From Glennen S, Church G: Adaptive toys and environmental controls. In Church G, Glennen S, editors: *The handbook of assistive technology,* San Diego, 1992, Singular Publishing Group; *C,* From Adaptivation Incorporated: *Recipes for success,* Sioux Falls, SD, 1999, Adaptivation.)

switch-latch timer, activation of the switch would result in music being played. When the music stops, the OT practitioner looks for signs that the user understands that the switch and the tape recorder are related somehow. For example, does the user reach for the

switch? Does the user reach for the tape-recorder? Does the user look at the switch? Does the user look at the tape-recorder? These are all signs that the user understands the relationship between the switch and what is being controlled and so can be taught to control devices and toys using switches.

Environmental Controls

Environmental control units (ECUs) are systems that allow an individual to control his or her environment. An ECU consists of an input device, a throughput method, and some form of output (see Table 26-2). Three common transmission methods can be used to purposefully manipulate and interact with the environment (Figure 26-7). ECUs offer a motivating option for increasing the functional independence of children with disabilities. ECUs are an important class of AT tools to keep in mind when considering user goals, as it is an area frequently overshadowed by adapted play technologies and communication technologies. It is important to note that infants as young as 9 months frequently reach for the remote control and proceed to aim it at the television!

Angelo suggested a number of questions be considered when making decisions about ECU options for clients.[1] These questions include asking what the user wants to be able to do, what the user's strengths and abilities are, the context(s) for ECU, and the type of feedback needed by the user. These questions are essentially the same as the ones we used in our assessment model. This model has merit regardless of the class of AT tools under consideration. The following case study illustrates the role of ECU options for pediatric clients with disabilities.

CASE *Study*

Sasha is a 4-year-old with spastic–quadriplegic cerebral palsy. She loves to listen to music and recently received a CD player for her birthday. Sasha's occupational therapist is interested in giving her the option of controlling her CD player when she is in her bedroom, where she usually plays her music. Sasha primarily uses a gross swipe toward objects. She has some visual acuity difficulties but has demonstrated the ability to discriminate line drawings 3 in. × 3 in. The OT practitioner decides to try the AirLink Cordless Switch from Ablenet. It has an angled base and a 2½-inch activation surface. It operates using infrared and so requires a control unit (Powerlink 3 by Ablenet). The surface area of the switch can accommodate a 2 in. × 2 in. line drawing of a CD player to help Sasha associate it with its purpose. The combination of four modes of control—direct, timed seconds, timed minutes, and latch—on the Powerlink 3, offers control

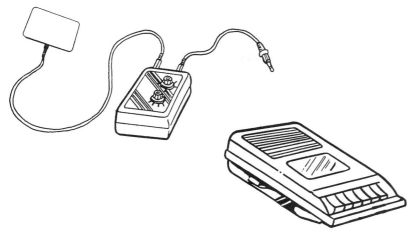

FIGURE 26-6 Switch-latch timer with switch (*on the left*) and toy tape recorder (*on the right*). (From Adaptivation Incorporated: *Recipes for success*, Sioux Falls, SD, 1999, Adaptivation.)

TABLE 26-2

Control Sequence for Environmental Control Systems

INPUT	THROUGHPUT	OUTPUT
Activates system by sending a signal	Receives and transmits signal	Receives signal and gives output
Examples include voice signal, switch activation, and button depression	Examples include radio frequency, ultrasound, and infrared transmission	Examples include lights being turned on or off, volume being turned up or down, CD player being turned on

X-	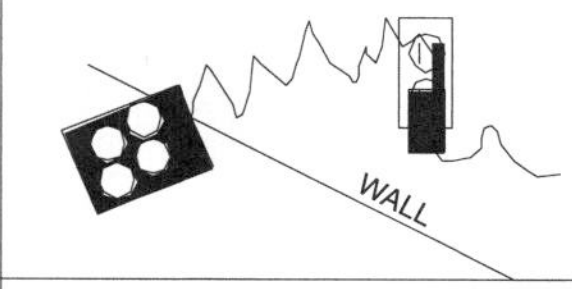	A transmitter sends radio frequency (RF) signals to a receiver (i.e., the module in the wall), and the appliance connected to the module turns on or off.
Ultrasound	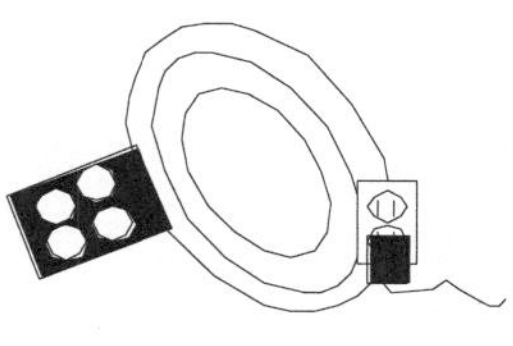	A transmitter sends ultrasound signals (sound waves) to a receiver (i.e., the module in the wall), and the appliance connected to the module turns on or off.
Infrared	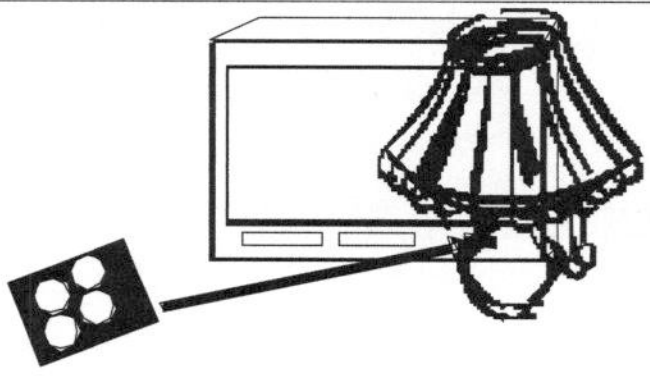	A transmitter sends infrared signals (IR) to a receiver that accepts infrared, and the corresponding unit is activated. Works like any household remote control.

FIGURE 26-7 Three common transmission methods for environmental control units.

flexibility. The OT practitioner decides to introduce the ECU using the timed mode in minutes; once Sasha gets the idea, she switches over to latched mode, which gives her complete control.

In summary, ECU systems for young children are generally straightforward and simple to operate. A list of potential ECU resources has been provided at the end of this chapter.

Simple Communication Technologies

Communication technologies (alternative augmentative communications [AAC]) are used in an area of clinical practice that attempts to compensate (either temporarily or permanently) for a person's difficulty using speech as a primary means of communication. It is important to understand that an AAC device is only *one* aspect of an individual's communication *system,* which could also include gestures, facial expressions, body language, and other nonsymbolic forms of communication.

A certified licensed speech–language pathologist (SLP) makes decisions about specific aids and devices for individual users. However, it is critical that all team members provide input regarding the specific strengths and abilities of a given user so that the SLP can make an informed decision. Moreover, it goes without saying that all persons involved in the care of an individual using an AAC device would need to understand how the system operates as well as how to interact with an individual using an AAC aid or device.

For the purposes of this chapter, we will focus on simple AAC technologies. These are systems that are either manual (i.e., have no electronic components) or simple electronic devices (i.e., use household batteries for operation). Referring back to the assessment model, the SLP looks to various team members to provide input regarding optimal seating and positioning for access to AAC devices, as well as a user's strengths and abilities relative to direct or indirect selection options and mounting needs. The remaining decisions focus specifically on the language options for AAC. These include how language will be represented (symbol type), what specific words or phrases need to be available to the user (vocabulary selection), what the user will see when they look at the aid or device (display organization), and finally, how messages will be stored and retrieved (message storage and retrieval).

For very young children, simple AAC technologies tend to be activity based. That is, children use specific displays to interact in the context of a specific activity such as snack time, playing with Play-Doh, blowing bubbles, or completing puzzles. Displays tend to include simple line drawings arranged in a row–column format

that includes anywhere from 2 to 32 vocabulary items, depending on a client's language ability. Manual displays might involve the use of a vest, eye gaze frame, or single sheet displays depending on individual motor abilities (Figure 26-8).

A number of simple battery-operated AAC systems that take advantage of human-recorded speech to transmit messages are available. The motivation of hearing a spoken message cannot be underestimated in young children for whom speech is difficult. Single message devices can give children an opportunity to request attention ("Please come here"), request assistance ("Can you help me?"), express a desire ("Please leave me alone"), express recurrence ("Let's do it again!"), or even saying that favorite toddler expression "NO!" Devices designed to present a series of messages (e.g., Step-by-Step Communicator by Ablenet, Inc.; Sequencer by Adaptivation, Inc.) can give children the opportunity to actively participate in story time ("He huffed, and he puffed, and he blew the house down!"), serve as the leader of an activity ("Ready, set, go!"), or tell Mom and Dad what happened at school that day ("I had pizza for lunch"; "We played musical chairs"; "I sat next to Billy on the bus.").

Simple battery-operated devices also come in more complex displays ranging from 2 to 16 possible messages. When using devices with limited messaging capability, SLPs make an effort to program messages that have applicability across a variety of contexts as opposed to those that are limited in use. For example, messages such as "I want a drink" or "I want to eat" are limited in scope. Mealtime and snack time are generally built into one's school day, so the need to request food or drink becomes

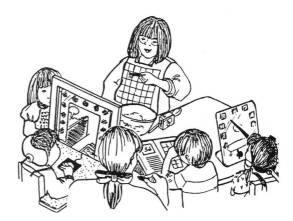

FIGURE 26- 8 Manual communication board display options. (From Goosens C, Crain SS, Elder PS: *Engineering the preschool environment for interactive communication: 18 months to 5 years developmentally,* ed. 2, Birmingham, 1994, Southeast Augmentative Communication Conference Publications, Clinician Series.)

somewhat moot. More powerful messages such as "my turn," "finished," "more," or "come here" are useful across a variety of activities and will give the child an opportunity to use his or her AAC device multiple times throughout the course of the day.

A recent addition to the technology options available to young children are Visual Scene Displays (VSDs). VSD refers to the way messages are stored and retrieved, and though they are created on high-technology devices, they are simple and intuitive to use. Instead of placing graphic symbols in a row–column format, VSDs use contextually rich visual images such as photographs or commercially available images of favorite characters (e.g., Dora Hannah Montana. Such displays provide communication partners with a greater context for interaction and language development. More information on VSDs can be found at http://www.imakenews.com/aac-rerc/e_article000676427.cfm

AAC devices have special cognitive, motor, perceptual, and learning requirements for the people that use them *and* their communication partners! It is for this reason that successful use of communication technologies involves a coordinated team approach focused on interactive communication and motivating activities. Careful planning and training are required for children to become competent users of AAC systems. Remember, the goal is to reinforce and facilitate *any* attempt at communication, since *what* a child has to say is more important than *how* he or she says it!

FUNDING FOR ASSISTIVE TECHNOLOGY

Federal legislation provides the foundation for funding for assistive technologies. In other words, lawmakers (senators and legislators) design bills (laws) using input from advocates (in this case, persons with disabilities, their caregivers, and professionals) that are designed to ensure *by law* that people have access to the equipment they need.

Prior to the 1970s, very little legislation addressed the needs of persons with disabilities (PWD). So they and their families relied on private and religious charities, fended for themselves, or just did not have the needed funding. The Rehabilitation Act of 1973 (referred to as *Section 504*) was the first major piece of legislation for PWD. It established the idea of "reasonable accommodation" (RA) and "least restrictive environment" (LRE). RA refers to the fact that the needs of persons with disabilities must be accommodated so as to not exclude them from the same experiences and opportunities as those of persons without disabilities. RA was written very vaguely and is essentially determined by courts (through law suits). LRE refers to the degree of

modifications in a job or academic program that is acceptable. The Rehab Act was patterned after Civil Rights Law. Simply stated, discriminating against individuals because of their disabilities became an act against the law. No person with any disability could be excluded from employment or secondary education solely on the basis of his or her condition. The Act mandated that employers and institutes of higher education receiving federal funds accommodate the needs of PWD.

In 1975, Congress enacted a major piece of legislation, also patterned after Civil Rights Law, this time protecting the rights of children with disabilities. The Education for All Handicapped Children Act, P.L. 94-142, later became known as the Individuals with Disabilities Act, or IDEA.[12] In this legislation, handicapped children were acknowledged as people with "certain inalienable rights," which are outlined in Box 26-2.

IDEA, as it pertains to AT, mandated that public schools (1) provide evaluation for assistive technology; (2) purchase, lease, or provide for acquiring aid or device; (3) select, design, fit, customize, adapt, repair, and replace aid or device; (4) coordinate and use other services with AT; (5) train child and family; and (6) train professionals.

Private insurance coverage of AT is dependent on individual policies. Often, a specific service such as assistive technology or rehabilitative technology may not be covered by the plan, but a provision for durable medical equipment (DME), which may or may not include the specific AT device or service that OT practitioners want to recommend, may be covered. Historically, private

---

BOX 26-2

IDEA Assistive Technology Mandates for Children With Disabilities

- A free, appropriate education regardless of handicapping condition
- Provision of educational services to the maximum extent appropriate in the least restrictive environment (LRE)
- The participation of parents in the educational process
- Due process procedures
- The right to related services (that's us!) to benefit from special education instruction
- The development of an individualized education program (IEP)—what is going to be done, who is going to do it, where it will be done, when it will be done, and how one will know that it has been completed (functional outcomes)

insurers have followed the lead of Medicare/Medicaid in detailing coverage for specific classes of AT tools. Service clubs, foundations, volunteer organizations, and low-interest bank loans should also be considered potential sources of full or supplemental funding for AT. Regardless of the source of funding, AT should be described in terms of the medical benefit to the client, which could include the prevention of secondary disability as well as the impact on quality of life. Specific details regarding expected outcomes and how those will be measured and documented should always be included in a request for funding.

SUMMARY

Assistive technology appliances and tools are an integral part of OT practice. AT fosters functional independence in persons with disabilities. The use of AT in pediatrics can motivate children with disabilities early on, and in so doing, it can ward off the negative impact of amotivation and learned helplessness. Because the range of AT products and devices is constantly changing, this chapter focused on best practice AT-related principles that will serve the OT practitioner regardless of the specific aid or device in question. Further, because of the dynamic nature of this field, it is imperative that the OT practitioner view his or her role as a member of a *team* of professionals that always includes family members and consider equipment manufacturers as potential sources of information about the complex and advancing field of assistive technology aids and devices.

References

1. Angelo J: *Assistive technology for rehabilitation specialists*, Philadelphia, 1997, F.A. Davis Company.
2. Capilouto G: Rehabilitation settings. In Kumar S, editor: *Multidisciplinary approach to rehabilitation*, Boston, 2000, Butterworth Heinemann.
3. Church G, Glennen S: *The handbook of assistive technology*, San Diego, 1992, Singular Publishing Group.
4. Clayton K, Mathena CT: Assistive technology. In Solomon J, editor: *Pediatric skills for occupational therapy assistants*, ed. 1, St. Louis, 2000, Mosby.
5. Cook A, Hussey S: *Assistive technologies: Principles and practices*, St. Louis, 1995, Mosby.
6. Fallon M., Wann J: Incorporating computer technology into activity-based thematic units for young children with disabilities, *Infants Young Child* 6:4, 1994.
7. Galvin J, Scherer M: *Evaluating, selecting and using appropriate assistive technology*, San Diego, 1996, Singular Publishing Group.
8. Glennen S, Church G: Adaptive toys and environmental controls. In Church G, Glennen S, editors: *The handbook of assistive technology*, San Diego, 1992, Singular Publishing Group.
9. Greenstein DB: It's child's play. In Galvin J, Scherer M: *Evaluating, selecting and using appropriate assistive technology*, San Diego, 1996, Singular Publishing Group.
10. Hollingsworth M: Computer technologies: A cornerstone for educational and employment equity, *Can J Higher Ed* 22:1, 1992.
11. Musselwhite C: *Adaptive play for special needs children*, San Diego, 1986, College-Hill Press.
12. P.L. 94-142: Individuals with Disabilities Act, 1975, US Congress.

Orthoses, Orthosis Fabrication, and Taping

ALLYSON BARRY

MELISSA M. STEVENS*

CHAPTER *Objectives*

After studying this chapter, the reader will be able to accomplish the following:

- Explain how orthoses and taping impact the occupational performance of children and adolescents
- Describe general considerations when fabricating and providing an orthosis
- Understand the goals of orthoses and taping for children and adolescents
- Define common orthosis options specific to upper and lower extremity problems
- Understand how orthoses and taping are used as intervention in pediatric practice
- Describe the role of a certified occupational therapy assistant (COTA) in fabricating and using orthoses and taping
- Explain strategies to increase the compliance of children and adolescents in using orthoses
- Describe terms, concepts, and trends in the use of Kinesio Tex taping method
- Discuss the best practice strategies for application, reassessment, and use of Kinesio Tex taping
- Provide concise information regarding the use, technique of application, and contraindications of Kinesio Tex tape

* We acknowledge the contributions of Melissa Fullerton from the second edition. We acknowledge the invaluable review by Chris Blake, CHT, OTR/L, during the preparation of the third edition.

KEY TERMS	CHAPTER OUTLINE

Orthoses or taping may help children and adolescents who have limited upper or lower extremity function. Both the occupational therapist and the occupational therapy assistant (OTA) have important roles in the fabrication and application of orthoses and taping for children and adolescents.

This chapter begins with a definition of the terms *orthosis*, *splint*, and *taping* and describes general considerations that OT practitioners rely on when fabricating **orthoses/splints** and applying taping. The authors outline the purpose of each technique and provide readers with an overview of application principles. A description of the materials used and an overview of some common types of orthoses used in pediatric practice are presented. Case examples illustrate the principles and concepts for using these techniques with children and adolescents.

DEFINITION

OT practitioners traditionally used the term *splint* to describe temporary devices fabricated to support a part of the body, whereas the term *orthotic* was used to refer to a more permanent device. To eliminate confusion in the use of terminology among orthotists, OT practitioners, and insurance companies, OT practitioners are now encouraged to use the term *orthosis* to refer to temporary and permanent devices that immobilize, restrain, or support a part of the body.[2] Therefore, this chapter will use the terms *splints* and *orthoses* interchangeably.

The purpose of an orthosis/splint is to protect, correct, or assist a joint, limb, or muscle to increase functional performance.[5] For example, an orthosis might protect an injured wrist from increased pain when a child or adolescent is playing or prevent deformity occurring during sleep. An orthosis might help support a child's wrist to make writing more efficient.

Orthoses may be classified as static or dynamic. *Static* orthoses prevent movement, promote functional position, and prevent deformity. *Dynamic* orthoses allow children to move the joints and assist with movement. Table 27-1 provides additional definitions of the types of orthoses in accordance with the Centers for Medicare and Medicaid (CMS).

Kinesio taping refers to a specialized taping procedure that is used to provide support to muscle and joint structures in the upper extremities, lower extremities, trunk, neck, and face. For example, taping may be used to cue a child to keep the shoulders depressed and the scapulae in the correct position so that he or she may use the arms more fully.

TABLE 27-1

Sample Types of Orthoses According to Centers for Medicare and Medicaid (CMS)

NAME	DESCRIPTION*	PURPOSE
Elbow orthosis	Rigid circumferential, dorsal, or volar framed orthosis with soft straps and closures for the arm, elbow, and forearm	Stabilizes and may limit motion of the elbow
Shoulder orthosis	Static, rigid circumferential, dorsal, or volar framed orthosis with soft straps and closures for the shoulder	Statically stabilizes or limits motion of the shoulder
Shoulder, elbow, wrist, hand, finger orthosis SEWHFO	Static, rigid anterior or posterior framed orthosis with soft straps and closures initiating proximal to the glenohumeral joint and axillary region, extending through the upper arm, crossing the elbow, wrists, and hand joints including fingers	Protects medical conditions of the shoulder, elbow, wrist, hand, and fingers during healing process and/or reduces contractures
Finger orthosis	Dynamic, rigid volar or dorsal orthosis with soft straps and closures. The orthosis may initiate at the proximal or middle digital crease and will extend to the tip of the finger/thumb	Protects medical conditions of the finger/thumb during healing process and/or reduces contractures and stiffness
Hand, finger orthosis	Dynamic, rigid volar, dorsal, radially or ulnar contoured orthosis with soft straps and closures; may initiate at the base of the hand and extend to the middle or distal digital crease or to the tip of the fingers	Protects medical conditions of the hand/finger/thumb during healing process and/or reduces contractures and stiffness

From CMS HCPCS Public Meeting Summary (by Chris Blake of the American Society of Hand Therapists), June 8, 2005.

GENERAL CONSIDERATIONS

Orthoses may stabilize, support, or protect body parts enabling children to use their hands (or legs in the case of lower extremity orthoses) during activities of daily living (ADLs), education, play, and social participation. OT practitioners consider many factors before designing and fabricating an orthosis to help a child engage in daily occupations. The OT practitioner considers the child's age, diagnosis, motivations, interests, habits, and routines, along with the context in which the orthosis will be worn. *Context* refers to the setting in which the child belongs, such as school, home, and his or her cultural, physical, temporal (i.e., time in child's life), and social environments.[1] The OT practitioner also considers the child's physical abilities (including range of motion [ROM], muscle tone, strength, endurance, and structural appearance). The OT practitioner uses clinical reasoning to determine the best solution for the child. For example, the OT practitioner may decide that a simple design is best to ensure proper wear and compliance or that a prefabricated orthosis will meet a particular child's temporary needs, whereas another child may need a custom-made orthosis for long-term wear.

Examples of the use of orthoses include the following:

- Orthoses sometimes provide children with external support necessary to improve ROM or to help the child compensate for lack of ROM. For example, a *universal cuff* allows a child who has a hand deformity to hold a spoon.
- Children who experience joint pain, such as children who have juvenile rheumatoid arthritis (JRA), may benefit from orthoses that will help them rest their joints. In this case, the purpose of the orthosis is to help children maintain ROM but rest the joint adequately during inflammatory periods of this disease (Figure 27-1).
- Children with muscle tone abnormalities may benefit from external support of the joints, which will provide them with stability that they typically lack. For example, an elbow orthosis may stabilize the elbow joint allowing the child or adolescent to focus on using his or her hands for holding objects more easily. A thumb splint may provide enough tactile input, sustained over time to open a fisted hand enough so that the child is able to pick up objects in the palm.

OT practitioners consider typical child and adolescent development (e.g., gross and fine motor skill development, age, and occupational roles) when fabricating an orthosis. (See Table 27-2 for a description of upper extremity development.) For example, 8-month-old

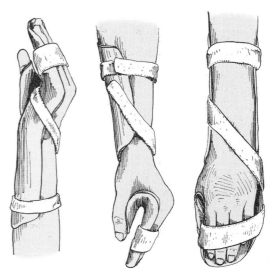

FIGURE 27-1 Static wrist hand finger orthosis (previously referred to as a resting hand splint) is an orthosis that promotes proper alignment of the wrist and hand used to prevent shortening of the long finger flexor tendons while the hand is at rest or not being used. (From Christensen, Barbara Lauristen. *Adult Health Nursing*, 5th Edition. Mosby, 2005.)

infants crawl on their hands and knees. Therefore, the OT practitioner making an orthosis for this infant wants to be sure that the splint allows the child to crawl.

Orthoses are customized to fit the individual and meet his or her occupational needs.[2,3,9] By positioning a limb in a functional position, the child or adolescent may engage in meaningful occupations such as play and ADLs. OT practitioners use their knowledge of anatomy, kinesiology, the child's medical condition(s) along with information about the child's age, developmental level, contexts, and, most importantly, the purpose of the orthosis. The OT practitioner uses all of these factors for clinical reasoning in order to design and fabricate the device. Generally, orthoses are recommended to improve function, promote proper position, and ensure hygiene.

GOALS OF ORTHOSIS FABRICATION

OT practitioners fabricate orthoses based on principles of anatomy and kinesiology. Box 27-1 provides an overview of these principles.

CLINICAL *Pearl*

The OT practitioner considers three points of pressure when designing an orthosis. The middle force is applied directly at the axis of the joint. Without crossing another joint, the two opposite forces are placed as far away from the middle force as possible for maximum efficiency.[4]

TABLE 27-2

Upper Extremity Development

AGE SKILL APPEARS (MONTHS)	UPPER EXTREMITY SKILLS
0–2	Physiologic flexion
2	Grasp reflex
3	Hands together on chest in supine position
4	Grasp reflex diminishing; objects held in both hands at midline; in supine position bears weight on forearm, with more weight on the ulnar than the radial side; pats sides of bottle with hands
5	Two-handed approach to objects, but grasp is unilateral; bilateral transfer; extended-arm weight bearing in prone position; places two hands on bottle, with some forearm supination
6	Weight shifts on extended arms in prone position; sits with a straight back; elbows fully extend when reaching
7	First purposeful release; pulls self to stand
8	Crawls on hands and knees
9	Active forearm supination when reaching
10	Pokes with index finger
12	Uses hands in coordinated manner in which one hand stabilizes and the other manipulates; begins to scribble
15	Releases a pellet with wrist extension and precision

Adapted from Jacobs ML, Austin N: *Splinting the hand and upper extremity: Principles and process,* Baltimore, MD, 2003, Lippincott Williams and Wilkins.

BOX 27-1

General Guiding Principles of Orthoses

- External stability may improve mobility and allow clients to engage in occupations.
- Orthoses provide continuous stretch to muscle.
- Orthoses position clients in a functional position.
- Orthoses should improve or maintain function.
- Orthoses should allow clients to participate in developmentally appropriate activities.

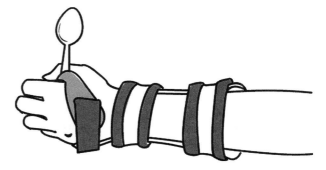

FIGURE 27-2 Functional orthosis—wrist extension orthosis with spoon attached. (Redrawn from Armstrong J: Splinting the pediatric patient. In Fess EE et al, editors: *Hand and upper extremity splinting: principles and methods,* ed 3, St. Louis, 2005, Mosby.)

Use of Orthoses to Improve Function

CASE *Study*

Kira is a 4-year-old girl with cerebral palsy (CP). She has decreased wrist stability, which makes it difficult for her to hold utensils. She is able to sit at a table but has poor coordination and is continuously dropping her spoon. A wrist extension splint was fabricated for Kira to help her hold the spoon (Figure 27-2).

A supported wrist orthosis was designed for Kira to wear while eating. This orthosis provides Kira with the wrist support she needs to increase hand control and be successful in this important ADL. The OT practitioner uses the principle that external stability may increase mobility. In this case, the orthosis allows Kira to use her hand and fingers to grasp the spoon. Therefore, creating stability around the wrist or elbow with the use of the orthosis may promote hand function.

A functional orthosis can substitute for weak or absent muscles, which may be caused by peripheral nerve dysfunction, neuromuscular disorders (e.g., CP), or spinal cord injuries.[2,4] Other examples of functional orthoses include those designed to help the child hold a pencil, toy, or eating utensil.

Several types of orthoses are used to improve hand function.

- **Serial static orthoses** immobilize joints in a stationary position.[6] The serial static orthosis applies continued force to maximize the length of the tissue and is worn for long periods allowing the tissue to adapt. Once the tissue has accommodated to the stretch, a new orthosis may be made, or the old orthosis is remolded, to hold the tissue at a new maximum length.[6]
- **Dynamic orthoses** apply force to one or more joints. These orthoses include a rubber band, pulley, spring, screw, hook, elastic, or other outriggers to provide the continuous force.[4] These types of orthoses are not worn as long as the serial orthoses. The force is continuous while the orthosis remains on, but the orthosis is removed periodically.[4]
- **Static progressive orthoses** are used to apply adjustable static force. The orthosis is applied as the joint is positioned at its maximum. The force is then adjusted when the tissue response allows repositioning to a new length.[4]

Three stages of healing follow tissue injury: (1) inflammatory (where the wound prepares to heal), (2) fibroplastic (the tissue structure is rebuilt), and (3) remodeling (configuration develops).[7] Edema can occur during any of these stages due to lack of functional use, which leads to stiffness and adherence and therefore continued inactivity.[4] Edema, or excess fluid build up, may develop due to increased capillary permeability, which results in leakage of fluid and protein into the tissue spaces.[13]

Elevation, active motion, gentle external massage, and compression may all help minimize edema. orthoses provide a form of compression and may decrease edema, reduce pain, and encourage tissue repair.[13] Applying orthoses during the early phase of healing allows the necessary rest and compression, as well as positioning, which protects the healing structures while maintaining a balanced, functional position.[13] Some health disorders cause edema and inflammation as well. Orthoses are an effective way to mobilize the stiff hand, but orthoses are most effective when combined with an exercise program.[4]

Use of Orthoses to Promote Proper Position

CASE *Study*

Timmy is an 8-year-old boy who is developing **contractures** (limitations in movement caused by soft tissue shortening, which may result in a "stiff" or fused joint that is unable to move) in his hands secondary to juvenile rheumatoid arthritis (JRA). His wrists are beginning to deviate in an ulnar direction; redness and swelling are present around the joints.

If a joint remains in an abnormal position, the risk of fusion and deformity increases, which may lead to limited use of the hands. Early use of an orthosis protects the affected joint and helps maintain the length of the soft tissue. The orthosis applies a continuous stretch to the muscles and promotes the performance of daily occupations.

Static orthoses serve the following purposes:

- They decrease or prevent contractures by maximizing range of motion (ROM), thus preventing muscle and tendon shortening.
- They provide stability to an unstable joint by giving external support to the joint.
- They improve joint alignment and prevent the progression of deformity. An orthosis may place the child's or adolescent's hand in the proper anatomical position.
- They provide rest to assist the healing process. (An orthosis will, for example, hold the hand in proper anatomic alignment, allowing the soft tissues to heal and edema and inflammation to diminish.[4])

The occupational therapist evaluated Timmy's hand function. The occupational therapist and OTA together designed a wrist extension orthosis with ulnar deviation block for Timmy (Figure 27-3). The wrist extension orthosis held Timmy's hand in slight wrist extension while providing a passive stretch to the wrist flexors. He wore his wrist extension orthosis with 2-hour increments to eliminate joint stiffness. See Figure 27-4 for Timmy's schedule for wearing the orthosis.

Some children require orthoses to protect them from injuring themselves. The OT practitioner must consider the safety of providing such orthoses and the consequences to the child and to others.

Use of Orthoses to Improve Hygiene and Prevent Skin Breakdown

CASE *Study*

Matt is a 10-year-old boy with pervasive developmental disorder (PDD). He continually picks at his scabs, increasing the risk of infection. The scabs fail to heal and bleed continuously, and they are beginning to scar. An orthosis is needed to protect Matt's fragile skin. The occupational therapist working with Matt decided on providing Matt with a protective covering for his skin.

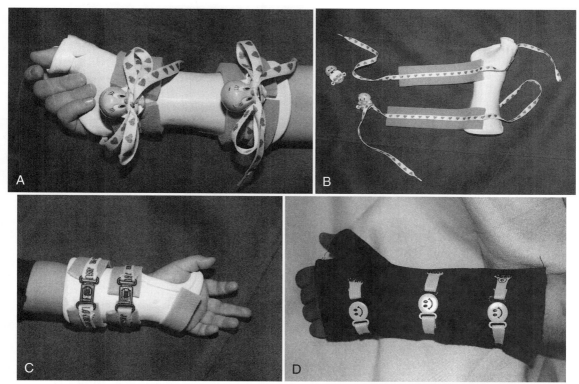

FIGURE 27-3 A, Wrist extension orthosis with thumb support made from thermoplastic material molded to the child. **B,** Wrist extension orthosis with thumb support made from thermoplastic material molded to the child. **C,** Wrist extension orthosis. **D,** Wrist extension orthosis is made of neoprene.

The OTA, under the supervision of the occupational therapist, fabricated a covering made of stockinette and terry cloth to provide comfort and also cover the existing scabs. However, after several weeks, it became apparent that Matt was able to pick at the scabs after biting through the covering. After collaboration with the occupational therapist, the OTA applied orthotic material over the stockinette so that Matt would be unable to pick at his scabs (Figure 27-5).

Using orthotic devices to prevent a child or adolescent from self-abuse and interfering behaviors or after a surgical procedure may be an adjunctive intervention provided by the OT practitioner.[2-4] For example, an orthosis can protect a postoperative area before complete healing has occurred.

CASE *Study*

Alex is a 10-year-old boy who has spastic–quadriplegic cerebral palsy. He keeps his left hand fisted with an indwelling thumb. His parents and teachers are concerned about his hands being sweaty and smelly because of the continuous fisting. The skin on Alex's hands is flaking, and food is being lodged in his hands. His fingernails have grown long and are digging into his palm. Furthermore, when Alex's hand is opened, his palm appears red and is bleeding. An orthosis is therefore needed to protect the palm from long and jagged fingernails.

The OTA and the occupational therapist collaborated to design a palm protector orthosis for Alex to improve hygiene and prevent his fingernails from cutting into his palm. He wore the orthosis during his waking hours, taking it off only for bathing and grooming. At night, Alex's hands were sufficiently relaxed and open, so he did not require a night orthosis.

An orthosis can be designed to help prevent or improve hygiene problems.[5-7] For example, a spastic hand that remains fisted is at high risk for skin breakdown. The inability to extend the fingers makes nail clipping difficult, and long or sharp fingernails can cut the skin, which may lead to infection. Orthoses are frequently fabricated to protect the palm and decrease the risk of skin breakdown (Figure 27-6). For example, an elbow extension orthosis may prevent a child from scratching his face.

Name: Timmy Smith Splint: Wrist cock up with ulnar deviation block	Schedule: 2 Hours ON 2 Hours OFF Purpose: Keep hand in a healthy position; stop stiffness and pain

I wear my splint for 2 hours.

Then, I keep it OFF for 2 hours. Then I put it back ON.

My splint helps my arthritis feel better. ☺

My schedule helps me and my OT know when I am wearing my splint.

I stop wearing my splint if I see any red areas or if it hurts.

	SUN.	MON.	TUES.	WED.	THURS.	FRI.	SAT.
8 - 10 am	ON ★	ON	ON ★	ON	ON ★	ON	ON
10 - 12 pm	OFF	OFF ✋	OFF ★	OFF ★	OFF ★	OFF ★	OFF
12 - 2 pm	ON ★	ON	ON	ON ★	ON	ON	ON
2 - 4 pm	OFF	OFF	OFF ★	OFF ★	OFF ★	OFF	OFF
4 - 6 pm	ON ★	★ ON	ON	ON	★ ON	★ ON	✋ ON
6 - 8 pm	OFF	OFF	OFF ★	✋ OFF	OFF ★	OFF ★	OFF
Bedtime	OFF						

★ = YES, I followed my schedule   ✋ = NO, I did not follow the schedule

FIGURE 27-4   Sample wear schedule.

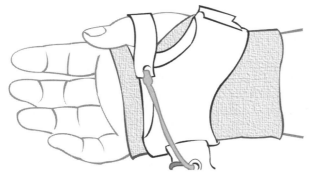

FIGURE 27-5 Orthosis for protection—elbow extension orthosis.

CONSIDERATIONS FOR PROVIDING ORTHOSES TO CHILDREN AND ADOLESCENTS

Prior to designing and fabricating an orthosis for a child or adolescent, the OT practitioner considers the occupations in which he or she engages and the purpose of the orthosis for that child. Understanding the desires of the

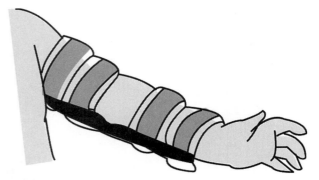

FIGURE 27-6   Hand orthosis to protect child's palm.

client helps the OT practitioner design an orthosis that is appealing and meaningful to the client, thereby increasing the chances that the orthosis will be worn. Compliance in wearing the orthosis is clearly related to how well the OT practitioner matches the interests and goals of the client. Consequently, the OT practitioner also considers the developmental and functional level as well as the ability to don and doff the orthosis. During consideration of the physical status, the OT practitioner examines skin integrity, edema, ROM, muscle tone, and current functional status. The OT practitioner must clearly evaluate how the client moves and functions to design an orthosis that does not interfere with the client's own techniques for moving. Since wearing an orthosis is key to the success of the intervention, OT practitioners use a variety of questions to guide decisions on orthoses, such as the following:[7]

1. What is the desired outcome of using the orthosis?
2. How will the orthosis have an impact on the client's ability to engage in occupations?
   - Will the orthosis improve the client's ability to perform?
3. What are the client's or the family's habits and routines? How will this have an impact on the wearing schedule and its use?
4. Will the orthosis "fit" within the context(s) of the client (e.g., physical, personal, social, cultural)? Are there any modifications that may make it a better fit (e.g., wearing the orthosis only at home)?
   - Will the splint be worn?
5. What are the client's primary, secondary, and associated problems?
   - How does the client feel about the orthosis?
   - Are there any associated sensory needs?
   - What are the client's physical needs?
6. Will the associated problems affect the orthosis?
   - What biomechanical principles are being addressed (e.g., stretch, position, alignment, stability)?

7. What orthotic design will best address the client's needs?
   - Should the orthosis be static or dynamic? If dynamic, what components should be used?
   - Should the orthosis be serial or static progressive?
   - Should the base be dorsal or volar?

8. What orthotic components are integral to meeting the purpose?
   - What joints should be included in the orthosis?
   - Is the orthosis easy to don and doff?

Table 27-3 lists common pediatric diagnoses and orthotic interventions that may prove beneficial.

Understanding the client better and designing an orthosis that meets the client's needs is the best way to ensure that the orthosis will be used. Compliance with the wear schedule and use of the orthosis is necessary to meet the stated goals.

Compliance

The motivation to wear an orthosis depends on how well the OT practitioner has addressed the client's concerns. Generally, children and adolescents will wear an orthosis that helps them do the things they want to do. Thus, taking the time to explain this to the children and their family members is important in ensuring their compliance with the wear schedule. Children and adolescents who do not understand the purposes and benefits of orthoses are apt to remove them. The OT practitioner should always take the time to describe the purpose, the schedule, and precautions for wearing the orthosis. OT practitioners should use simple language at the client's level of understanding.

Some children and adolescents may see orthoses as something that makes them "different" from their peers; they may feel as though the orthosis makes them "stand out." These individuals may not want to wear orthoses because of social factors. Therefore, it is advantageous for OT practitioners to consider the client's concerns regarding the appearances of orthoses. Sometimes adding interchangeable colorful Velcro bands or using bright-colored (or school-color) orthotic material is enough to increase compliance.

The following strategies may increase compliance in following an orthosis protocol:

- Educate the client and his or her caregiver regarding the purposes and goals of the orthosis/splint.[2] The client may be more apt to wear the orthosis

TABLE 27-3

Common Pediatric Diagnoses Utilizing Splinting Interventions

DIAGNOSIS	SPLINTING INTERVENTIONS
Cerebral palsy Hemiplegia—involvement on one side of the body	Functional orthoses that facilitate proper positions of arms, e.g., wrist/hand orthoses, neoprene orthoses, thumb abduction orthoses
Quadriplegia	Wrist/hand immobilization orthoses, antispasticity orthoses, neoprene orthoses, wrist/finger orthoses
Duchenne muscular dystrophy	Functional orthoses that promote stability in weak joints for increased function, e.g., wrist/hand orthoses, elbow orthoses
Rett syndrome	Orthoses designed to protect clients from self-abusive behaviors, e.g., elbow extension orthoses
Osteogenesis imperfecta	Orthoses designed to protect clients from frequent fractures due to decreased stability and structure of the bones, e.g., wrist/hand immobilization orthoses
Arthrogryposis	Functional orthoses fabricated to promote engagement in functional activities and prevent further contractures, e.g., wrist extension orthoses, neoprene orthoses, and elbow extension orthoses
Brachial plexus palsy	Functional orthoses fabricated to inhibit stretching and facilitate protection of the muscles and nerves, e.g., wrist extension orthoses, elbow extension orthoses, neoprene orthoses
Juvenile rheumatoid arthritis	Functional orthoses fabricated to promote ROM for engagement in functional activities and for protection and to decrease deformities, e.g., wrist extension orthoses, MP joint extension orthoses

ROM, range of motion; *MP*, Metacarpal phalanges.
Adapted from Jacobs ML, Austin N: *Splinting the hand and upper extremity: Principles and process*, Baltimore, MD, 2003, Lippincott Williams and Wilkins.

if he or she understands why it is necessary. For example, if a client understands that wearing the orthosis will help him or her play video games with friends, he or she might be more likely to wear it.

- Provide simple written, verbal, and pictorial instructions.
- Use positive reinforcement (e.g., verbal praise, stickers) for following the orthosis/splint schedule.
- Design orthoses that are attractive and pleasing to clients.
- Demonstrate the proper orthosis application to a client and his or her caregiver.[5]
- In a hospital setting, correlate the orthosis/splint schedule with staff shift changes and include the schedule into the hospital care plan.
- Label orthoses/splints clearly. Color coding or using a number system to show clients and caregivers how to don and doff them might prove helpful.[5]

CLINICAL *Pearl*

Children and adolescents may be more likely to wear orthoses that they find aesthetically pleasing and functional. Allowing clients to choose the color of the orthosis or strapping may increase compliance in wearing it. Encouraging clients and responding to their feedback on how an orthosis feels and looks increases compliance as well. The client may like the orthosis better if it is personalized. Personalizing an orthosis/splint includes allowing the client to attach stickers or write, draw, or paint on the orthosis. See Figure 27-7, which shows a festive Halloween drawing.

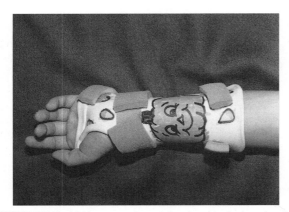

FIGURE 27-7 Wrist extension orthosis with festive drawing. (From Armstrong J: Splinting the pediatric patient. In Fess EE et al, editors: *Hand and upper extremity splinting: principles and methods*, ed 3, St. Louis, 2005, Mosby.)

Precautions

Children, adolescents, and their caregivers must know what signs to look for while checking for skin breakdown. These signs include redness, soreness, and broken skin. Skin breakdown can lead to **pressure sores**, which can develop relatively quickly when the skin is compromised. Improperly fitting orthoses or those that have been applied incorrectly may cause skin breakdown.

To prevent skin breakdown caused by wearing an orthosis, the OT practitioner notes the location of a bony prominence (e.g., the ulnar styloid process) and takes care to ensure that there is sufficient padding around that area or that it is not in contact with the orthotic material.[5] The OT practitioner examines the orthosis to make sure that its edges are rolled upward and not digging into the skin.

The padding may include self-sticking foam or gel padding. Including padding for bony prominences during the fabrication of the orthosis helps protect them. Stockinette can also be used to protect the integrity of the skin. Additional care should be taken to prevent pressure sores in a child or adolescent who has decreased sensation or decreased ability to communicate. Careful inspection of the skin by both caregivers and OT practitioners is necessary.

CLINICAL *Pearl*

Padding can actually create pressure points in other places. OT practitioners need to carefully and frequently inspect all areas of the skin for redness as well as educate caregivers on how to inspect the skin.

CLINICAL *Pearl*

Velcro can rub onto the skin and create pressure sores. OT practitioners should carefully inspect the orthosis to make sure that the Velcro is not rubbing on the client's skin.

Evaluation

The occupational therapist receives the referral, assesses the need for an orthosis, and decides which type of orthosis will address the client's needs and best meet intervention goals. The OTA assists the occupational therapist in fabricating the orthosis or may fabricate the orthosis, depending on his or her skill level, setting of care, and reimbursement/funding sources. Medicare does not permit OTAs to fabricate orthoses independently.

After determining the goal of the orthosis, the OT practitioner considers the following factors when designing the orthosis:

- *Anatomic structures.* The OT practitioner examines structures to determine if deformities or abnormalities are present (Figure 27-8).
- *Abnormal muscle tone.* Spasticity may influence orthoses in different ways. For example, an orthosis applied to one area may change the muscle tone and affect the other joints of that extremity.[6]
- *Time frames for healing.* Healing rates differ among adults, children, and adolescents. Children tend to heal more quickly but may remain in an orthosis for longer periods. Some clients have a difficult time adhering to their orthosis protocol, which may influence healing time.
- *Swelling.* Managing edema (swelling) remains the same in children, adolescents, and adults (e.g., using ice, elevation, compression). Careful observation and management by caregivers are very important. The orthosis may need to be remolded or refitted if a client develops edema, which may cause the skin to be more sensitive to pressure and lead to skin breakdown or pressure sores.
- *Compliance.* Compliance can affect the length of time an orthosis needs to be prescribed and may also affect intervention planning and goal setting. See Figure 27-9 for creative ideas to help with compliance while working with children and adolescents.
- *Sensory factors.* Some children and adolescents are hypersensitive to touch and may not tolerate an orthosis. Nonverbal clients may have difficulty indicating they are in pain or discomfort. Careful fabrication of the orthosis, padding around bony prominences, the use of a stockinette, and careful monitoring help the client with sensory issues tolerate the orthosis.
- *Cognition and developmental age.* The client's age will affect the design and fabrication of the orthosis. For example, if a child is still "mouthing" objects, the orthosis should not have small pieces or contain glue or adhesive that is toxic. Also, some physicians may order an orthosis that will "overprotect" an active child. For example, instead of fabricating a hand-based orthosis for a proximal phalanx fracture, a forearm-based orthosis that provides more durability and protection during play and other daily occupations may be prescribed.
- *Latex allergies and precautions.* Many children and adolescents with special needs develop latex allergies. Some orthotic materials or attachments (rubber bands) may contain latex. OT practitioners need to be aware of these potential reactions and use alternative materials.
- *Home environment.* Children or adolescents who live in geographic areas with warm climates may need to use perforated thermoplastic material to allow airflow, decrease sweating, and prevent melting of the orthotic material.

FABRICATION TIPS

The occupational therapist and the OTA often assist each other during the fabrication of pediatric orthoses because of the special issues in this population. Orthoses are fabricated from a pattern or protocol. OT practitioners may modify a pattern, design a pattern unique to the client, or use a prefabricated pattern (Box 27-2).

OT practitioners must ensure that the orthosis fits properly and achieves the desired outcome. Box 27-3 provides some tips for achieving a pleasing cosmetic appearance of an orthosis. The material should not cause any irritation or rubbing. OT practitioners must check to determine that the client or his or her caregiver is able to apply the orthosis properly and that it fits (sometimes it is necessary to make marks on the orthosis). The straps keeping the orthosis in place should be long enough to hold the orthosis in place, but not so long as to cause extraneous material to be left hanging. Edges should be rounded to make sure that they do not rub against the client and create pressure sores. The OT practitioner carefully analyzes how well the orthosis meets its stated goal. For example, a dynamic orthosis allows the child to move, whereas a static orthosis promotes resting function (not movement).

Orthotic Material

The OT practitioner selects the type of material depending on the client's age, muscle tone, level of cooperation, and level of pain.[2] Table 27-4 provides the reader with properties of specific materials.

The weight of the material needs to be taken into consideration, especially with very young children or adolescents with weak muscles. The thinner materials ($\frac{1}{16}$" to $\frac{3}{32}$") often provide adequate positioning while minimizing weight. They also allow for better conformability to smaller hands.[4,8]

Neoprene orthoses may be more comfortable for children or adolescents with contractures because of the soft nature of the material (Figure 27-10). However, severe spasticity and rigid deformity cannot be controlled with neoprene.[4,8]

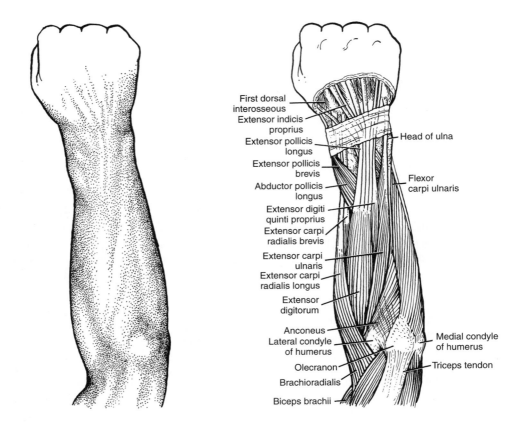

First dorsal interosseous
Extensor indicis proprius
Extensor pollicis longus
Extensor pollicis brevis
Abductor pollicis longus
Extensor digiti quinti proprius
Extensor carpi radialis brevis
Extensor carpi ulnaris
Extensor carpi radialis longus
Extensor digitorum
Anconeus
Lateral condyle of humerus
Olecranon
Brachioradialis
Biceps brachii

Head of ulna
Flexor carpi ulnaris
Medial condyle of humerus
Triceps tendon

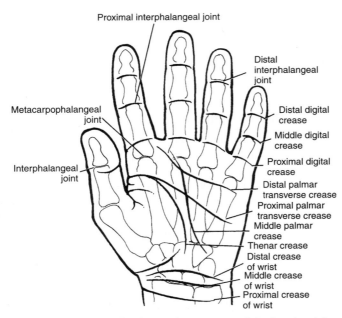

Proximal interphalangeal joint
Metacarpophalangeal joint
Interphalangeal joint

Distal interphalangeal joint
Distal digital crease
Middle digital crease
Proximal digital crease
Distal palmar transverse crease
Proximal palmar transverse crease
Middle palmar crease
Thenar crease
Distal crease of wrist
Middle crease of wrist
Proximal crease of wrist

FIGURE 27-8 Anatomic structures of the hand and forearm. (From Fess EE et al: *Hand and upper extremity splinting: principles and methods*, ed 3, St. Louis, 2005, Mosby.)

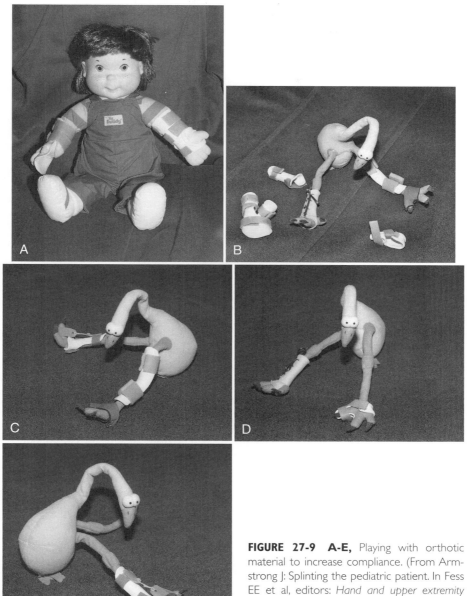

FIGURE 27-9 A-E, Playing with orthotic material to increase compliance. (From Armstrong J: Splinting the pediatric patient. In Fess EE et al, editors: *Hand and upper extremity splinting: principles and methods*, ed 3, St. Louis, 2005, Mosby.)

Table 27-4 lists a variety of orthotic material, associated handling characteristics, and examples of how the material is used.

Congenital Hand Differences

Some children and adolescents are born with deformities of the hand or upper extremity, known as congenital hand differences. When fabricating orthoses for children with congenital hand differences, the OT practitioner looks at the child's development and current functioning, determines the purpose of the orthosis, and considers the context in which the child will use the orthosis. The goal of orthoses for children who have congenital hand differences is to improve functional ability for engagement in daily activities.

See Table 27-5 for descriptions of common pediatric congenital hand differences and orthosis options.

ORTHOSES FOR THE LOWER EXTREMITIES

OT practitioners often work with physical therapy (PT) personnel to fabricate orthoses for the lower extremities for children and adolescents. Children and adolescents

BOX 27-2

Orthosis Fabrication Tips

1. If a client does not like to be touched or is in pain but remains cooperative, the OT practitioner may use a drapable plastic-like material. In order to minimize contact with the client's skin, double-sided tape can be used to stabilize the position of the forearm trough until the orthosis cools and hardens. Before the orthosis is fabricated, the client's arm can be positioned in supination, with the wrist in extension over the table edge or wedge. In this position, gravity helps maintain the wrist in the desired position during orthosis fabrication.

2. For a client who is squirming around during fabrication but not in pain, a more forgiving material, such as one in the rubber category, which allows the OT practitioner to hold on to the orthosis and the client limb with more force while molding, can be used.

3. A perforated material should be used with a client who tends to perspire excessively or lives in climates that are hot and humid. A stockinette sleeve/glove may help absorb the moisture from the perspiration.

4. With few exceptions, outriggers and orthotic attachments are not recommended for children because these attachments tend to have small pieces that may become detached and consequently be a choking hazard; they could also cause injury to the eyes, ears, and other areas of the body if the child is running and falls on the orthosis.

BOX 27-3

A Checklist for Enhancing Cosmesis

- No pen marks
- No rough edges
- No surface impressions (fingerprints, nail lines, etc.)
- Moleskin to cover ragged edges
- No rolling or folding back of material around the thenar eminence or bony prominences
- Well-secured Velcro (does not appear to be peeling off)
- Use of D-ring closure if the child is unable to remove Velcro easily
- Round edges of Velcro
- Flair edges
- Correct length of straps

with abnormal tone, burns, fractures, or other injuries or conditions affecting the lower extremities may benefit from orthoses for the lower extremities. See Table 27-6 for descriptions of common lower-extremity orthoses. The same precautions and considerations that are taken with orthoses for the upper extremities must also be applied to splinting the lower extremities.

Once the orthosis has been fabricated, the OT practitioner analyzes its usefulness by determining if the orthosis meets its stated goal. The OT practitioner checks the structural components of the orthosis, demonstrates to the client and his or her parents or caregivers how to don and doff the orthosis and reviews the wear schedule. The OT practitioner answers any questions the client and his or her parents may have and observes the client donning and doffing the orthosis. Adjustments may be made if the OT practitioner is not satisfied with the orthosis or if any red areas on the client's skin are noted. (OT practitioners may ask the client to wear the splint for 15 to 30 minutes in the clinic so that any skin redness can be noted). Box 27-4

provides questions the OT practitioner considers before giving the orthosis to the client.

KINESIO TAPING

The *Kinesio Tex tape* is a type of tape that can be used as an adjunct to therapy. Utilizing the Kinesio tape during intervention has many different advantages. The Kinesio tape can be applied to protect weakened limbs and also used as a conservative treatment or alternative treatment to surgery.

The original Kinesio Tex and Kinesio taping method was invented by Dr. Kenzo Kase. Dr. Kase developed the technique as an intervention modality for pain relief and to treat sports-related injuries.[9,10] The primary goal of taping as an adjunct to intervention is to aid the body in self-healing.[9,10] The Kinesio taping method activates the neurologic and circulatory systems by mimicking human kinesiology and normal muscle activity.[9,10] Muscles play a primary role in stabilizing body structures, venous circulation throughout the body, lymphatic drainage, and body temperature. Imbalance between muscles and joints may cause movement deficits, pain, and injury.[9] Taping provides the stability that is needed to move effectively.

Kinesio taping addresses the following areas (Table 27-7):

- Muscular functions
- Joint functions
- Lymphatic functions
- Skin functions

Muscular Functions

The Kinesio tape provides external support to the muscles. The tape is applied in specific directions, which encourages normal movement in muscle activity. The

TABLE 27-4

Handling Characteristics of Orthotic Material and Examples

THERMOPLASTIC NAME	HANDLING CHARACTERISTICS	RECOMMENDED USE
Aquaplast	Latex-free Nondraping 100% memory Translucent when heated	Large orthoses Serial orthoses Orthoses for spasticity Elbow orthoses Ankle/foot orthoses
EZ form	Latex-free Low-temperature thermoplastic Maximum resistance to stretch Excellent draping abilities Extremely rigid Bonds to itself when heated Remains in place while molding (good for using to contour the palmar arches) Can be ordered with an Antimicrobial factor to reduce odors Heats slowly and cools quickly	For patients who are unable to cooperate Adapting ADL equipment Antispasticity orthoses Functional positioning orthoses such as resting hand orthoses, resting pan mitt orthoses, elbow orthoses
Fabric-form	Latex-free Thin material Great for lightweight orthoses Low profile material Moderate drapability Heats and cools quickly	Finger/gutter orthoses
Flex-form	Increased rigidity Easy to mold Maximum resistance to stretch Resistant to finger printing Requires no reinforcing Self-bonding Heats at 160–170 degrees with a working time of 3–5 minutes.	Elbow orthoses Gutter orthoses
Orthoplast	Latex-free Excellent durability Nondraping May be molded without finger printing Resistant to stretch Adheres to itself when heated	Static or functional positioning orthoses Antispasticity orthoses
Orthoplast II	Low temperature thermoplastic Excellent drapability Drapes well for a close fit Adheres to self; however requires solvent for bonding Edges trim and finish well	Ideal for static or dynamic orthoses Finger orthoses Small hand orthoses Wrist orthoses
Silon-LTS	Latex-free Combines a low-temperature thermoplastic with a therapeutic surface of silicone	Indications for use are with hypertrophic scars* Use as a prophylaxis** after surgery

Continued

TABLE 27-4

Handling Characteristics of Orthotic Material and Examples—cont'd

THERMOPLASTIC NAME	HANDLING CHARACTERISTICS	RECOMMENDED USE
Synergy	Retains shape after setting Conforms to small contours Approximately 3–5 minutes working time Moderately resistant to stretch	Neurologic circumferential orthoses Ball orthoses Lower-limb-positioning orthoses Body jackets

X-Lite	Low-temperature thermoplastic has an open
	  weave design for lightweight application
	Well-ventilated decreasing skin breakdown due to
	  limited breathability
	Material is self-bonding
	Rigidity is increased by the addition of multiple
	  layers
		Positioning and for building up
		  tool handles for activities of
		  daily living, self-feeding.

*Hypertrophic scars: scar tissue or areas of fibrous tissue that replaces normal tissue after injury.
**Prophylaxis: a measure taken for the prevention of disease or injury.

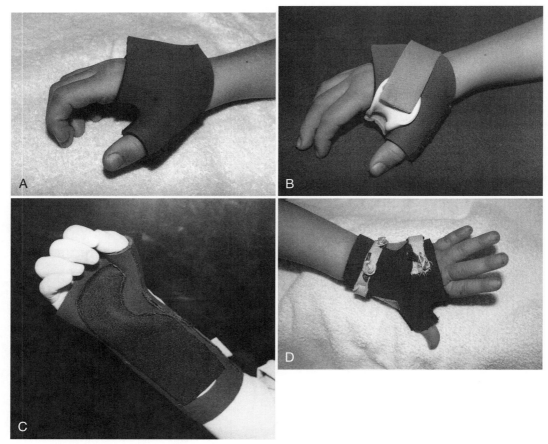

FIGURE 27-10   Neoprene orthosis. (From Armstrong J: Splinting the pediatric patient. In Fess EE et al, editors: *Hand and upper extremity splinting: principles and methods*, ed 3, St. Louis, 2005, Mosby.)

TABLE 27-5

Common Pediatric Congenital Hand Differences

SPECIFIC DIAGNOSIS	TYPES	DESCRIPTIONS	DEVELOPMENTAL ISSUES	ORTHOSIS OPTIONS
Camptodactyly	Infant	Congenital flexion of PIP	Lack of full finger opening	Serial orthosis
	Adolescent	Nontraumatic PIP flexion contracture		
	Syndromic	Congenital flexion of PIP		
Syndactyly	Simple	Only skin is involved	Limited finger use	Postoperative orthosis
	Complex	Fusion of bone and skin	Limited grasp	
Radial ray deficiencies: hypoplastic thumbs	1st Degree	Slim thumb	May avoid use of thumb	Soft neoprene orthosis
	2nd Degree	Poor thenars Unstable MP Tight web		Soft or rigid orthosis Postoperative protective orthosis
	3rd Degree	Absent thenars Unstable MP	Uses scissor grasp	Rigid orthosis Postoperative protective orthosis
	4th Degree	Floating thumb	Nonfunctional thumb Uses scissor grasp	Postoperative protective orthosis
	5th Degree	Absent thumb	Uses scissor grasp	Protective orthosis
Radial ray deficiencies: radial club hands	Type 1	Short radius Hypoplastic thumbs	Normal use, except thumbs	Orthosis as needed for thumbs
	Type 2	Hypoplastic radius	Lack of crawling Difficulty weight bearing	Radial- or ulnar-based orthosis Postoperative protective and night orthosis
	Type 3	Absent distal radius	Little finger prehension	Radial- or ulnar-based orthosis Postoperative protective and night orthosis
	Type 4	Aplastic radius	Little finger prehension	Radial- or ulnar-based orthosis Postoperative protective and night orthosis
Thumb-in-palm deformity	Type 1	Extensor pollicis brevis and longus deficiencies	Poor prehension	Soft orthosis for day Rigid orthosis for night
	Type 2	Extensor pollicis brevis and longus deficiencies Contractures	Poor prehension	Soft orthosis for day Rigid orthosis for night Postoperative protective orthosis
	Type 3	MP instability	Minimum thumb use	Soft orthosis for day Rigid orthosis for night Postoperative protective orthosis
	Type 4	Miscellaneous deformities	Minimum thumb use	Orthosis as needed

Continued

TABLE 27-5

Common Pediatric Congenital Hand Differences—cont'd

SPECIFIC DIAGNOSIS	TYPES	DESCRIPTIONS	DEVELOPMENTAL ISSUES	ORTHOSIS OPTIONS
Trigger thumb/ fingers		Triggering/crepitus Palpable nodule	May resist use due to pain Limited grasp and release	Orthosis as needed
Arthrogryposis	Distal	Flexed, webbed, and overlapping fingers MP joints in ulnar deviation Adducted thumbs	Limited grasp and release Poor prehension	Static progressive Postoperative

ADLs, activities of daily living; *MP*, metacarpophalangeal; *PIP*, proximal interphalangeal.
Adapted from Peck-Murray J, Gibson G: Rising to the challenge: Children with congenital hand differences, Presentation at the American Occupational Therapy Association Annual Conference and Expo, Long Beach, CA, May 13, 2005.

TABLE 27-6

Common Lower Extremity Orthoses

TYPE OF DEVICE	OBJECTIVES	INDICATIONS
Posterior ankle-foot orthosis	To rest the ankle in order to relieve pain To immobilize the ankle To correct or prevent contractures	For non–weight-bearing situations including the following: Mild to moderate spastic hemiparesis Injuries to distal tibia/fibula or ankle Clients at risk of developing ankle flexion contractures Congenital foot differences Cerebral palsy Acute burns Nerve injuries Flaccid hemiparesis
Static hip-stabilizing orthosis for hip dysplasia	To maintain proper position of a displaced hip in order to allow for hip stabilization	Unilateral or bilateral hip dysplasia
Spiral dynamic hip-knee-ankle-foot strap	To promote proper positioning of lower extremity To improve gait pattern To normalize tone To stabilize the head of the femur in the acetabulum	Head injury Spina bifida Cerebral palsy Lower-extremity paralysis
Posterior knee orthosis	To prevent or reduce knee flexion contracture To stabilize the knee during ambulation To rest the knee	Burns Knee fracture Flexion contracture
Circumferential tibia-stabilizing orthosis	To stabilize a tibia fracture For protection	Midshaft tibial fractures Osteogenesis imperfecta

Data from McKee P, Morgan L: *Orthotics in rehabilitation: Splinting the hand and body*, Philadelphia, 1998, F.A. Davis.

movement increases blood flow to the muscle spindles and fibers, thus creating stronger contractions. These contractions reduce muscle fatigue, reduce pain, and improve ROM.[9,10] For example, a child with a winged scapula may benefit when the tape is applied in a specific manor, mimicking the normal movement of the serratus anterior muscle, rhomboids, or middle fibers of the trapezius to facilitate normal ossicilation of the scapulo-humeral rhythm. The taping provides enough support to encourage the child to continue to use the muscle, thereby strengthening the muscle function and decreasing the winging in the scapular.

Orthosis Checklist

- Does the orthosis achieve its purpose?
- Does the orthosis maintain the proper position and angles for which it was designed?
- Does the orthosis fit the contours of the foot without causing discomfort, redness, irritation?
- Does the orthosis immobilize any joints unnecessarily?
- Is the orthosis long enough to provide proper support?
- Are all edges smooth and all pressure points relieved?
- Can the client or caregiver properly don and doff the orthosis?
- Does the client or caregiver understand the purpose and wear schedule of the orthosis?
- Is the orthosis cosmetically acceptable to the client?

Joint Functions

Taping is also used to correct misalignment of the joint(s).[9,10] Abnormal muscle tone or muscle weakness may interfere with joint alignment and movement. The Kinesio tape provides external support to help correct abnormal muscle tone or muscle weakness, which may provide enough support to align the joint for better movement. Positioning joints in correct alignment promotes movement and subsequently decreases edema (swelling), improves ROM, and decreases pain.[9,10]

Lymphatic Functions

Kinesio taping helps reduce excess heat and therefore decreases inflammation and pain.[14] The tape allows the lymphatic fluid that may get trapped under the skin to drain and thus improves blood circulation.[10] When the Kinesio Tex tape is applied with no stretch to the skin, it enables the fascia (i.e., fibrous connective membrane that covers, supports, and separates muscles) layers to spread out, allowing for less resistance of fluid, increasing blood flow, and decreasing excess heat or inflammation, and thus facilitates movement within pain-free parameters to participate in ADLs.

Skin Functions

The skin houses sensory and mechanical receptors that relay impulses of pain, temperature, and pressure to the central nervous system (CNS). The Kinesio tape applied to the skin stimulates these sensory receptors and serves to relieve pain, tension, and tightness of the skin that may be causing discomfort.[9,10]

CLINICAL *Pearl*

The Kinesio Tape Gold was used in the 2008 Olympic Games in Beijing. Many athletes wore the tape, which highlighted the use of the tape in many different ways and consequently increased its popularity.

Four Functions of Kinesio Tape

MUSCLE	JOINT	LYMPHATIC	SKIN
Supports muscles	Improves the relationships of joint surfaces	Improves circulation by removing congestion under skin layers	Activates the CNS to decrease pain, temperature, and pressure
↓	↓	↓	↓
Avoids injury by preventing muscle cramps	Reduces pain and inflammation	Removes excess heat and chemical substances	Gently separates the skin layers to reduces inflammation
↓	↓	↓	↓
Improves ROM	Improves ROM	Improves ROM	Improves ROM
↓	↓	↓	↓

Benefits to Treatment

Adapted from The Kinesio Taping Association, 2003.

Properties of the Kinesio Tape

Elastic Tape

The Kinesio tape (Figure 27-11) is latex free and consists of highly elastic fibers woven together in such a way that they stretch and recoil with memory.[10] The tape stretches along the longitudinal axis, thus allowing movement to occur while providing external stability.[9,10] The underside, or the skin side, has an adhesive backing that includes a heat-sensitive acrylic adhesive. The tape mimics the thickness of the top layer of the skin and thus is comfortable, light weight, and breathable.[9,10] The Kinesio tape stays on the skin even when in water or when in contact with sweat. The tape may be worn for 3 to 5 days before it may need to be replaced or removed.[10]

Rigid Tape

The rigid tape (i.e., McConnell brand) can also be used to provide external stability to joints (Figure 27-12). The rigid tape immobilizes joints and consequently prevents movement. The McConnell tape comprises two layers of tape. The top layer of tape (cover roll) protects the skin from direct contact with the inner layer (leukotape), which contains the adhesive latex material, which, in some individuals, can create blisters, redness, irritation or rash when in contact with the skin.

Refer to the chart (Table 27-8) to compare and contrast the elastic tape versus the rigid tape.[12]

Application of the Kinesio Tape

OT practitioners use their knowledge of kinesiology, anatomy, and occupational therapy when using taping with clients (Figure 27-13). Children and adolescents who are very active may not be good candidates for

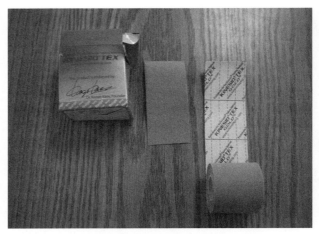

FIGURE 27-12 Kinesio tape.

taping, since the tape may wear off quickly or fail to stay adhered to the skin.

Strategies and techniques for applying the Kinesio tape include the following:

- Advise children, adolescents, and caregivers about the contraindications to wearing the tape. Provide a clear wear schedule.
- The tape should be applied 30 minutes prior to an activity to allow the skin, muscle, joint, and lymphatic systems ample time to adjust and accommodate the tape and its effects.[9,10]
- The skin should be dry, free of lotion, and free of excess hair before the tape is applied.[11]
- The tape should be applied in the direction of the movement that is being facilitated or inhibited. For example, when the goal of the tape is to support a weakened muscle, the tape should be placed at the origin of the muscle and end at the insertion of the muscle. To inhibit spasticity in a muscle, the tape should be applied in an insertion-to-origin fashion.[10]
- Once the direction of light pull (e.g., 10%, 20%, etc.) is determined, the center of the tape should be laid over the center of the muscle belly that has to be influenced (i.e., supported, facilitated, or inhibited). After the tape is applied to the muscle belly, it should then be applied proximally to distally.
- The tape should be gently rubbed onto the skin creating a light neutral warmth effect, which will activate the heat-sensitive adhesive property of the tape.[10]
- The tape should be blotted dry if it has been immersed in water. Rubbing the tape with a towel creates friction and will peel the edges of the tape from the skin.[10]

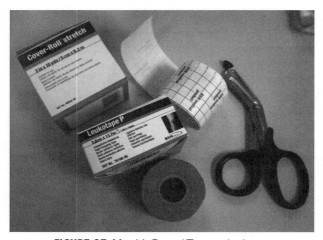

FIGURE 27-11 McConnel Tape and scissors.

TABLE 27-8

Elastic Tape versus Rigid Tape

ELASTIC	RIGID
Reduces muscle spasms and cramping/muscle tone by relaxing the muscle and providing mobility through stability	Reduces pain through immobilizing structures
Prevents overcontraction of a muscle by providing proprioceptive input on the intended muscle	Reduces muscle spasms/contraction by unloading the muscles through passive contraction of designated muscles by accommodating joint structures
Provides input to weakened muscles through proprioceptive input	Mechanically supports weakened muscles
Reduces pain through stimulation of muscle fibers and interstitial layers of skin	Inhibits maladaptive movements of muscles and joints

Adapted from The Kinesio Taping Association, 2003.

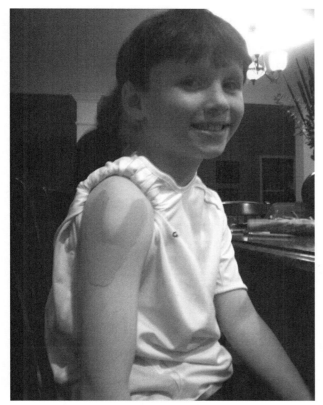

FIGURE 27-13 Child with Kinesio tape on deltoid.

Removing the Kinesio tape

- After 6 to 7 days, the tape should be removed by pulling slowly (unlike a bandaid) in the direction of hair growth.[9,10]
- Removal should begin with the upper portion of the tape; the tape should be rolled off the skin with the index and middle fingers as if the fingers were walking backward. Lotion, baby oil, canola oil, or medical tape remover may be used over the tape for easy removal.
- The tape can be taken off even while the client is in the shower or swimming pool.
- The tape should stay off for 8 to 24 hours prior to applying new tape.
- A warm cloth soaked in soapy water should be used to remove any residue. Care should be taken not to scrub abrasively against the skin. The skin should be allowed to breathe and the tape reapplied as needed.

Contraindications for Use of the Kinesio Tape

The following are the contraindications for the use of the Kinesio tape:

- Lack of skin integrity: open wounds, infections, scrapes, cuts, burns, newly granulated scars, and cancers or any metastatic diseases
- Poor client compliance
- High activity level of the patient
- Allergies to adhesives
- Application of tape over pain patches such as Lidoderm patches

Origin to Insertion

A muscle should be taped by beginning at the origin of the muscle and going to the insertion to facilitate or support weakened muscles for chronic conditions or deficits.[9,10] For example, children with cerebral palsy may have scapular winging due to abnormal muscle tone. The abnormal muscle tone can be attributed to low muscle tone or high muscle tone, either of which can create imbalance of the scapulohumeral rhythm by applying forces on specific muscles in opposing directions.

Insertion to Origin

This application technique is recommended to stabilize joints and relax contracted or overused muscles. It also aids in relaxing the muscles that spasm or muscles that are edematous due to acute injury.[9,10]

SUMMARY

The OT practitioner uses knowledge of anatomy, physiology, kinesiology, and biomechanics in his or her practice. An understanding of the variety of pediatric conditions and OT principles help design and fabricate orthoses and apply taping. Careful analysis of the many factors influencing the client's occupational performance is necessary when designing an orthosis. OT practitioners work together with clients and their families to design and fabricate orthoses that meet the clients' goals. Orthoses can be used to promote function, prevent deformity, and improve hygiene. Kinesio taping can be used as an **adjunctive therapy** with orthoses to provide support and stability to the extremity to maximize functional participation in daily occupations.

References

1. American Occupational Therapy Association: Occupational therapy practice framework: domain and process, ed 2. *Am J Occup Ther* 62:625–703, 2008.
2. Colditz JC: Efficient mechanics of PIP mobilization splinting. *Br J Hand Ther* 5:65, 2000.
3. Colditz JC: Principles of orthoses and splint prescription. In Peimer CA, editor: *Surgery of the hand*, New York, 1996, McGraw-Hill.
4. Colditz JC: Therapist's management of the stiff hand. In Mackin EJ et al, editors: *Rehabilitation of the hand and upper extremity*, St. Louis, 2002, Mosby, pp 1021–1047.
5. Footer CB: The effects of therapeutic taping in gross motor function in children with cerebral palsy. *Pediatr Phys Ther* 18:245–52, 2006.
6. Gossman M, Sahrmann S, Rose S: Review of the length-associated changes in muscle: experimental evidence and clinical implications. *Phys Ther* 62:1799–1808, 1982.
7. Hardy MA: The biology of scar formation. *Phys Ther* 69:1014–1024, 1989.
8. Jacobs M, Austin N: *Splinting the hand and upper extremity*, Baltimore, 2003, Lippincott Williams & Wilkins.
9. Kase K, Hashimoto T, Okane T: *Kinesio taping: perfect manual*, Durham, NC, 1998, Universal Printing and Publishing.
10. Kase K, Martin P, Yasukawa A: *Kinesio taping in pediatrics*, Tokyo, 2006, Kinesio USA, LLC.
11. Martin P, Yasukawa A: *Use of Kinesio tape in pediatrics to improve oral motor control, 18th Annual Kinesio Taping International Symposium Review*, Tokyo, 2003, Kinesio Taping Association.
12. Sackos DT et al: *The effects of McConnell taping technique on strength and pain in subject with symptoms of patellafemoral pain syndrome, Proceedings of the 12th Internal Congress of the World Confederation for Physical Therapy*, Washington, DC, 1995, World Confederation for Physical Therapy.
13. Sorenson MK: The edematous hand. *Phys Ther* 69:1059–1064, 1989.
14. Kase K, Stockheimer KR: *Kinesio taping for lymphoedema and chronic swelling*, Albuquerque, NM, 2006, Kinesio USA.

Internet Resources

Kinesio Taping Association.
www.kinesiotapingassociation.com
Kinesio Tape in the Olympics.
www.kinesiotape.ca
Kinesio Tape Official Web site.
http://www.nbcolympics.com/handball/photos/galleryid=214080.html
Kinesio Tape Official Website.
http://www.nbcolympics.com/waterpolo/photos/galleryid=213069.html
Kinesio Tape Official Website.
http://www.nbcolympics.com/basketball/photos/galleryid=211541.html
Progressive Rehab Concepts.
http://www.ProRehabConcepts.com

REVIEW *Questions*

1. What are the principles of orthosis fabrication for a child or adolescent?
2. What is the role of the OTA in applying orthoses for children and adolescents?
3. How can the OT practitioner improve the compliance of a child or adolescent in the use of an orthosis?
4. What are some of the properties of different orthotic materials?
5. How does taping benefit children and adolescents?
6. What are the goals of orthoses?
7. How are orthoses fabricated, and what questions should OT practitioners consider when fabricating them?
8. What are the different types of orthoses?

SUGGESTED *Activities*

1. Fabricate an orthosis for protection, hygiene, position, and function.
2. Locate the bony prominences on the elbow, wrist, and hand.
3. Demonstrate the anatomic positions of the elbow, wrist, and hand.
4. Create a schedule for splint wearing for an adolescent.
5. Ask a child or adolescent about his or her preferences regarding an orthosis.
6. Make a compliance checklist for a wear schedule for Kinesio taping.

Animal-Assisted Services

JEAN W. SOLOMON

JANE CLIFFORD O'BRIEN

CHAPTER *Objectives*

After studying this chapter, the reader will be able to accomplish the following:

- Identify organizations that promote animal and human interactions
- Define and distinguish between animal-assisted activities and animal-assisted therapy
- Describe the types of small and large animals that might be used during animal-assisted activities and animal-assisted therapy
- Define and distinguish between therapeutic horseback riding and hippotherapy
- Describe the mission and function of the North American Riding for the Handicapped Association
- Discuss incorporating animals into pediatric occupational therapy practice

Do you have a pet? If so, take a moment to think about how your pet makes you feel. What is the first pet that you remember having? One of the authors of this chapter had a lightning bug that was kept in a vented jar by the bed. The light from this little bug helped the author go to sleep at night. It gave a sense of security.

Research supports the conclusion that animals can reduce social stress, increase motivation, and offer unconditional love (Box 28-1).[1] The focus of this chapter is on animal-assisted services. Two types of animal-assisted services will be discussed: (1) animal-assisted activities, and (2) animal-assisted therapy. The chapter also describes ways to incorporate animals into occupational therapy (OT) intervention and the benefits of using animals. A variety of examples of intervention activities using animals is provided throughout to provide some ideas and possibilities.

SELECTED ORGANIZATIONS

Numerous national and international organizations are concerned with the interactions between animals and humans and animal-assisted services. The International Association of Human–Animal Interaction Organizations (IAHAIO), the Delta Society, and Assistance Dogs International (ADI) will be discussed (see Resources at the end of this chapter for a list of organizations).

The IAHAIO was founded in 1990 to provide a forum for national and international associations or related organizations interested in understanding and appreciating human–animal interactions. The primary purpose of the organization is to coordinate its structure nationally and internationally. Its mission is to promote research, education, and the sharing of information regarding the role of animals in human health and quality of life. The activities of the IAHAIO include sponsoring workshops, publishing information that adds to the body of knowledge on human–animal interactions, and influencing public policies that promote the integration of animals into human society.[6]

BOX 28-1

Positive Effects That Animals Have on Humans

- Decrease in social stress, thus improving social interaction
- Improvement in quality of life by increase in self-competence and control over the environment
- Improvement in cardiovascular health
- Increase in trust
- Acceptance of unconditional love

The Delta Society promotes human health and well-being through positive interactions with animals. It publishes guidelines for developing animal-assisted therapy programs, professional standards for dog trainers, and information regarding service dogs. It offers workshops and home study courses for registering clinicians who use animals during therapy. According to the Delta Society, approximately 2000 animal-assisted therapy programs are available in the United States. Dogs are the animals most often used during physical rehabilitation intervention.[6]

ADI is a coalition of nonprofit organizations dedicated to training, placing, and using assistance dogs. The organization publishes a newsletter to educate the public on the benefits of assistance dogs.

CLINICAL *Pearl*

The movement of a horse can help a child gain balance. Successful interaction with the horse promotes self-confidence. The disposition of the horse is critical to positive interaction.

ANIMAL-ASSISTED ACTIVITIES

Animal-assisted activities are those activities that involve human and animal interactions. Examples of animal-assisted activities include the use of assistance dogs, taking cats to visit residents in a nursing home, keeping fish in a kindergarten classroom, and participation in a therapeutic horseback riding class (Figure 28-1). These activities offer opportunities for children and adolescents to care for as well as to interact with animals while grooming, feeding, and petting them. For example, during therapeutic horseback riding, the child or adolescent learns not only to ride the horse but also to take care of it.

ANIMAL-ASSISTED THERAPY

Animal-assisted therapy uses animals to improve the medical, developmental, physical, and mental conditions of children or adolescents. **Hippotherapy**, or therapy using horses, is one of the most popular types of animal-assisted therapy. Dogs are also frequently involved in animal-assisted therapy (Figure 28-2).[6] Animal-assisted therapy is carried out by a qualified OT practitioner. This type of therapy includes the evaluation of the child's body functions and structure, the design and implementation of an intervention plan, documentation of goals and progress, as well as re-evaluation and planning for the discontinuation of services.[3] In both animal-assisted activities and animal-assisted therapy, the welfare and safety of people and animals are top priorities. The following example illustrates animal-assisted therapy.

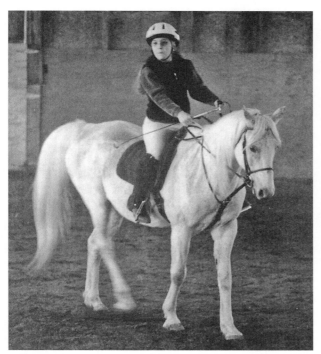

FIGURE 28-1   A girl is having a lesson in horse riding. (Photo by Donald W. Smith, from Crawford JJ, Pomerinke KA: *Therapy pets: the animal-human healing partnership,* Amherst, NY, 2003, Prometheus Books.)

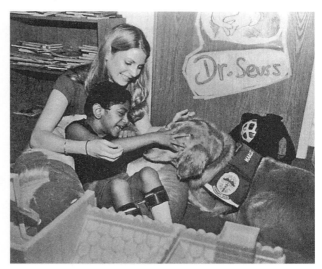

FIGURE 28-2   A dog provides the incentive for a boy to stretch tight muscles. (Photo by Dick Dressel, from Crawford JJ, Pomerinke KA: *Therapy pets: the animal-human healing partnership,* Amherst, NY, 2003, Prometheus Books.)

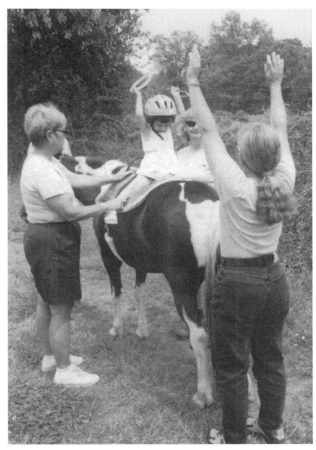

FIGURE 28-3   A hippotherapy session in which a girl participates in balance activities while she is sitting on a horse. (Photo by Nicholas McIntosh, from Crawford JJ, Pomerinke KA: *Therapy pets: the animal-human healing partnership,* Amherst, NY, 2003, Prometheus Books.)

CASE *Study*

Henry is a 6-year-old child who has spastic–quadriplegic cerebral palsy. He attends hippotherapy sessions on a weekly basis during the spring and fall seasons. Carl, the OT practitioner, has set the following goals or anticipated outcomes for this intervention (Figure 28-3).

Long-Term Goals

- Henry will demonstrate functional trunk control while sitting during leisure time.
- Henry will reach for objects while sitting to perform occupations of activities of daily living (ADLs).

Short-Term Goals

- Henry will maintain the upright position while sitting on the horse for 2 minutes.
- Henry will maintain his sitting balance as the horse walks one fourth of the distance of the riding arena.
- Henry will touch the horse's ears with each hand, alternating individually and simultaneously (unilaterally and bilaterally), in three out of four sequence trials.

During Henry's hippotherapy session, Carl engages him in stretching activities while Henry is seated bareback and backward on the horse. Carl assists Henry to reach for the horse's ears and hindquarters. While Carl is assisting Henry with his arms, Becki, a physical therapy assistant, stabilizes Henry's trunk and legs. After the stretching activities, two volunteers join the team to serve as helpers as the horse begins to move under the direction of the trainer/instructor. Carl facilitates upper trunk and arm control, and Becki facilitates pelvic mobility with leg stability. In each of the four corners of the riding arena, the following therapeutic activities are located: (1) a pressure switch that activates a tape playing Henry's favorite music, (2) a beanbag toss, (3) a punching bag to encourage arm and leg movement, and (4) a ring tree game. Carl, Becki, and Henry work together at each of the stations as the volunteers manage the horse and offer extra help as needed.

In the above scenario, the emphasis of the animal-assisted session is to improve Henry's postural control (i.e., sitting posture) for ADLs and leisure activities. These therapeutic goals are addressed during the riding session. This differs from therapeutic riding, in which program the goal of the session is to help the child engage in horseback riding. The following example provides readers with an example of goals that emphasize riding as the outcome (versus motor performance as the outcome).

CASE *Study*

Galen lives on a farm, where his family regularly ride horses (Figure 28-4). He is a 7-year-old child with spastic–quadriplegic cerebral palsy. The OT practitioner has recommended a therapeutic riding program and has set the following goals and objectives for intervention.

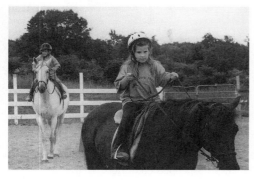

FIGURE 28-4 Two girls enjoy learning to ride horses at summer camp. For some children, riding is an occupation. (Courtesy: Cheryl Joyce.)

Long-Term Goals

- Given adaptive equipment for safety, Galen will ride a horse for 20 minutes on trails.
- Galen will be able to mount his horse with moderate physical assistance.

Short-Term Goals

- Galen will maintain the upright position while sitting on the horse for 5 minutes.
- Galen will maintain the upright position while sitting on the horse as the horse walks one fourth of the distance of the riding arena.

In this scenario, the OT intervention is similar to Henry's; however, the goals of Galen's and Henry's sessions differ. The goal of Galen's sessions is for him to be a competent rider so that he can participate in the occupations of his family. The goal of Henry's sessions is for him to gain skills that may be used in other occupations (e.g., improved sitting balance, improved reaching). Therapeutic riding often becomes a leisure activity for children, thus allowing the intervention to become occupation based.

SMALL ANIMALS

Small animals are those that typically weigh less than 40 pounds. Dogs, which are mammals, are one type of small animal. Other types include reptiles such as snakes; amphibians such as frogs; fish; and invertebrates such as hermit crabs and worms (Table 28-1). This chapter discusses the different types of small animals, with special attention devoted to dogs.

Mammals are animals that have a backbone and are characterized by hair on the skin and mammary glands that produce milk in females. They are warm-blooded animals that maintain a relatively warm body temperature independent of the environmental temperature. Examples of animals that are classified as mammals are dogs, cats, rabbits, and guinea pigs.

Dogs are one of the most popular pets and the most frequently used small mammal for animal-assisted services (Figure 28-5). They offer a large variety of choices. Dogs are small, medium, or large in size and may be purebred or a mix of breeds. Examples of small purebred dogs are dachshunds, Chihuahuas, and cocker spaniels. Large dog breeds include chows, German shepherds, Saint Bernards, Great Pyrennes, and standard poodles. Mixed breeds (also known as "mutts") can be small, medium, or large in size.

The characteristics of the breed and the individual personality of the dog are both considered when selecting a dog for animal-assisted services or to be a pet. One

TABLE 28-1

Types of Small Animals

CLASSIFICATION	DEFINITION	EXAMPLES
Mammal	Warm blooded with backbone	Dog, cat, rabbit, guinea pig
Reptile	Cold blooded with horny or scaly skin	Snake
Amphibian	Cold blooded with smooth skin	Frog, toad, salamander
Fish	Cold blooded with fins and gills	Goldfish, beta fish
Invertebrate	Cold blooded without backbone	Worm, snail, hermit crab

aspect of a dog's personality is *temperament*, which refers to the dog's natural or instinctive behavior. When stressed, a dog will respond according to its temperament, and frequently this is characteristic of its breed. For example, chows are known to show an aggressive response under stress.

Training involves teaching a dog to follow commands while being controlled or led by a person. Although a dog can be trained to be obedient, the temperaments of certain breeds may override their training during stressful situations. For example, in crowds of people with a lot of noise and movement, chows tend to growl and become "snappy."

A service dog is one that assists people who have physical or sensory disabilities.[1] **Service dogs** are legally defined in the Americans with Disabilities Act (ADA). According to ADA, the three types of service dogs are (1) guide dogs, (2) hearing dogs, and (3) medical alert dogs (Box 28-2). A *guide dog* is one that assists a person who has a visual impairment or is blind. A *hearing dog* is one that assists a person who has a hearing loss or is deaf. A *medical alert dog* is one that assists a person in a medical emergency by detecting specific physiologic changes and locating assistance during medical emergencies.[1]

CLINICAL *Pearl*

Cats are the most suitable institutional pets because of their lifestyles (eating and toileting habits, exercise requirements) and independence (Figure 28-6).

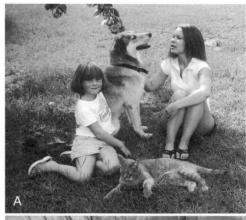

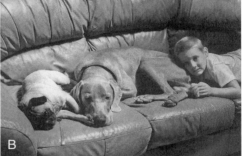

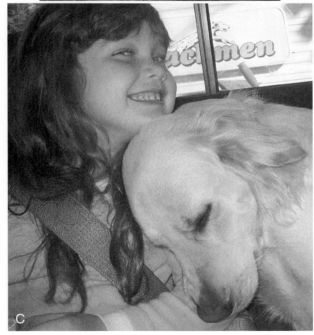

FIGURE 28-5 **A,** Two girls relax in the shade with their pets. **B,** A boy relaxes with his pets. **C,** A girl cuddles with her pet. (**A,** Courtesy: Susan Gentry. **B,** Courtesy: Cheryl Joyce. **C,** Courtesy: Debbie Dewitt.)

BOX 28-2

Types of Service Dogs

- A *guide dog* is one that assists a person who has a visual impairment or is blind.
- A *hearing dog* is one that assists a person who has a hearing loss or is deaf.
- A *medical alert dog* is one that assists a person in a medical emergency by detecting specific physiologic changes and locating assistance during medical emergencies.

CLINICAL *Pearl*

A child or adolescent must have a certain level of maturity to benefit from having a service dog.

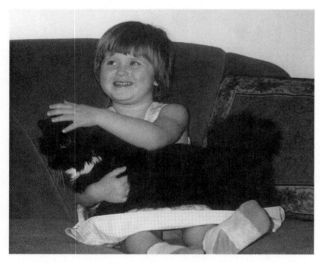

FIGURE 28-6 A girl enjoys the softness of her cat. (Courtesy: Jan Froehlich.)

Another way to categorize dogs is as companions or pets, which may include personal as well as institutional pets. A *personal pet* lives with an individual or family and is a part of that individual's or family's life. An *institutional pet* resides in a facility or institution such as a skilled nursing facility.

Reptiles are animals that have a backbone and horny or scaly skin. Reptiles have lungs to breathe. They are cold-blooded animals that do not have a constant body temperature. Legless lizards and turtles are examples of reptiles that intrigue children. A wide range of nonpoisonous snakes may serve as pets or social companions.

Reptilian pets tend to require less human attention and care than do other small animals. They require less frequent feeding and handling, which is a consideration in choosing the best animal to be used for animal-assisted services.

Amphibians are cold-blooded animals that have a backbone and smooth skin. All amphibians have gills because at some point in their development, an aquatic environment is required. Amphibians lay eggs to reproduce. Examples of amphibians are frogs, toads, and salamanders. Children and adolescents are usually fascinated by amphibians in their natural environments. Catching, trapping, and releasing frogs or other amphibians in their natural environments require problem-solving, timing, sequencing, and precise motor skills (Figure 28-7).

Fish are also cold-blooded animals with backbones, fins for mobility, and gills for breathing. They live in water and require minimum human attention and interaction. Fish that are popular as home and classroom pets include goldfish, beta fish, and kissing fish. Animal-assisted activities involving fish might include increasing independence in instrumental ADLs (IADLs) through caring for them. Fish are not an appropriate choice for animal-assisted therapy, although decorating a fish tank and caring for fish are pleasant activities for children. Furthermore, many children enjoy the occupation of fishing.

Invertebrates are animals that do not have a backbone. Examples of invertebrates are worms, snails, insects, and hermit crabs (Figure 28-8). As mentioned at the beginning of the chapter, one of the authors had a lightning bug as the first pet; a lightning bug is another example of this type of animal. Children who live in rural areas have wonderful opportunities to interact with invertebrates. Hermit crabs and snails are favorites among this class of animal to be kept as pets at home or in a classroom setting.

LARGE ANIMALS

Large animals are those that typically weigh more than 40 pounds. Horses are one of the most frequently used large animals in animal-assisted services. Other large animals that might be considered for human–animal interactions include farm animals, exotic animals, and marine mammals.

Most farm animals are large and live on a tract of land that is being cultivated for food for human consumption. Examples of large farm animals are horses or mules, pigs, goats, cows, and sheep. Farm animals may have monetary value to the person caring for them. A special relationship of mutual respect is often obvious between the animal and the human caregiver (Figure 28-9).

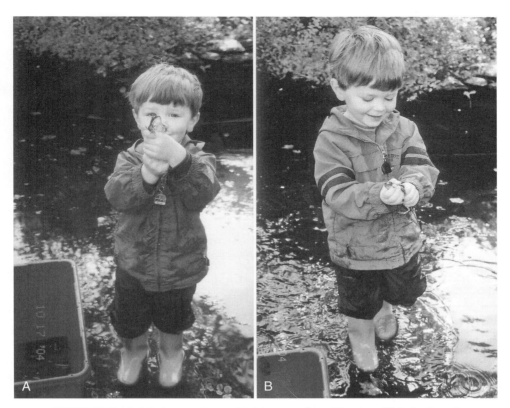

FIGURE 28-7   A little boy catches and holds onto a frog. (Courtesy: Michelle Stone.)

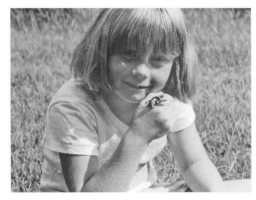

FIGURE 28-8   A girl plays with her pet hermit crab. (Courtesy: Susan Gentry.)

CLINICAL *Pearl*

Keeping goldfish in a horse's 75- to 100-gallon water tank can help control algae, especially during the hot months. Horses and goldfish coexist well in this situation. Goldfish require minimum or no care, especially if the water tank has an automatic system to refill it to the maximum water level.

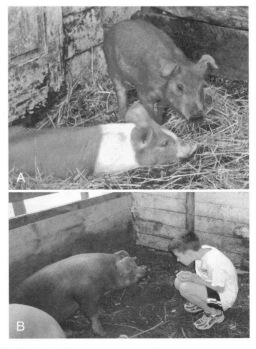

FIGURE 28-9   A, Two piglets allow children to learn responsibility. **B,** A boy learns how to care for and train his pet pig. (**A,** Courtesy: Cheryl Joyce. **B,** Courtesy: Mike O'Brien.)

Exotic animals such as llamas, peacocks, and emus are considered foreign to the United States, or from another part of the world. Interest in raising exotic animals is growing in many areas of the United States. The potential to incorporate exotic animals into animal-assisted activities and therapy has not been fully explored.

CLINICAL *Pearl*

Horses will often lick before they bite another horse or a person. Cows also enjoy licking the salt from human hands. Cows do not have upper teeth and so have no inclination to bite. A horse's tongue is smooth, whereas a cow's tongue is lumpy and coarse.

CLINICAL *Pearl*

Pigs can be trained to "come" and "sit" as one would train a dog. Young pigs may be trained by using a harness and leading them. Just like other animals, pigs' temperaments vary, although most pigs are typically not mean. Pigs will bite to the side if provoked.

Marine mammals (e.g., dolphins, whales, seals) are warm-blooded animals that live in salty or brackish water. Although they are available for animal-assisted activities (enjoyment or play) on a commercial basis, no known programs incorporating them into animal-assisted therapy exist currently.

Horses are one of the most widely used large animals for animal-assisted services. According to the American Hippotherapy Association (AHA), **therapeutic riding** is an animal-assisted activity for humans who have physical, emotional, and/or mental disabilities. Hippotherapy refers to animal-assisted therapy in which an OT clinician or occupational therapist uses the movement of the horse as an intervention tool to improve the client's body function. The horse's walk is rhythmic and repetitive, similar to the pattern of movement in the human pelvis during walking (per the AHA). In addition to the input from the movement of the horse, the human–horse interaction offers a wide range of sensory experiences that have an impact on the tactile, olfactory, visual, and vestibular sensory systems.

As previously stated, therapeutic riding encompasses a variety of horse-related activities for people with disabilities. An example of an adolescent engaged in therapeutic horseback riding is described below (Figure 28-10).

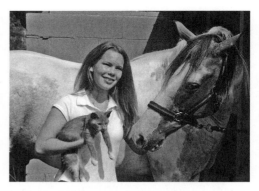

FIGURE 28-10 While preparing the horse for an afternoon ride, a girl picks up and holds the barn cat. (Courtesy: Susan Gentry.)

CASE *Study*

Julia is a 12-year-old girl who has osteoporosis of unknown etiology. Her mother Peg takes her to the local stable on the recommendation of the OT practitioner that Julia would benefit from therapeutic horseback riding. Julia has been involved in this program for 18 months and enjoys riding her favorite horse Scotty. On their arrival at the barn, they are greeted by Toni, who is the barn manager, riding instructor, and trail guide. Toni assists Julia with haltering Scotty and leading him to the tack area, and Peg gets another horse Ace and leads him to the tack area as well. Once Scotty's and Ace's lead ropes are secured, both are groomed and their hooves picked. The benefits for Scotty and Ace are obvious. The benefits for Julia include weight bearing while shifting weight with the use of a wide range of movements with both arms as she reaches to the top of Scotty's hindquarters and the peaks of his ears. The resistance of the tangles in his mane, forelocks, and tail provide strengthening exercises for Julia's arms and a challenge to her trunk balance and leg stability.

After the riders tack their horses, everyone mounts, and the trail ride begins. The horse is now doing the work by carrying its rider on its back. The rider and the instructor/guide have a mutual responsibility to ensure the safety and well-being of the rider and the horse. The trail ride lasts for an hour, during which time the group encounters narrow paths in the woods to negotiate and small trees to maneuver around. The therapeutic benefits for Julia include lower extremity resistive exercise while maintaining trunk and upper extremity stability to remain seated on Scotty while reining and steering him. The emphasis in therapeutic horseback riding is on the ride, during which the child gains certain skills.

The goal of therapeutic riding differs from that of hippotherapy, in which a licensed medical professional incorporates a horse into the therapy session as an intervention tool. Children and adolescents with health disorders involving the neuromusculoskeletal system benefit from hippotherapy. Examples of specific conditions include cerebral palsy, developmental delay, and pervasive developmental delay or autism. Box 28-3 lists objectives for the outcomes of hippotherapy, and Box 28-4 lists objectives for hippotherapy as an occupation.

In hippotherapy, a licensed physical therapist, occupational therapist, speech/language pathologist, physical therapy assistant, or occupational therapy assistant (OTA) uses the movement of the horse to improve an individual's body function and structure. The goals and objectives of the professionals listed above differ. A therapeutic riding instructor (TRI) often participates in hippotherapy sessions. The TRI will have goals and objectives that concentrate on teaching a child or adolescent to ride a horse. The goals and objectives of the physical therapist will emphasize improving the client's overall mobility and quality of movement. The speech/language pathologist will focus on communication skills. The OT practitioner will concentrate on the underlying performance skills necessary for the client to successfully participate in daily occupations. The following case

---

BOX 28-3

Sample Objectives for Hippotherapy Outcomes

Improvement in functioning in all areas of occupation by developing the following:
- Muscle tone for improved motor control
- Balance and equilibrium responses
- Gross and fine motor coordination
- Symmetry of motor functions
- Postural control
- Speech and language skills
- Self-efficacy and self-concept
- Body awareness
- Emotional well-being
- Regulation of behavior
- Sense of success

BOX 28-4

Sample Objectives for Hippotherapy Outcomes Based on Occupation

- Improvement in the child's ability to engage in the occupations involved in the care and maintenance of horses
- Participation in riding sessions
- Grooming and caring for the horse
- Participation in social activities (e.g., 4-H)

---

study describes the roles, goals, and objectives of the OT practitioner in hippotherapy.

CASE *Study*

Juan is a 6-year-old child who has a medical diagnosis of autism. He receives OT services through the local school district. He also receives outpatient OT services through a private practice located in the community. For 6 months of the year, Juan participates in weekly hippotherapy sessions with Rita, the occupational therapy assistant (OTA) assigned to his case.

Juan's long-term OT goal is that he will ride a horse for 20 minutes as a leisure activity, with stand-by assistance. His short-term goals are that he will hold onto the reins with both hands while receiving verbal cueing and follow verbal one-step commands while riding the horse.

A physical therapist participates in the session on alternative weeks. The goal of physical therapy is to improve body functions (e.g., improve bilateral coordination, strength, and endurance for riding). Another member of the team is a speech therapist. The goal of speech therapy is to improve the communication required while riding a horse. The unique nature of OT is shown by the goal of improving the child's ability to engage in the riding session. The OT practitioner may make accommodations to assist Juan in being successful at riding. In addition, the OT practitioner may consult with and educate the riding staff to optimize Juan's time and success on the horse.

The North American Riding for the Handicapped Association (NARHA) is a membership organization that promotes safe, professional, ethical, and therapeutic horse riding activities through education, communication, standards (see Box 28-4), and research for people with or without disabilities.[2,4] The NARHA has certification from the AHA to ensure the professionalism of practicing clinicians and detailed standards to keep participating clients safe.[2,4] Selecting and training horses for hippotherapy is one of the purposes of NARHA-certified centers (Box 28-5). The NARHA's mission is to foster positive human- and equine-assisted activities and therapy (EAAT). A relatively new NARHA program, Horses for Heroes, provides EAAT services for veterans. The NARHA centers also offer opportunities for hippotherapy education and research.

INCORPORATING ANIMALS INTO PEDIATRIC OCCUPATIONAL THERAPY PRACTICE

Incorporating animals into the OT process involves several occupations or life activities in which individuals participate (Figure 28-11). Engagement in IADLs such

Selected Standards or Guidelines in Choosing a Horse for Animal-Assisted Services

- At least 8 years of age
- Extensive training and riding time (quantified in miles)
- Good conditioning
- Good performance skills (i.e., symmetrical and balanced movement, voice trained [obedient to the trainer's or OT practitioner's voice], tolerant of the rider's unexpected behaviors)
- Excellent temperament

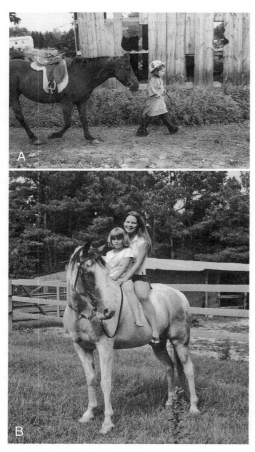

FIGURE 28-11 A, A girl brings a horse back to her stall. **B,** The horse stands patiently as two girls pose for a picture. (**A,** Courtesy: Cheryl Joyce. **B,** Courtesy: Susan Gentry.)

as care of pets, health management and maintenance, safety procedures, and informal personal education participation might be the outcomes of animal-assisted activities and animal-assisted therapy. The OT practitioner may also decide to use animal-assisted therapy to improve a child's ability to perform certain client

factors needed for successful participation in occupations. Children may need to develop problem-solving and fine motor skills or the balance to care for pets or interact with an animal. The OT practitioner needs to consider the cultural, physical, spiritual, and virtual contexts of the client when incorporating animals into activities and therapy.[3] The activity demands and individual client factors will have an impact on the decision-making process.[3] Questions to guide practitioners in decision-making concerning animal-assisted therapy include the following.

- Who are your clients?
- Where will the animal-assisted services be provided?
- Are you considering a large animal or a small animal for these services?
- What characteristics are you looking for in the animal?
- What type of human–animal interaction will be involved?
- What are the potential health hazards?
- What pets or other animals are present at the client's home? Does the client have access to them?
- What are the goals of incorporating an animal into the therapy sessions?
- What is the best fit between the animal and the client?

Intervention Planning

Animals can be used in therapy as a modality (i.e., the animal is the tool to improve the skill) or as the goal itself (i.e., caring for the animal is the occupation that the person is trying to master) (Figures 28-12 and 28-13). For either reason, the OT practitioner must carefully analyze the tasks required for client participation in the activity in order to use the animal effectively in therapy sessions. Once the OT practitioner has established the goals of the therapy session, a decision on the type of animal activity is required, as illustrated by the case study below.

CASE *Study*

George is a 5-year-old boy who has limited use of his right arm. He loves animals and has a pet cat that he has been unable to see since his hospitalization. The OT practitioner decides to surprise George in the therapy session and bring in a cat for him to brush using both of his arms and hands. The OT practitioner positions the cat so that George has to reach for and hold it. This is a natural activity for him because it emphasizes his love of animals.

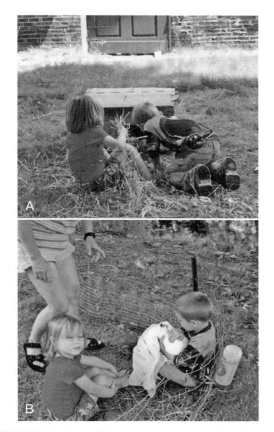

FIGURE 28-12 A and B, A boy and a girl care for their bunnies as part of their daily chores. (Courtesy: Cheryl Joyce.)

The goal of the session is to help George improve motor skills (e.g., the use of his right hand). Therefore, throughout the session, the OT practitioner skillfully adapts the activity in such a way that George has to use his right arm. In this example, brushing the cat is an activity that promotes right arm movement.

Brushing the cat could also be considered the goal of the session (e.g., the occupation itself is the goal) in this scenario because George has a cat at home. Therefore, if one of his chores is to brush his cat, the OT practitioner may want to focus the session on how he will be able to do this despite limited movement in his right arm. In this case, the OT practitioner would position the cat in such a way that George would be successful in the task. This would help George adapt and compensate for the limited use of his right arm to be able to effectively fulfill his role as caregiver for the pet.

OT practitioners may decide to help children explore their environments in visual, auditory, and/or tactile modalities through animals. Exploration of their environments helps children develop sensory and problem-solving skills.

CASE *Study*

Seth, a 2-year-old boy with developmental delays, lived in the inner city. When his OT practitioner proposed using insects and animals in therapy sessions, Seth's parents

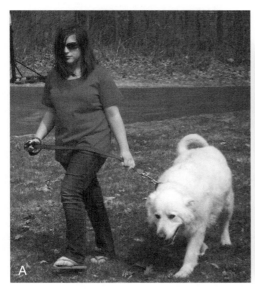
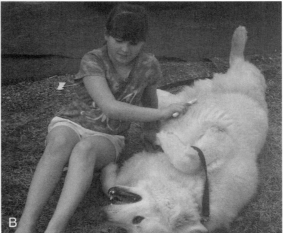

FIGURE 28-13 A, A girl takes her pet dog for a walk as part of her daily chores. **B,** Another girl grooms the dog, as part of her chores. (Courtesy Scott O'Brien)

smiled and stated that unlike his older brother, Seth had never explored a sandbox or the ground. The parents had not realized before that because of his delays, he had never felt the ground or grass. The OT practitioner planned a session in which sand, worms, ants, and plants would be used. While Seth was playing during this session, his mother pointed out the various objects. The OT practitioner also placed small toys in the sand and allowed Seth to determine whether or not each toy was an animal. Seth smiled and laughed when he picked up a worm and observed its movements. His mother enjoyed teaching her son about the animals and insects and told him stories about her own childhood experiences. This session empowered the mother and reminded her in a subtle way that children at all levels of ability value exploration. Furthermore, Seth was able to experience typical sensations, although they were somewhat different from those of his inner city environment.

Animal-assisted therapy can help children with emotional and/or behavioral difficulties. Animals have a calming effect and are responsive to humans. Therefore, children can be taught to read the cues of animals, and this new skill may transfer to reading the cues of people in their lives. Caring for animals can be satisfying to children, and teaching them to perform simple commands to animals can be rewarding. The bond between the child and his or her pet is beneficial, especially in the case of a child who experiences behavioral and/or emotional difficulties. The nurturing nature of animals and the feeling of acceptance created by them help these children. The OT practitioner may need to model the appropriate way to touch an animal and thus help the child bond with the animal. The session may focus on reading the animal's cues, caring for it, or teaching it to do a trick. Through these sessions, the child must learn patience, understanding, timing, caring, and perseverance. Caring for animals requires consistency in performance and organization.

Animals may be used as a modality to improve the social participation of children. A child may show his or her pet to friends, meet other children with the same type of pet, or join clubs that discuss the care of animals (e.g., a 4-H club, riding organization, fair). These groups help children learn about and gain interest in their pets and develop a sense of belonging. The OT practitioners can help children with special needs participate in these groups by helping them adapt or compensate as needed.

OT practitioners may find that animal-assisted therapy helps children develop interests, motivations, belief in their skills. For example, Taylor and colleagues found preliminary evidence that with hippotherapy, **volition** (one's interests, self-efficacy, and motivation) may improve in children with autism.[5] The authors used the Pediatric Volitional Questionnaire to measure volition in three children with autism before, during, and after 16 weeks of hippotherapy.[5]

The activities described above are just a few of the many possibilities that animal-assisted therapy offers to children and OT practitioners. Intervention must be centered on the child's and his or her family's needs. OT practitioners should understand the family's culture and attitude toward animals. Many of these activities can be tailored to meet the needs of children with special needs.

SUMMARY

Use of animals can be a creative and interesting modality for OT intervention. Furthermore, many children participate in occupations involving animals, making this a natural fit for OT. Children of all ages enjoy interactions with animals and occupations that involve them. We urge OT practitioners to continue to explore this area.

References

1. Crawford JJ, Pomerinke KA: *Therapy pets: the animal–human healing partnership,* Amherst, NY, 2003, Prometheus Books.
2. Hulchanski C: Horsing around. *Advance for Occupational Therapist* 24:50, 2008.
3. American Occupational Therapy Association: Occupational therapy practice framework: domain and process, ed 2. *Am J Occup Ther* 62:625–703, 2008.
4. Sherer-Silkwood D: The difference lies in the perspective. *NARHA Strides* 9:14–16, 2003.
5. Taylor R et al: Volitional change in children with autism: a single case design study of the impact of hippotherapy on motivation. *Occup Ther Mental Health* 25:192–200, 2009.
6. Winkle M: Dogs in practice: beyond pet therapy. *OT Practice* 8:12–17, 2003.

Recommended Reading

Britton W: *The legend of rainbow bridge,* Morrison, CO, 1994, Savannah Publishing. (Age 8 to adult.)
Brown M: *The dead bird,* New York, 1983, HarperCollins. (Ages 4 to 7)
Calmenson S: *Rosie, a visiting dog story,* New York, 1994, Clarion Books. (Ages 4 to 10)
Coudert J: The *good shepherd: a special dog's gift of healing,* Salt Lake City, 1998, Andrews McMeel Publishing. (Age 12 to adult)

This bibliography was formerly part of catalog item PET400. Other parts of PET400 are available: *Pet Loss and Bereavement Bibliography* and *Healthy Reasons to Have a Pet.*

Curtis P: *Animal partners: training animals to help people,* New York, 1982, EP Dutton. (Age 8 to adult)

Curtis P: *Cindy, a hearing-ear dog,* New York, 1981, EP Dutton. (Ages 4 to 10)

Davis C: *For every dog an angel: the forever dog,* Portland, 1997, Lighthearted Press. (Age 4 to adult)

Disalvo-Ryan D: *A dog like Jack,* New York, 1999, Holiday House. (Ages 4 to 8)

Duncan S: *Joey Moses,* Seattle, 1998, Storytellers Ink. (Age 10 to adult)

Fine A, Eisen C: *Afternoons with puppy: inspirations from a therapist and his animals,* Lafayette, IN, 2007, Purdue University Press. (Age 10 to adult)

Fine A: *Handbook on animal-assisted therapy: theoretical foundations and guidelines for practice,* ed 2, New York, 2006, Academic Press.

Golder S: *Buffy's orange leash,* Washington, DC, 1988, Kendell Green Publications. (Ages 4 to 8)

Garfield J: *Follow my leader,* New York, 1994, Puffin. (Ages 9 to 12)

Hocken S: *Emma and I,* New York, 1978, EP Dutton. (Age 10 to adult)

Hubbard C: *One golden year: a story of a golden retriever,* New York, 1999, Apple. (Ages 9 to 12)

Kennedy P, Christie R: *Through Otis' eyes: Lessons from a guide dog puppy,* New York, 1998, Howell Book House. (Ages 3 to 7)

Kerswell J: *The complete book of horses,* Avenel, NJ, 1993, Crescent Books. (Age 8 to adult).

McGinty AB: *Guide dogs: seeing for people who can't,* New York, 1999, PowerKids Press. (Ages 8 to 10)

Mooney S: *A snowflake in my hand,* New York, 1983, Delacorte. (Age 12 to adult)

Moore E: *Buddy, the first seeing-eye dog (Hello Reader! Level 4),* New York, 1996, Scholastic. (Ages 4 to 8)

Morehead D: *A special place for Charlee: a child's companion through pet loss,* Broomfield, CO, 1996, Partners in Publishing. (Ages 3 to 6)

Nieburg H: *Pet loss: a thoughtful guide for adults and children,* New York, 1982, Harper & Row. (Age 10 to adult)

Ogden P: *Chelsea: the story of a signal dog,* Boston, 1992, Fawcett. (Age 12 to adult)

Okimoto JD: *A place for Grace,* Seattle, 1993, Sasquatch Books. (Ages 4 to 8)

Osofsky A: *My buddy,* New York, 1992, Henry Holt. (Ages 4 to 8)

Rogers F: *When a pet dies,* New York, 1988, GP Putnam's Sons. (Ages 3 to 5)

Rossite NP: *Rugby and Rosie,* New York, 1997, Dutton/Penguin. (Ages 5 to 9)

Rylant C: *Dog heaven,* New York, 1995, Scholastic. (Ages 4 to 8)

Rylant C: *Cat heaven,* New York, 1997, Scholastic. (Ages 4 to 8)

Sibbitt S: *"Oh, where has my pet gone?" A pet loss memory book,* Wayzata, MN, 1991, B Libby Press. (Ages 3 to 13)

Siegel ME, Koplin HM: *More than a friend: dogs with a purpose,* New York, 1984, Walker and Co. (Age 10 to adult)

Smith ES: *A service dog goes to school,* New York, 1988, Morrow Junior Books. (Ages 4 to 8)

Vinocur T: *Dogs helping kids with feelings,* New York, 1999, PowerKids Press. (Ages 4 to 13)

Viorst J: *The tenth good thing about Barney,* New York, 1971, Macmillan. (Ages 4 to 8)

White B, Sullivan T: *The leading lady: Dinah's story,* New York, 1991, Bantam Books. (Age 12 to adult)

Wilhelm H: *I'll always love you,* New York, 1985, Crown Publishing Group. (Ages 4 to 8)

Wilson MS: *No ordinary dog,* Claremont, CA, 1995, Wilson Publishing. (Ages 8 to 12)

Yates E: *Sound friendships: the story of Willa and her hearing-ear dog,* Woodstock, VT, 1987, Countryman Press. (Age 10 to adult)

Resources

Assistance Dogs International
http://www.adionline.org
American Hippotherapy Association (AHA)
http://www.americanhippotherapyassociation.org/

The Delta Society
www.deltasociety.org
c/o Delta Society, USA
580 Naches Avenue SW, No. 101
Renton, WA 98055-2297

International Association of Human-Animal Interaction Organizations
www.iahaio.org

North American Riding for the Handicapped Association (NARHA)
http://narha.org/
PAWS for Health
www.vcu.edu/paws/benefit.htm

Resources for Games and Activities During Hippotherapy Sessions

Adapted Physical Education catalogs
http://www.flaghouse.com
Educational catalogs such as Nasco
http://www.nascofa.com
Freedom Riders
http://www.freedomrider.com
Lorrie Renker
http://www.educationequine.com
Sportsmark by Signam
http://www.sportsmark.co.uk

REVIEW QUESTIONS

1. List specific organizations and associations concerned with the positive effects of human–animal interactions.

2. What is an animal-assisted activity?
3. What is animal-assisted therapy?

SUGGESTED ACTIVITIES

1. Volunteer at your local Society for the Prevention of Cruelty to Animals (SPCA).
2. Volunteer with a therapeutic horseback riding and/or hippotherapy program.
3. Visit a local zoo and list and categorize the animals that you see. Describe their behaviors in terms of the humans who are observing them.
4. Go camping near a river or lake. Record and categorize the animals that you interact with in that area.
5. Develop a list of activities involving pets that could be used in OT practice. Use the OTPF to analyze client factors and activity demands.

Glossary

Abduction: Moving away from the body; movement away from the midline of the body

Accommodation: Automatic adjustment of the lens of the eye to permit the retina to focus of objects at varying distances; adaptation or special consideration

Achievement stage: The late childhood stage (6 to 11 years of age) in which children successfully accomplish movements and skills. Refers to the refinement of movements and skills

Acknowledgment: Providing feedback to individuals, which assures them that they have been "heard"

Acquired condition/Acquired disorder: An illness or state of health that is not inherited and interferes with an individual's ability to be functionally independent

Acquired immune deficiency syndrome (AIDS): A severe immunologic disorder caused by the retrovirus HIV (human immunodeficiency virus) that is characterized by increased susceptibility to infections and certain rare cancers; transmitted primarily through body fluids

Active ROM (AROM): Movement at a joint that occurs because of the contraction of skeletal muscle

Activities of daily living (ADLs): Self-maintenance activities such as dressing and feeding; also called *basic activities of daily living (BADLs)* or *personal activities of living (PADLs)*

Activity: Specified pursuit in which an individual participates

Activity analysis: A tool that helps occupational therapy practitioners prioritize, plan, and implement effective treatment; involves identifying every characteristic of a task and examining each client factor, performance component, performance area, and performance context

Activity configuration: The process of selecting specific activities to use during an intervention

Activity demands: Those things which are needed to carry out an activity

Activity synthesis: Modifying, grading, and/or changing the structure or steps of an activity into a whole; includes adapting, grading, and reconfiguring activities

Acute: Extremely severe symptoms or conditions; having a rapid onset and following a short but severe course

Adaptation: Adjustment or change to suit a situation

Adapting activities: Modifying or changing a task or using adaptive equipment to make a task easier

Adaptive response: The ability of the brain to receive, interpret, and respond effectively to sensory information

Addiction: An intense psychological and physiologic craving

Adduction: Movement toward the midline of the body

Adjunctive therapy: An intervention used to assist with the primary intervention and intervention outcomes

Agonist: Prime mover, or the primary muscle, that creates movement at a joint

Agoraphobia: Fear of public places and open spaces

Akinesis: Absent or reduced control of voluntary muscles

Alignment: To move toward a straight line; posturally, to keep body segment bones and joints correctly oriented toward each other, particularly in the proximal areas of the head, neck, trunk, and pelvis

Allergen: A substance (such as pollen or mold) that causes an allergic reaction or sneezing, wheezing, itching, or skin rashes because of an abnormally high sensitivity to the substance

Alveolus (plural: alveoli): Terminal sac-like structures of the lungs, which are the sites of gas exchange between the respiratory and circulatory systems

Amputation: The loss of a body part, often all or part of an arm or leg

Antagonist: Opposite of the agonist in action (i.e., lengthens in order to allow shortening of the agonist)

Anatomic position: The upright position with the palms facing forward and the arms resting by the sides of the body, legs slightly spread apart, and toes pointing outward

Anterior/ventral: Front

Antibody: A Y-shaped protein that is secreted into the blood or lymph in response to the presence of an antigen or invading microorganism

Antifat: A negative attitude toward persons who are obese or overweight

Antigen: Toxins, bacteria, foreign blood cells, or cells from transplanted organs that cause the body to produce antibodies

Anxiety: A state of uneasiness, apprehension, uncertainty, and fear resulting from the anticipation of a threatening event or situation

Areas of occupation: Daily activities in which people engage, including activities of daily living (ADLs), instrumental activities of daily living (IADLs), education, work, play, leisure, and social participation

Arteriole: Small artery

Artery: Vessel that moves blood away from the heart

Arthrogryposis: A congenital disorder marked by generalized stiffness of the joints; often accompanied by nerve and muscle degeneration, resulting in impaired mobility

Articulation: Juncture between bones or cartilage

Assistive technology (AT): A concept that encompasses the process by which an individual with disabilities acquires or sustains independence by using assistive technology devices

Assistive technology device (AT device): A piece of equipment that assists individuals with disabilities in performing occupations or daily activities and is used on a daily basis

Assistive technology service (AT service): Any service that directly assists an individual with disabilities in the selection, acquisition, and/or use of an assistive technology device

Assistive technology team (AT team): A group of professionals who make recommendations and carry out the training of an individual with a disability by using an assistive technology device

Asymmetrical: Not symmetrical or balanced

Ataxia: Abnormal fluctuation of muscle from normal to hypertonic (increased muscle tone); loss of the ability to coordinate muscular movement; loss of the ability to coordinate movements, usually due to fluctuations in muscle tone from normal to abnormally high

Athetosis: A type of cerebral palsy characterized by involuntary writhing movements, particularly of the hands and feet; loss of ability to coordinate movement due to the fluctuation of muscle tone form abnormally low to abnormally highmuscle; writhing movements

Attention deficit hyperactivity disorder (ADHD): A neurobehavioral disorder characterized by difficulty with attention, hyperactivity, distractibility, and impulsivity

Atom: Smallest unit of matter with subatomic parts of electrons, protons, and neutrons. Protons and neutrons are located in the nucleus of an atom. The electrons circle around in the valence(s) that surround the atom's nucleus. The number of electrons in an atom's outermost valence determines how that element bonds with other elements.

Autism: A disorder characterized by severe and complex impairments in reciprocal social interaction and communication skills and the presence of stereotypical behavior, interests, and activities

Automatic reflex movement: Movement that is instinctual, which assists in an individual's development and survival

Backward chaining: A way to grade an activity in which an individual learns the last step first; begins with the individual completing the last step after watching the occupational therapy practitioner perform the first few steps and progresses to the individual learning the next to the last step (and so on) until the whole sequence is independently performed

Ball and socket or triaxial joint: A freely moving joint such as the hip and shoulder joints; movement occurs in all three cardinal planes

Base of support: The body structure that carries the weight during static and dynamic balancing

Bathing and showering: Typical skills involving soaping, rinsing, and drying the body, which are learned in early childhood

Bilateral motor control: Both sides of the body working together during an activity; ability to use two sides of the body in smooth movements simultaneously

Biomechanical frame of reference: A framework in which the evaluation and intervention focuses on range of motion, strength, endurance, and preventing contractures and deformities; used primarily with orthopedic disorders

Blood pressure: The pressure that the circulating blood puts on the walls of the vessels

Body awareness: Internal sense of body structures and their relationships to each other

Body image: An attitude toward one's own body

BMI (body mass index): Measurement based upon one's height and weight and calculated based on (weight/[height]^2 $\times$ 703)

Bolus: Solids and semisolids that have been chewed (masticated) and mixed with saliva prior to being swallowed

Bone: Dense, semirigid, porous, calcified connective tissue that forms the major portion of the skeletal system in the human body and other vertebrates

Bone density: Thickness of bone

Brain plasticity: Lifelong ability of the brain to reorganize neural pathways

Burn: An injury to body tissue caused by thermal, electrical, chemical, or radioactive agents

Capacity: Ability to perform

Capillary: A thin-lined blood vessel that connects arterial blood supply with venous blood supply; exchange of nutrients and waste products occurs in the capillary beds

Carbon: An abundant, nonmetallic element that is found in inorganic and organic compounds; highly reactive in binding with other elements because of the number of electrons in its outer valence or shell

Carbon dioxide (CO$_2$): A compound that consists of one atom of carbon and two atoms of oxygen that is necessary for photosynthesis in plants and is a waste product of cellular respiration in animals

Cardiac disorders: Conditions that involve the heart and/or blood vessels

Care of others: Refers to the physical upkeep and nurturing of pets or other human beings

Cardiovascular system/Circulatory system: Organ system consisting of the heart, blood vessels, and blood that functions in the transport and exchange of nutrients and waste products throughout the body

Cartilage: Tough, elastic, fibrous connective tissue found in various parts of the body

Cellular respiration: Process that takes place in the mitochondria of cells, during which chemical reactions result in the production of adenosine triphosphate (ATP), which is the source of energy for other chemical reactions

Center of gravity: The midpoint or center of the weight of a body or object (In standing adult, this is midpelvic region)

Central nervous system (CNS): Brain and spinal cord

Central vision: "Center of gaze"; straight-ahead vision

Cerebral palsy (CP): A motor function disorder caused by a permanent, nonprogressive brain defect or lesion; characterized by a disruption in the volitional control of posture and movement; produces atypical muscle tone and unusual ways of moving

Cerebrovascular accident (CVA or stroke): Condition that involves the disruption of blood flow to the brain, which may result from a blockage or rupture of an artery resulting in partial or total loss of motor and sensory control on one side of the body.

Child-directed: The child takes the lead or initiates the movement, activity, or goals

Chromosome: A threadlike, linear strand of deoxyribonucleic acid (DNA) and its associated proteins that carry genes and pass along genetic information

Circumduction: Combination of flexion, abduction, extension, and adduction in such a way that the distal aspect of the extremity moves in a circle

Client-centered: An approach to treatment whereby the occupational therapy practitioner includes the client in every part of the evaluation and intervention programs, including the decision about the plan of action

Client factors: Components of activities required that affect performance and are specific to each client

Coactivation: Secondary to reciprocal innervations that means that two or more muscles are sent a message from the nervous system to become active or to contract/relax simultaneously

Co-contraction: Contraction of both the agonist and the antagonist to provide stability at a joint

Cognition: The mental processes of the construction, acquisition, and use of knowledge, as well as perception, memory, and the use of symbolism and language

Cognitive memory: Recall of thought

Cognitive sequencing: Mentally perceiving the steps of an activity

Collaboration: Working cooperatively with others to achieve a mutual goal

Comorbidities: Two or more existing medical or health conditions

Communication/interaction skill: A performance skill involving language and psychosocial skills

Community: A "person's natural environment, that is, where the person works, plays and performs other daily activities"; "an area with geographic and often political boundaries demarcated as a district, county, metropolitan area, city, township, or neighborhood . . . . a place where members have a sense of identity and belonging, shared values, norms, communication, and helping patterns"; locality in which a group lives and participates in daily occupations

Community-based practice: A practice with a public health perspective that focuses on health promotion and education; a practice within a community

Community mobility: Mobility in the community or outside the home

Compensatory movement patterns: Patterns of movement used because of reduced control of voluntary muscle

Competency stage: The toddler or middle childhood stage (2 to 6 years of age), in which children learn basic motor and performance skills

Compliance: Cooperation with recommended regimen, e.g., wearing an orthosis or changing positions

Compound: Consisting of two or more substances or elements

Consultation: The act or process of providing advice or information

Context: Conditions, including physical, personal, temporal, social, cultural, and virtual conditions, surrounding the client that influence performance

Contraction: Movement of the myofibrils (actin and myosin) in such a way that shortening of the muscle or increased tension in the muscle occurs

Contracture: Soft tissue tightness that interferes with movement at a joint or joints; a limitation in movement caused by soft tissue shortening that may result in a "stiff" or fused joint

Contusion: An injury that does not disrupt the integrity of the skin and is characterized by swelling, discoloration, and pain

Cri-du-chat syndrome: A rare genetic condition caused by the absence of part of chromosome 5; also known as *cat's cry syndrome* because it is recognized at birth by the presence of a kitten-like cry

Crush wound: A break in the external surface of the bone caused by severe force applied against tissues

Cultural considerations: Thoughtful consideration of the client's customs, beliefs, and expectations, which may be part of the larger society to which the individual belongs

Decubitus ulcer: A pressure sore caused by lying in the same position; *decubitus* means "to lie down"; sores that result from pressure on the skin over a bony prominence or as the result of continuous pressure on any area

Deformity: Bony fixation of a joint

Deltoid tuberosity: Bony landmark on the proximal, lateral aspect of the humerus which is the location of insertions for anterior, middle, and posterior muscles

Demyelinization: Destruction of the myelin sheaths that surround nerve fibers

Deoxyribonucleic acid (DNA): A nucleic acid that carries genetic information and is made of nucleotides and repeating sugar-phosphate groups

Development: The act or process of growth and/or maturation

Developmental coordination disorder (DCD): Disorder characterized by motor coordination that is markedly below the chronological age and intellectual ability and significantly interferes with activities of daily living

Developmental disorder: A mental and/or physical disability that arises before adulthood and lasts throughout one's life

Developmental dyspraxia: Neurologic disorder of motor coordination manifested by difficulty thinking out, planning out, and executing planned movements; difficulty with motor planning that is the result of sensory processing problems

Developmental frame of reference: A framework in which intervention is provided at the level at which the child is currently functioning and requires that the OT clinician provide a slightly advanced challenge

Developmental milestones: Skills that are common at different stages in development

Diaphragm: Dome-shaped muscle that separates the thorax from the abdomen and functions during inhalation/exhalation

Digestion: Mechanical and chemical processing of food

Digestive system: Organ system consisting of the digestive tract and associated body structures that functions in the mechanical and chemical breakdown of what is eaten into nutrients that the body can use at the cellular level

Diplegia: A term describing the distribution of affected muscles in individuals with cerebral palsy, in which the musculature of the lower extremities is more affected than that of the upper extremities

Dislocation: Displacement of the normal relationship of bones at a joint

Disruptive behavior disorder: A mental disorder characterized by socially disruptive behavior that is typically more distressing to others than to the individual with the disorder

Distal: Farther away from the body

Domain: A sphere of knowledge, influence, or activity

Down syndrome: A genetic disorder caused by the presence of an extra chromosome 21, which results in mental and motor delays in dressing and undressing—putting on (donning) and taking off (doffing) one's clothes—which are essential, basic self-care skills learned in infancy and early childhood

Duchenne muscular dystrophy: The most common form of muscular dystrophy; characterized by pseudo-hypertrophy of muscles, especially of the calf muscles; seen in males only

Due process: Parents' ability to take legal action against a school if their child's educational rights are violated; derived from the words *due*—owed or owing as a natural or moral right—and *process*—to proceed against by law

Dynamic balance (dynamic equilibrioception): Ability to move through the environment without falling over

Dynamic orthosis: An orthosis that allows movement in desired joint(s); a splint that assists an individual with movements

Dysphagia: Difficulty with swallowing

Dyspraxis: Difficulty with motor planning

Dystonia: Neurologic movement disorder, in which sustained muscle contractions result in twisting and/or repetitive movements and abnormal postures

Eating: The ability to keep food and fluids in the mouth, move them around inside the mouth, and swallow them

Eating disorder: A mental disorder characterized by a disturbance in eating behavior

Ecologic model: A model that studies the relationship between humans and their physical and social environments

Edema: Swelling or increased fluid secondary to an inflammatory response

Educational activities: Those tasks that promote learning, especially in academic areas such as reading, writing, and math

Efficacy: Capacity for beneficial change

Element: Substance composed of atoms; each element on the periodic chart has a consistent number of protons equal to the number of electrons

Endocrine system: Organ system comprising the endocrine glands located throughout the body that controls body functions through the secretion of hormones

Endometrium: Inner lining of the uterus that is shed during menstruation

Endurance: Activity tolerance; capacity to perform exercises or activities over time

Environment: The physical and social features of the specific context in which a child or adolescent engages in occupations

Environmental control unit (ECU): A system that allows an individual with limited motor control to operate electrical devices such as telephones, room lights, and televisions

Environmental impact: The extent to which physical or social aspects of an environment provide a specific child or adolescent with opportunities, supports, demands, or constraints

Environmentally induced disorder: An atypical condition that results from an environmental toxin (such as lead)

Equifinality: The inability to predict how a given situation or event in the present will develop in the future

Equilibrium reactions/Equilibrium responses: Automatic, reflexive, compensatory movements of body parts that restore and maintain the center of gravity over the base of support when either the center of gravity or the supporting surface is displaced; complex postural reactions that involve righting reactions with rotation and diagonal patterns and are essential for volitional movement and mobility; responses that begin at 6 months and persist throughout one's life

Esotropia: Type of strabismus in which one or both eyes turn inward

Eukaryotic cell: a cell that has a membrane-bound nucleus that contains genetic information

Evaluation: The process of using formal and informal measures to quantify an individual's performance in areas of occupation

Evidenced-based practice: Practice based on review and critique of research and proof of efficacy

Exceptional educational need (EEN): The determination that a disability or handicapping condition exists and interferes with the child's or adolescent's ability to participate in an educational program

Exotropia: Type of strabismus in which one or both eyes turn outward

Exploration stage: The infancy or early childhood stage (0 to 2 years of age), in which the child seeks out stimuli; the child is just beginning to move and perform skills

Extension: Straightening a joint increasing the angle

Fading assistance: A method of grading an activity by gradually reducing the level of assistance given until the individual performs the activity independently

Facilitation/Excitation: Planned, graded physical guidance techniques used to improve movement coordination by increasing inadequate muscle tone, altering sensory responsiveness, and/or altering behavioral states (e.g., hands-on facilitation techniques that are targeted at key postural points such as the shoulders, trunk, and hips)

Feed backward: Reflective movements in response to stimuli (e.g., throwing ball at a target and reflecting on where it hit).

Feed forward: Anticipatory movement to prepare for a motor response (e.g., deciding where to run to catch a ball)

Feeding: The process of bringing food and fluids to the mouth from containers such as plates, bowls, and cups

Fetal alcohol syndrome: A disorder that occurs as a result of excessive alcohol consumption by the mother during pregnancy; includes birth defects such as cardiac, cranial, facial, and neural abnormalities, with associated delays in physical and mental growth

Fine motor skill: The ability to use the small muscles of the body, especially those of the hands, to perform tasks

Fixation: Contraction of muscle(s) to create stability at a joint; may be normal or abnormal

Flexion: Bending a joint decreasing the angle

Forward chaining: A way to grade an activity in which an individual learns each step from the beginning; begins with the individual starting the sequence and ends with the occupational therapy practitioner finishing what the individual has not yet learned

Fracture: A break, rupture, or crack in bone or cartilage

Fragile X syndrome: A disorder characterized by a nearly broken X chromosome; the signs and symptoms may include an elongated face, prominent jaw and forehead, hypermobile or lax joints, flat feet, and intellectual disability

Frame of reference: Framework that helps the occupational therapy practitioner identify problems, evaluate, develop intervention, and measure outcomes

Free, appropriate public education (FAPE): Free public education that is mandated for all children, adolescents, and young adults who have disabilities and are between 3 and 21 years of age

Freedom to suspend reality: The ability to participate in "make-believe" or activities in which the participants pretend; the ability to create new play situations and interact with materials, space, and people in ways that are fluid, flexible, and not bound to the constraints of real life

Functional support capacities: Represent secondary neurobehavioral, motor, social-emotional, and/or cognitive proficiencies that are not functional in the occupational sense but are considered prerequisites for the end products to develop normally

Fussy baby syndrome: Condition in which the infant is easily upset and given to bouts of ill temper; associated with infants who have sensory regulatory disorders

Gastroesophageal reflux disease (GERD)/Gastric reflux: Condition in which the acid chyme from the stomach is regurgitated into the esophagus

Gene: A hereditary unit with a specific sequence of DNA that occupies a specific space on a chromosome and determines a specific characteristic of an individual

General sensory disorganization: Disorders in which sensory systems are providing inaccurate information; may be associated with impairments in the tactile, vestibular, and/or auditory systems; also associated with infants who are characterized as "fussy babies"

Genetic conditions: Disorders that occur as a result of abnormal or absent genes

Guillain-Barré syndrome: A syndrome that is characterized by the demyelinization of the peripheral nerves, which causes temporary paresis or paralysis

Glenohumeral joint: The articulation between the head of the humerus and the glenoid fossa of the scapula

Global mental functions: Refers to consciousness, orientation, sleep, temperament and personality, and energy and drive

Gradation: A systematic progression of activities

Grading activities: Changing one or more aspects of a task (usually by increasing or decreasing demands) to make it easier or harder to perform; modifying activities

Gravitational insecurity: Extreme fear or anxiety that one will fall when the feet are not in contact with a supporting surface

Gross motor skills: Activities that require the use of the larger body muscles (e.g., shoulders, hips, and knees)

Growth: Development; increase in size

Habits: Acquired tendencies to respond and perform in consistent ways in familiar or common environments or situations.

Habituation: The internal readiness a child or an adolescent has to demonstrate a consistent pattern of behavior guided by habits and roles; this readiness is associated with specific temporal, physical, or social environments

Hair: Filament mostly made of protein that grows from follicles located in the dermis

Half-kneeling: A resting position supported by the knee of one leg and the foot of the other leg with the thighs and trunk somewhat upright

Handling: Methods of providing specific sensory input to individuals with atypical muscle tone, posture, and movement; touching and manipulating with the hands

Health (World Health Organization [1948]): "Health is a state of complete physical, mental and social well-being and not merely the absence of disease or infirmity"; condition of optimal well-being of an organism

Hearing impairment: A disorder in the auditory system that may be a sensorineural or conductive disorder; relationships exist among hearing impairments and the vestibular system, balance, and chronic otitis

Heart rate (pulse): Beats of the heart per minute

Hemiplegia: A term describing the distribution of affected muscles in individuals with cerebral palsy, in which only the musculature on one side of the body is affected

High technology: Technology that is expensive and not readily available, such as computers, environmental control units, and powered wheelchairs

Home health company: An agency that contracts with nurses and occupational therapy and other practitioners to provide home-based services

Home management activities: Tasks that are necessary to obtain and maintain personal and household possessions

Homeostasis: Tendency of maintaining a relatively stable internal environment

Horizontal abduction: Moving the body part in the horizontal or transverse plane such that the distal aspect of the extremity moves *away* from the midline of the body

Horizontal adduction: Moving the body part in the horizontal or transverse plane such that the distal aspect of the extremity moves *toward* the midline of the body

Hydrogen: The lightest and most abundant element in the universe; one of the most abundant elements found in living matter

Hypersensitive: Increased sensitivity or awareness

Hypertonicity: Abnormally increased muscle tone associated with atypical postural alignment and decreased range of motion at joints; also known as *high tone* or *spasticity*

Hypertropia: Type of strabismus in which there is a permanent upward deviation of one eye

Hyposensitive: Decreased sensitivity or sensory awareness

Hypotonicity: Abnormally decreased muscle tone associated with atypical postural alignment and excessive range of motion at joints; also known as *low tone or flaccidity*

Hypotropia: Type of strabismus in which a permanent downward deviation of one eye is present

Hypoxia ischemia: Lack of oxygen due to lack of blood supply

Ideation: The ability to conceptualize internal representations of purposeful actions

Ideational praxis: A higher-level cognitive function; a component of praxis (a process that includes developing a concept or idea, planning, and executing a motor action)

Identity: The individual and contextual factors that constitute self-perception

Immobilization: Fixing a position of a joint to prevent movement at that joint

Immune system: Not a distinct organ system, but rather a coordination of the interaction of many of the organ systems in response to inflammation or infection; activated by the presence of potentially pathogenic organisms or substances

Inclusion: Models that are based on the premise that children with special needs should be educated in a regular classroom (instead of a self-contained classroom), with support personnel or services provided in that classroom (instead of pull-out services)

Incontinence: Inability to control bowel and/or bladder

Individualized education program (IEP): The written educational plan developed by a team, which includes the student's strengths and weaknesses as well as annual goals and short-term objectives

Individualized education program team: The team of parents, teachers, special educators, occupational therapy clinicians, and others, which determines a student's need for services

Individual family service plan (IFSP): The written intervention plan that is developed by the IFSP team and has as its focus family priorities and resources

Individuals with Disabilities Act (IDEA): Encourages occupational therapy practitioners to work with children in their classroom environments and provide support to the regular education teacher (integration); it also encourages schools to allow students with disabilities to meet the same educational standards as their peers

Inferior/Caudal: Toward the feet or tail

Inflammatory response: A localized protective reaction in response to irritation, injury, or infection, which is characterized by redness, pain, swelling, and sometimes reduced movement or function; an immune system response

In-hand manipulation: Moving objects within the hand

Inhibition: Planned, graded physical guidance techniques used to reduce excessive muscle tone, calm overly excited behavioral states, and decrease sensory hypersensitivity; suppression

Innervation: The distribution of nerve supply

Insertion of a muscle: The opposite end of a muscle relative to the origin that moves during a muscle contraction

Instrumental activities of daily living (IADLs): The complex activities of daily living that are needed to function independently in the home, at school, and in the community

Integumentary system: Organ system consisting of the skin and associated structures and functions as the first line of defense against potential invading microbes

Intellectual disability: Below-average cognitive functioning that causes developmental delays and impairments in multiple areas of occupation, including social participation, education, ADL and IADL skills, and play/leisure

Intelligence quotient (IQ): A ratio of tested mental age to chronologic age that is usually expressed as a quotient (i.e., the result of dividing one number by another) and multiplied by 100; determined by using a standardized test that measures an individual's ability to form concepts, solve problems, acquire information, reason, and learn

Interactive model: A model in which the service provider and the recipient of the services act upon each other in such a way that the services provided meet the needs of the recipient

Interest: What a child or adolescent finds enjoyable or satisfying

Internal control: The extent to which individuals are in charge of their own actions and the outcome of an activity

Intervention plan: A detailed description of the goals, methods, and expected outcomes of therapy

Intrinsic motivation: A prompt to action that comes from within the individual; drive to action that is rewarded by doing the activity itself, rather than deriving some external reward from it

Involuntary: Under smooth muscle or cardiac muscle control

Joint: Articulation between two or more bones at which movement may occur

Juvenile rheumatoid arthritis: A chronic disorder that begins in childhood and is characterized by stiffness and inflammation of the joints, weakness, loss of mobility, and deformity

Key points of control: The body structures used during handling to promote active movement

Kinesio taping: Taping of joints and muscles to provide support and stability without affecting circulation of movement or range of motion

Kinesthesia: Sense that detects weight and movement in muscles, tendons, and joints

Kneeling: A resting position supported by the knees with the thighs and trunk somewhat upright

Kyphoscoliosis: A condition in which both kyphosis and scoliosis of the vertebral column are present

Larynx: "Voice box"; a cartilaginous organ of the respiratory system located between the pharynx and the trachea that houses the vocal cords

Lateral: Farther away from the midline of the body

Lateral or external rotation: Moving a body part away from midline; only possible in triaxial joints or the hip and shoulder joints; during this rotation, the head of the femur or the head of the humerus moves out of the articulating fossa

Lateral weight shift: Transferring the body's weight away from the midline or laterally

Learned helplessness: Condition in which one has learned to behave as if helpless or unable to perform activities/occupations

Least restrictive environment (LRE): A classroom setting with minimum limitations; associated with the premise that children with disabilities have the right to be with nondisabled children

Legitimate tools: Instruments that are in accordance with the established and accepted standards of a profession or discipline

Leisure: Freedom from the demands of work; engaging in a nonobligatory activity that is intrinsically motivating during free time

Leisure activities: Activities that are not associated with time-consuming duties and responsibilities

Leukemia: A group of pediatric health conditions involving various acute and chronic tumor disorders of the bone marrow

Level of arousal: The amount of alertness and attention needed for an activity; must be at the optimum level for learning to take place

Levels of supervision: Refers to the amount of oversight required for the occupational therapy practitioner to perform duties

Life cycle: The events that typically occur during one's life

Ligament: Sheet or band of tough fibrous tissue that connects muscle to bone or supports an organ

Linguistic skills: Language abilities

Living matter: Organic matter (matter containing carbon)

Long-term care: Care that is provided in a residential facility when a family or primary caregiver is unable to meet an individual's medical needs; includes the goals of providing appropriate medical care and therapeutic intervention

Low technology: Technology that is inexpensive, easy to obtain, and simple to produce

Lymph: Watery fluid found in lymph vessels and nodes

Lymph nodes: Small bodies located on the lymphatic vessels that filter bacteria and other foreign materials from the lymph fluid

Lymphatic system: Organ system consisting of lymphatic vessels and associated structures that functions in transport and exchange as well as responding to an immune response

Matter: Anything that takes up space and has mass or weight

Media: An intervening substance through which something else is transmitted or carried on; an agency by which something is accomplished, conveyed, or transferred

Medial or internal rotation: Moving a body part toward the midline or medially; only occurs in the hip and shoulder joints during which the head of the femur or the head of the humerus turns inward

Medial: Closer to the midline of the body

Memory: The ability to store, retain, and retrieve information

Metabolism: Sum of all chemical reactions that occur in an organism

Method: A means or manner of procedure, especially a regular and systematic way of accomplishing something

Mild intellectual disability: A category of intellectual disability in which an individual has a below-average IQ (ranging from 55 to 69) and typically requires intermittent support; generally allows the individual to master academic skills ranging from Grades 3 to 7, though more slowly than other students

Misalignment: Misplacement

Model of practice: Framework that helps occupational therapy practitioners organize their thinking

Moderate intellectual disability: A category of intellectual disability in which an individual has a below-average IQ (ranging from 40 to 54) and typically requires some level of support as an adult; generally allows the individual to master academic skills at Grade 2 level, though significantly more slowly than other students

Molecule: Smallest part of a substance that retains the chemical and physical properties of the substance and is composed of two or more atoms

Monoplegia: One extremity involvement

Mood disorder: A mental disorder characterized by a disturbance in mood

Morphogenetic principle: The theory that systems tend to evolve and adapt to the larger environment

Morphostatic principle: The theory that systems tend to maintain the status quo (i.e., stay the same)

Motor control: Ability to move smoothly and efficiently

Motor control frame of reference: Follows a task-oriented approach that encourages the repetition of desired movements in a variety of settings and circumstances

Motor learning: Refers to the techniques to teach someone how to move

Motor memory: Recall of action patterns within body structures such as muscles and joints

Motor neuron: Also known as *effector neuron,* as it causes a motor response at the effector site

Motor skill: A performance skill involving objects; includes gross and fine motor skills

Multidisciplinary: Relating to multiple fields of study involved in the care of clients; suggests that although the various disciplines are working in collaboration, they are also working in parallel, with each distinct discipline being accountable and responsible for its tasks and functions regarding client care

Muscle tone: The degree of tension in muscle fibers while a muscle is at rest; the degree of elasticity and contractility in the muscle tissue; the resting state of a muscle in response to gravity and emotion

Muscular system: Organ system consisting of skeletal, smooth, and cardiac muscles that functions in the movement of the body or materials through the body by the contraction and relaxation of muscles; additional functions include maintenance of posture and heat production

Nails: Horn-like envelopes, made of the protein *keratin,* which engulf the distal aspect of the phalanges of the digits of the fingers and toes known as *fingernails* and *toenails*

Natural environment: Usual or ordinary environment

Negotiation: Process of making decisions and resolving disputes

Neurobiology: Biology that focuses on the nervous system

Neurodevelopmental treatment (NDT): A therapeutic approach used when working with clients who have neurologic disorders and have difficulty controlling movements, which interferes with function; occupational therapy clinicians providing NDT treatment need to have advanced training; techniques include direct handling techniques to increase a client's independence

Neurologic conditions: Congenital or acquired disorders such as spina bifida and Erb's palsy, which affect the central or peripheral nervous system

Neurologic rehabilitation: Restoration intervention that focuses on treating neurologic impairment(s)

Neuron: Smallest unit of the nervous system that consists of a cell body, dendrites (which carry impulses *to* the cell body) and axons (which carry impulses *away* from the cell body) with myelin sheaths that increase the rate of impulse propagation

Nervous system: Organ system consisting of the brain, spinal cord, and peripheral nerves that regulates the responses to internal and external stimuli; functions in communication within and without and controlling the response to stimuli

Nitrogen: A nonmetallic element that is found in all proteins; one of the most abundant elements found in living matter

No Child Left Behind: Established in 2001 to increase the standards for teaching and improve the results of student learning; supports the use of scientifically based practices by occupational therapy professionals working in the educational setting

Non-normative life cycle events: The unanticipated events of life, such as the frequent hospitalization of a young child or premature death of a child or parent

Nonprogressive: Not getting worse

Normal: Occurring naturally; not deviating from the standard

Normative life cycle events: The usual and expected events of life, such as birth, starting school, and adolescence

Nystagmus: Unintentional jittering of one or both eyes

Obesity: Excessive body weight caused by an accumulation of adipose tissue or fat

Obligation: Social, legal, or moral requirement

Occupation: An activity that has unique meaning and purpose for a person

Occupational forms/Tasks: Conventionalized sequences of action that are coherent, oriented to a purpose, sustained in collective knowledge, culturally recognizable, and named

Occupational therapy intervention process model (OTIPM): A model for occupational therapy evaluation and intervention in which a client-centered, top-down, occupation-based approach is used

Occupational Therapy Practice Framework: Terminology developed to assist occupational therapy practitioners in defining the process and domains of occupational therapy

Optimize: Maximize

Oral defensiveness: Aversion to harmless oral sensations

Oral hygiene: Typical skills that are learned in early childhood, such as brushing the teeth

Oral–motor development: Maturation of the oral–motor structures

Origin of a muscle: Part of the muscle that attaches to bone or muscle and is stationary during a muscle contraction

Organ: Aggregate of several different types of tissues to perform a particular function

Organ system: Aggregate of organs that perform specific function(s)

Orthopedic condition: A disorder that involves the skeletal system and associated muscles (i.e., joints and ligaments)

Orthosis: Refers to an orthotic device; a term used interchangeably with splint; a bracing system designed to control, correct, and/or compensate for bony deformities or muscle imbalance; an external orthopedic appliance

Oxygen: A nonmetallic element that is necessary for cellular respiration; one of the most abundant elements found in living matter

Paraplegia: Paralysis or loss of motor and sensory control in both legs

Passive ROM (PROM): Movement that occurs at a joint secondary to an outside force

Pathologic fracture: Broken bone caused by a disease or health condition

Pediatric medical care system: A group of individuals (professional, paraprofessional, and nonprofessional) who form a complex and unified whole dedicated to caring for children who have health disorders

Perception: Process of understanding sensory information

Perceptual coping strategies: Defining events, situations, and crises in ways that promote adaptation

Performance capacity: The ability of a child or adolescent to do things provided by the status of his/her underlying objective physical and mental components; also influenced by the child's or adolescent's subjective experience.

Performance skills: The observable elements of action, including motor skills, process skills, and communication/interaction skills

Periods of development: Specific developmental stages categorized by age, including infancy, early childhood, middle childhood, adolescence, and adulthood

Peripheral nervous system (PNS): All nerves located outside the brain and spinal cord that connect the central nervous system to body structures such as limbs and internal organs; peripheral nerves, spinal nerves, cranial nerves, and nerves associated with the autonomic nervous system

Peripheral vision: "Side vision"; the ability to see objects outside of the line of vision or center of gaze

Peristalsis: Involuntary movement of food through the digestive tract

Personal causation: A child's or an adolescent's sense of capacity and efficacy for occupations

Personal hygiene and grooming skills: Typical skills such as face washing, hand washing, and hair care that are learned in early childhood

Pervasive developmental disorder (PDD): A collection of disorders marked by delays in communication and social development; difficulties understanding language relating to events, objects, and/or people; atypical play skills and transitions; and repetitive movements or maladaptive behavior patterns; a group of pediatric health conditions affecting a variety of body functions and structures with a wide range of severity

Pharynx: Muscular organ that connects the mouth to the esophagus; movement of the bolus in pharynx occurs secondary to peristalsis

Phosphorus: A nonmetallic and highly reactive element found in phosphates; most abundant salt found in living matter

Phosphate: An inorganic chemical that is a salt

Physiological flexion: Total body flexion of a neonate primarily due to the position in utero

Pica behavior: Craving and eating inedible items such as plaster and dirt

Play: Any spontaneous or organized activity that provides enjoyment, entertainment, amusement, and/or diversion; an experience that involves intrinsic motivation, with emphasis on the process rather than product and internal rather than external control; a make-believe experience that takes place in a safe, nonthreatening environment

Play adaptations: Changes in materials or activities to promote successful play for children who have disabilities

Play assessment: Observations of children during play by the occupational therapy practitioner

Play environment: The setting in which the occupational therapy practitioner assesses children at play; consists of child-friendly toys and materials

Play goals: Outcomes of play during the occupational therapy process

Playfulness: Abstract noun derived from the adjective *playful*; a behavioral or personality trait characterized by flexibility, manifest joy, and spontaneity

Positioning: Specific ways of placing an individual to maintain postural alignment, provide postural stability, facilitate normal patterns of movement, and increase interaction with the environment; can include the use of adaptive equipment; placing the body in a position usually with the aid of equipment to maintain the position

Posterior/Dorsal: Back

Postural (skeletal) alignment: Mechanically efficient position or alignment of joints of the neck and trunk

Postural mechanism: A term used to encompass muscle tone, postural tone, equilibrium, and righting responses, as well as protective extension reactions

Postural-ocular and bilateral integration dysfunction: Sensory-based motor dysfunction characterized by a cluster of several sensory, behavioral, and motor characteristics

Postural stability: Equilibrium in the neck and trunk that provides a base of support in such a way that controlled mobility of the arms and legs is possible; the ability to maintain equilibrium and balance or return to the original position after displacement from that position

Postural tone: Underlying contraction of skeletal muscles that allows the body structures to maintain their position in space

Prader-Willi syndrome: A genetic health disorder that involves chromosome 15; characterized by varying degrees of intellectual disability, overeating habits, and self-mutilating behavior

Praxis: The ability to conceptualize, organize, and execute nonhabitual, novel motor tasks; motor planning

Prematurity: Being born prior to full term; a baby born after less than 37 weeks' gestation from the mother's last menstrual day (per the World Health Organization [WHO])

Prescriptive: The role of the occupational therapist in working with a child in a directive manner, providing the family and the child with a plan

Pretend play: Play that involves symbolic games, imagination, and suspension of reality

Pressure sore: An ulceration caused by the death of cells due to lack of blood supply

Prevocational skills: Abilities that are needed for a vocational or work setting

Primitive reflexes: A group of movement patterns that begin emerging at birth and continue until approximately 4 to 6 months of age; reflexes that are controlled primarily by the lower brain centers; reflexes that enable the body to respond to influences such as head or body position mechanically and automatically with a change in muscle tone; reflexes that provide the developing infant with numerous consistent posture and movement patterns for early interaction with the environment

Principles of development: Refers to the guidelines and general progression of growth and performance skill attainment

Process skill: A performance attribute involving cognition

Profound intellectual disability: A category of intellectual disability in which an individual has a below-average IQ (25 or lower) and requires pervasive support throughout life and extensive assistance with ADLs; physical disorders generally accompany cognitive limitations

Pronation: In an erect (sitting or standing) position turning the palm down to face the floor

Prone: Positioned on stomach

Proprioception: A sensory system having receptors in the muscles, joints, and other internal tissues that provide internal awareness about the positions of body parts

Proprioceptive feedback: Muscle–joint input that provides information regarding position in space and/or in relation to objects

Protective extension reactions: Postural responses that are used to stop a fall or prevent injury when equilibrium reactions cannot do so; responses that involve straightening of the arms and/or legs toward a supporting surface

Proximal: Closer to the body

Psychogenic: Originating in the mind or in emotions

Psychosocial occupational therapy: The area of clinical practice that provides services to children and adolescents with mental health problems

Psychosocial skills: Performance components that refer to an individual's ability to interact in society and process emotions; include psychological, social, and self-management skills

Public health approaches: Approaches with a focus on health promotion and prevention in populations

Quadriplegia (tetraplegia): A term describing the distribution of affected muscles in individuals with cerebral palsy, in which the musculature of all four extremities is affected; may also affect the musculature of the neck and facial areas

Radial deviation: Moving the wrist radially or toward the thumb

Range of motion (ROM): The amount of movement available at a specified joint; measured with a goniometer by occupational therapy practitioners

Readiness skills: Those abilities in the performance components and areas that are necessary for engaging in activities related to education, home management, care of others, and vocation

Reading the child in context: A moment-to-moment observation and analysis of a child's relationship to the social and physical environments and the child's responses to the therapeutic process; a tool that helps occupational therapy practitioners plan and implement treatment

Reciprocal innervation: The distribution of nerve supply to antagonistic muscles, which allows one muscle to be excited and contract while the other muscle is inhibited, thus relaxing the muscle(s); excitation of the agonist with inhibition of the antagonist thus allowing movement at a joint

Referral: A request for a screening or evaluation to determine whether one would benefit from occupational therapy services

Relaxation: Lengthening of a muscle; loosening up

Reproductive system: Organ system of female and male reproductive organs that function in sexual reproduction

Resources: Support in the form of time, money, friends, and family; supplies, equipment, and personnel that provide support

Respiratory distress syndrome (RDS): A disease in newborns (especially premature neonates) characterized by difficulty breathing, cyanosis, and formation of a glossy membrane over the alveoli of the lungs

Respiratory rate: Number of breaths per minute

Respiratory system (Pulmonary system): Organ system consisting of the lungs and associated structures that functions in gas exchange with the environment

Righting reactions: Responses that maintain the alignment of body parts; postural reactions that occur in response to a change in the position of the head and body in space; reactions that bring the head and trunk back into an upright position

in space; involve extension, flexion, abduction, adduction, and lateral flexion; begin to emerge between 6 and 9 months of age and persist throughout life

Robotics: Engineering science and technology of robots, including the design and manufacturing of robots

Roles: A socially or personally defined status that is associated with actions or attitudes

Role delineation: The clear separation of responsibilities between the registered occupational therapist and the certified occupational therapy assistant

Rote learning: The acquisition of behaviors that become routine, though not always fully understood or carried out with sincerity; learning that usually occurs through memorization and repetition

RUMBA criteria: Method of writing and evaluating goals; RUMBA stands for *r*elevant, *u*nderstandable, *m*easurable, *b*ehavioral, and *a*chievable (attainable)

Scapular elevation: Upward movement of the scapula

Scapular depression: Downward movement of the scapula

Scapular protraction: Movement of the scapula *away* from the midline of the body

Scapular retraction: Movement of the scapula *toward* the midline of the body

Scapular winging: A condition in which the vertebral borders of the scapulae move away from the thoracic wall, especially during weight-bearing through the arm as result of muscle weakness

Screening: An informal or formal measure that determines an individual's need for occupational therapy evaluation and intervention

Sebaceous glands: Microscopic exocrine glands found in the dermis of the skin that secrete sebum to lubricate the skin and hair

Seizure: A condition in which an individual has sudden convulsions, as in individuals with epilepsy

Self-concept: The total person that the child or adolescent envisions himself or herself to be

Self-efficacy: The individual's perception of his or her own capabilities

Self-esteem: Pride in oneself; self-respect

Self-regulation: Ability to calm self

Sensorimotor frame of reference: An intervention approach that focuses on using sensory input to change muscle tone or movement patterns; used with children and adolescents who have disorders of the central nervous system

Sensory diet: A carefully designed activity plan for sensory input a person needs to stay focused and organized

Sensory discrimination: Ability to discern and assign meaning to specific sensory stimuli

Sensory input: The basic sensations of touch, sound, and movement that influence the parts of the central nervous system that govern and produce skilled, automatic movements

Sensory integration (SI): The organization of sensory input to produce an adaptive response; a theoretical process and treatment approach; addresses the processing of sensory information from the environment; includes discriminating, integrating, and modulating sensory information in order to produce meaningful, adaptive responses; occupational therapy clinicians may have advanced training and certification in *Ayres Sensory Integration®* (ASI) through Western Psychological Services and the University of Southern California

Sensory integration frame of reference: An approach to intervention developed by A.J. Ayres that utilizes suspended equipment and child-directed activity to facilitate adaptive responses and thereby improve central nervous system processing

Sensory modulation: Interpreting and filtering sensory information

Sensory modulation disorder: Impairment in the ability to regulate incoming sensations or failure to detect and orient to novel or important sensory information

Sensory neuron: Also known as *affector neuron*; sends sensory information to be processed by the central nervous system

Sensory processing: The means by which the brain receives, detects, and integrates incoming sensory information for use in producing adaptive responses to one's environment

Sensory system conditions: Diseases, impairments, or deficits in visual, auditory, vestibular, gustatory/olfactory, or tactile functioning

Service competency: The process ensuring that two individual occupational therapy practitioners will obtain equivalent results (i.e., replication) when administering a specific assessment or providing intervention

Severe intellectual disability: A category of intellectual disability in which an individual has a below-average IQ (ranging from 25 to 39) and typically requires extensive support throughout life; generally, individuals may be able to learn basic self-care skills, although they are unable to live independently as adults

Shaken baby syndrome: A cluster of impairments resulting from an infant being jerked violently back and forth. A severe type of head injury; occurs when an infant and/or child is shaken violently resulting in the brain hitting against the skull. Symptoms include lethargy, tremors, vomiting, coma, and/or death, depending on the extent of the damage.

Side-lying: Position referring to lying on one's side

Sitting: A resting position supported by the buttocks and thighs with the trunk somewhat upright

Skeletal system: Organ system consisting of bones, cartilage, and joints that protects and supports internal organs and other body structures; works with the muscular system to create movement at joints

Skill: Observable, goal-directed action that a person uses or demonstrates while performing a task

Skin: Largest organ in the human body; first line of defense for the immune system to guard against potentially harmful invading microbes

Skin integrity: Condition of the skin

Skin irritation: Painful reaction of the skin to chemical or mechanical forces

SOAP note: A method of documentation that contains the following subject areas: subjective (thoughts, feelings, and verbalizations), objective (session goal and what occurred), assessment (summary of objectives), and plan (future objectives and session goals)

Social groups: Collections of people who come together for formal and/or informal purposes and who influence the things a child or adolescent does when interacting within those social groups

Social participation: Associated with the organized patterns of behavior that are expected of a child interacting with others within a given social system, such as the family, peers, or community

Social skills: Skills that promote effectively living and interacting within a community

Soft tissue injury: Damage to muscles, nerves, skin, and/or connective tissue

Somatodyspraxia: Inadequate processing of tactile, proprioceptive, and kinesthetic information that causes difficulty in motor planning

Somatosensory system: Sensory system that processes tactile, proprioceptive, and kinesthetic information

Spasticity: A state of increased tone in a muscle with associated exaggerated deep tendon reflex; increased muscle tone; hypertonicity; often occurs when a stretch reflex is activated in a muscle

Specific mental functions: Factors that refer to attention, memory, perception, thought, higher-level cognition, language, calculation, sequencing complex movements, psychomotor capacity, emotion, and experience of self and time

Spina bifida: Split spine (a common disorder seen by the occupational therapy practitioner); comprises three types: occulta, meningocele, and myelomeningocele; common to treat children with myelomeningocele-type spina bifida because of its associated sensory and motor deficits

Splint: A device that immobilizes, restrains, or supports a part of the body

Splinter skill: A specific, often complex task mastered by a child who lacks the underlying developmental capabilities to perform it; usually attained through compensatory methods and practice rather than by remediating the underlying developmental components

Spontaneity: Acting without effort or premeditation; driven by internal forces

Sprain: A traumatic injury to the tendons, muscle, or ligaments around a joint and characterized by pain, swelling, and discoloration

Standing: A resting position supported by the feet with the legs, thighs, and trunk somewhat upright

Static balance (static equilibrioception): Ability to maintain a posture or position without falling over

Static orthosis: An orthosis that prevents movement in a desired joint

Stereognosis: The ability to identify objects through touch

Strabismus: "Crossed eyes"; condition in which the eyes do not line up while focusing

Strength: Ability of a muscle or muscle group to move against gravity and additional resistance; power

Subacute: Condition between acute and chronic

Subluxation: An incomplete or partial dislocation of a bone below the joint

Substance abuse: A pattern of behavior in which the use of substances has adverse consequences

Substance dependence: A pattern of behavior in which substances continue to be used despite serious cognitive, behavioral, and physiologic symptoms

Substance-related disorder: A mental disorder resulting from the inappropriate use of drugs, medications, or toxins

Suck–swallow–breathe (s-s-b) synchrony: A skill used continuously throughout life that allows an individual to breathe while simultaneously and unconsciously sucking in and swallowing food, drink, and saliva; its disruption can interfere profoundly with development

Superior/Cephalad: Towards the head

Supination: Turning the palm up toward the ceiling

Supine: Position referring to being on one's back

Switch: A device used to break or open an electric circuit; an item that connects, disconnects, or diverts an electric current; used with children who have disabilities in order to promote successful interaction with computers, battery-operated toys, and powered mobility systems

Symmetrical: Balanced or evenly distributed, such as weight through the trunk and hips while sitting in chair

Symmetry: Alignment of the body in such a way that the head is in the midline position, the trunk is straight, and the weight is distributed equally on both sides of the body

Tactile defensiveness: Aversion to touch

Teratogen: Anything that causes the development of abnormal structures in an embryo and results in a severely deformed fetus

Therapeutic media: Activities that are meaningful and motivating to clients and address their goals

Therapeutic use of self: The occupational therapy practitioner's "planned use of his or her personality, insights, perceptions, and judgments as part of the therapeutic process" (Punwar & Peloquin, 2000, p. 285) and conscious use of self in therapy as "the use of oneself in such a way that one becomes an effective tool in the evaluation and intervention process" (Mosey); the art of using oneself to successfully promote engagement in chosen daily activities

Tic disorder: A mental disorder characterized by tics or involuntary muscle contractions

Tissue: Aggregate of cells to perform a particular function

Top-down teaching: Teaching that begins with the whole and works down to the individual components

Touch: Information received via skin receptors; includes light touch, deep pressure touch, pain, and temperature

Toilet hygiene: Typical skills that are learned in early childhood such as clothing management, maintaining toileting position, transferring to and from toileting, and cleaning the body

Tongue thrust: A movement in which the tongue extends outside the lips, interferes with swallowing, and causes food to be pushed outside the mouth; often seen in individuals with cerebral palsy or Down syndrome

Top-down approach: Focuses on occupations as the means and ends and emphasizing client-centered care

Trachea: "Wind pipe"; a cartilaginous tube that connects the larynx to the bronchi of the lungs through which oxygen and carbon dioxide flow

Transdisciplinary: Refers to "across" disciplines; this approach involves a variety of professionals who work closely with children and may, in fact, share roles. Team members may work on goals of another profession

Transition plan: Plan for change, refers to going to another stage, such as moving from middle to high school or high school to independent living

Transitional movement: Movement from one position to another

Traumatic brain injury (TBI): Condition in which there is serious injury to the brain that causes neurologic impairment; a result of acute trauma to the brain; multiple symptoms are associated with the diagnosis of TBI which vary widely, from mild to severe; mild symptoms include loss of consciousness, headache, and blurred vision; moderate or severe TBI symptoms include similar symptoms, in addition to vomiting or nausea, pupil dilation, seizures, slurred speech, weakness or numbness in the extremities, and agitation

Typical: Exhibiting qualities, traits, or characteristics that identify a group; not deviating from the standard or norm

Ulnar deviation: Moving the wrist ulnarly or toward the little finger

Unilateral: Involving one side of the body or one arm/leg

Universal precautions: Use of protective barriers such as gloves, gowns, aprons, masks, and/or protective eyewear to decrease risk of exposure to diseases and/or infections

Urinary system: Organ system consisting of the kidneys and associated body structures that function to filter nutrients and waste products from blood and other fluids that circulate throughout the body; additional functions include resorption of nutrients and elimination of waste products

Validation: Process of establishing evidence

Value: Things that a child or adolescent finds important and meaningful

Vein: Vessel that moves blood to the heart

Venule: Small vein

Vertebral column: Part of the axial skeletal system that comprises vertebrae and functions to protect the spinal cord and to support the body

Vestibular input: Linear and/or rotational movement information received in the inner ear

Visuodyspraxia: Visual constructive and praxis deficits

Visuomotor integration: Ability to coordinate movements through vision

Visuomotor skills: Coordination of the eyes with the hands or other body parts in such a way that the eyes guide precisely controlled movements; also referred to as *visuomotor integration skills* and *eye–hand skills* or *eye–foot skills*

Visual accommodation: The ability of the eyes to change optical power to maintain focus on an object

Vision impairment: A condition of decreased visual acuity or impaired processing of visual input

Visual perception: The ability to interpret and use what is being or has been seen

Vocational activities: Work-related activities that typically have a monetary incentive or salary; abilities/skills needed for an occupation, trade, or profession

Volition: A child's or adolescent's pattern of thoughts and feelings about himself or herself that occur as he or she anticipates, chooses, experiences, and interprets his or her engagement in occupations

Voluntary: Under skeletal muscle control

Weight shift: Transferring of body weight from one structure to another

Whole skills: Those occupations or activities that can be done automatically (i.e., without thinking)

Willbarger protocol: Intervention regimen designed to reduce sensory hypersensivity

Work: An area of occupation that includes employment and volunteer activities

Work simplification/Energy conservation techniques: Analyzing and dividing tasks to a simple level to conserve energy; use of large versus small muscle groups

World Health Organization (WHO): Specialized agency within the United Nations that acts as the coordinating authority on international public health

Bibliography

Ayres J: *Sensory integration and learning disorders*, Los Angeles, CA, 1972, Western Psychological Services.

Ayres J: *Developmental dyspraxia and adult-onset apraxia*, Torrance, CA, 1985, Sensory Integration International.

Cornelia de Lange syndrome: United States National Library of medicine: http://ghr.nlm.nih.gov/condition=corneliadelangesyndrome: Accessed February 2010.

Mckinley, W., Silver, T, Santos, K., Pai, A: Functional outcomes per level of spinal cord injury, 2008, http://emedicine.medscape.com/article/322604-overview. Accessed October 6, 2010.

May-Benson T A, Cermak S A: Development of an assessment for ideational praxis, *Am J Occup Ther* 61:148–153, 2007.

NINDS Pervasive Developmental Disorders, 2009: adapted from the National Institutes, of Neurological Disorders and Stroke, National Institutes of Health: http://www.ninds.nih.gov/disorders/pdd/pdd.htm: Accessed October 6, 2010.

Stroke: http://www.nlm.nih.gov/medlineplus/ency/article/000726.htm: Accessed October 6, 2010.

NINDS: *Traumatic brain injury: Hope through research*, NIH Publication No. 02-2478, February 2002.

Rothmund-Thomson syndrome (RTS): Http://ghr.nlm.nih.gov/condition-rothmundthomson-syndrome: Accessed October 6, 2010.

"What is NDT?": www.ndta.org/whatisndt.php: Accessed October 6, 2010.

The American Heritage Dictionary of the English Language
World Health Organization (WHO)